Pathology of the Mediastinum

Pathology of the Mediastinum

Edited by

Alberto M. Marchevsky, MD
Director of Pulmonary and Mediastinal Pathology,
Department of Pathology and Laboratory Medicine, Cedars-Sinai Medical Center, Los Angeles;
Clinical Professor of Pathology, David Geffen UCLA School of Medicine, Los Angeles, CA, USA

Mark R. Wick, MD
Professor of Pathology, Department of Pathology,
University of Virginia Health System, Charlottesville, VA, USA

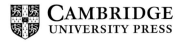

CAMBRIDGE
UNIVERSITY PRESS

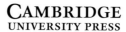

CAMBRIDGE
UNIVERSITY PRESS

University Printing House, Cambridge CB2 8BS, United Kingdom

Published in the United States of America by Cambridge University Press, New York

Cambridge University Press is part of the University of Cambridge.

It furthers the University's mission by disseminating knowledge in the pursuit of education, learning and research at the highest international levels of excellence.

www.cambridge.org
Information on this title: www.cambridge.org/9781107031531

© Cambridge University Press 2014

First published 2014

Printed in Spain by Grafos SA, Arte sobre papel

A catalogue record for this publication is available from the British Library

Library of Congress Cataloging in Publication data
Pathology of the mediastinum / edited by Alberto M. Marchevsky, Mark R. Wick.
    p. ; cm.
Includes bibliographical references and index.
ISBN 978-1-107-03153-1
I. Marchevsky, Alberto M., editor of compilation.   II. Wick, Mark R., 1952– editor of compilation.
[DNLM: 1. Mediastinal Diseases–pathology–Atlases.   2. Mediastinum–pathology–Atlases. WF 17]
RC280.M35
616.2′707–dc23
2013047253

ISBN 978-1-107-03153-1 Mixed Media

ISBN 978-1-107-05430-1 Hardback

ISBN 978-1-107-67630-5 CD-ROM

Contents

List of contributors   *page* vi
Preface   vii

1. **The mediastinum**   1
   Alberto M. Marchevsky and Mark R. Wick

2. **Imaging of the mediastinum**   4
   Xiaoqin Wang and Ajay Singh

3. **Inflammatory diseases of the mediastinum**   25
   Alberto M. Marchevsky and Mark R. Wick

4. **The thymus gland**   37
   Alberto M. Marchevsky and Mark R. Wick

5. **Pathology of non-neoplastic conditions of the thymus**   51
   Alberto M. Marchevsky and Mark R. Wick

6. **Low-grade and intermediate-grade malignant epithelial tumors of the thymus: thymomas**   65
   Alberto M. Marchevsky, Saul Suster, and Mark R. Wick

7. **High-grade malignant epithelial tumors of the thymus: primary thymic carcinomas**   104
   Mark R. Wick, Alberto M. Marchevsky, and Saul Suster

8. **Neuroendocrine carcinomas of the thymus**   131
   Alberto M. Marchevsky, Saul Suster, and Mark R. Wick

9. **Germ cell of the mediastinum**   146
   Sean R. Williamson and Thomas M. Ulbright

10. **Parathyroid lesions, paragangliomas, thyroid tumors, and pleomorphic adenomas of the mediastinum**   169
    Mark R. Wick and Alberto M. Marchevsky

11. **Hematopoietic neoplasms of the mediastinum**   199
    Serhan Alkan

12. **Cystic lesions of the mediastinum**   211
    Mark R. Wick and Alberto M. Marchevsky

13. **Mesenchymal tumors of the mediastinum**   226
    Bonnie Balzer, Mark R. Wick, and Susan Parson

14. **Tell me what you need, so I'll know what to say**   270
    Frank C. Detterbeck

15. **Clinical pathology of disorders of the mediastinum**   276
    Kent Lewandrowski

16. **Surgical pathology of the heart**   285
    Gregory A. Fishbein, Atsuko Seki, and Michael C. Fishbein

17. **Morphologic alterations of serous membranes of the mediastinum in reactive and neoplastic settings**   317
    Aliya N. Husain and Thomas Krausz

Index   344

Contributors

Serhan Alkan, MD
Professor of Pathology; Director of Clinical Pathology; and
Director of Hematopathology and Personalized Medicine
Diagnostics,
Cedars-Sinai Medical Center, Los Angeles, CA, USA

Bonnie Balzer, MD, PhD
Director of Surgical Pathology,
Dermatopathology and Musculoskeletal Pathology Services,
Cedars-Sinai Medical Center, Los Angeles, CA, USA

Frank C. Detterbeck, MD
Professor and Chief, Yale Thoracic Surgery,
Yale University School of Medicine, New Haven, CT, USA

Gregory A. Fishbein, MD
Resident Physician, Anatomic Pathology,
Department of Pathology and Laboratory Medicine,
David Geffen UCLA School of Medicine,
Los Angeles, CA, USA

Michael C. Fishbein, MD
Piansky Professor of Pathology and Medicine;
Head, Cardiovascular and Autopsy Pathology,
Department of Pathology and Laboratory Medicine,
David Geffen UCLA School of Medicine,
Los Angeles, CA, USA

Aliya N. Husain, MD
Professor of Pathology, University of Chicago,
Chicago, IL, USA

Thomas Krausz, MD
Professor of Pathology, University of Chicago,
Chicago, IL, USA

Kent Lewandrowski, MD
Associate Chief of Pathology, Director of Pathology
Laboratories and Molecular Medicine,
Massachusetts General Hospital; Professor of
Pathology, Harvard Medical School, Boston, MA, USA

Alberto M. Marchevsky, MD
Director of Pulmonary and Mediastinal Pathology,
Department of Pathology and Laboratory Medicine,
Cedars-Sinai Medical Center, Los Angeles;
Clinical Professor of Pathology,
David Geffen UCLA School of Medicine,
Los Angeles, CA, USA

Susan Parson, MD
Anatomic and Clinical Pathology Resident,
Cedars-Sinai Medical Center, Los Angeles, CA, USA

Atsuko Seki, MD
Department of Pathology, National Hospital Organization,
Tokyo Medical Center, Tokyo, Japan

Ajay Singh, MD
Assistant Professor, Department of Radiology,
Massachusetts General Hospital, Boston, MA, USA

Saul Suster, MD
Professor and Chairman, Department of Pathology and
Laboratory Medicine, Medical College of Wisconsin,
Milwaukee, WI, USA

Thomas M. Ulbright, MD
Lawrence M. Roth Professor of Pathology, Department of
Pathology and Laboratory Medicine, Indiana University
School of Medicine, Indianapolis, IN, USA

Xiaoqin Wang, MD
Radiology President, Department of Radiology,
University of Kentucky, Lexington, KY, USA

Mark R. Wick, MD
Professor of Pathology, Department of Pathology,
University of Virginia Health System,
Charlottesville, VA, USA

Sean R. Williamson, MD
Senior Staff Pathologist, Department of Pathology
Henry Ford Hospital, Detroit, MI, USA

Preface

The mediastinum is an anatomical area of great interest to pathologists, pulmonologists, radiologists, thoracic surgeons, and oncologists as it can be the site of origin of a surprisingly large number of neoplastic and non-neoplastic conditions. The two editors and several other surgical pathologists with many years of experience in the diagnosis of thymic neoplasms, malignant mesothelioma, soft tissue lesions, lymphomas, cardiac lesions, and other mediastinal lesions have collaborated with a multidisciplinary team of physicians that includes an experienced thoracic surgeon, cardiac pathologists, radiologists, and a clinical pathologist to provide a comprehensive review of mediastinal pathology.

The book includes a review of the anatomy of the mediastinum and its various structures and a concise yet informative discussion of the diagnosis of various mediastinal lesions by imaging methods. The embryology, anatomy, and pathophysiology of the thymus are reviewed in detail, followed by a comprehensive and well-illustrated description of the various non-neoplastic conditions that can arise in the thymus.

A significant portion of the book is dedicated to a comprehensive review of the pathology of thymomas, thymic carcinomas, thymic neuroendocrine carcinomas, and other thymic neoplasms. Although thymomas and other thymic neoplasms are relatively uncommon, they have been the subject of great interest because of their association with myasthenia gravis and many other para-neoplastic conditions. In addition, the pathologic classification of thymomas has stimulated heated controversy in the literature with multiple articles extolling the advantages of certain classification systems and strongly criticizing others. Indeed, there has been so much disagreement in the terminology necessary to categorize thymomas that the World Health Organization (WHO) has proposed as a compromise a classification scheme that categorizes thymomas in an unprecedented manner with various letters such as A, B1, B2, and others rather than with descriptive terminology or nomenclature that reflects their histogenesis.

The book includes a novel classification scheme of thymic epithelial malignancies that correlates closely with the WHO system. The two editors, who have been interested in the pathology of thymic neoplasms for over three decades, were fortunate to be able to collaborate with Dr. Saul Suster, one of the most experienced international experts in the pathology of thymomas, in the development of this classification. It emphasizes that all thymic epithelial neoplasms are malignant and stratifies thymomas and thymic carcinomas into three levels of malignancy, underscoring that certain thymomas share similar prognosis with selected thymic carcinomas. The classification scheme uses simple descriptive terminology that underscores the most important morphological features of each thymic epithelial lesion variant and emphasizes the frequent presence of heterologous morphological features in thymomas and thymic carcinomas. The clinical significance of these and other classifications of thymoma and thymic carcinomas is discussed in detail, followed by a description of the Masaoka-Koga and Moran staging systems and a brief discussion of the treatment of patients with these malignancies.

The pathology of neuroendocrine and germ cell tumors of the tumor is described in detail. Neuroendocrine tumors of the thymus are classified as neuroendocrine carcinomas, a terminology that has become standard in various locations other than the thorax. The fact that mediastinal "carcinoid tumors" have a more aggressive clinical behavior that their counterparts arising from the lungs is discussed together with a critical review of current best evidence underscoring the classification of these lesions into typical and atypical carcinoid tumors by WHO.

The three chapters describing thymic neoplasms are followed by two chapters providing a concise yet comprehensive review of mediastinal germ cell tumors, parathyroid and thyroid lesions, paragangliomas, and pleomorphic adenoma of the mediastinum. Another chapter is devoted to describing in detail the pathology of the multiple non-neoplastic and neoplastic cystic lesions of the mediastinum.

The book does not intend to review the pathology of malignant lymphomas in detail, but it includes a chapter written by an experienced hematopathologist who provides a brief description of the most frequent hematopoietic lesions of the mediastinum and various algorithms to guide general pathologists in the interpretation of these lesions. Likewise, although this is not intended to be a "sarcoma," cardiac pathology or pleural pathology book, three other chapters provide concise and quite comprehensive review of the pathology of multiple neoplastic and non-neoplastic mesenchymal, cardiac and pleural lesions. These chapters provide a comprehensive review of the use of immunohistochemistry in the diagnosis of these lesions.

In summary, the book is intended to provide a concise, comprehensive, and well-illustrated review of mediastinal pathology. We hope that it will provide readers with a practical and extensively illustrated reference that will assist them during their daily diagnostic work and help surgical pathologists and their clinical colleagues become familiar with the most important aspects of the biology, clinico-radiologic, and therapy of thymomas and many other mediastinal lesions.

Alberto M. Marchevsky, MD
Mark R. Wick, MD

The mediastinum

Alberto M. Marchevsky, MD, and Mark R. Wick, MD

The mediastinum is the chest cavity region located as a "septum" between the two pleural cavities [1-5]. It is an area of great interest to internists, pulmonologists, imaging specialists, thoracic surgeons, and pathologists because it can be the site of origin of numerous pathologic processes [6]. Indeed, the mediastinum has been compared to a "Pandora's box" full of surprises for physicians concerned with chest diseases.

Many interesting clinical problems associated with mediastinal lesions have become apparent in the last few decades with the development of very sensitive new radiologic techniques such as computerized tomography (CT scan), magnetic resonance imaging (MRI), and the extensive use of invasive diagnostic procedures such as mediastinoscopy, limited thoracotomy, transthoracic fine needle aspiration biopsy, ultrasound guided transesophageal fine needle aspiration biopsy (EUS), and ultrasound guided transbronchial fine needle aspiration biopsy [7-10]. These techniques enable the detection, localization and biopsy of mediastinal lesions hitherto located in "blind spots" of chest X-rays. However, the diagnosis of most mediastinal lesions is often rendered pathologically, a task that is often not simple, as the mediastinum contains numerous organs such as the thymus, lymph nodes, ganglia, ectopic thyroid and parathyroid tissues, soft tissues, and others that can become involved in various pathologic processes [6].

The aim of this volume is to review the clinicopathologic aspects of all mediastinal lesions of interest to the surgical pathologist, with the exception of pathologic processes in the esophagus. Although the esophagus is located in the mediastinum, a detailed description of its pathology is generally included in books dealing with the gastrointestinal tract.

Anatomy of the mediastinum

The mediastinum extends anteroposteriorly from the sternum to the spine and sagitally from the thoracic inlet to the diaphragm (Fig. 1.1) [1,2,5,9,11,12]. Its boundaries include the sternum anteriorly, the thoracic vertebra posteriorly, the first thoracic rib, first thoracic vertebra, and manubrium superiorly, and the diaphragm inferiorly. It contains the thymus, the heart and other structures shown in Figs 1.1 and 1.2.

Anatomic classifications of the mediastinum

It has become customary in clinical practice to divide the mediastinum into anatomic compartments separated by arbitrary lines. There are several anatomic classifications of the area, but the most widely used scheme is a simple one that divides the mediastinum into four compartments: superior, anterior, middle, and posterior (Fig. 1.3) [1-3]. This classification is useful in that certain pathologic lesions are most frequently located in particular compartments [3-5,11]. For example, thymic and thyroid tumors are usually in the anterior mediastinum, whereas most neurogenic lesions are found in the posterior compartment [3]. This scheme, however, has several drawbacks such as the fact that there is no agreement in the literature on whether the posterior mediastinum should extend backward only to the anterior margins of the vertebral bodies or more posteriorly into what some authors term the paraspinal area.

Heitzman tried to overcome the limitations of this oversimplified view of the mediastinum by proposing a much more detailed classification of the area based on anatomic landmarks that can be recognized on chest roentgenograms. In his scheme, the mediastinum can be divided into thoracic inlet, anterior mediastinum, supraaortic area, infraaortic area, supraazygous area, infraazygous area, and hila [7].

The *thoracic inlet* marks the cervicothoracic junction and is the area above and below a plane drawn transversely through the first rib. The *anterior mediastinum* is the region extending from the thoracic inlet to the diaphragm in front of the pericardium, ascending aorta, and superior vena cava. The *supraaortic area* is the region located behind the left side of the anterior mediastinum. It extends from the aortic arch to the thoracic inlet. The *infraaortic area* is the region located behind the left side of the anterior mediastinum. It extends from below the aortic arch to the diaphragm. The *supraazygous area* is the region located behind the right side of the anterior mediastinum. It extends from the arch of the azygous vein to the thoracic inlet. The *infraazygous area* is the region extending behind the right side of the anterior mediastinum from below the arch of the azygous vein to the diaphragm. The

---

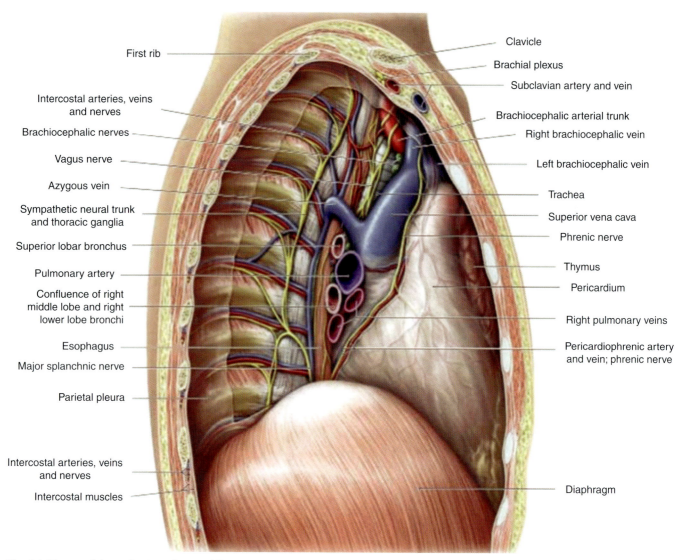

First rib

Clavicle

Brachial plexus

Subclavian artery and vein

Intercostal arteries, veins and nerves

Brachiocephalic arterial trunk

Brachiocephalic nerves

Right brachiocephalic vein

Vagus nerve

Left brachiocephalic vein

Azygous vein

Trachea

Sympathetic neural trunk and thoracic ganglia

Superior vena cava

Phrenic nerve

Superior lobar bronchus

Pulmonary artery

Thymus

Confluence of right middle lobe and right lower lobe bronchi

Pericardium

Right pulmonary veins

Esophagus

Major splanchnic nerve

Pericardiophrenic artery and vein; phrenic nerve

Parietal pleura

Intercostal arteries, veins and nerves

Intercostal muscles

Diaphragm

Fig. 1.1 Diagram of the mediastinum showing different structures.

- Heart (H)
- Trachea (T)
- Great vessels (GV)
- Thymus gland (G)
- Sympathetic nerves and ganglia
- Thoracic duct, lymphatic ducts, and lymph nodes

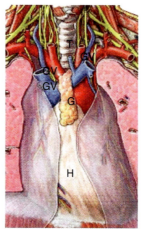

Fig. 1.2 Diagram of the mediastinum showing the heart and other mediastinal structures of interest.

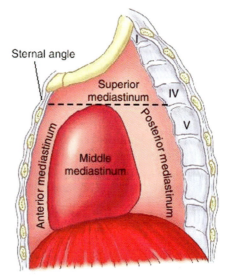

Sternal angle

Superior mediastinum

Anterior mediastinum

Posterior mediastinum

Middle mediastinum

Fig. 1.3 Diagram of the mediastinum illustrating the various mediastinal compartments.

hila include both major bronchi and surrounding bronchopulmonary structures.

This classification is useful from the imaging point of view because it enables imaging specialists to localize lesions with accuracy and aids in suggesting differential diagnosis, but is of relatively little value to a surgical pathologist faced with the task of establishing the pathologic diagnosis of a particular mediastinal lesion that could arise in more than one area. Therefore, throughout this volume we utilize the simpler and more widely used classification of the mediastinum into four compartments: superior, anterior, middle, and posterior.

Anatomic compartments

The *superior mediastinum* extends above a line drawn from the manubrium of the sternum through the lower edge of the fourth thoracic vertebral body (Fig. 1.3)[5,12]. The *anterior mediastinum* lies below the superior compartment, between the sternum and the pericardium. The *posterior mediastinum* extends behind a coronal plane through the posterior aspect of the pericardium. The *middle compartment* lies between the anterior and posterior divisions of the mediastinum.

The superior mediastinum contains the phrenic nerves and the superficial and deep cardiac plexuses (Fig. 1.1). In addition, the superior and middle mediastina contain a large number of structures that can be explored with the mediastinoscope and are usually classified according to their relationship to the trachea, as the mediastinoscopist follows its pathway in order to explore the paratracheal areas[8,9,13–16]. They include (a) the soft tissues anterior to the trachea, thyroid isthmus and blood vessels (superior vena cava, pulmonary artery, aortic arch, anterior communicating jugular vein, thyroid veins, and thyroidea ima artery and vein); (b) to the right of the trachea, blood vessels (right carotid artery, right subclavian artery, azygous vein, pulmonary artery, and superior division of the right pulmonary artery), nerves (right recurrent laryngeal nerve, vagus nerve), and bronchi (right main bronchus and right upper lobe bronchus); (c) to the left of the trachea, blood vessels (thoracic duct, aortic arch, bronchial artery, pulmonary arteries), left recurrent laryngeal nerve, esophagus, and left main bronchus; and (d) inferior to the trachea, carinal lymph nodes, esophagus, and tracheal bifurcation.

The middle mediastinum strictly should include only the pericardium and its contents. For convenience, however, most anatomy textbooks describe the hila of the lungs in this compartment and include in the middle mediastinum important bronchopulmonary lymph nodes classified by Nagaishi as follows: bronchopulmonary, pulmonary ligament, Botallo's ligament, tracheal bifurcation, tracheobronchial, paratracheal, pretracheal, aortic arch, and innominate vein angle nodes[1–3].

The anterior mediastinum merges at its upper end with the superior compartment and reaches inferiorly to the diaphragm. It contains the thymus gland, blood vessels (e.g., the internal mammary artery and vein), lymph nodes (internal mammary and diaphragmatic lymph nodes), connective tissue, and fat. Occasionally it can contain thyroid and parathyroid tissue.

The posterior mediastinum is the space located behind the pericardium and above the diaphragm. It merges directly with the superior mediastinum and includes important structures such as the descending portion of the thoracic aorta, esophagus, veins of the azygous system (azygous and superior and inferior hemiazygous veins), thoracic duct, lymph nodes (pre-aortic, paraaortic, posterior intercostal, middle diaphragmatic, and descending intercostal nodes), and ganglia and nerves of the thoracic sympathetic trunk.

References

1. Ugalde PA, Pereira ST, Araujo C et al. Correlative anatomy for the mediastinum. *Thorac Surg Clin.* 2011;21:251–72, ix.

2. Deslauriers J. Preface. Thoracic anatomy: pleura and pleural spaces, mediastinum, diaphragm, and esophagus. *Thorac Surg Clin.* 2011;21:xiii–xxiv.

3. Esposito C, Romeo C. Surgical anatomy of the mediastinum. *Semin Pediatr Surg.* 1999;8:50–3.

4. Heap SW. The sectional anatomy of the mediastinum. *Australas Radiol.* 1984;28:208–18.

5. Carter DR. The anatomy of the mediastinum. *Ear Nose Throat J.* 1981;60:153–7.

6. Marchevsky AM, Kaneko M. *Surgical Pathology of the Mediastinum.* 1991; New York: Raven Press.

7. Heitzman ER. *The Mediastinum: Radiologic Correlations with Pathology.* 2012; New York: Springer.

8. Vilmann P, Puri R. The complete "medical" mediastinoscopy (EUS-FNA + EBUS-TBNA). *Minerva Med.* 2007;98:331–8.

9. Priola SM, Priola AM, Cardinale L et al. The anterior mediastinum: anatomy and imaging procedures. *Radiol Med.* 2006;111:295–311.

10. Sarrazin R, Le Bas JF, Coulomb M. The mediastinum in sagittal sectioning. Anatomy and magnetic resonance imaging (MRI). *Surg Radiol Anat.* 1987;9:95–105.

11. Drake RL, Vogl W. *Gray's Anatomy for Students.* 2009; New York: Churchill Livingstone.

12. Last RJ. *Anatomy, Regional and Applied.* 1978; New York: Churchill Livingstone/Elsevier.

13. Zakkar M, Tan C, Hunt I. Is video mediastinoscopy a safer and more effective procedure than conventional mediastinoscopy? *Interact Cardiovasc Thorac Surg.* 2012;14:81–4.

14. Venissac N, Alifano M, Mouroux J. Video-assisted mediastinoscopy: experience from 240 consecutive cases. *Ann Thorac Surg.* 2003;76:208–12.

15. Mentzer SJ, Swanson SJ, DeCamp MM et al. Mediastinoscopy, thoracoscopy, and video-assisted thoracic surgery in the diagnosis and staging of lung cancer. *Chest.* 1997;112:239S–241S.

16. Kirschner PA. Cervical mediastinoscopy. *Chest Surg Clin N Am.* 1996;6:1–20.

Imaging of the mediastinum

Xiaoqin Wang, MD, and Ajay Singh, MD

Introduction

Chest radiography is widely used as the initial imaging study in patients with suspected thoracic disease. Mediastinal abnormality is often manifested as unexpected findings on plain radiography performed for unrelated indications. Computed tomography (CT) is the imaging modality of choice for further characterization of suspected mediastinal masses because it can define the anatomy and characterize the tissues. CT is also a popular imaging modality for the evaluation of the mediastinum because of its wide availability and rapid image acquisition ability. Magnetic resonance imaging (MRI) can allow further soft tissue characterization and functional studies. MRI is often used to evaluate soft tissue pathologies, cardiovascular function, and spinal abnormalities.

Although there is no physical boundary to separate the compartments, the mediastinum is often arbitrarily divided into compartments to develop a differential diagnosis. Disease processes can easily spread across contiguous compartments [1]. There are many ways of dividing the mediastinal compartments on images, which have been attempted by radiologists Felson, Zylak, and Heitzman [2–4]. Felson's approach divides the mediastinum into anterior, middle, and posterior compartments, based on two imaginary lines drawn on a lateral chest radiograph. The first line is drawn from the thoracic inlet to the diaphragm along the posterior heart border and anterior tracheal wall, dividing the anterior and middle mediastinum. The second line is drawn 1 cm posterior to the anterior margin of the dorsal vertebrae, and separates the middle and posterior mediastinum (Fig. 2.1) [2].

Anterior mediastinal mass

The anterior mediastinum mainly contains the thymus gland, fatty tissues, anterior mediastinal lymph nodes, and pericardium. The differential diagnosis of the anterior mediastinal mass includes thymic, thyroid, lymphoid, and germ cell tumors.

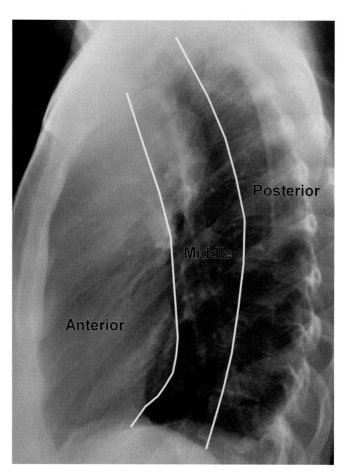

Fig. 2.1 Felson's division of the mediastinum.
The anterior line drawn posterior to the pericardium and anterior to the trachea divides the anterior from the middle mediastinum. The posterior line drawn 1 cm posterior to the anterior margin of the vertebral bodies separates the middle and posterior mediastinum.

Thymic abnormalities

Both composition and configuration of a normal thymus gland changes with age. The thymus is mainly composed of lymphocytes and epithelial cells at birth, but is replaced by fat by the age of 40 years [5]. The thymus appears largest in size in

Pathology of the Mediastinum, ed. Alberto M. Marchevsky and Mark R. Wick. Published by Cambridge University Press.
© Cambridge University Press 2014.

(a)

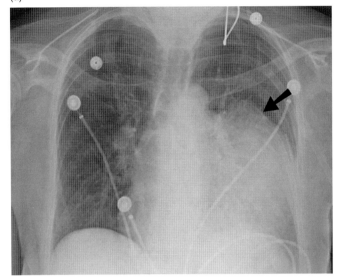

(b)

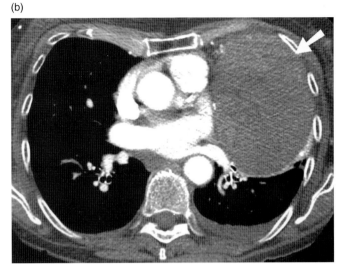

(c)

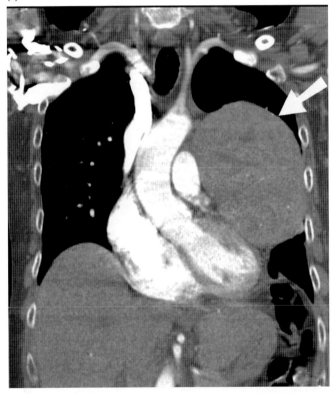

Fig. 2.2 Thymoma in a 74-year-old female.
(a) Chest radiograph, frontal view, shows a large left anterior mediastinal mass (arrow), silhouetting the left heart border.
(b) and (c) Axial and coronal reformation CT images show a well-defined soft tissue mass (arrow) along the left heart border.

proportion to the chest at birth, and starts to decrease in size after puberty, progressively undergoing fatty infiltration [6]. The thymus is not commonly visualized on CT in healthy adults.

A variety of pathologic conditions arise from cells of thymic origin, including thymoma, thymic carcinoma, thymolipoma, and thymic hyperplasia. Both thymoma and thymic carcinoma are tumors arising from the thymic epithelial cells and therefore located in the anterior mediastinum. Thymoma is a low-grade malignant thymic tumor which can be invasive or non-invasive. On CT scans a thymoma is seen as a homogeneous enhancing lobulated soft-tissue mass in the anterior mediastinum (Fig. 2.2). There is frequent association between thymoma and myasthenia gravis [7].

Thymic carcinoma is a malignant thymic tumor, which is almost indistinguishable in CT appearance from thymoma. It can invade the mediastinal fat and adjacent structures or pleura (Fig. 2.3). The relatively new World Health Organization classification scheme for thymic epithelial tumors

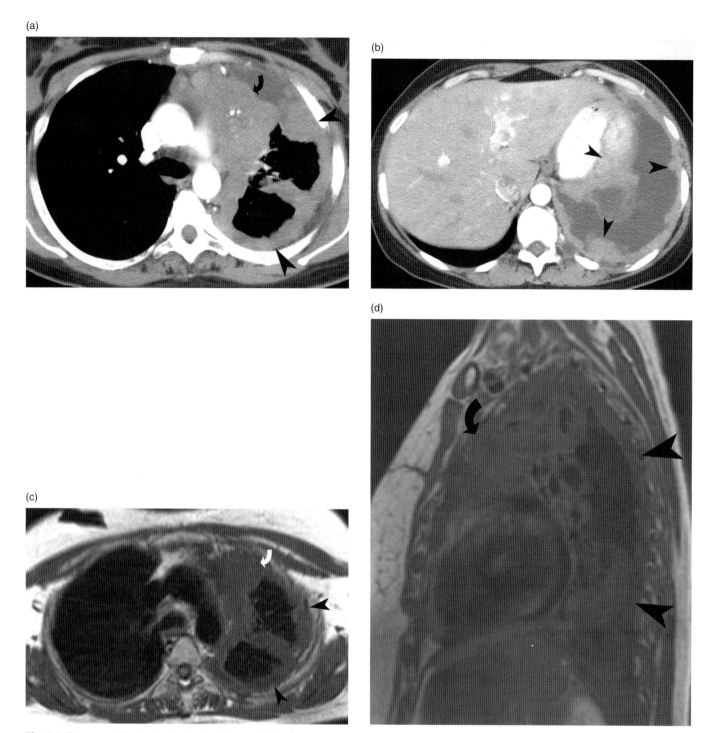

Fig. 2.3 Thymoma with pleural extension in a 36-year-old female.
Contrast-enhanced CT **(a–b)** and T1-weighted MR **(c–d)** shows a soft tissue mass (curved arrows) with calcifications in the anterior mediastinal, extending lateral to the aortic arch and aortopulmonary window. There is direct extension in to the pleural, indicated by nodular enhancing pleural thickening (arrowheads).

correlates with the invasiveness and clinical behavior of the tumors [8]. Although this classification is based on histology, familiarity with the correlation between this classification and CT findings will help the radiologist with the diagnosis.

Thymic hyperplasia is the abnormal diffuse enlargement of thymus due to either true thymic hyperplasia or lymphoid hyperplasia. Lymphoid hyperplasia is caused by chronic inflammation and proliferation of lymphoid follicles [9]. Lymphoid hyperplasia can be seen in patients with autoimmune diseases or endocrine diseases such as systemic lupus erythematosus, Addison's disease, and myasthenia gravis. Mendelson *et al.* reported that lymphoid hyperplasia is seen in up to two

(a)

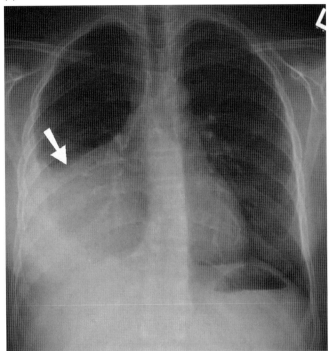

(b)

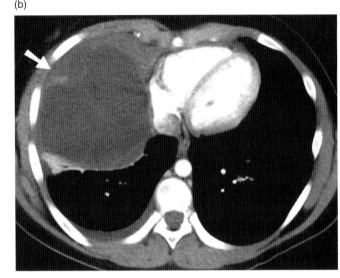

Fig. 2.4 Mature cystic teratoma in an 11-year-old female.
(a) Chest radiograph shows a large right anterior medistinal mass (arrow), silhouetting the right heart border with right pleural effusion.
(b) Contrast-enhanced CT demonstrates a septated cystic mass (arrow) with soft tissue component along the right heart border.

thirds of patients with myasthenia gravis disease [10]. True thymic hyperplasia is often seen in young patients after resolution of severe illness, steroid treatment, chemotherapy, thyrotoxicosis, and Graves' disease [10]. It is not possible to distinguish between the two types solely on the basis of imaging findings. On imaging studies, both types of thymic hyperplasia show diffuse homogeneous thymic enlargement with normal thymic tissue and shape. Awareness of the imaging features of thymic hyperplasia can help the radiologist to distinguish them from thymic neoplasm, which presents with focal mass on CT or MRI.

Thymolipoma is a rare, slow-growing, benign thymic tumor composed of mature adipose tissue and thymic tissue. It often affects young adults asymptomatically. Thymolipoma is often seen incidentally on chest radiograph as mediastinal widening. CT and MR imaging shows a large fatty mass anterior to the heart, with fibrous septa. The recurrence after surgical resection is rare [11].

Germ cell tumor

Germ cell tumors account for a fifth of all mediastinal tumors, most commonly located in the anterior mediastinum [12]. In general, germ cell tumors most often occur in the gonads, with the thorax being a rare site. It often affects children and young adults without sex predilection. Although benign germ cell tumors affect male and female patients with equal frequency, malignant germ cell tumors have predilection for male patients. Based on the cell types, germ cell tumors are usually categorized into teratomas, seminomas and non-seminomatous germ cell tumors [13].

Mediastinal teratoma is the most common mediastinal germ cell neoplasm. It is a slow-growing benign tumor that often occurs in children and young adults (less than 40 years). It is most often asymptomatic and has no sex predilection. Radiographically, the teratoma appears as a loculated cystic or solid mass with variable wall thickness in the anterior mediastinum near or within the thymus (Fig. 2.4). It may contain fluid, soft tissue, calcium, or fat attenuation, which are features of mature hematoma. Mature teratoma often has excellent prognosis and recurrence after surgical resection is rare [13].

Mediastinal seminoma is the second most common mediastinal germ cell tumor and the most common malignant mediastinal germ cell tumor. It often affects young white males and may be associated with elevated β human chorionic gonadotropin (β-HCG). CT typically shows large bulky homogeneous soft tissue attenuation mass in the anterior mediastinum, which may locally invade adjacent structures or metastasize to the lungs. Seminoma is highly sensitive to both radiotherapy and Cisplatin-based chemotherapy, with good long-term survival rate [13].

Mediastinal non-seminomatous germ cell tumors are malignant and include yolk sack tumor, embryonal carcinoma, and choriocarcinoma, as well as mixed germ cell neoplasm.

These tumors typically affect young adult men and are usually symptomatic. They often secrete the tumor markers, such as lactate dehydrogenase, alpha fetoprotein, and β-HCG, which can be used for diagnosis or follow up. On CT, non-seminomatous malignant germ cell tumors are often seen as large irregular heterogeneous density soft tissue mass with necrosis, hemorrhage, cyst formation, and peripheral contrast enhancement. They may show local invasion, lymph nodal or hematogenous metastasis [14]. The non-seminomatous germ cell tumors have poor prognosis and can be treated with Cisplatin-based chemotherapy or surgery [13].

Thyroid abnormalities

Goiter accounts for the majority of mediastinal thyroid mass. It almost always presents as a unilateral anterior mediastinal mass with glandular or fibrous continuity with the thyroid gland [15]. An ectopic primary intrathoracic thyroid mass is extremely rare. It is often an incidental finding in a female patient. However, large mediastinal goiter may have mass effects upon the adjacent structures causing tracheal or esophageal deviation or compression [15]. On CT without intra-venous iodinated contrast, thyroid mass is seen as a homogeneous, smoothly marginated, space-occupying lesion with high attenuation, due to the iodine content. It shows intense and prolonged contrast enhancement with intravenous contrast [16]. Goiter may contain cystic or calcific foci. Radionuclide scintigraphy is important in confirming the diagnosis. A CT scan of the neck is often obtained to define the extent of disease [15]. Please be aware that iodinated contrast can delay the radionuclide imaging.

Mediastinal lymphoma

Mediastinal lymphoma mainly arises from the lymph node or thymus with anterior and middle mediastinal predilection. Although both Hodgkin's and non-Hodgkin's lymphoma can cause mediastinal masses, Hodgkin's lymphoma more commonly involves the mediastinum than the non-Hodgkin's lymphoma [17]. The patients with lymphoma often have hilar adenopathy and splenomegaly.

The typical CT appearance for Hodgkin's lymphoma is multiple smooth rounded homogenous or heterogeneous soft tissue density mass in the anterior mediastinum (Fig. 2.5) [18]. It tends to spread contiguously along lymph node chains, commonly affecting the prevascular and paratracheal nodes. It can cause mass effect on the adjacent mediastinal structures. Pleural or pulmonary involvement is not very common [17]. Calcifications in Hodgkin's lymphoma are rare but may be seen after therapy.

Non-Hodgkin's lymphoma is a diverse group of disease with variable histology, clinical course, and radiographic appearance. Compared with Hodgkin's disease, non-Hodgkin's disease is more likely to spread to the extranodal sites and often skip the lymph node groups [19]. Isolated pulmonary, pleural, or pericardial diseases are sometimes seen

with non-Hodgkin's lymphoma. Although thoracic CT is often used as the initial imaging modality to evaluate the lymphoma, it is not an ideal imaging tool in assessing treatment response because not all effectively treated lymphoma decrease in size. It has been reported that positron emission tomography with 2-[fluorine-18]fluoro-2-deoxy-D-glucose can detect tumor viability following treatment [20].

Middle mediastinal masses

The most common abnormalities of the middle mediastinum are lymphadenopathy, cystic lesions, esophageal disease, tracheal abnormalities, diaphragmatic hernia, and vascular abnormalities.

Lymphadenopathy

The common causes of enlarged mediastinal lymph nodes are lymphoma, leukemia, metastasis, infection, sarcoidosis, and Castleman's disease.

On CT, normal lymph nodes manifest as discrete elliptical soft tissue with central hilar fat. Morphology, calcification, and contrast enhancement are used to characterize the lymph node, but lymph node size is the most important measurement to assess the lymph node. Lymph nodes with short axis diameter greater than 10 mm are generally considered to be pathologically enlarged [21,22]. The size criteria for normal lymph nodes also depends on the location. Some lymph nodes, such as the subcarinal lymph node with short axis measurement of up to 15 mm, can be normal. Internal mammary nodes, paracardiac nodes, and paravertebral nodes are not often visible on CT in a healthy subject [23].

Calcified lymph nodes are most often due to prior granulomatous disease, including histoplasmosis, tuberculosis, and sarcoidosis. Less commonly they may also be seen in silicosis, coal workers' pneumoconiosis, mucinous adenocarcinoma, treated lymphoma, or metastatic osteosarcoma.

Low attenuation in lymph nodes often reflects necrosis and can be seen in active tuberculosis, fungal infections, lymphoma, and neoplasm. Marked enhancement of an enlarged lymph node can indicate Castleman's disease, papillary thyroid disease, or hypervascular metastasis [24,25].

Other than the characteristics of the lymph node, the differential considerations in radiology are also based on the patient's clinical presentation, age, and immune status. For example, in a young African American female adult without symptoms, the presence of symmetric bilateral hilar and mediastinal lymphadenopathy favors the diagnosis of sarcoidosis. In a patient with pulmonary infection, the hilar and mediastinal masses are likely reactive lymphadenopathy. Enlarged mediastinal lymph nodes in a patient with a known history of cancer will be concerning for metastasis. Leukemia and chronic lymphocytic lymphoma patients often present with middle mediastinal and hilar lymphadenopathy.

Metastatic cancers, especially from the lung, head, neck, breast, and upper gastrointestinal tract are the major causes of

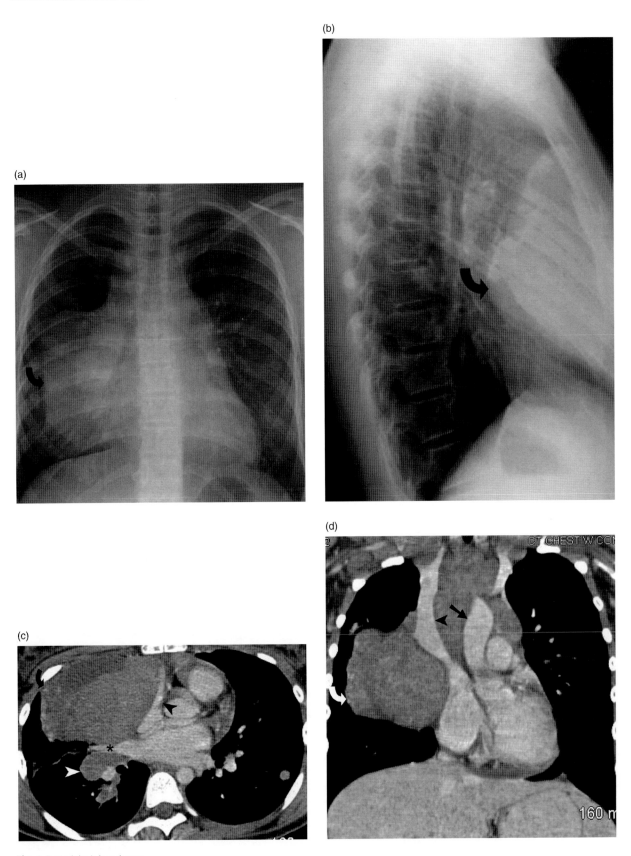

Fig. 2.5 Hodgkin's lymphoma
(a) and (b) Chest radiograph, frontal and lateral views, show a large anterior mediastinal mass (curved arrow) with right-sided extension anterior to the right lung. The bilobed density projecting through the center of the mass represents the right hilar lymphadenopathy.
(c) and (d) Axial CT image and coronal reformat shows a large heterogeneous mass (curved arrow) in the anterior mediastinal compressing the superior vena cava (black arrowhead), right pulmonary vein (asterisk), and main pulmonary artery (straight arrow). There is right hilar lymphadenopathy (white arrowhead).

mediastinal lymphadenopathy [12,26]. The revised Response Evaluation Criteria in Solid Tumor (RECIST), version 1.1 provides standards about how to measure and assess lymph nodes. Lymph nodes with a short axis of more than 15 mm are considered measurable and assessable as target lesions whereas lymph nodes with a short axis more than 10 mm but less than 15 mm are considered as non-target but assessable lesions [22].

Sarcoidosis is a systemic non-caseating granulomatous disease of unknown cause that affects almost any organ in the body. It has predilection for young African American females. The most common CT findings are bilaterally symmetric hilar lymphadenopathy and pulmonary infiltrates in characteristic perivascular distribution (Fig. 2.6) [27]. Mediastinal adenopathy without hilar involvement is rare [28].

Acute or chronic infection including viral, bacterial, or fungal infection is another important cause of middle mediastinal lymphadenopathy. There is often associated cough, fever, chills, or elevated white blood count. In patients with tuberculosis, enlarged lymph nodes often show rim enhancement and central necrosis (Fig. 2.7). In patients with chronic fungal or tuberculous infections, the lymph nodes are often calcified [29].

Histoplasma capsulatum is a well-recognized cause of mediastinal and hilar disease, particularly in the endemic central United States. It has a broad spectrum of imaging findings, ranging from clinically insignificant adenopathy to fibrosing mediastinitis. The adenopathy caused by histoplasma often calcifies during the healing phase of the disease (Fig. 2.7) [30].

Castleman's disease, also known as angiofollicular lymph node hyperplasia, is a lymphoproliferative disorder of unknown etiology [31]. It can present as a benign localized form with single mediastinal mass, or a progressive diffuse form with generalized lymphadenopathy. Due to its highly vascular nature, Castleman's disease is typically manifested as

Fig. 2.6 Sarcoidosis in a 45-year-old male.
Chest radiograph, frontal view, shows bilateral hilar masses (arrowheads) proven to be sarcoidosis.

(a)

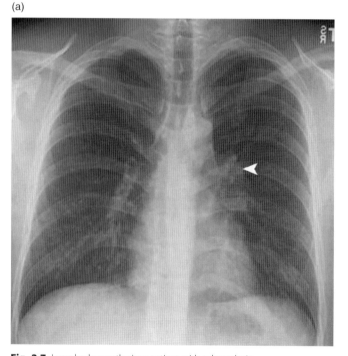

(b)

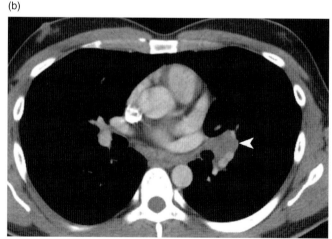

Fig. 2.7 Lymphadenopathy in a patient with tuberculosis.
(a) Chest radiograph, frontal and lateral views, show left hilar mass (arrowheads) proven to be lymphadenopathy.
(b) Axial contrast-enhanced CT confirms the left hilar lymphadenopathy (arrowhead).

marked homogeneous enhancement on CT after intravenous contrast administration [32].

Mediastinal cysts

Mediastinal cysts occur in all compartments of the mediastinum. Major mediastinal cystic masses include bronchogenic cysts, duplication cysts, pericardial cysts, pancreatic pseudocysts, and tumors with cystic degeneration, especially after treatment. On CT, mediastinal cysts are round, fluid attenuation masses which do not enhance on contrast CT or MR. MRI is very useful for evaluation of mediastinal cystic masses and demonstrates high signal intensity on T2-weighted sequences. The cysts are seen on cross-sectional imaging as round or oval, thin-walled and well defined lesions with no infiltration of surrounding structures. Hemorrhage and infection in benign cysts may complicate the imaging appearance and make it sometimes difficult to distinguish them from neoplastic cystic masses on the CT or MRI scan [33]. Clinical history and laboratory tests can help narrow down the diagnosis in many cases. We are going to focus on the major congenital mediastinal cysts, including bronchogenic cysts, duplication cysts, and pericardial cysts in the mediastinum.

Bronchogenic cysts result from abnormal budding from the embryonic foregut. They are the most common congenital cysts in the middle mediastinum and are often adjacent to the trachea or carina [34]. Most bronchogenic cysts are asymptomatic and may occasionally cause chest pain or dyspnea due to compression upon the adjacent structures. They may increase in size due to superimposed infection or hemorrhage. Bronchogenic cysts demonstrate characteristic homogeneous, non-enhancing, sharply marginated masses on CT or MRI.

Duplication cyst is another less common congenital foregut cyst with clinical symptoms and imaging appearance similar to bronchogenic cyst. It is usually located within or adjacent to the esophageal wall. Approximately 50% of pediatric patients with thoracic duplication cysts contain ectopic gastric mucosa which may cause hemorrhage or perforation of the cyst. Ectopic gastric mucosa in duplication cysts can be detected with Tc-99m sodium pertechnetate radionuclide scanning [35].

Pericardial cysts are always connected to the pericardium, but rarely communicate with the pericardial sac [36]. Most pericardial cysts occur in the right anterior cardiophrenic angle and manifest as anterior mediastinal masses blunting the pericardiophrenic angle. They have CT and MR imaging features similar to those of other congenital mediastinal cysts (Fig. 2.8a). Ultrasound can help to characterize the cysts.

Neuroenteric cysts are congenital abnormalities due to failure of complete separation of the notochord from the foregut. Neuroenteric cysts are usually located in the posterior mediastinum, but can be found in the spinal column, brain, abdomen, pelvis, or subcutaneous tissue [37]. Neuroenteric cysts

are benign cysts with the typical appearance of simple cysts as described earlier (Fig. 2.8b–c).

Esophageal abnormalities

Esophageal tumor, dilatation, esophagitis or varices can present as mediastinal mass on cross-sectional imaging. Endoscopy of the esophagus can provide direct visualization of the mucosal lining, but may not allow accurate evaluation of more extrinsic pathologies. CT is often used to evaluate extramucosal extension and disease complications. An esophagram allows the assessment of esophageal mobility and distensibility.

Esophageal cancer is often classified into two groups: squamous cell carcinoma, which occurs most commonly in the proximal esophagus, and adenocarcinoma, which occurs most commonly in the distal esophagus. Barium studies and endoscopy of the esophagus are most commonly used in the initial evaluation of patients with suspected esophageal cancer. CT is a complimentary imaging tool in oncologic workup, used mainly for disease staging, surgical planning, and treatment. Esophageal cancer may appear as abnormal wall thickening with direct outside extension or lymphadenopathy on CT. The normal thickness of the esophageal wall measures between 1 and 3 mm, depending on the distention of the esophagus [38]. Positron emission tomography (PET) using 2-[fluorine-18] fluoro-2-deoxy-D-glucose (18F-FDG) is being used to stage patients with esophageal cancer [39].

The prognosis of esophageal cancer is often poor because there is frequent direct focal tumor invasion of periesophageal soft tissues secondary to the lack of serosa in the esophageal wall [40]. Surgery, radiation, and chemotherapy are the treatment options, which depend on the cancer stage.

Esophageal dilatation can be caused by abnormal esophageal motility (e.g. achalasia or scleroderma), or distal obstruction secondary to benign or malignant lesions [40].

Hiatal hernia is most commonly seen as lower middle mediastinal mass on radiograph (Fig. 2.9a). The sliding type with migrated gastroesophageal junction is seen more often than the paraesophageal type.

Esophageal varices are abnormally dilated veins in the esophageal wall which may appear as middle mediastinal masses in patients with portal hypertension (uphill varices) or superior vena cava compression or narrowing (downhill varices). This can be easily appreciated on CT with intravenous contrast (Fig. 2.9b) or barium study.

Diaphragmatic hernia

Diaphragmatic hernia, either congenital or acquired, may also appear as mediastinal mass on a screening chest radiograph. The most common congenital diaphragmatic hernia is the Bochdalek hernia, which often occurs along the left posterior costodiaphragmatic margin and may contain retroperitoneal fat and abdominal viscera (Fig. 2.10). The less common congenital type is the Morgagni hernia, which occurs on the right

(a)

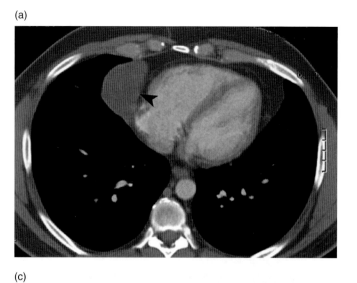

(b)

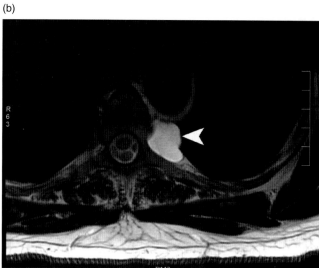

(c)

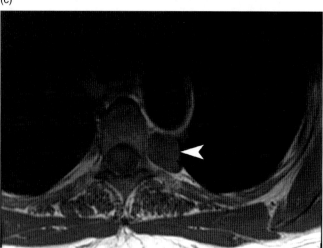

Fig. 2.8 Mediastinal cysts.
(a) Contrast-enhanced CT shows a well-defined pericardial cyst (arrowhead) at the anterior cardiophrenic angle.
(b)–(c) Neuroenteric cyst in a 53-year-old female. Axial T1-weighted **(b)** and T2-weighted **(c)** MR image at the T4 vertebrae level shows a cystic lesion (arrow) lateral to the pedicle.

(a)

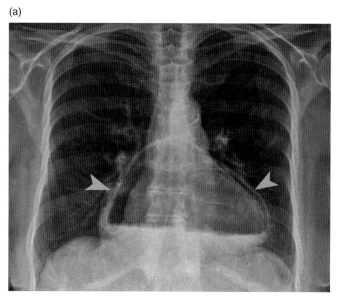

(b)

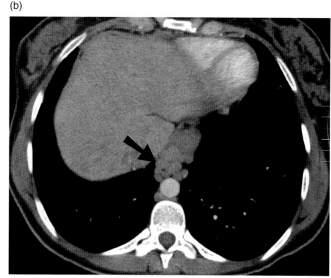

Fig. 2.9 Hiatus hernia (a) and esophageal varices (b).
(a) Frontal radiograph demonstrates a large hiatus hernia (arrowheads), containing an air-fluid level.
(b) Contrast-enhanced CT demonstrates multiple esophageal varices (arrow) at the gastroesophageal junction

(a)

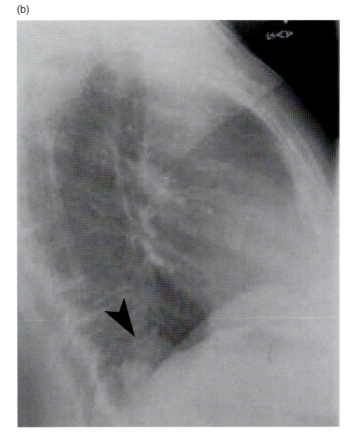

(b)

(c)

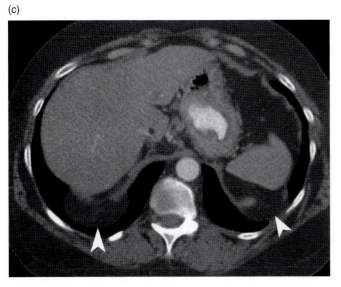

Fig. 2.10 Bochdalek diaphragmatic hernia.
(a) and (b) Chest radiograph, frontal and lateral views, demonstrate hemispherical mass projecting over the left dome of the diaphragm.
(c) Contrast-enhanced CT shows bilateral Bochdalek diaphragmatic hernias, containing fat (arrowheads).

side and may contain omentum, liver, or bowel. Morgagni hernia, in contrast to Bochdalek hernia, often manifests as anterior mediastinal mass causing blunting of the right pericardiphrenic angle (Fig. 2.11a–b). The acquired diaphragmatic hernia often results from trauma or iatrogenic causes (Fig. 2.11c). CT scan with coronal and sagittal reformatted images is the most effective and useful imaging technique on diaphragmatic hernia [41]. The imaging findings include discontinuity of the diaphragm, CT collar sign, dependent viscera sign, thick crus sign, and absent diaphragm sign.

Posterior mediastinal mass

The posterior mediastinum contains the vertebral column, connective tissue, sympathetic nerve chains, and peripheral nerves. Neurogenic tumors are the most common causes of

(a)

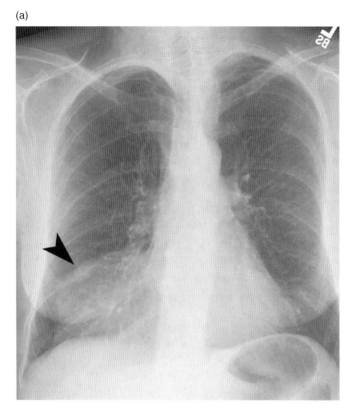

(b)

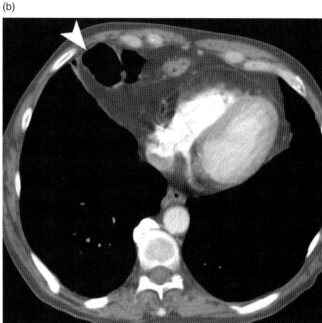

(c)

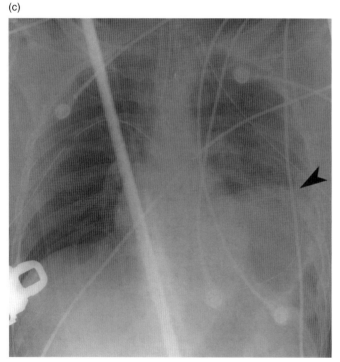

Fig. 2.11 Morgagni hernia **(a–b)** and traumatic diaphragmatic rupture **(c)**.
(a) Morgagni hernia in a 65-year-old female. Chest radiograph, frontal view,
shows well defined density mass (arrowhead) at the right cardiophrenic angle.
(b) Contrast-enhanced CT of the same patient demonstrates Morgagni hernia
(arrowhead), containing colonic loop and fat.
(c) Frontal chest radiograph in a patient with traumatic diaphragmatic rupture
demonstrates intrathoracic herniation of the stomach, as indicated by the
position of the nasogastric tube tip (arrowhead).

posterior mediastinal masses [29]. Depending on the tissue of origin, the neurogenic neoplasm can be divided into three groups: neoplasm of the nerve sheaths (neurofibroma or schwannoma), neoplasm of the sympathetic ganglion cells (neuroblastoma, ganglioneuroma, or ganglioneuroblastoma), and neoplasm of the paraganglia (paraganglioma) [29]. In pediatric patients, neurogenic tumors are usually malignant, like neuroblastoma. In adult patients, they are usually benign (ganglioneuroma, neurofibroma, schwannoma). MRI plays an important role in imaging evaluation of neurogenic tumors.

Schwannoma

Schwannoma is an encapsulated benign nerve sheath tumor which is the most common neurogenic tumor of the posterior mediastinum. Schwannoma has different variants and is associated with neurofibromatosis type II [42]. Prognosis is excellent and recurrence is rare after surgical resection [43]. This mass has high cellular components and often contains calcification. It can also undergo cystic and myxomatous degeneration as well as bleeding. The tumors can grow through the adjacent intervertebral foramen or spinal canal, and manifest as a "dumb-bell" shape. This tumor demonstrates homogeneous or heterogeneous high signal intensity on T2 weighted images (Fig. 2.12a–c) [44]. Unless it has undergone degeneration, it strongly enhances on MRI or CT.

Neurofibroma

Neurofibroma is an uncommon spinal tumor, and most commonly affects 20–40-year-old male patients. The patients are typically younger than those with spinal schwannomas. It may manifest as a sporadic solitary tumor with a capsule or pseudocapsule, or as a component of neurofibromatosis type I [29]. Unlike schwannoma, this tumor is hypocellular and contains myxomatous and fibrous tissues.

On imaging neurofibromas typically show gradual and weak contrast enhancement. Neurofibroma can manifest as a homogeneous or heterogeneous high signal intensity mass on T2-weighting MRI, like schwannoma, or as diffuse involvement of the long nerve segment with "bag of worms" appearance, as in plexiform neurofibroma [44]. The recurrence rate after resection is generally low but higher in patients with neurofibromatosis type I, compared to non-familial form [45].

Neuroblastoma

Neuroblastoma is an uncapsulated malignant sympathetic ganglion tumor found in children with a median age at diagnosis of 22 months [46]. It can occur in the adrenal gland, extradrenal retroperitoneum, and thoracic, pelvic, or neck paraspinal ganglia. Approximately 20% of neuroblastomas occur in the posterior mediastinum [47]. This tumor contains neuroblasts, their derivatives (ganglion cells and Schwann cells), and stroma. Necrosis, hemorrhage, and calcification are common in this tumor. Most neuroblastoma (90–95%) can secrete catecholamines, including vanillylmandelic acid and homovanillic acid, which can be used to assist in staging and prognosis [48]. Neuroblastoma often manifest as a calcified mass with heterogeneous signal density and varying contrast enhancement [44]. It often runs along the anterolateral surface of several vertebrae with tapering [49].

Paraganglioma

Paraganglioma (chemodectoma) is a rare neural tumor arising from the paraganglion cells that lie adjacent to the sympathetic ganglia or plexuses throughout the body. In the thorax, it often arises near the base of the great vessels or adjacent to the heart [50]. Paragangliomas contain a well-developed vascular network, hemorrhage, and cystic degeneration [51]. This tumor often manifests as a well- or ill-defined heterogeneous mass "salt-and-pepper" appearance on T2-weighted MRI due to the signal voids related to its hypervascularity [51].

Extramedullary hematopoiesis

Extramedullary hematopoiesis is a rare cause of mass in the posterior mediastinum. It often results from compensatory formation of blood elements outside of the bone marrow due to inadequate production or excessive destruction of blood cells. It can be associated with severe anemia, thalassemia, sickle cell disease, osteopetrosis, myelofibrosis, or congenital hemolytic anemia. This tumor-like condition can also occur in the liver, spleen, kidney, or lymph node.

On imaging it appears as a mass adjacent to the vertebrae (frequently bilaterally) or ribs (commonly multiple ribs) in the thorax (Fig. 2.12d) [52]. CT shows a well-defined, heterogeneous paravertebral mass with often homogeneous and intense enhancement owing to the high vascularity [53]. This often occurs with coarse bone trabeculation in the adjacent vertebra. Calcification in this tumor is extremely rare. Extramedullary hematopoiesis often regresses or disappears after the underlying causes have been corrected [54].

Mediastinal injury

Mediastinal injury may result from a variety of causes, with trauma or iatrogenic injuries being the most common. Chest radiography is the first imaging examination that is performed to evaluate patients with suspected mediastinal injury. However, findings on chest radiograph are non-specific and require further workup with contrast-enhanced CT. The most common post-traumatic vascular injury is to the aorta. The non-vascular post-traumatic injury can involve the tracheobronchial tree, esophagus, or thoracic duct.

Thoracic aortic injury is the major concern in mediastinal injuries because of the high mortality and need for quick diagnosis as well as intervention. Approximately 75–90% of all traumatic aortic injury cases are immediately fatal [55–7]. Traumatic aortic injury can be caused by motor vehicle collisions, falls from height, and penetrating injuries [58]. Although traumatic aortic injury can occur in any portion of the aorta, it most often occurs in the aortic isthmus or 2 cm distal to the origin of the left subclavian artery [57,58].

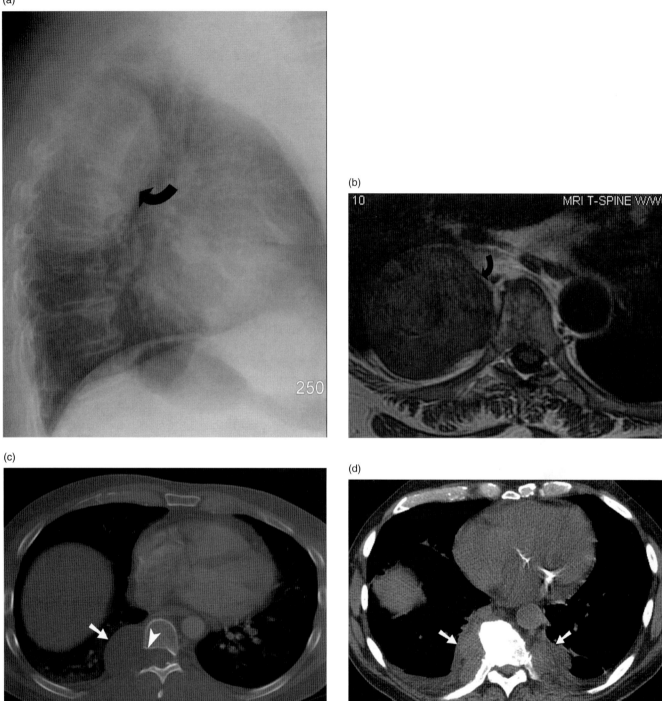

Fig. 2.12 Posterior mediastinal masses.
(a) Schwannoma. Lateral view of the chest shows a large posterior mediastinal mass (curved arrow).
(b) Axial T1-weighted MR image of the same patient demonstrates a well-defined mass paraspinal (curved arrow) of low intensity.
(c) Contrast-enhanced CT in bone window setting demonstrates a paraspinal schwannoma (arrow) in a different patient, causing a widening of the adjacent neural foramina (arrowhead).
(d) Extramedullary hematopoiesis: axial non-contrast CT of the chest demonstrates bilateral paraspinal masses (arrows) due to extramedullary hematopoiesis.

The initial chest radiograph may show abnormal aortic contour, tracheal deviation, mediastinal widening, tracheal deviation, and rightward deviation of the nasogastric tube at level of T4 [56]. However, these findings on chest radiograph are neither sensitive nor specific. Although in the past, conventional aortography was used to diagnose traumatic aortic injury, over the last decade CT angiography has become the imaging modality for definite diagnosis. The advantages of CT angiogram include rapidity of evaluation, high sensitivity, and high negative predictive value [59,60].

(a)

(b)

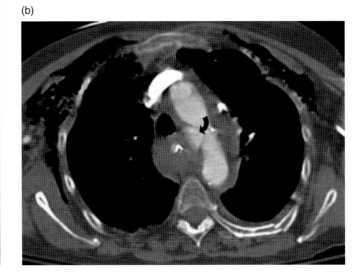

(c)

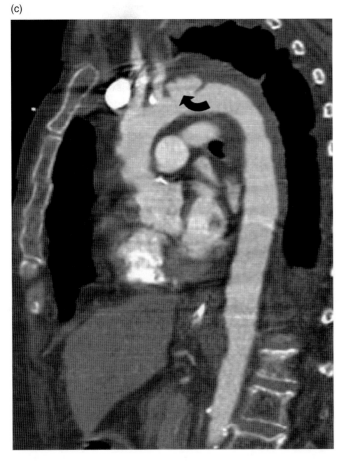

Fig. 2.13 Traumatic aortic injury.
(a) Frontal chest radiograph shows non-specific mediastinal widening and extensive air in the chest wall.
(b) and (c) Axial contrast-enhanced CT and sagittal reformation demonstrates superior hematoma and traumatic pseudoaneurysm (curved arrow) arising from the aortic arch. Soft tissue emphysema is also noted in the bilateral chest wall.

The CT signs of thoracic aortic injury include mediastinal hematoma, change in aortic contour, intimal irregularity, pseudoaneurysm, or intramural hematoma (Fig. 2.13) [58]. Traumatic aortic injury is treated urgently with surgical repair (open thoracotomy) or endovascular stent-grafting [58]. The patient who survives traumatic aortic injury without surgery may go on to develop a chronic pseudoaneurysm [56].

(a)

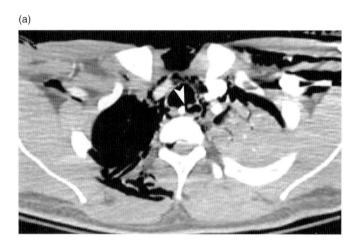

(b)

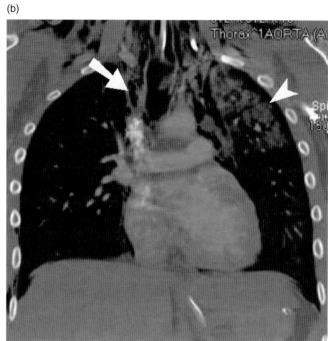

(c)

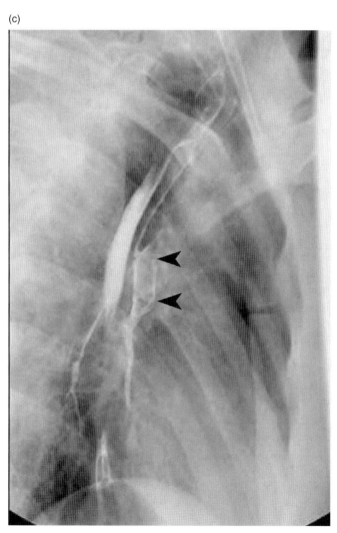

Fig. 2.14 Tracheoesophageal fistula.
(a) Contrast-enhanced axial CT shows communication between the trachea and esophagus (arrowhead).
(b) Coronal reformation demonstrates extensive pneumomediastinum (arrow) and left upper lobe consolidation (arrowhead).
(c) Esophagram confirms the contrast leakage from the esophageal lumen to the trachea (arrowheads).

(a)

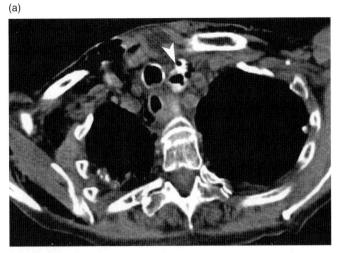

(b)

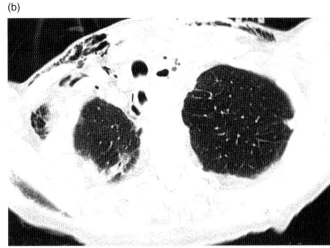

Fig. 2.15 Esophageal perforation (iatrogenic).
(a)–(b) Axial contrast-enhanced CT in soft tissue and lung windows demonstrate esophageal wall thickening, extraluminal gas collection, as well as oral contrast.

Tracheobronchial injury

Tracheobronchial injury is uncommon in patients with thoracic trauma. The diagnosis of tracheobronchial injury is often delayed because the damaged airway column can be maintained by peritracheobronchial tissue and the radiographic imaging findings are non-specific.

Common CT manifestations include pneumomediastinum, pneumothorax, pneumoretroperitoneum, cervical subcutaneous emphysema, atelectasis, and overdistension of the endotracheal tube balloon cuff. The late complications of this injury include bronchopleural fistula, tracheoesophageal fistula (Fig. 2.14), and tracheobronchial stenosis [61]. Bronchoscopy with direct visualization of the tracheobronchial tear is important for the prompt diagnosis of tracheobronchial injury.

Esophageal perforation

Esophageal perforation is a surgical emergency as it can lead to acute mediastinitis and rapid patient deterioration. It can be caused by trauma, iatrogenic injuries (Fig. 2.15), or neoplasm. Approximately 10% of cases of esophageal perforation can be secondary to vomiting and are described as Boerhaave's syndrome (Fig. 2.16) [62].

On the initial chest radiograph, esophageal perforation may show air collections in the mediastinum and subcutaneous soft tissues (Fig. 2.15a and Fig. 2.16a). While injury to the superior two thirds is usually associated with right pleural effusion, injury of the lower one third results in left pleural effusion [63]. CT with oral contrast is often used to assess the esophageal perforation. The CT findings of esophageal injury include esophageal wall thickening or defect, periesophageal fluid, mediastinal air, and oral

contrast leakage (Fig. 2.15 and Fig. 2.16) [61]. Esophagram under fluoroscopy with water soluble contrast is often used to confirm the diagnosis.

Mediastinum inflammation

Mediastinitis refers to inflammation of the connective tissues or fat surrounding the mediastinum. Acute mediastinitis is a life-threatening condition, often presenting with acute onset of fever, chill, and retrosternal pain. The etiologies include esophageal or airway perforation, thoracic surgery, or direct extension of infection from the pharynx, pleura, lung, chest wall, paraspinal region, or retroperitoneum (e.g. pancreatitis) [62,64].

CT is the imaging modality of choice for diagnosis and assessment of mediastinitis. On CT, it can manifest as increased mediastinal fat attenuation, free mediastinal gas, localized fluid collection, pleural effusion, mediastinal lymph node, pulmonary opacity, and empyema (Fig. 2.17) [64,65]. Acute mediastinitis is often treated with both surgical and medical methods, depending on the cause and complication of this condition. Mediastinal abscess often requires surgical drainage (Fig. 2.18).

Chronic mediastinitis is an uncommon benign disorder characterized with excessive fibrosis in the mediastinum soft tissues. It is also known as fibrosing mediastinitis, sclerosing mediastinitis, or mediastinal fibrosis [66]. Most cases of chronic mediastinitis are caused by granulomatous disease, such as histoplasmosis, tuberculosis, or other fungal infections. Less common causes include sarcoidosis, cancer, or autoimmune disease [62]. Most cases of chronic mediastinitis in the United States are caused by *Histoplasma capsulatum*. Chronic mediastinitis can cause compression of the mediastinal structures, including the superior vena cava,

(a)

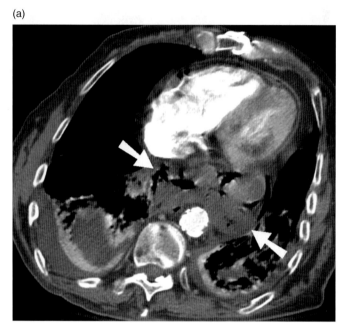

(b)

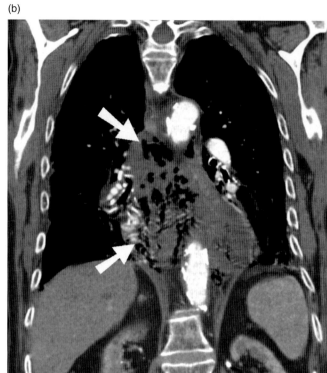

(c)

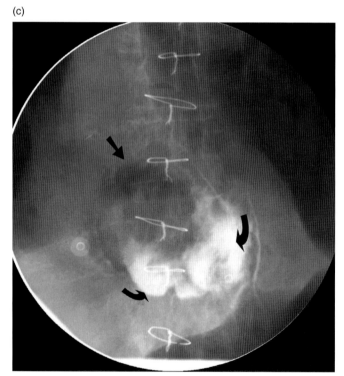

Fig. 2.16 Boerhaave's syndrome (spontaneous esophageal rupture) in a 91-year-old male.
(a)–(c) Axial contrast-enhanced CT and coronal reformation demonstrates abnormal gas and fluid collection (arrows) adjacent to the distal esophagus.
(c) Esophagram with water soluble contrast confirms extraluminal contrast (curved arrows) and air (straight arrow) around the distal esophageal leak.

(a)

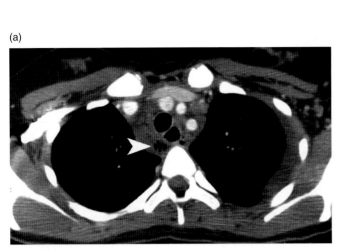

(b)

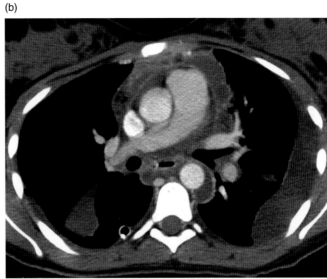

Fig. 2.17 Acute mediastinitis in an 18-year-old female.
(a)–(b) Axial CT images demonstrate the abnormal mediastinal fat stranding, pericardial effusion, pericardial enhancement, and extraluminal gas collection (arrowhead) in the mediastinum, secondary to duodenal perforation.

(a)

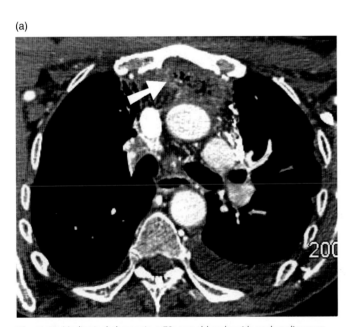

(b)

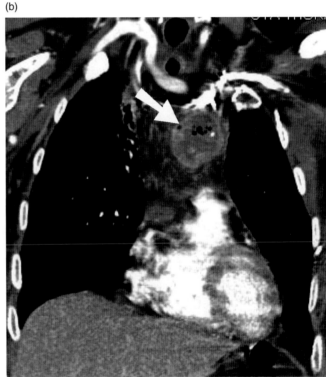

Fig. 2.18 Mediastinal abscess in a 70-year-old male with neck malignancy.
(a)–(b) Contrast-enhanced CT and coronal reformation demonstrates loculated air and fluid containing collection (arrow) in the anterior mediastinum.

pulmonary veins or arteries, central airways and bronchi, or esophagus [67].

On CT, chronic mediastinitis often manifests as diffuse or focal infiltrative soft tissue attenuation that obscures the normal adjacent mediastinal structures. It often occurs in the bilateral hilar regions and anterior to tracheal bifurcation. The presence of localized calcified mediastinal soft tissue mass with suspected chronic mediastinitis in young patients is diagnostic

(a)

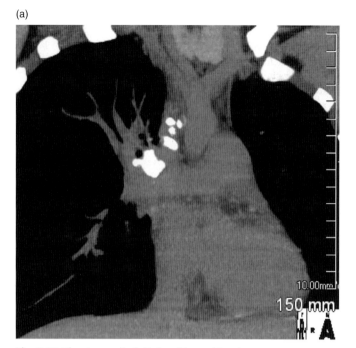

(b)

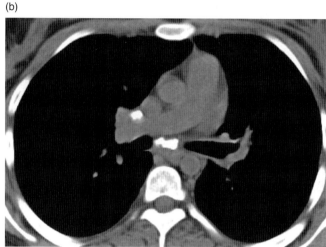

Fig. 2.19 Fibrosing mediastinitis in a 17-year-old male.
(a)–(b) Axial CT scan and coronal reformation show calcified granulomas in the right perihilar and subcarinal regions likely secondary to histoplasmosis.

of fibrosing mediastinitis caused by previous histoplasmosis or tuberculosis (Fig. 2.19). MRI can provide assessment of the vascular patency as well as evaluation of the extent of chronic mediastinitis [67].

References

1. Whitten CR, Khan S, Munneke GJ, Grubnic S (2007) A diagnostic approach to mediastinal abnormalities. *Radiographics* 27: 657–671

2. Felson B (1969) The mediastinum. *Seminars Roentgenology* 4: 41–58

3. Zylak CJ, Pallie W, Jackson R (1982) Correlative anatomy and computed tomography: a module on the mediastinum. *RadioGraphics* 2: 592

4. Heitzman ER, Goldwin RL, Proto AV (1977) Radiologic analysis of the mediastinum utilizing computed tomography. *Radiol Clin North Am* 15: 309–29

5. Suster S, Rosai J (1990) Histology of the normal thymus. *Am J Surg Pathol* 14: 284–303

6. Jacobs MT, Frush DP, Donnelly LF (1999) The right place at the wrong time: historical perspective of the relation of the thymus gland and pediatric radiology. *Radiology* 210: 11–16

7. Lewis JE, Wick MR, Scheithauer BW, Bernatz PE, Taylor WF (1987) Thymoma. A clinicopathologic review. *Cancer* 60: 2727–43

8. Han J, Lee KS, Yi CA, Kim TS, Shim YM, Kim J, Kim K, Kwon OJ (2003) Thymic epithelial tumors classified according to a newly established WHO scheme: CT and MR findings. *Korean J Radiol* 4: 46–53

9. Restrepo CS, Pandit M, Rojas IC, Villamil MA, Gordillo H, Lemos D, Mastrogiovanni L, Diethelm L (2005) Imaging findings of expansile lesions of the thymus. *Curr Probl Diagn Radiol* 34: 22–34

10. Mendelson DS (2001) Imaging of the thymus. *Chest Surg Clin N Am* 11: 269–93

11. Bogot NR, Quint LE (2005) Imaging of thymic disorders. *Cancer Imaging* 5: 139–49

12. Strollo DC, Rosado-de-Christenson ML, Jett JR (1997) Primary mediastinal tumors. Part 1: tumors of the anterior mediastinum. *Chest* 112: 511–22

13. Nichols CR (1991) Mediastinal germ cell tumors. Clinical features and biologic correlates. *Chest* 99: 472–9

14. Rosado-de-Christenson ML, Templeton PA, Moran CA (1992) From the archives of the AFIP. Mediastinal germ cell tumors: radiologic and pathologic correlation. *Radiographics* 12: 1013–30

15. Buckley JA, Stark P (1999) Intrathoracic mediastinal thyroid goiter: imaging manifestations. *AJR Am J Roentgenol* 173: 471–5

16. Bashist B, Ellis K, Gold RP (1983) Computed tomography of intrathoracic goiters. *AJR Am J Roentgenol* 140: 455–60

17. Diehl LF, Hopper KD, Giguere J, Granger E, Lesar M (1991) The pattern of intrathoracic Hodgkin's disease assessed by computed tomography. *J Clin Oncol* 9: 438–43

18. Tecce PM, Fishman EK, Kuhlman JE (1994) CT evaluation of the anterior mediastinum: spectrum of disease. *Radiographics* 14: 973–90

19. Hopper KD, Diehl LF, Lesar M, Barnes M, Granger E, Baumann J (1988) Hodgkin's disease: clinical utility of CT in initial staging and treatment. *Radiology* 169: 17–22

20. Okada M, Sato N, Ishii K, Matsumura K, Hosono M, Murakami T (2010) FDG PET/CT versus CT, MR imaging, and 67Ga scintigraphy in the post-therapy evaluation of malignant lymphoma. *Radiographics* 30: 939–57

21. Schwartz LH, Bogaerts J, Ford R, Shankar L, Therasse P, Gwyther S, Eisenhauer EA (2009) Evaluation of lymph nodes with RECIST 1.1. *Eur J Cancer* 45: 261–7

22. Eisenhauer EA, Therasse P, Bogaerts J, Schwartz LH, Sargent D, Ford R, Dancey J, Arbuck S, Gwyther S, Mooney M *et al.* (2009) New response evaluation criteria in solid tumours: revised RECIST guideline (version 1.1). *Eur J Cancer* 45: 228–47

23. Muller NL, Silva CIS (2008) *Imaging of the chest*. Philadelphia: Elsevier

24. Suwatanapongched T, Gierada DS (2006) CT of thoracic lymph nodes. Part I: anatomy and drainage. *Br J Radiol* 79: 922–8

25. Suwatanapongched T, Gierada DS (2006) CT of thoracic lymph nodes. Part II: diseases and pitfalls. *Br J Radiol* 79: 999–1000

26. Mahon TG, Libshitz HI (1992) Mediastinal metastases of infradiaphragmatic malignancies. *Eur J Radiol* 15: 130–4

27. Koyama T, Ueda H, Togashi K, Umeoka S, Kataoka M, Nagai S (2004) Radiologic manifestations of sarcoidosis in various organs. *Radiographics* 24: 87–104

28. Conant EF, Glickstein MF, Mahar P, Miller WT (1988) Pulmonary sarcoidosis in the older patient: conventional radiographic features. *Radiology* 169: 315–19

29. Strollo DC, Rosado-de-Christenson ML, Jett JR (1997) Primary mediastinal tumors: part II. Tumors of the middle and posterior mediastinum. *Chest* 112: 1344–57

30. Goodwin RA, Lloyd JE, Des Prez RM (1981) Histoplasmosis in normal hosts. *Medicine (Baltimore)* 60: 231–66

31. Castleman B, Iverson L, Menendez VP (1956) Localized mediastinal lymph node hyperplasia resembling thymoma. *Cancer* 9: 822–30

32. McAdams HP, Rosado-de-Christenson M, Fishback NF, Templeton PA (1998) Castleman's disease of the thorax: radiologic features with clinical and histopathologic correlation. *Radiology* 209: 221–8

33. Jeung MY, Gasser B, Gangi A, Bogorin A, Charneau D, Wihlm JM, Dietemann JL, Roy C (2002) Imaging of cystic masses of the mediastinum. *Radiographics* 22 Spec No: S79–93

34. McAdams HP, Kirejczyk WM, Rosado-de-Christenson ML, Matsumoto S (2000) Bronchogenic cyst: imaging features with clinical and histopathologic correlation. *Radiology* 217: 441–6

35. Ferguson CC, Young LN, Sutherland JB, Macpherson RI (1973) Intrathoracic gastrogenic cyst: preoperative diagnosis by technetium pertechnetate scan. *J Pediatr Surg* 8: 827–8

36. Feigin DS, Fenoglio JJ, McAllister HA, Madewell JE (1977) Pericardial cysts. A radiologic-pathologic correlation and review. *Radiology* 125: 15–20

37. Aydin K, Sencer S, Barman A, Minareci O, Hepgul KT, Sencer A (2003) Case report: Spinal cord herniation into a mediastinal neuroenteric cyst: CT and MRI findings. *Br J Radiol* 76: 132–4

38. Reinig JW, Stanley JH, Schabel SI (1983) CT evaluation of thickened esophageal walls. *AJR Am J Roentgenol* 140: 931–4

39. Iyer R, Dubrow R (2004) Imaging of esophageal cancer. *Cancer Imaging* 4: 125–32

40. Kawashima A, Fishman EK, Kuhlman JE, Nixon MS (1991) CT of posterior mediastinal masses. *Radiographics* 11: 1045–67

41. Eren S, Ciris F (2005) Diaphragmatic hernia: diagnostic approaches with review of the literature. *Eur J Radiol* 54: 448–59

42. Kurtkaya-Yapicier O, Scheithauer B, Woodruff JM (2003) The pathobiologic spectrum of Schwannomas. *Histol Histopathol* 18: 925–34

43. Safavi-Abbasi S, Senoglu M, Theodore N, Workman RK, Gharabaghi A, Feiz-Erfan I, Spetzler RF, Sonntag VK (2008) Microsurgical management of spinal schwannomas: evaluation of 128 cases. *J Neurosurg Spine* 9: 40–7

44. Nakazono T, White CS, Yamasaki F, Yamaguchi K, Egashira R, Irie H, Kudo S (2011) MRI findings of mediastinal neurogenic tumors. *AJR Am J Roentgenol* 197: W643–52

45. Seppala MT, Haltia MJ, Sankila RJ, Jaaskelainen JE, Heiskanen O (1995) Long-term outcome after removal of spinal neurofibroma. *J Neurosurg* 82: 572–77

46. Brossard J, Bernstein ML, Lemieux B (1996) Neuroblastoma: an enigmatic disease. *Br Med Bull* 52: 787–801

47. Morris JA, Shcochat SJ, Smith EI, Look AT, Brodeur GM, Cantor AB, Castleberry RP (1995) Biological variables in thoracic neuroblastoma: a Pediatric Oncology Group study. *J Pediatr Surg* 30: 296–302

48. Lonergan GJ, Schwab CM, Suarez ES, Carlson CL (2002) Neuroblastoma, ganglioneuroblastoma, and ganglioneuroma: radiologic-pathologic correlation. *Radiographics* 22: 911–34

49. Ikezoe J, Sone S, Higashihara T, Morimoto S, Arisawa J, Kuriyama K, Monden Y, Nakahara K, Ogawa Y, Shiozaki H (1986) CT of intrathoracic neurogenic tumours. *Eur J Radiol* 6: 266–9

50. Balcombe J, Torigian DA, Kim W, Miller WT, Jr. (2007) Cross-sectional imaging of paragangliomas of the aortic body and other thoracic branchiomeric paraganglia. *AJR Am J Roentgenol* 188: 1054–8

51. Lee KY, Oh YW, Noh HJ, Lee YJ, Yong HS, Kang EY, Kim KA, Lee NJ (2006) Extra-adrenal paragangliomas of the body: imaging features. *AJR Am J Roentgenol* 187: 492–504

52. Al-Marzooq YM, Al-Bahrani AT, Chopra R, Al-Momatten MI (2004) Fine-needle aspiration biopsy diagnosis of intrathoracic extramedullary hematopoiesis presenting as a posterior mediastinal tumor in a patient with sickle-cell disease: Case report. *Diagn Cytopathol* 30: 119–21

53. Berkmen YM, Zalta BA (2007) Case 126: extramedullary hematopoiesis. *Radiology* 245: 905–8

54. Georgiades CS, Neyman EG, Francis IR, Sneider MB, Fishman EK (2002) Typical and atypical presentations of extramedullary hematopoiesis. *AJR Am J Roentgenol* 179: 1239–43

55. Frick EJ, Cipolle MD, Pasquale MD, Wasser TE, Rhodes M, Singer RL, Nastasee SA (1997) Outcome of blunt thoracic aortic injury in a level I trauma center: an 8-year review. *J Trauma* 43: 844–51

56. Creasy JD, Chiles C, Routh WD, Dyer RB (1997) Overview of traumatic injury of the thoracic aorta. *Radiographics* 17: 27–45

57. Dosios TJ, Salemis N, Angouras D, Nonas E (2000) Blunt and penetrating trauma of the thoracic aorta and aortic arch branches: an autopsy study. *J Trauma* 49: 696–703

58. Steenburg SD, Ravenel JG, Ikonomidis JS, Schonholz C, Reeves S (2008) Acute traumatic aortic injury: imaging evaluation and management. *Radiology* 248: 748–62

59. Steenburg SD, Ravenel JG (2008) Acute traumatic thoracic aortic injuries: experience with 64-MDCT. *AJR Am J Roentgenol* 191: 1564–9

60. Melton SM, Kerby JD, McGiffin D, McGwin G, Smith JK, Oser RF, Cross JM, Windham ST, Moran SG, Hsia J *et al.* (2004) The evolution of chest computed tomography for the definitive diagnosis of blunt aortic injury: a single-center experience. *J Trauma* 56: 243–50

61. Euathrongchit J, Thoongsuwan N, Stern EJ (2006) Nonvascular mediastinal trauma. *Radiol Clin North Am* 44: 251–8

62. Akman C, Kantarci F, Cetinkaya S (2004) Imaging in mediastinitis: a systematic review based on aetiology. *Clin Radiol* 59: 573–85

63. Kshettry VR, Bolman RM, (1994) Chest trauma. Assessment, diagnosis, and management. *Clin Chest Med* 15: 137–46

64. Exarhos DN, Malagari K, Tsatalou EG, Benakis SV, Peppas C, Kotanidou A, Chondros D, Roussos C (2005) Acute mediastinitis: spectrum of computed tomography findings. *Eur Radiol* 15: 1569–74

65. Katabathina VS, Restrepo CS, Martinez-Jimenez S, Riascos RF (2011) Nonvascular, nontraumatic mediastinal emergencies in adults: a comprehensive review of imaging findings. *Radiographics* 31: 1141–60

66. Goodwin RA, Nickell JA, Des Prez RM (1972) Mediastinal fibrosis complicating healed primary histoplasmosis and tuberculosis. *Medicine (Baltimore)* 51: 227–46

67. Rossi SE, McAdams HP, Rosado-de-Christenson ML, Franks TJ, Galvin JR (2001) Fibrosing mediastinitis. *Radiographics* 21: 737–57

Inflammatory diseases of the mediastinum

Alberto M. Marchevsky, MD, and Mark R. Wick, MD

Acute and chronic mediastinitis are relatively infrequent conditions that are usually diagnosed and treated clinically. Indeed, most cases of mediastinitis are seen by pathologists at autopsy, following descending infections from the neck, complications of endoscopy, ingestion of foreign objects and complications of cardiac surgery or other surgical procedures [1–4]. Mediastinal biopsies are usually performed to diagnose mediastinal neoplasms but occasionally show only variable amounts of inflammation and/or fibrosis. The diagnosis of mediastinitis should be rendered cautiously in these instances, as the inflammatory reaction may be secondary to an adjacent neoplasm (e.g. Hodgkin's lymphoma) that was not properly sampled [5,6].

The inflammatory conditions of the mediastinum can be classified according to their clinical course and histologic characteristics into acute and chronic mediastinitis, granulomatous lymphadenitis, and sclerosing mediastinitis [7–11]. They can also be classified according to their etiology as idiopathic, infectious (e.g. fungi, mycobacteria, other), autoimmune conditions (e.g. Riedel's thyroiditis, IgG4 disease, Behcet's disease) and other conditions such as sarcoidosis, and Wegener's granulomatosis [12–23].

Acute mediastinitis

Etiology

Acute mediastinitis is an uncommon and potentially lethal clinical condition that is almost always secondary to a complication of other clinical problems such as sternal osteomyelitis, dental abscess, esophageal perforation, or cardiac surgery and other invasive diagnostic or surgical procedures [1,4]. Multiple reports have characterized the development of acute mediastinitis following sternotomy, cardiac surgery, and mediastinal biopsies [1,4,24,25]. Acute mediastinitis following esophageal perforation frequently results from postoperative dehiscence of intrathoracic esophageal anastomoses and can also develop after endoscopy and/or therapeutic dilatation of the esophagus, blunt or penetrating trauma, ingestion of foreign body, emesis (Boerhaave's syndrome), radiation-associated necrosis, or erosion of the esophageal wall by malignant tumors (Table 3.1) [1,4,26].

Table 3.1. Etiologic factors in acute mediastinitis

Cardiac surgery and other thoracic surgical procedures

Esophageal perforation caused by
Postoperative dehiscence of esophageal anastomoses
Endoscopy
Therapeutic dilatation of esophagus
Blunt or penetrating trauma
Ingestion of foreign body
Boerhaave's syndrome
Tumors

Extension of infectious processes in adjacent areas
Cervical cellulitis caused by odontogenic and other infections
Lung abscess
Vertebral osteomyelitis
Sternal osteomyelitis
Subphrenic abscess

The development of infection following esophageal perforation is potentiated by the dynamics of respiration, as the fluctuations in negative intrathoracic pressures tend to suck esophageal contents including air, saliva, enzymes, bile, acid food, and bacteria into the mediastinum. The usual result is a highly virulent necrotizing mediastinitis.

Infrequently, acute necrotizing mediastinitis develops as the result of direct penetration through soft tissue planes, usually anterior to the prevertebral fascia, or lymphatic spread of infections present in structures such as the neck, pleura, lung, subphrenic spaces, and vertebrae adjacent to the mediastinum [13,27]. Descending necrotizing mediastinitis is an unusual, usually lethal condition that follows cervical cellulitis secondary to odontogenic infections, tonsillitis, or pharyngitis that extend into the mediastinum [28–31].

Clinical findings

Patients with acute mediastinitis present with fever to 102°F, pain that varies in location according to the area of inflammation, respiratory distress, and dysphagia [1].

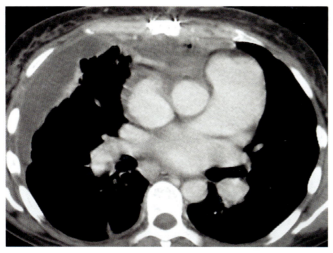

Fig. 3.1 Acute mediastinitis. Chest CT shows widening of the anterior mediastinum with ill-defined borders in a patient that presented with high fever, respiratory distress, and some dysphagia.

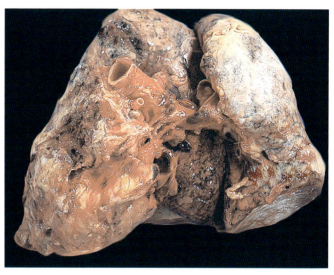

Fig. 3.2 Acute mediastinitis at autopsy showing a diffuse fibrinous exudate in the mediastinum and pleural surfaces.

(a)

(b)

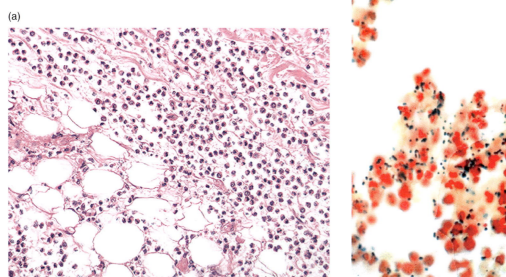

Fig. 3.3 (a) Acute mediastinitis. The patient developed acute mediastinitis following cardiac surgery and underwent re-exploration and debridement. Adipose tissue shows fat necrosis and extensive acute inflammation (H&E 100x). **(b)** Gram stain shows numerous gram positive cocci (Gram stain 1000x).

Respiratory distress occurs when the pleura is involved by extension of the acute inflammatory process from the mediastinum. Pain is usually present at the site of perforation. This lateralization is often useful in defining the site of esophageal perforation [2].

Severe dyspnea appears in patients with severe necrotizing mediastinitis, usually as a result of airway compression by the inflammatory process or because of massive pleural effusions and/or pneumothorax. Dysphagia accompanies perforation of the esophagus or the pharynx and is manifested by pain and distress while swallowing that can also help to localize the site of perforation [1,2,4].

The physical examination is usually not diagnostic in patients with acute mediastinitis, but there may be cervical tenderness in cases with cervical cellulitis and subcutaneous emphysema in cases of esophageal perforation. Chest roentgenograms and computerized scans (CT scans) are essential for the diagnosis of acute mediastinitis [4,32–34]. They usually show mediastinal widening with ill-defined borders and/or pleural effusion (Fig. 3.1). Occasionally the chest

(a)

(b)

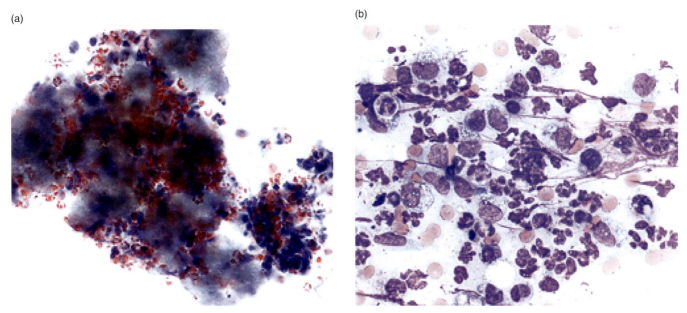

Fig. 3.4 (a) Fine-needle aspiration biopsy from a patient with acute mediastinitis. Smears show numerous acute inflammatory cells (DiffQuick 1000x). **(b)** Fine-needle aspiration from a patient with acute mediastinitis showing acute inflammatory cells and bacteria (DiffQuick 1000x).

roentgenogram may be normal. Esophagoscopy is contraindicated except when necessary to remove a foreign body.

Pathology

The pathology of acute mediastinitis is that of severe inflammation in the mediastinal soft tissues, often with abscess formation and is usually seen by pathologists at autopsy (Fig. 3.2). Occasionally, biopsies or debridement specimens are received in the surgical pathology laboratory and show fibroadipose tissue with severe acute inflammation (Fig. 3.3a). Gram stains can show bacteria (Fig. 3.3b). Infrequently, patients with acute mediastinitis undergo transthoracic fine needle aspiration biopsies (FNA) that show numerous acute inflammatory cells (Fig. 3.4a) and bacteria (Fig. 3.4b).

Aerobic and anaerobic bacteria such as β-hemolytic *Streptococcus, Staphylococcus aureus,* anaerobic *Streptococcus,* and *Bacteroides* can be isolated from FNA, resected tissues, and/or autopsy [11].

Treatment

The treatment of acute mediastinitis includes surgery for the correction of the pathogenetic factors and drainage of abscesses as well as appropriate antibiotic therapy and electrolyte, ventilatory, and nutritional support [1–4].

Chronic mediastinitis
Sclerosing mediastinitis

A number of infectious and non-infectious diseases can lead to the development of sclerosing mediastinitis characterized by the presence of chronic mediastinal inflammation with fibrosis accompanied in some instances by granuloma formation [5,10,12,16,18,23,32,35,36–38].

Sclerosing mediastinitis can be visualized on chest roentgenograms, chest CT or magnetic resonance imaging (MRI) as mass densities that compress various mediastinal structures and closely simulate a malignant process [39–43].

This syndrome has been reported with various names, such as fibrous mediastinitis, sclerosing mediastinitis, granulomatous mediastinitis, mediastinal fibrosis complicating healed primary histoplasmosis and tuberculosis, as well as others [23,36,44–56]. More recently, clinico-pathologic findings overlapping with those of sclerosing mediastinitis have been described in patients with IgG4-related sclerosing disease [47,57,58].

Etiology

The etiology and pathogenesis of chronic mediastinitis remain enigmatic in many instances. Oulmont described the first patient with this syndrome in 1855 and classified it as idiopathic fibrous mediastinitis [59]. Osler in 1903 described several additional patients with mediastinal fibrosis of unclassified etiology and superior vena cava obstruction [60]. The disease was thought to be secondary to tuberculosis or syphilis until 1925, when Knox reported cases associated with fungal infections [61]. Among the various etiologies currently proposed are infections by fungi (histoplasmosis, aspergillosis, mucormycosis, and cryptococcosis) and mycobacteria (tuberculous and non-tuberculous) and non-infectious factors such as IgG4-related disease, sarcoidosis, rheumatic fever, neoplasms, traumatic hemorrhage, and drugs (methysergide) (Table 3.2) [12,15,16,19–22,36,37,47,62–66]. In rare instances, the disease is familial and multifocal, and patients present with

Table 3.2. Etiologic factors of sclerosing mediastinitis

Fungal infections
    Histoplasmosis
    Aspergillosis
    Mucormycosis
    Cryptococcosis

Mycobacterial infections
    Tuberculosis
    Non-tuberculous infections

Bacterial infections
    Nocardiosis
    Actinomycosis

Autoimmune disease
    Behcet's syndrome
    Riedel's thyroiditis
    IgG4-related syndrome

Sarcoidosis

Rheumatic fever

Neoplasms

Trauma

Drugs

Idiopathic

retroperitoneal and mediastinal fibrosis, sclerosing cholangitis, Riedel's thyroiditis, and pseudotumor of the orbit [67].

Histoplasmosis is the most frequently implicated infectious etiology of granulomatous mediastinitis with fibrosis in the United States, but in many instances the cause of the disease remains undetermined, and the process is classified as idiopathic sclerosing mediastinitis [8,9,17,68–73].

Patients with bacterial infections caused by *Nocardia* or *Actinomyces* have been cited as examples of chronic mediastinitis with granuloma formation but usually develop extensive areas of mediastinal fibrosis and present with clinical manifestations similar to other instances of sclerosing mediastinitis [17].

Pathogenesis

The pathogenesis of the development of extensive, progressive fibrosis in some patients with mediastinal granulomas remains unclear, and several theories have been proposed to explain this complication [74–76].

Kunkel and associates suggested that mediastinal fibrosis resulted from traumatic rupture of granulomatous lymph nodes with spread of their irritating contents into adjacent soft tissues [77]. However, there are reported instances of accidental spillage of granulomatous tissues into the mediastinum at surgery without any evidence of subsequent dissemination of the disease [78]. Mathisen and Holta demonstrated lymph stasis and vein obstruction in patients with retroperitoneal fibrosis and suggested that the transudation of protein-rich fluid

resulted in progressive fibrous organization [79]. This theory fails to explain why chronic edema in other parts of the body does not result in fibrosis that extends progressively into adjacent tissues.

Baum and associates and Goodwin and collaborators proposed the most interesting and currently accepted hypothesis [80]. They suggested that sclerosing mediastinitis results from a delayed hypersensitivity reaction. They demonstrated the development of progressive fibrosis in granulomas caused by histoplasmosis and postulated the presence of an unidentified antigen that stimulated fibroblastic activity at the periphery of the granulomas. This antigen, in their concept, could diffuse into adjacent tissues and stimulate the development of an enlarging histoplasmoma that extends from areas of caseous necrosis in mediastinal lymph nodes into adjacent soft tissues. Known findings that support this hypothesis include the presence of strongly positive skin reactivity and serologic reactivity to histoplasma in some patients with sclerosing mediastinitis and hypergammaglobulinemia and hypercomplementemia in others. The infiltration of the fibrous mass by extensive aggregates of plasma cells also suggests an immunologic reaction [14,74,76,81,82].

Moreover, antinuclear antibodies and deposits of IgA, IgG, and IgM have been demonstrated on the surface of collagen fibers of patients with retroperitoneal fibrosis, a disorder thought to be related to sclerosing mediastinitis [57,67,79,83].

Clinical findings

Sclerosing mediastinitis is usually self-limiting and tends to regress with time, but it can be a serious clinical problem resulting in permanent incapacity or even death. All age groups may be affected, but the condition is found most often in white (90%), young (average age 19 to 25 years) females (female/male ratio of 3:1).

The clinical manifestations of this disorder vary considerably depending on the presence of an infectious process or the development of an expanding fibrous mass that can slowly infiltrate, surround, and compress various mediastinal structures such as blood vessels, trachea, esophagus, heart, and nerves [51]. Thin-walled veins are most commonly affected, and superior vena cava obstruction is a common complication (Fig. 3.5). Indeed, mediastinal granuloma with fibrosing mediastinitis is the most common benign cause of superior vena cava obstruction [19,48,84].

About 40% of patients with sclerosing mediastinitis are asymptomatic at the time of the initial diagnosis and are found to have abnormal chest roentgenograms with mediastinal densities suggesting the presence of a neoplasm. However, most patients present with non-specific complaints such as cough, dyspnea, chest pain, fever, wheezing, dysphagia, and/or hemoptysis [85].

Imaging findings in sclerosing mediastinitis include asymmetric widening of the mediastinum with distortion

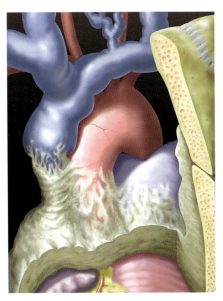

Fig. 3.5 Schematic representation of sclerosing mediastinitis presenting as ill-defined gray tissue compressing the mediastinal great vessels.

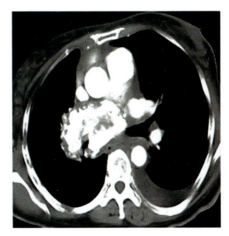

Fig. 3.6 Chest CT with contrast of a patient with sclerosing mediastinitis showing a large middle mediastinal mass and pleural effusion.

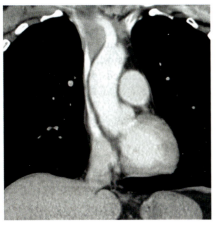

Fig. 3.7 MRI of a patient with sclerosing mediastinitis showing compression of the superior vena cava by the fibrotic process.

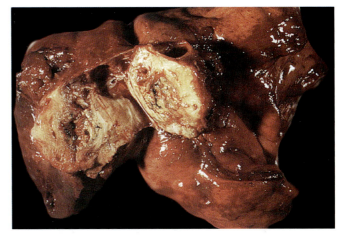

Fig. 3.8 Sclerosing mediastinitis presenting as a firm gray-tan mass that grossly simulated a neoplasm infiltrating the mediastinum and peribronchial soft tissues.

and obliteration of the tissue planes, recognizable in frontal and lateral chest roentgenographs and chest CT scans (Fig. 3.6) [46,51]. The process may also be seen as a diffuse mass with lobulated contours. Calcification of mediastinal lymph nodes, particularly in endemic areas, is a strong indication of histoplasmosis [70]. A small number of patients also have pulmonary reticular and nodular interstitial infiltrates that appear to originate from the hilar areas and are related to congestion, lymphatic stasis, and/or interstitial fibrosis [46]. Rarely, wedge-shaped areas of consolidation suggestive of pulmonary infarcts have been seen. Tomograms and CT scans are useful in order to study airways and to demonstrate areas of narrowing of the trachea and/or bronchi. Angiograms, venograms and MRI are helpful to detect compression of arteries and veins by the fibrosing process (Fig. 3.7) [46,51]. Upper gastrointestinal X-ray studies can demonstrate esophageal narrowing.

Pathology

Sclerosing mediastinitis is characterized by a diffuse or localized ill-defined infiltration of mediastinal structures by dense fibrous tissue that can closely simulate a neoplasm on gross examination (Fig. 3.8). Microscopically it shows varying degrees of infiltration by chronic inflammatory cells, dense fibrosis, and occasional microcalcifications (Fig. 3.9a–c) [86–88]. Epithelioid granulomas with or without central necrosis are often seen (Fig. 3.10). Granulomas and/or multinucleated giant cells may be encountered, however, only in focal areas encased by dense fibrous tissue, and their detection may require the study of multiple histologic sections. Special stains such as Gomori methenamine silver (GMS) and periodic acid Schiff (PAS) are useful for the detection and morphologic characterization of fungi such as *Histoplasma* (Fig. 3.11), *Aspergillus*, *Cryptococcus*, and others. Acid-fast bacilli, either *Mycobacterium tuberculosis* or atypical mycobacteria, may be found.

(a)

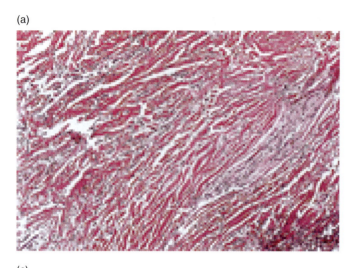

(b)

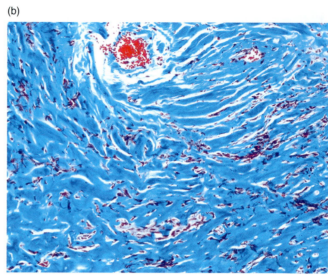

(c)

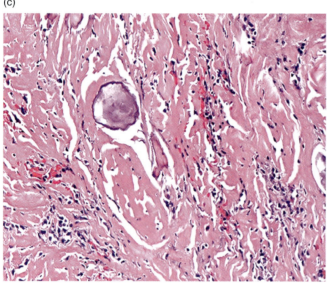

Fig. 3.9 (a) Biopsy of a patient with sclerosing mediastinitis showing dense fibrosis with collagenization (H&E 40x). **(b)** Trichrome stain of 9A highlights the presence of dense fibrosis with collagenization (trichrome stain 40x). **(c)** Focal microcalcifications can also be seen in sclerosing mediastinitis.

Lymph nodes with active granulomatous infections may also be present. These lymph nodes as well as other areas of caseating necrosis are ideal sites to biopsy and should be looked for by thoracic surgeons at the time of thoracotomy.

The infiltration of mediastinal structures in patients with sclerosing mediastinitis can be extensive, closely simulating a malignant neoplasm on imaging studies [76,84,89]. Infiltration of the superior vena cava results in superior vena cava syndrome, which can worsen considerably when secondary thrombosis of the stenosed vein ensues [48,60]. Invasion of the pulmonary veins usually occurs around the left atrium and results in a clinical syndrome that closely mimics mitral valve stenosis with pulmonary hypertension [90,91]. This complication is usually fatal. Secondary thrombosis of the pulmonary veins may be associated with pulmonary infarcts [92]. Pulmonary artery involvement with secondary pulmonary infarction and coronary artery involvement resulting in myocardial infarction have also been described [92,93]. Histologically, the arteries have infiltration of their media and adventitia by fibrous tissue and intimal proliferation that results in thrombosis secondary to irregular blood flow. Thrombosis of the pulmonary arteries can also result in pulmonary infarcts.

Bronchial and tracheal obstruction is a rare complication in patients with sclerosing mediastinitis, since the airway cartilage usually acts as a barrier against fibrous tissue invasion. When invasion occurs, it is usually accompanied by a secondary ectasia of veins and lymphatic vessels in the airway lamina propria, which in turn leads to hemoptysis, dyspnea, and markedly abnormal pulmonary function tests. This complication is usually fatal.

The esophagus is rarely compressed in sclerosing mediastinitis, since it is a freely movable structure that can be displaced by the fibrous mass without being infiltrated by it. However, in patients with severe forms of the disease in which the entire mediastinum is encased by the fibrosing process, esophageal obstruction does occur.

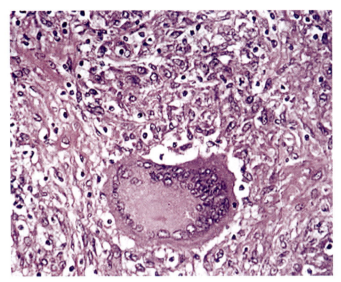

Fig. 3.10 Granuloma with multinucleated giant cell in a biopsy from a patient with sclerosing mediastinitis (H&E 100x).

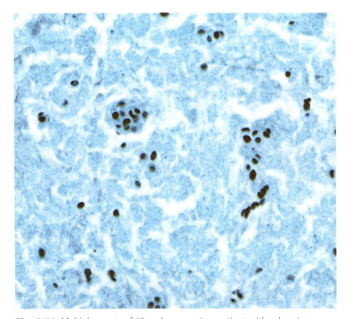

Fig. 3.11 Multiple yeasts of *Histoplasma* sp in a patient with sclerosing mediastinitis (Gomori methenamine silver stain 1000x).

Rarely, mediastinal fibrosis is complicated by a syndrome of left vocal cord paralysis as a result of involvement of the recurrent laryngeal nerve and esophageal diverticulum formation [94].

The lung may exhibit pathologic changes secondary to pulmonary venous or arterial obstruction in patients with sclerosing mediastinitis [14,92,95,96]. They include medial hypertrophy and intimal proliferation of pulmonary medium and small arteries and arterioles, pulmonary edema, and intra-alveolar accumulations of hemosiderin-laden macrophages, as seen in patients with pulmonary hypertension secondary to mitral stenosis [95,97–99]. Secondary thrombosis can ensue in these small vessels and contribute to a more severe degree of pulmonary hypertension. Rare instances of pulmonary infarcts following arterial or venous thrombosis have also been reported [92]. A more frequent complication in patients with sclerosing mediastinitis is pulmonary interstitial fibrosis, which can follow a clinical and pathologic course similar to that in patients with usual interstitial pneumonitis (UIP) [70,100].

In isolated instances, sclerosing mediastinitis may be associated with a similar fibrotic process in the retroperitoneum, thyroid, and other organs [57,67].

Prognosis and treatment

In most patients with sclerosing mediastinitis, the disease follows a slow, self-limiting clinical course [48,101,102]. For example, only one of 31 patients studied at the Mayo Clinic with this syndrome died of cardiorespiratory failure 26 years after the initial diagnosis [87]. It is controversial whether the evolution of the disease can be altered by corticosteroid therapy [102–104]. Few patients with presumed histoplasmosis have received amphotericin B therapy, but most cases have no evidence of active infection, and it is not known whether antifungal therapy has a useful role in the treatment of this syndrome [51]. Surgery is indicated in patients that develop complications as a result of compression of mediastinal structures, and thoracotomy and biopsy are frequently needed to establish the diagnosis [51]. In approximately 25% of patients with localized granulomas, complete excision of the lesion can be achieved. It appears that in at least some cases excision of local granulomas prevented the development of subsequent progressive fibrosis [71,87,105,106]. In patients with symptoms secondary to compression of mediastinal vessels or other structures, balloon angioplasty, stents, and reconstructive surgery are necessary to alleviate vascular, esophageal, or airway obstruction [48,54,107,108].

Sclerosing mediastinitis in IgG4-related sclerosing disease

IgG4-related sclerosing disease is a recently characterized syndrome identified by the presence of fibrotic mass lesions in patients with an elevated serum titer of immunoglobulin G4 (IgG4) (normal <135 mg/dL) [109,110].

Pathogenesis

IgG4 is the least common of the four subclasses of IgG (IgG1–IgG4), it does not activate complement, has a low affinity for target antigens, and is a T-helper cell 2-dependent isotype [109].

The etiology and pathogenesis of IgG4 remains unknown. The purported autoimmune etiology was first recognized in patients with chronic pancreatitis that presented with a mass lesion that narrowed the pancreatic duct creating painless obstructive jaundice and responded favorably to steroid therapy. These patients frequently had other autoimmune conditions such as Sjogren syndrome, sclerosing cholangitis, primary biliary cirrhosis, and inflammatory bowel

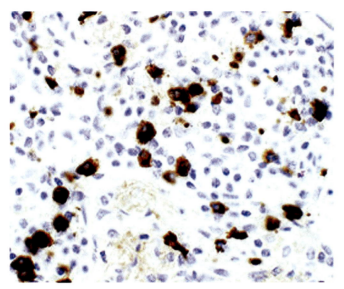

Fig. 3.12 Sclerosing mediastinitis in a patient with IgG4-related sclerosing disease. Immunostain for IgG4 shows multiple cells with intracytoplasmic immunoreactivity (PAP Immunostain 200x).

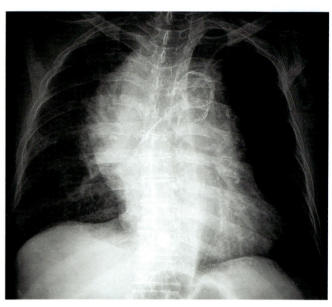

Fig. 3.13 Massive mediastinal hemorrhage presenting on chest CT scan as an anterior mediastinal mass with left pleural effusion.

(b)

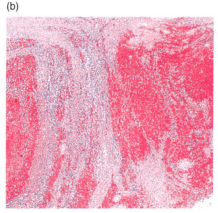

Fig. 3.14 (a) Large organizing blood clot evacuated surgically from a patient with massive mediastinal hemorrhage. **(b)** Microscopy of the lesion shown in Fig. 3.14a shows a recent clot (H&E 20x).

(a)

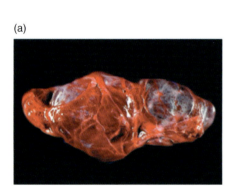

disease [47,57,58,83,109–112]. They also had elevated autoantibodies such as antinuclear antibodies (ANA), rheumatoid factor, anticarbonic anhydrase II, and antilactoferrin. An association with HLA DRB1*405-DQB1*0401 has also been described [109].

Clinical manifestations

Patients with IgG4-related sclerosing disease usually present with no fever or constitutional symptoms and develop various manifestations secondary to the presence of fibrotic mass lesions at various sites such as the pancreas, hepatobiliary tract, salivary gland, orbit, retroperitoneum, mediastinum, soft tissue, skin, central nervous system, breast, kidney, prostate, lung, and other locations [109]. The syndrome affects mostly middle-aged and elderly patients with a male predominance. Laboratory tests usually show increased immunoglobulins IgG,

IgG4, and IgE and variable titers of various autoantibodies such as ANA and rheumatoid factor.

The mass lesions develop over time at multiple sites, sometimes after many years, although the syndrome can remain localized to one site in some patients.

Pathology

Sclerosing mediastinitis associated with IgG4-related sclerosing disease shows similar gross pathologic features to those described above for other patients with idiopathic sclerosing mediastinitis [47]. Microscopically, the lesions overlap with those seen in sclerosing mediastinitis and are characterized by the presence of prominent lymphoplasmacytic infiltration, lymphoid follicle formation, fibrosis and/or obliterative phlebitis [47,111]. According to the relative predominance of the lymphoplasmacytic and sclerotic

components the histologic patterns can be classified as pseudo-lymphomatous, mixed, and sclerosing. Immunostains for immunoglobulins show the presence of IgG4+ plasma cells, > 50 per high power field, and an IgG4/IgG ratio > 40% (Fig. 3.12).

Prognosis and treatment

Patients are usually treated with steroid therapy, with excellent response [83,109,112]. Response to therapy is manifested by a progressive decline in serum IgG4 levels and a decrease in lymphoplasmacytic tissue infiltrates. Fibrotic and sclerotic masses may not respond to steroids and may require surgery to treat local complications secondary to compression of mediastinal structures.

Mediastinal hemorrhage

Patients with massive mediastinal hemorrhage that can simulate a rapidly growing malignant tumor or a cyst on chest roentgenograms or CT scan (Fig. 3.13) have been described [113–115]. Mediastinal hemorrhage can develop spontaneously or following trauma, extracorporeal membrane oxygenation, treatment of hyperthyroidism, uremia, anticoagulation therapy, and intravenous drug abuse [113,114,116–119]. Grossly the lesions appear as large anterior or middle mediastinal hematomas that can be drained surgically (Fig. 3.14a). Histologically they show recent hemorrhage with variable degrees of hemosiderosis and organization (Fig. 3.14b).

References

1. Pierce TB, Razzuk MA, Razzuk LM, Luterman DL, Sutker WL. Acute mediastinitis. *Proc (BaylUniv Med Cent)* 2000;13(1):31–3.

2. Payne WS, Larson RH. Acute mediastinitis. *Surg Clin North Am* 1969; 49(5):999–1009.

3. Liu J, Zhang X, Xie D *et al.* Acute mediastinitis associated with foreign body erosion from the hypopharynx and esophagus. *Otolaryngol Head Neck Surg* 2012;146(1):58–62.

4. Jablonski S, Brocki M, Kordiak J, Misiak P, Terlecki A, Kozakiewicz M. Acute mediastinitis: evaluation of clinical risk factors for death in surgically treated patients. *ANZ J Surg* 2012;19: 308–15.

5. Zisis C, Kefaloyannis EM, Rontogianni D *et al.* Asymptomatic chest wall Hodgkin disease mimicking fibrosing mediastinitis. *J Thorac Cardiovasc Surg* 2006;131(2): e1–e2.

6. Flannery MT, Espino M, Altus P, Messina J, Wallach PM. Hodgkin's disease masquerading as sclerosing mediastinitis. *South Med J* 1994; 87(9):921–3.

7. Smith SJ, Vyborny CJ, Hines JL. Chronic superior vena cava occlusion related to fibrosing mediastinitis treated with self-expanding shunts. *Cardiovasc Intervent Radiol* 1997; 20(2):161–2.

8. Salyer JM, Harrison HN, Winn DF, Jr., Taylor RR. Chronic fibrous mediastinitis and superior vena caval obstruction due to histoplasmosis. *Dis Chest* 1959;35(4):364–77.

9. Lull GF, Jr., Winn DF, Jr. Chronic fibrous mediastinitis due to *Histoplasma capsulatum* (histoplasmal mediastinitis). Report of three cases with different presenting symptoms. *Radiology* 1959;73: 367–73.

10. Lagerstrom CF, Mitchell HG, Graham BS, Hammon JW, Jr. Chronic fibrosing mediastinitis and superior vena caval obstruction from blastomycosis. *Ann Thorac Surg* 1992;54(4):764–5.

11. Marchevsky AM, Kaneko M. *Surgical Pathology of the Mediastinum*, 2nd ed. New York: Raven Press; 1991.

12. Wightman SC, Kim AW, Proia LA *et al.* An unusual case of Aspergillus fibrosing mediastinitis. *Ann Thorac Surg* 2009;88(4):1352–4.

13. Allotey J, Duncan H, Williams H. Mediastinitis and retropharyngeal abscess following delayed diagnosis of glass ingestion. *Emerg Med J* 2006; 23(2):e12.

14. Light AM. Idiopathic fibrosis of mediastinum: a discussion of three cases and review of the literature. *J Clin Pathol* 1978;31(1):78–88.

15. Cartier Y, Nogueira HA, Muller NL. Fibrosing mediastinitis associated with Riedel's thyroiditis–computed tomographic findings: case report. *Can Assoc Radiol J* 1998;49(6): 408–10.

16. Zhang C, Yao M, Yu Z, Jiang L, Jiang X, Ni Y. Rare fibrosing granulomatous mediastinitis of tuberculosis with involvement of the transverse sinus. *J Thorac Cardiovasc Surg* 2007; 133(3):836–7.

17. Schowengerdt CG, Suyemoto R, Main FB. Granulomatous and fibrous mediastinitis. A review and analysis of 180 cases. *J Thorac Cardiovasc Surg* 1969;57(3):365–79.

18. Lee JY, Kim Y, Lee KS, Chung MP. Tuberculous fibrosing mediastinitis: radiologic findings. *AJR Am J Roentgenol* 1996;167(6):1598–9.

19. Esquivel L, az-Picado H. Fibrosing TB mediastinitis presenting as a superior vena cava syndrome: a case presentation and echocardiogram correlate. *Echocardiography* 2006; 23(7):588–91.

20. Atasoy C, Fitoz S, Erguvan B, Akyar S. Tuberculous fibrosing mediastinitis: CT and MRI findings. *J Thorac Imaging* 2001;16(3):191–3.

21. Kanne JP, Mohammed TL. Fibrosing mediastinitis associated with Behcet's disease: CT findings. *Clin Radiol* 2007; 62(11):1124–6.

22. Harman M, Sayarlioglu M, Arslan H, Ayakta H, Harman E. Fibrosing mediastinitis and thrombosis of superior vena cava associated with Behcet's disease. *Eur J Radiol* 2003; 48(2):209–12.

23. Matousovic K, Martinek V, Spatenka J, Stejskal J, Chadimova M. Malignant Wegener's granulomatosis with fibrosing mediastinitis and vena cava superior syndrome. *Ren Fail* 2012; 34(2):244–6.

24. Tiveron MG, Fiorelli AI, Mota EM *et al.* Preoperative risk factors for mediastinitis after cardiac surgery: analysis of 2768 patients. *Rev Bras Cir Cardiovasc* 2012;27(2): 203–10.

25. Risnes I, Abdelnoor M, Veel T, Svennevig JL, Lundblad R, Rynning SE. Mediastinitis after coronary artery

bypass grafting: the effect of vacuum-assisted closure versus traditional closed drainage on survival and reinfection rate. *Int Wound J* 2012 27.

26. Divisi D, Di TS, Garramone M, Crisci E, Crisci R. Necrotizing mediastinitis linked to Boerhaave's syndrome: a surgical approach. *J Thorac Cardiovasc Surg* 2009;57(1):57–8.

27. Benezra C, Spurgeon L, Light RW. Mediastinal abscess secondary to vertebral osteomyelitis. *Postgrad Med* 1982;71(3):220–3.

28. Saute M. Descending necrotizing mediastinitis: an old issue with a new approach. *Eur J Cardiothorac Surg* 2012;42(4):e73.

29. Sarna T, Sengupta T, Miloro M, Kolokythas A. Cervical necrotizing fasciitis with descending mediastinitis: literature review and case report. *J Oral Maxillofac Surg* 2012; 70(6):1342–50.

30. Kocher GJ, Hoksch B, Caversaccio M, Wiegand J, Schmid RA. Diffuse descending necrotizing mediastinitis: surgical therapy and outcome in a single-centre series. *Eur J Cardiothorac Surg* 2012;42(4):e66–e72.

31. Ishinaga H, Otsu K, Sakaida H et al. Descending necrotizing mediastinitis from deep neck infection. *Eur Arch Otorhinolaryngol* 2013;207(4):1463–6.

32. Zorn SK, Schachter EN, Smith GJ, McLoud T. Pulmonary artery obstruction with fibrosing mediastinitis. *Lung* 1978; 155(2):91–100.

33. Cortez-Escalante JJ, Dos Santos AM, Garnica GC, Sarmento AL, Castro CN, Romero GA. Mediastinitis and pericardial effusion in a patient with AIDS and disseminated Mycobacterium avium infection: a case report. *Rev Soc Bras Med Trop* 2012;45(3): 407–9.

34. Cogan IC. Necrotizing mediastinitis secondary to descending cervical cellulitis. *Oral Surg Oral Med Oral Pathol* 1973; 36(3):307–20.

35. Yangui F, Battesti JP, Valeyre D, Kheder AB, Brillet PY. Fibrosing mediastinitis as a rare mechanism of pulmonary oedema in sarcoidosis. *Eur Respir J* 2010; 35(2):455–6.

36. Toonkel RL, Borczuk AC, Pearson GD, Horn EM, Thomashow BM.

Sarcoidosis-associated fibrosing mediastinitis with resultant pulmonary hypertension: a case report and review of the literature. *Respiration* 2010; 79(4):341–5.

37. Rossi SE, McAdams HP, Rosado-de-Christenson ML, Franks TJ, Galvin JR. Fibrosing mediastinitis. *Radiographics* 2001;21(3):737–57.

38. Makhija Z, Murgatroyd F, Gall N, Marrinan MT, Deshpande R, Desai SR. Fibrosing mediastinitis and occlusion of pulmonary veins after radiofrequency ablation. *Ann Thorac Surg* 2009; 88(5):1674–6.

39. Worrell JA, Donnelly EF, Martin JB, Bastarache JA, Loyd JE. Computed tomography and the idiopathic form of proliferative fibrosing mediastinitis. *J Thorac Imaging* 2007; 22(3):235–40.

40. Weinstein JB, Aronberg DJ, Sagel SS. CT of fibrosing mediastinitis: findings and their utility. *AJR Am J Roentgenol* 1983;141(2):247–51.

41. Takalkar AM, Bruno GL, Makanjoula AJ, El-Haddad G, Lilien DL, Payne DK. A Potential Role for F-18 FDG PET/CT in Evaluation and Management of Fibrosing Mediastinitis. *Clin Nucl Med* 2007;32(9):703–6.

42. Sherrick AD, Brown LR, Harms GF, Myers JL. The radiographic findings of fibrosing mediastinitis. *Chest* 1994; 106(2):484–9.

43. Rodriguez E, Soler R, Pombo F, Requejo I, Montero C. Fibrosing mediastinitis: CT and MR findings. *Clin Radiol* 1998;53(12):907–10.

44. Koksal D, Bayiz H, Mutluay N et al. Fibrosing mediastinitis mimicking bronchogenic carcinoma. *J Thorac Dis* 2013;5(1):E5–E7.

45. Posligua W, Zarrin-Khameh N, Tsai P, Lakkis N. Fibrosing mediastinitis causing ostial coronary artery compression in a young woman. *J Am Coll Cardiol* 2012;60(25): 2693.

46. McNeeley MF, Chung JH, Bhalla S, Godwin JD. Imaging of granulomatous fibrosing mediastinitis. *AJR Am J Roentgenol* 2012;199(2):319–27.

47. Peikert T, Shrestha B, Aubry MC et al. Histopathologic overlap between fibrosing mediastinitis and IgG4-related disease. *Int J Rheumatol* 2012; 207–56.

48. Phillips PM, Mallette AC, Aru GM, Mitchell ME. The treatment of superior vena cava syndrome secondary to idiopathic fibrosing mediastinitis with balloon angioplasty and stenting. *Am Surg* 2012;78(12):1405–6.

49. Gustafson MR, Moulton MJ. Fibrosing mediastinitis with severe bilateral pulmonary artery narrowing: RV-RPA bypass with a homograft conduit. *Tex Heart Inst J* 2012;39(3):412–15.

50. Tancredi A, Cuttitta A, Del NC, Scaramuzzi R. Fibrosing mediastinitis as a cause of right claudication. *Updates Surg* 2012;64(1):63–7.

51. Peikert T, Colby TV, Midthun DE et al. Fibrosing mediastinitis: clinical presentation, therapeutic outcomes, and adaptive immune response. *Medicine (Baltimore)* 2011; 90(6):412–23.

52. Joskin J, Ghaye B. Focal fibrosing mediastinitis. *JBR-BTR* 2011; 94(3):124–5.

53. Albers EL, Pugh ME, Hill KD, Wang L, Loyd JE, Doyle TP. Percutaneous vascular stent implantation as treatment for central vascular obstruction due to fibrosing mediastinitis. *Circulation* 2011;123(13):1391–9.

54. Smith JS, Kadiev S, Diaz P, Cheatham J. Pulmonary artery stenosis secondary to fibrosing mediastinitis: management with cutting balloon angioplasty and endovascular stenting. *Vasc Endovascular Surg* 2011;45(2): 170–3.

55. Goo DE, Kim YJ, Choi DL, Kwon KH, Yang SB. Bilateral breast enlargement: an unusual presentation of superior vena cava obstruction in a hemodialysis patient with fibrosing mediastinitis. *Cardiovasc Intervent Radiol* 2011; 34 Suppl 2: S195–S197.

56. Addatu DT, Jr., Tan HC. Fibrosing mediastinitis causing acute ostial left main myocardial infarction. *J Invasive Cardiol* 2010;22(9):456–60.

57. Taniguchi T, Kobayashi H, Fukui S, Ogura K, Saiga T, Okamoto M. A case of multifocal fibrosclerosis involving posterior mediastinal fibrosis, retroperitoneal fibrosis, and a left seminal vesicle with elevated serum IgG4. *Hum Pathol* 2006;37(9): 1237–9.

58. Zen Y, Sawazaki A, Miyayama S, Notsumata K, Tanaka N, Nakanuma Y. A case of retroperitoneal and

mediastinal fibrosis exhibiting elevated levels of IgG4 in the absence of sclerosing pancreatitis (autoimmune pancreatitis). *Hum Pathol* 2006; 37(2):239–43.

59. Oulmont N. *Des Obliterations de la Veine Cave Superier.* Paris: JB Baillere; 1855.

60. Osler W. On obliteration of the superior vena cava. *Bull Johns Hopkins Hosp* 1903;14:169–82.

61. Knox LB. Chronic mediastinitis. *Am J Med Sci* 1925;169:807–20.

62. Toonkel RL, Borczuk AC, Pearson GD, Horn EM, Thomashow BM. Sarcoidosis-associated fibrosing mediastinitis with resultant pulmonary hypertension: a case report and review of the literature. *Respiration* 2010; 79(4):341–5.

63. Leong DP, Dundon BK, Steele PM. Unilateral pulmonary vein stenosis secondary to idiopathic fibrosing mediastinitis. *BMJ Case Rep* 2009; bcr2007124404.

64. Cheng YJ, Hsieh KC, Hwang JC. Fibrosing mediastinitis as a rare sequel of iatrogenic rupture of bronchogenic cyst: a case report. *Int J Surg* 2008;6(6): e100–e102.

65. Robertson BD, Bautista MA, Russell TS *et al.* Fibrosing mediastinitis secondary to zygomycosis in a twenty-two-month-old child. *Pediatr Infect Dis J* 2002; 21(5):441–2.

66. Cooper JA. Fibrosing mediastinitis. *Radiographics* 2001;21(3):736.

67. Comings DE, Skubi KB, Van EJ, Motulsky AG. Familial multifocal fibrosclerosis. Findings suggesting that retroperitoneal fibrosis, mediastinal fibrosis, sclerosing cholangitis, Riedel's thyroiditis, and pseudotumor of the orbit may be different manifestations of a single disease. *Ann Intern Med* 1967; 66(5):884–92.

68. Park HM, Jay SJ, Brandt MJ, Holden RW. Pulmonary scintigraphy in fibrosing mediastinitis due to histoplasmosis. *J Nucl Med* 1981; 22(4):349–51.

69. Lloyd TV, Johnson JC. Pulmonary artery occlusion following fibrosing mediastinitis due to histoplasmosis. *Clin Nucl Med* 1979; 4(1):35–6.

70. Wieder S, Rabinowitz JG. Fibrous mediastinitis: a late manifestation of

mediastinal histoplasmosis. *Radiology* 1977;125(2):305–12.

71. Strimlan CV, Dines DE, Payne WS. Mediastinal granuloma.*Mayo Clin Proc* 1975;50(12):702–5.

72. Goodwin RA, Nickell JA, Des Prez RM. Mediastinal fibrosis complicating healed primary histoplasmosis and tuberculosis. *Medicine (Baltimore)* 1972;51(3):227–46.

73. Lull GF, Jr., Winn DF, Jr. Chronic fibrous mediastinitis due to *Histoplasma capsulatum* (histoplasmal mediastinitis). Report of three cases with different presenting symptoms. *Radiology* 1959;73: 367–73.

74. Afrin LB. Sclerosing mediastinitis and mast cell activation syndrome. *Pathol Res Pract* 2012;208(3):181–5.

75. Miyata T, Takahama M, Yamamoto R, Nakajima R, Tada H. Sclerosing mediastinitis mimicking anterior mediastinal tumor. *Ann Thorac Surg* 2009;88(1):293–5.

76. Mole TM, Glover J, Sheppard MN. Sclerosing mediastinitis: a report on 18 cases. *Thorax* 1995;50(3):280–3.

77. Kunkel WMJ, Claggett OT, McDonald JR. Mediastinal granulomas. *J Thorac Surg* 1954;27:565–74.

78. Friedman JL, Baum GL, Schwarz J. Primary pulmonary histoplasmosis: associated pericardial and mediastinal manifestations. *Am J Dis Child* 1965; 109:298–303.

79. Mathisen W, Holta AL. Idiopathic retroperitoneal fibrosis. *Surg Gynecol Obstet* 1966;122:1278–82.

80. Baum GL, Green RA, Schwartz J. Enlarging pulmonary histoplasmoma. *Am Rev Respir Dis* 1960;82:721–6.

81. Urschel HC, Jr., Razzuk MA, Netto GJ, Disiere J, Chung SY. Sclerosing mediastinitis: improved management with histoplasmosis titer and ketoconazole. *Ann Thorac Surg* 1990; 50(2):215–21.

82. Dunn EJ, Ulicny KS, Jr., Wright CB, Gottesman L. Surgical implications of sclerosing mediastinitis. A report of six cases and review of the literature.*Chest* 1990;97(2):338–46.

83. Gill J, Taylor G, Carpenter L, Lewis C, Chiu W. A case of hyperIgG4 disease or IgG4-related sclerosing disease presenting as retroperitoneal fibrosis, chronic sclerosing sialadenitis and

mediastinal lymphadenopathy. *Pathology* 2009;41(3):297–300.

84. Bays S, Rajakaruna C, Sheffield E, Morgan A. Fibrosing mediastinitis as a cause of superior vena cava syndrome. *Eur J Cardiothorac Surg* 2004; 26(2):453–5.

85. Hoogsteden HC, Zondervan PE, van Hezik EJ, Dijksterhuis EK, Hilvering C. Fibrosing mediastinitis. *Neth J Med* 1988;33(3–4):182–6.

86. Hewlett TH, Steer A, Thomas DE. Progressive fibrosing mediastinitis. *Ann Thorac Surg* 1966;2(3):345–57.

87. Dines DE, Payne WS, Bernatz PE, Pairolero PC. Mediastinal granuloma and fibrosing mediastinitis. *Chest* 1979; 75(3):320–4.

88. Beekman JF, Weled BJ. Mediastinal granuloma and fibrosing mediastinitis. *Chest* 1979;76(6):714.

89. Kang DW, Canzian M, Beyruti R, Jatene FB. Sclerosing mediastinitis in the differential diagnosis of mediastinal tumors. *J Bras Pneumol* 2006; 32(1):78–83.

90. Trinkle JK. Fibrous mediastinitis presenting as mitral stenosis. *J Thorac Cardiovasc Surg* 1971;62(1):161–2.

91. Chazova I, Robbins I, Loyd I, Newman J, Tapson V, Zhdaov V, Mayrick B. Venous and arterial changes in pulmonary veno-occlusive disease, mitral stenosis and fibrosing mediastinitis. *Eur Respir J* 2000; 15(1):116–22.

92. Katzenstein AL, Mazur MT. Pulmonary infarct: an unusual manifestation of fibrosing mediastinitis. *Chest* 1980; 77(4):521–4.

93. Addatu DT, Jr., Tan HC. Fibrosing mediastinitis causing acute ostial left main myocardial infarction. *J Invasive Cardiol* 2010;22(9):456–60.

94. Cohn M, Giuffra L, Demos N. Temporary vocal cord paralysis in fibrosing mediastinitis. *J Med Soc N J* 1983;80(10):841–3.

95. Arnett EN, Bacos JM, Marsh HB, Savage DD, Fulmer JD, Roberts WC. Fibrosing mediastinitis causing pulmonary arterial hypertension without pulmonary venous hypertension. Clinical and necropsy observations. *Am J Med* 1977;63(4):634–43.

96. Routsi C, Charitos C, Rontogianni D, Daniil Z, Zakynthinos E. Unilateral

pulmonary edema due to pulmonary venous obstruction from fibrosing mediastinitis. *Int J Cardiol* 2006; 108(3):418–21.

97. Botticelli JT, Schlueter DP, Lange RL. Pulmonary venous and arterial hypertension due to chronic fibrous mediastinitis. Hemodynamics and pulmonary function. *Circulation* 1966; 33(6):862–71.

98. Berry DF, Buccigrossi D, Peabody J, Peterson KL, Moser KM. Pulmonary vascular occlusion and fibrosing mediastinitis. *Chest* 1986; 89(2):296–301.

99. Ahmad S. Pulmonary hypertension secondary to fibrosing mediastinitis. *Cleve Clin J Med* 1991;58(6):475.

100. Ryu DS, Cheema JI, Costello P. Fibrosing mediastinitis with peripheral airway dilatation and central pulmonary artery occlusion. *J Thorac Imaging* 2004;19(3): 204–6.

101. Thiessen R, Matzinger FR, Seely J, Aina R, Macleod P. Fibrosing mediastinitis: successful stenting of the pulmonary artery. *Can Respir J* 2008; 15(1):41–4.

102. Lal C, Weiman D, Eltorky M, Pugazhenthi M. Complete resolution of fibrosing mediastinitis with corticosteroid therapy. *South Med J* 2005;98(7):749–50.

103. Ikeda K, Nomori H, Mori T *et al.* Successful steroid treatment for fibrosing mediastinitis and sclerosing cervicitis. *Ann Thorac Surg* 2007; 83(3):1199–201.

104. Ichimura H, Ishikawa S, Yamamoto T *et al.* Effectiveness of steroid treatment for hoarseness caused by idiopathic fibrosing mediastinitis: report of a case. *Surg Today* 2006;36(4):382–4.

105. Ferguson TB, Burford TH. Mediastinal Granuloma. A 15-Year Experience. *Ann Thorac Surg* 1965;24:125–41.

106. Strimlan CV, Khasnabis S. Primary mediastinal myelolipoma. *Cleve Clin J Med* 1993;60(1):69–71.

107. Ferguson ME, Cabalka AK, Cetta F, Hagler DJ. Results of intravascular stent placement for fibrosing mediastinitis. *Congenit Heart Dis* 2010;5(2): 124–33.

108. Nakanishi R, Nishikawa H. Successful management of idiopathic fibrosing mediastinitis with superior vena cava thrombosis. *J Cardiovasc Surg (Torino)* 2005;46(1):95.

109. Cheuk W, Chan JK. IgG4-related sclerosing disease: a critical appraisal of an evolving clinicopathologic entity. *Adv Anat Pathol* 2010;17(5): 303–32.

110. Stone JH, Khosroshahi A, Deshpande V *et al.* Recommendations for the nomenclature of IgG4-related disease and its individual organ system manifestations. *Arthritis Rheum* 2012; 64(10):3061–7.

111. Deshpande V, Zen Y, Chan JK *et al.* Consensus statement on the pathology of IgG4-related disease. *Mod Pathol* 2012;25(9):1181–92.

112. Inoue M, Nose N, Nishikawa H, Takahashi M, Zen Y, Kawaguchi M. Successful treatment of sclerosing mediastinitis with a high serum IgG4 level. *Gen Thorac Cardiovasc Surg* 2007; 55(10):431–3.

113. Gomelsky A, Barry MJ, Wagner RB. Spontaneous mediastinal hemorrhage: a case report with a review of the literature. *Md Med J* 1997;46(2): 83–7.

114. Lawler SS, Reeve R. Mediastinal hemorrhage: diagnostic and therapeutic problems. *Hawaii Med J* 1984; 43(5):152, 154.

115. Prenger KB, Poeschmann PH, Smits PH, Eygelaar A. Massive mediastinal hemorrhage following treatment of hyperthyroidism with radioactive iodine. *Thorac Cardiovasc Surg* 1984; 32(2):122–3.

116. Piers DA, Janssen S, Oosten HR, Prenger KB. Mediastinal hemorrhage after treatment of thyrotoxicosis using radioiodine. *Clin Nucl Med* 1988; 13(8):574–6.

117. Singh S, Ptacin MJ, Bamrah VS. Spontaneous mediastinal hemorrhage. A complication of intracoronary streptokinase infusion for coronary thrombosis. *Arch Intern Med* 1983; 143(3):562–3.

118. Epstein AM, Klassen KP. Spontaneous superior mediastinal hemorrhage. *J Thorac Cardiovasc Surg* 1960; 39:740–5.

119. Brown N, Tomsykoski AJ, Stevens RC. Mediastinal hemorrhage secondary to uremia. *Am J Med* 1953;15(4): 588–90.

The thymus gland

Alberto M. Marchevsky, MD, and Mark R. Wick, MD

The thymus gland is a central organ of the immune system, essential for the development of cell-mediated immunity [1]. It can be the site of origin of numerous pathologic conditions including tumors, cysts, and developmental abnormalities described in the subsequent chapters of this volume [2].

Anatomy

The thymus is located in the anterior mediastinum in front of the great vessels and superior to the base of the pericardium and the heart [1,3,4]. It has a pyramidal shape and is composed of two closely apposed lobes, each completely covered by a fibrous capsule that extends into the parenchyma in the form of connective tissue septa (Fig. 4.1). These septa divide the thymic tissue into many lobules measuring from 0.5 to 2 mm in greatest dimension composed of cortical and medullary elements (Fig. 4.2).

Embryology

The thymus arises as paired structures from the endoderm of the third and, to a lesser and inconstant degree, fourth branchial pouches during the sixth intrauterine week [5,6]. Recent studies provide support for an endoderm-centric model and it remains controversial whether the ectoderm of the third branchial clefts also contributes to its origin [7]. The mesoderm contributes the thymic vascular stroma and mesenchymal cells.

The thymus shares a common embryologic origin with the lower pair of parathyroid glands. From each side of the neck, the embryonal thymic anlagen migrate downward and medially into the anterosuperior mediastinum as epithelial tubules or cords, while the inferior parathyroid glands remain in contact with the lower poles of the thyroid. Only the upper pole of each thymic lobe remains in the neck. The thymic epithelial elements proliferate in the mediastinum, and by the eighth intrauterine week, they lose contact with the branchial clefts.

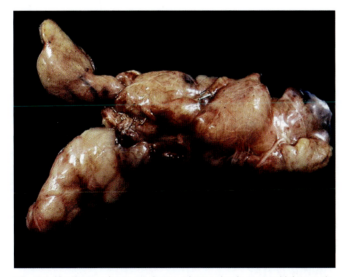

Fig. 4.1 The thymus shows a Y shape with two closely apposed lobes, each covered by a fibrous capsule and superior "horns".

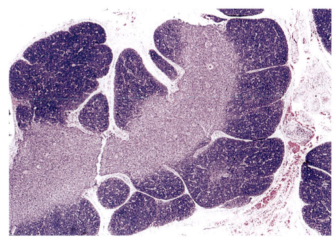

Fig. 4.2 Photomicrograph of the thymus at low-power microscopy shows a lobule composed of an external cortical area that is darker blue as a result of higher cellularity and an internal medullary area (H&E 20x).

Table 4.1. Approximate thymic weights by age

Age	Weight
Newborn	~ 10–25 grams
1 year old	~ 15–25 grams
7–27 years old	~ 18–35 grams
27–66 years old	< 15 grams

The embryogenesis and development of thymic epithelial cells was studied by German pathologists in the early twentieth century, generating different theories regarding how the primitive epithelial structures of the thymus develop. Hammar maintained that the thymic epithelial cells increase in size and number in an onion-layer fashion and form solid thymic corpuscles that by the thirteenth to fourteenth week of intrauterine life become Hassall's corpuscles [5]. Schambacher had a different view based on the examination of lymphocyte-depleted thymus glands, and suggested that Hassall's corpuscles derive from a system of discontinuous epithelial tubules whose epithelium proliferates in concentric layers [6]. A more recent study by Shier supports Schambacher's view [8].

The thymus is an epithelial organ during the second month of intrauterine life, but by the end of this month, the proliferating epithelial tubules and cords become infiltrated by lymphocytes and mesenchymal elements [8].

Thymic lymphocytes develop from hematopoietic stem cell precursors that develop into thymocytes through a maturation and differentiation process described later on in the chapter [9,10]. Most thymic lymphocytes have a very short life span and die *in situ*. A few others, however, have a long life span and are seeded into peripheral lymphoid tissues during late fetal and early postnatal life [10].

The origin of thymic myoid cells is unknown [11–19]. They may be derived from the mesenchyme surrounding the thymic epithelium, or they may arise directly from the epithelial reticular cells.

The thymus grows rapidly in embryonic life. By the ninth to tenth week of intrauterine life, the two lobes become apposed, and the gland increases in size to reach a mean weight of 15 g at birth [20]. In the neonatal period, the thymus reaches its largest relative size. It continues to grow until puberty to reach a mean weight of 18–35 g and then begins a gradual process of involution (Table 4.1).

Multiple signaling molecules such as bone morphogenic protein 4 (Bmp4), fibroblast growth factor 8 (Fgf8), sonic hedgehog (SHH) and Wnt-gene Sb (WntSb) and transcription factors such as eyes absent homolog 1 (EYA1), forkhead box protein n1 (FOXn1), homeobox protein a3 (HOXa3), paired box protein 1 (PAX1), paired box protein 9 (PAX9), sine oculis homolog ¼ (SIX ¼) and T-box 1 (Tbx1) have been implicated in thymic development [7]. A discussion of experimental evidence supporting their respective roles in thymic development is beyond the scope of this chapter.

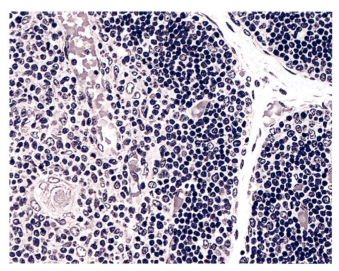

Fig. 4.3 The thymic cortex and medulla are shown at higher magnification than in Fig. 4.2. The medulla shows Hassall's corpuscles with keratinization (H&E 40x).

Ectopic thymic tissue

Small islands of ectopic thymic tissue can be found outside the capsule of the gland in the neck, tympanic cavity, different areas of the mediastinum (posterior and anterior compartments and hilum), and the lung [21–27]. These islands most likely represent remnants of thymic tissue incorporated in ectopic locations during embryologic development at the time when the thymic anlagen migrated from the branchial clefts into the mediastinum.

In rare instances, these islands of ectopic thymic tissue become hyperplastic, cystic, or neoplastic [28,29].

Histology

The thymic lobules are incompletely surrounded by fibrous septa and are composed of two areas that can be distinctly recognized in histologic sections: the cortex and medulla (Fig. 4.3) [30]. The medulla extends continuously from one lobule into others, giving the organ a characteristic "branching" configuration when viewed by low-power microscopy. The thymic cortex and medulla are composed of various types of epithelial cells described below, closely admixed with lymphocytes. Thymic lymphocytes are generically designated as thymocytes, although some investigators restrict the term to immature thymic T lymphocytes [9].

Thymic cortex

The thymic cortex is the peripheral portion of thymic lobules [30]. It is more cellular than the medulla and appears darker than the medulla under low-power microscopy (Fig. 4.3). It is composed of two antigenically distinct types of epithelial cells: the subcapsular and the cortical cells (Table 4.2) [31–33]. These epithelial cells share several structural

Table 4.2. Antigenic characteristics of thymic epithelial cells

Antigen	Secretory ("endocrine")* epithelium		Non-secretory epithelium	
	Subcapsular cortical cells	Medullary cells	Inner cortical cells	Hassall's corpuscles
Polyclonal keratin	+	+	+	+ +**
Keratin AE-1	+	−	+	−
Keratin AE-2	−	−	−	+
Keratin AE-3	+	+	+	−
A2B5	+	+	−	−
TE-4	+	+	−	−
Anti-p19	+	+	−	−
HLA Class I	+	+	+	−
HLA-DR	+	−	+	−
TE-3	−	−	+	−
Leu-7	+	−	−	−
PE-35	−	+	−	−

* Immunocytochemical studies have demonstrated intracytoplasmic thymulin, thymosin α-1, thymosin β-3, and thymopoietin in these cells.
A2B5: Monoclonal antibody against complex ganglioside present in neuroendocrine cells and neurons.
TE-4: Monoclonal antibody to thymic epithelial cells.
Anti-p19: Antibody to core protein of the human T-cell lymphoma virus (HTLV).
TE-3: Monoclonal antibody to thymic stroma.
Leu-7: Differentiation antigen present also in neuroendocrine cells and human null/killer lymphoid cells.
** Hassall's corpuscles react strongly with antibodies to high molecular weight keratin (AE-2), a finding characteristic of mature epithelial cells.
PE-35: Monoclonal antibody to medullary epithelium.

and immunophenotypic features such as the presence of tonofilaments and desmosomes under electron microscopy and reactivity with antibodies to keratin AE1/AE3 and monoclonal antibodies such as anti-KiM3 [17,30,34–42].

The subcapsular thymic epithelial cells form an almost continuous row at the periphery of the thymic cortex [43]. They have a stellate cytoplasm with a large round to oval nucleus exhibiting a clear chromatin pattern and a medium to large central nucleolus. Subcapsular epithelial cells express cytoplasmic immunoreactivity with antibodies to class I (A,B,C) and II (DR) HLA antigens, Leu7, and other antigens listed in Table 4.1[30]. An interesting feature of these cells is their capacity to secrete hormones such as thymosin α-1 (Fig. 4.4), thymosin β-3, and thymopoietin, which are able to induce TdT positivity in TdT-prothymocytes derived from the bone marrow [31–33,44–46]. Some large subcapsular cortical epithelial cells of the thymus enclose numerous immature thymocytes with active mitotic activity and are thought to represent the thymic "nurse"cells [44]. These cells exhibit immune reactivity with antibodies to neuropeptides [47–49].

The cortical epithelial cells are difficult to visualize on light microscopy as they have round to oval nuclei, clear chromatin pattern, inconspicuous nucleoli, and scanty cytoplasm (Fig. 4.5), features similar to those seen in histiocytes [30]. They

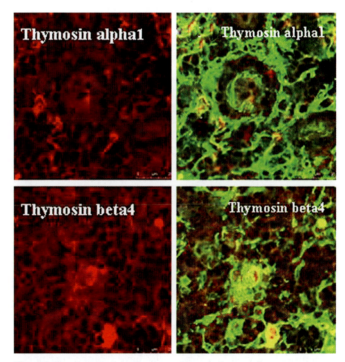

Fig. 4.4 Thymic epithelial cells secrete thymosin (Immunofluorescence. Green: fluorescein isothiocyanate; red: tetramethylrhodamine-5 and 6-isothyocyanide 20x).

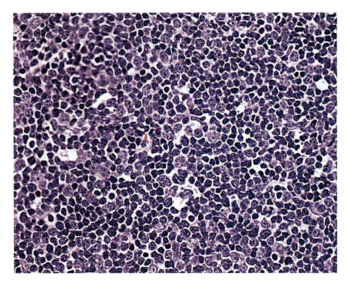

Fig. 4.5 Thymic cortex. Epithelial cortical cells are slightly larger and have more open chromatin pattern than thymocytes (H&E 100).

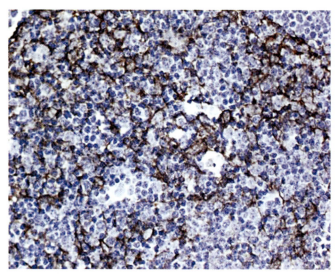

Fig. 4.6 Thymic cortex. The cortical epithelial cells can be better visualized with Immunostains for keratin AE1/AE3. They form a mesh of interconnected cells with scanty cytoplasm. (PAP Immunostain 40x).

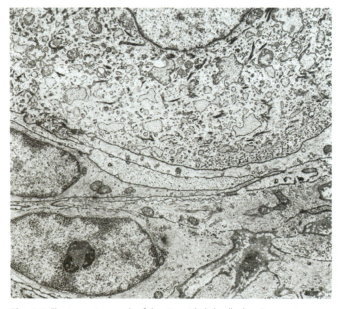

Fig. 4.7 Electron micrograph of thymic epithelial cells showing scanty organelles, intermediate filaments, and long cytoplasmic projections covered by a basement membrane.

are closely admixed with large lymphoid cells (lymphoblasts) and smaller lymphocytes. The cortical epithelial cells can be readily identified using keratin antibodies such as AE1/AE3 (Fig. 4.6). The inner cortical epithelial cells of the thymus have morphologic features similar to subcapsular cortical epithelial cells but exhibit distinct antigenic determinants such as a Leu-7–phenotype and strong immunoreactivity to the monoclonal antibody TE-3 (Table 4.2). In contrast to the thymic subcapsular epithelial cells they lack secretory characteristics. Ultrastructurally, thymic cortical cells have scanty, peripheral organelles, intermediate filaments, and long cytoplasmic projections covered by basal lamina material (Fig. 4.7).

The thymic cortex has medium or large lymphoblasts with a round nucleus and a narrow cytoplasmic rim that are in close contact with epithelial cells [38,44,50]. The nucleus of these thymocytes has an open chromatin structure without a prominent nucleolus. Mitoses are frequent. Thymic lymphoblasts represent up to 5% of thymocytes and exhibit the antigenic characteristics listed in Table 4.3 [9,31]. The thymic cortex also has smaller, more mature thymocytes with the phenotypic features listed in Table 4.3. An interesting feature of thymic cortical lymphocytes is the presence of double positive (DP) cells with simultaneous T4 and T8 nuclear immunoreactivity and TdT nuclear immunoreactivity (Fig. 4.8) [9]. Cortical thymocytes comprise the majority (60–80%) of thymic lymphoid cells [30].

The thymic cortex has numerous degenerating thymocytes that undergo lympholysis and phagocytosis by cortical macrophages that stain strongly with reagents to α-naphtyl acetate esterase and acid phosphate [30]. The presence of phagocytosis becomes prominent in patients with acute thymic involution resulting in a "starry-sky" pattern, discussed in Chapter 5.

Thymic medulla

The medulla is the central portion of thymic lobules and appears lighter than the cortex on low power microscopy, reflecting the presence of smaller densities of epithelial and lymphoid cells [30]. It contains characteristic epithelial structures known as Hassall's corpuscles, reticular medullary epithelial cells, and lymphocytes [51,52].

Hassall's corpuscles are complex tubular structures composed of mature epithelial cells aggregated in concentric layers (Fig. 4.9). They exhibit varying degrees of central keratinization and/or calcification and occasionally may become cystic. Cystic Hassall's corpuscles have a central space containing proteinaceous material and degenerated lymphocytes and eosinophils. The epithelium of Hassall's corpuscles secretes a

Table 4.3. Immunophenotype at different stages of T-cell development

Antigen	Thymic stem cells	Myeloid precursors	T/NK precursors	Pre-T1	Pre-T2	Early double +	Double +
CD34	++	+	++	+	−	−	−
CD1A	−	−	−	+	+	+	+
CD2	−	?	+	+	+	+	+
CyCD3	−	−	Low	+	+	+	+
CD4	−	Low	−	−	+	+	+
CD5	−/low	−	+	+	+	+	+
CD7	++	?	++	+	+	+	+
CD8α	−	−	−	−	−	−	+
CD8β	−	−	−	−	−	−	+
CD44	++	++	+	+	−	−	−
CD45RA	+	+	++	+	−	−	−
GM-CSFR	−	+	−	−	−	−	−

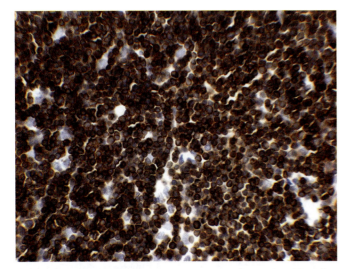

Fig. 4.8 Thymic cortex showing numerous immature thymocytes with nuclear TdT+ immunoreactivity (PAP Immunostain 40x).

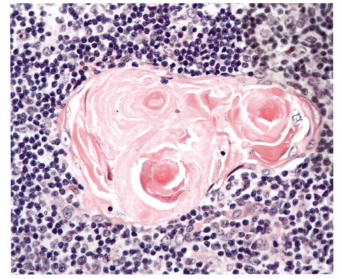

Fig. 4.9 Hassal's corpuscle in thymic medulla. It is composed of keratinized thymic medullary in a tight aggregate (H&E 20x).

sulfated acid mucopolysaccharide and is continuous with the medullary reticular cells. Ultrastructurally, the epithelial cells of Hassall's corpuscles have features similar to those of the "reticular" cells present in the cortex and medulla of the thymus, and they exhibit complex interdigitating cell processes bound by prominent desmosomes [52].

Hassall's corpuscles stain strongly with antibodies to keratin, particularly with a monoclonal antibody to high-molecular keratin (AE2) that is considered a marker of mature epithelial cells [30,53]. Immunoglobulins have been described in Hassall's corpuscles [54].

The reticular epithelial cells of the thymic medulla have a fusiform shape with an oval or spindle nucleus [30]. The nuclear chromatin is slightly more hyperchromatic than that of cortical epithelial cells. The cytoplasm has numerous tonofilaments, prominent desmosomes, and shorter cytoplasmic projections. Medullary epithelial cells are keratin AE1/AE3+ (Fig. 4.10), HLA-DR⁻, TE-4⁺, and A2B5⁺ and exhibit other phenotypic characteristics listed in Table 4.2. They also secrete thymosin α-1, thymopoietin, and other thymic hormones [44,53]. Medullary lymphocytes (Fig. 4.10) are more mature than cortical thymocytes and express CD3+ immunoreactivity (Fig. 4.11), negative TdT immunoreactivity, and the other phenotypic features listed in Table 4.3 [30].

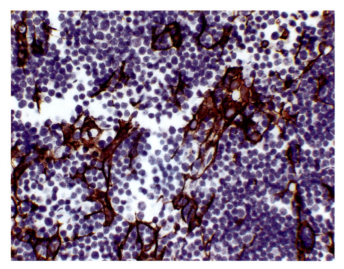

Fig. 4.10 Thymic medulla. The reticular epithelial cells exhibit keratin AE1/AE3 immunoreactivity (PAP Immunostain 40x).

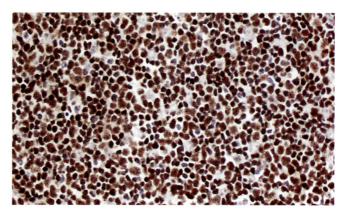

Fig. 4.11 Thymic medulla. Lymphoid cells are more mature single positive lymphocytes (PAP Immunostain for CD4 40x).

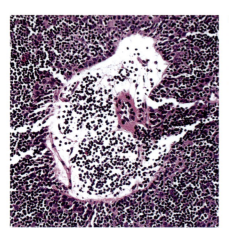

Fig. 4.12 Medullary perivascular space showing a central venule, a space with lymphocytes, and peripheral thymic tissue (H&E 40x).

Thymic vasculature: perivascular spaces

The vasculature of the thymus derives from branches of the internal mammary, inferior thyroid, and pericardiophrenic arteries [3,4,55,56]. Thymic veins are located in the so-called extraparenchymal compartment, separate from the cortex and medulla. They characteristically exhibit perivascular spaces that are difficult to recognize in sections of the normal gland but become prominent in certain histologic types of thymomas, such as thymomas B2, providing a helpful diagnostic clue [30,57]. Thymic veins and perivascular spaces exhibit thin-walled venous structures surrounded by clear spaces containing a variable number of lymphocytes (Fig. 4.12). The clear spaces are separated from the thymic cortex and the medulla by a basal lamina that can be visualized by immunocytochemistry using antibodies to laminin and collagen IV [52]. The basement membrane of perivascular spaces can also be demonstrated ultrastructurally [58].

Detailed ultrastructural studies with electron-opaque tracers have demonstrated the presence of a blood-thymus barrier [59].

Thymic innervation

The thymus is innervated by small nerves derived from the vagus nerve and sympathetic nerves [4].

B lymphocytes in the thymus

The large majority of thymic lymphoid cells are T-cells, but a smaller number of B lymphocytes are present within germinal centers and as individual B cells [43,60–64]. Thymic B lymphocytes are present primarily in the fibrous septa and in perivascular spaces, although they have been described within the medulla. Intramedullary B cells are particularly prominent in the thymus glands of fetuses, newborns, and children and tend to cluster around Hassall's corpuscles. Thymic B lymphocytes exhibit immunoreactivity for IgG, IgA, and IgM in the fetal and adult thymus [43,54]. In the fetal thymus, IgM cells predominate, while IgG positive cells are more frequent in the adult thymus.

Immunocytochemical studies have also demonstrated the presence of immunoglobulins in Hassall's corpuscles and in other thymic areas [54].

Rare plasma cells can be seen in the connective tissue septa of the thymus and occasionally within the medulla.

Other cell types in the thymus

In addition to the cell types already described, the thymus has interdigitating dendritic cells, Langerhans cells, mast cells, eosinophils, neuroendocrine cells, and myoid or striated cells [15,17,18,30,35,47–49,65–74].

Thymic dendritic cells are a heterogenous population of cells that are antigen presenting cells and play an important role in immune surveillance and tolerance [75–77]. Immature dendritic cells with ultrastructural and immunohistochemical features of Langerhans cells are usually found in the dermis but have also been described in the thymus [73,74]. They are considered as the precursors of more mature dendritic cells. The current model is that hematopoietic stem cells differentiate in the thymus into DN1 lymphoid cells, dendritic cells, or natural killer cells. Precursor dendritic cells develop into a

heterogeneous population of up to five different phenotypic variants of antigen presenting cells [75]. They can be broadly grouped into a major CD123+ plasmacytoid (pDC) population and a smaller CD11c+ myeloid (mDC) population. The function of thymic pDC remains unknown but it has been suggested that they play a role in the development of thymocytes through the secretion of interferon-alpha and may help protect the thymus against viral infections.

Eosinophils are present in the normal thymus of infants and children but are infrequent in adults [30].

Myoid or striated cells are prominent in the thymus of birds and reptiles but are infrequent in the human thymus [12]. In humans they are found in small groups adjacent to Hassall's corpuscles and are more frequent in the thymus of newborns and infants [11–18]. Although infrequent, these cells have generated great interest because of their potential role in the pathogenesis of myasthenia gravis [13]. They increase in density in patients with myasthenia gravis and true thymic hyperplasia.

Myoid cells are characterized by an acidophilic cytoplasm that contains cross striations identical to those seen in skeletal muscle. These striations cross exhibit immunoreactivity for actin and myosin, troponin, and acetylcholine receptor (AChR) [13,78]. Ultrastructurally, the striations of thymic myoid cells exhibit thick actin and myosin myofilaments arranged in a haphazard fashion with focal dense Z-band formation as seen in immature skeletal muscle [12,14,16,52]. These striations have, however, no organized sarcomere formation. Myoid cells have no visible cell-to-cell attachments to reticular epithelial cells or Hassall's corpuscles.

The thymus gland also has neuroendocrine cells that secrete hormones and are influenced by circulating hormones [47–49,65–71,79]. Thymic neuroendocrine cells can be readily identified in birds, reptiles, and other animals but are sparse in the human thymus, where they can be found in the subcapsular epithelium, medulla, and rarely, the cortex. They exhibit immunoreactivity with antibodies to oxytocin, vasopressin, neurophysin, and other neuropeptides [47,65]. Thymic neuroendocrine cells may be related embryologically to the C cells of the thyroid gland.

Thymic hormones

The thymus gland produces several polypeptide hormones that are thought to regulate specific immunological roles of lymphoid cells and induce lymphocyte differentiation *in vivo* and *in vitro* [80–85]. A few of these polypeptides have been characterized chemically, and some have been synthesized. The best-known thymic hormones are thymosin fraction V, thymosin α-1 (Fig. 4.4), thymopoietin II, thymic humoral factor (THF), thymulin, and serum thymic factor (FTS).

The secretion of these peptides is thought to be modulated by the neuroendocrine network, comprising the thyroid, hypophisis, adrenals, gonads, and other glands [71,80].

These systemic hormones also exert their physiologic effects on so-called post-thymic lymphoid precursor cells found in the neonatal spleen and on mature T-cells through cellular processes that involve binding to specific membrane receptors, interaction with adenylate cyclase, and an increase in GMP levels [82,83].

A. Goldstein and associates isolated from calf thymus the first thymic hormone, thymosin, in 1966 [86]. This protein fraction has lymphopoietic activity. In 1972, thymosin was further purified and characterized, and one of its active components was isolated: thymosin fraction V [85–91]. This component of thymosin is a family of 20 or more heat-stable polypeptides with molecular weights ranging from 1,000 to 5,000 that are divided into three regions according to their isoelectric point (pI): α region (pI below 5.5), β (pI 5.5–7), and γ (pI above 7) [87]. Thymosin α-1 consists of 28 amino acid residues, has a molecular weight of 3,108, and has been synthesized in the laboratory. It has 10 to 100 times more biologic activity than thymosin fraction V.

Thymosin can induce multiple functional changes in lymphocytes, such as production of macrophage migratory inhibitory factor (MIF), increased formation of antibody-forming cells, development of functional suppressor T-cells, and induction of TdT formation by immature lymphoid cells [87,88]. Thymosin is also capable of restoring certain immune functions in thymus-deprived or immunodeficient patients or animals. For example, it increases cytotoxic-suppressor T-cell numbers and stimulates the development of delayed hypersensitivity reactions in immunosuppressed children and cancer patients.

Thymopoietin was isolated by G. Goldstein and associates as a polypeptide fraction present in calf thymus that interfered with neuromuscular transmission [92]. It is a polypeptide composed of 49 amino acids and is present in two forms: thymopoietin I and II [81,89,93]. These two forms differ by only two amino acids.

Thymopoietin has been synthesized chemically and is known to be capable of inducing the production of various T-cell antigens *in vitro* and restoring immunological functions of aged mice [81]. Its probable role in the pathogenesis of myasthenia gravis is discussed in Chapter 5.

Thymic humoral factor (THF) was isolated by Trainin and associates and is a small peptide with a molecular weight of 3,230 and 31 amino acid residues [81–84,94]. It is capable of restoring the immunocompetence of lymphoid cells from neonatal athymic mice and of inducing these cells in culture to participate in mixed lymphocyte reactions, develop inducer activities, and acquire graft-versus-host capabilities. Thymic humoral factor also restores cellular immunocompetence to patients suffering from primary or secondary immunodeficiencies and has been used experimentally in the treatment of immune disorders.

Serum thymic factor (FTS) was isolated by Bach. It is a nonapeptide with a molecular weight of 857 [81,95]. It is capable of inducing lymphoblasts to form T-cell antigens such as θ, Ly 1-2-3, and TL (81). It also retards the growth of Moloney sarcoma virus-induced tumors *in vivo* and enhances T-cell-mediated cytotoxicity in thymectomized mice [81].

Thymulin was discovered in the early 1970s and is a hormone nonapeptide secreted by thymic epithelial cells involved in several aspects of intrathymic and extrathymic T-cell differentiation [66]. It also has anti-inflammatory and analgesic properties in the brain, raising the potential to be used as a therapeutic agent.

Thymic hormones have been under intense investigation during the past decades. Indeed, several hormones such as thymosin and FTS have been localized to the thymic epithelium in immunocytochemical studies [96–98]. In addition, thymosin, FTS, and THF have been utilized in clinical trials for the treatment of patients with immunodeficiency, malignancy, viral and fungal infections, and autoimmune disorders [80,87]. Results from these trials are encouraging but difficult to evaluate, given the small number of patients treated with hormonal therapy and the complex nature of their clinical problems.

The thymus and immunity

The thymus has an important role as a central organ of the immune system [9,99–102]. The importance of the thymus in the development of immunity was recognized in the 1960s by Miller and associates and other investigators demonstrating that the removal of the gland from neonatal mice rendered the animals severely immune deficient and prone to infections [101–110]. Neonatal thymectomy also resulted in lymphopenia in blood and thoracic duct lymph and in marked lymphoid depletion in the paracortical areas of lymph nodes. Additional experiments with thymectomy preceded by sublethal irradiation demonstrated similar defects in adult mice. Moreover, the immune defects produced by these experimental conditions could be restored by grafts of thymic epithelial anlage or of thymic tissue enclosed in cell-impermeable Millipore® diffusion chambers, by infusion of thymic lymphocytes, and by the injection of thymic extracts.

These experimental data were also supported by the report by Di George and associates in 1967 of patients with congenital absence of the thymus and immunologic abnormalities such as a marked impairment in their capacity to develop delayed hypersensitivity reactions and ability to reject allografts [111].

Currently, the thymus is viewed as one of the two primary or central lymphoid organs. As such, it is not primarily involved in antibody production, and its development does not appear to be dependent on antigenic stimulation [101].

T-cell development in the thymus: thymopoiesis

The thymic epithelial cells create a microenvironment that plays a key role in T-cell maturation [40,42,44,46,112]. They induce the proliferation and differentiation of hematopoietic stem cells into thymocytes and post-thymic T-cells through direct contact and through the secretion of thymic hormones and various cytokines [113]. In turn, the thymocytes induce thymic epithelial cell proliferation through the secretion of interleukin-1 (IL-1) and other cytokines, as shown in tissue culture models [114]. As part of this interaction between thymic epithelial cells and thymocytes, there is a process of adhesion of both cell types, mediated through adhesion molecules such as ICAM-1 and LFA-1 that are expressed on the surface of the epithelial cells [115–117].

Active T-cell development occurs in the thymic epithelial space composed of the cortical and medullary compartments described above. [99,113,118,119]. Hematopoietic CD34+, CD1A- stem cells, or progenitor cells from the bone marrow migrate from the bloodstream and undergo P-selectin-mediated homing in the thymic cortex (Fig. 4.13). They begin their thymic differentiation as triple negative CD3- CD4- CD8- cells, acquire CD3+ antigenicity evolving into double negative (DN) cells, and undergo a process of chemokine-driven outward cortical migration and maturation as DN1, DN2 and DN3 cells [113]. In the subcapsular area of the thymic cortex they undergo different stages of T-cell development as pre-T1, pre-T2, early double positive (EDP), and double positive (DP) thymocytes (Table 4.3) that can differentiate into natural killer T-cells (NKT cells), become apoptotic, or undergo CCR-7 regulated migration from the cortex to the medulla (Fig. 4.13 and Fig. 4.14). During this migration process from the cortex to the medulla, the DP cells have intimal contact with subcapsular cortical thymic epithelial cells that secrete the various hormones discussed above. In the medulla the DP thymocytes differentiate into CD4+ or CD8+ single positive (SP) lymphocytes and get exposed to various antigens by antigen presenting dendritic cells, developing into memory T-cells that are important in the process of immunologic self-tolerance.

DN cells lack CD4 and CD8 co-receptors and undergo four successive maturation stages that can be characterized by the cell surface expression of CD117, CD44, and CD25 receptors [120]. The stages are: DN1 (CD117+ CD44+ CD25-), DN2 (CD117+ CD44+, CD25+), DN3 (CD117 low or negative CD44- CD25+), and DN4 (CD117- CD44- CD25-). DN1 cells are not committed T-cell precursors and can develop into T-cells, dendritic cells, and natural killer cells. Differentiation from DN1 to DN2 triggers a developmental program leading to diverse expressions of the T-cell receptor (TCR). Thymocyte survival in this stage is regulated by cytokines secreted by thymic stromal cells, particularly interleukin-7 (IL-7). During the DN3 stage the thymocytes generate pre-T1 and pre-T2 cells through a rearranged beta chain and a pre-alpha chain (Fig. 4.14). During the DN IV precursor stage, thymocytes become DP thymocytes (CD4+, CD8+) for 3–4 days [99]. Thereafter there is T-cell antigen receptor rearrangement in the thymic medulla resulting in the development of single positive (SP) CD4 or CD8 naïve T-cells. These cells further differentiate after interaction with antigen presenting dendritic cells into T helper or T cytotoxic cells that leave the thymus and are exported to the periphery.

Thymic epithelial cells secrete various cytokines that regulate the maturation and education of lymphocytes, such as granulocyte-colony stimulating factor (G-CSF), granulocyte-monocyte CSF (CSF-GM-CSF), interleukins 1, 2 and 3, macrophage-colony stimulating factor (M-CSF), stem cell

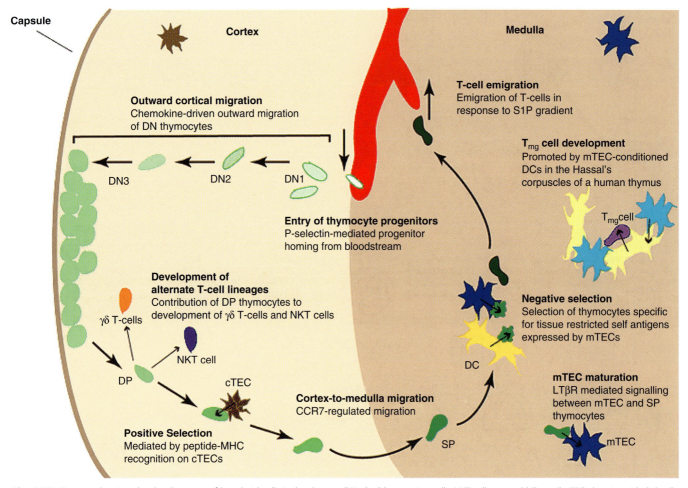

Capsule

Cortex

Medulla

Outward cortical migration
Chemokine-driven outward migration
of DN thymocytes

DN3   DN2   DN1

T-cell emigration
Emigration of T-cells in
response to S1P gradient

T$_{mg}$ cell development
Promoted by mTEC-conditioned
DCs in the Hassal's
corpuscles of a human thymus

T$_{mg}$cell

Entry of thymocyte progenitors
P-selectin-mediated progenitor
homing from bloodstream

**Development of
alternate T-cell lineages**
Contribution of DP thymocytes to
development of γδ T-cells and NKT cells

Negative selection
Selection of thymocytes specific
for tissue restricted self antigens
expressed by mTECs

γδ T-cells

NKT cell

DC

DP   cTEC

Cortex-to-medulla migration
CCR7-regulated migration

mTEC maturation
LTβR mediated signalling
between mTEC and SP
thymocytes

Positive Selection
Mediated by peptide-MHC
recognition on cTECs

SP

mTEC

Fig. 4.13 Diagram showing the development of lymphoid cells in the thymus. DN: double negative cells; NKT cells: natural killer cells; TEC: thymic epithelial cells; DP: double positive cells; SP: single positive cells; DC: dendritic cells.

factor (SCF), transforming growth factor beta (TGF-beta), keratinocyte growth factor (KGF), oncostatin M (OSM) and leukemia inhibitory factor (LIF) [9,118,119]. It is beyond the scope of this volume to discuss the mechanism of action of these various cytokines.

The thymus and immunologic self-tolerance

The thymus also serves as the central organ of immunologic self-non-self-discrimination and the development of tolerance [121]. The maintenance of immunologic self-tolerance requires the coordination of multiple complementary systems and the Autoimmune Regulator (AIRE) gene [122]. The AIRE gene is primarily but not exclusively expressed by medullary thymic epithelial cells [122]. A discussion of the role of the thymus in tolerance is beyond the scope of this volume and has been recently reviewed by Griesemer *et al.* [121].

Thymic involution

The thymus undergoes marked morphologic and physiologic changes with aging [80,99,123–127]. The size of the gland increases from birth until puberty and decreases later in life

until the age of 50. Histologically, the involuting thymus exhibits a marked decrease in lymphocyte and Hassall's corpuscle numbers, epithelial elements become clumped, cystic changes appear, secretory granules are depleted, and tissues are replaced by lipid-laden macrophages and adipose cells.

However, the widespread belief that the thymus disappears in adult life is no longer accepted, and several anatomic studies have shown that the gland, although atrophic, persists throughout life [125].

Approximate thymic weights at different ages are 12 to 15 g at birth, 30 to 40 g at puberty, and 10 to 15 g at age 60 [20]. The thymic size varies a great deal in different individuals, and at any given age a patient may have a gland that is either larger or smaller than expected from published tables.

A detailed anatomic study of human thymus glands at necropsy by Kendall and associates has demonstrated a gradual age-related decrease in thymus wet weight after puberty and a significant increase in extractable lipid up to the age of 50, supporting the notion of replacement of thymic elements by adipose tissue [20]. This study reported significantly lower wet and lipid thymic

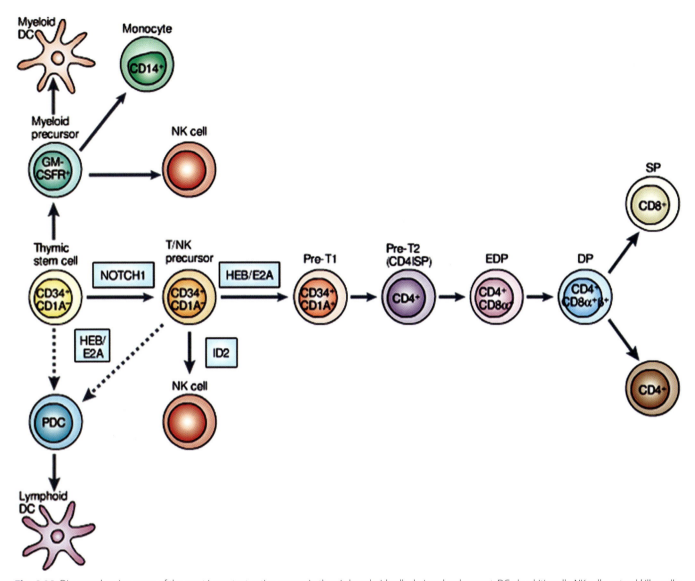

Fig. 4.14 Diagram showing some of the most important antigens seen in thymic lymphoid cells during development. DC: dendritic cells; NK cells: natural killer cells; GM-CSFR: granulocyte-macrophage colony-stimulating factor; PDC: plasmacytoid dendritic cells; EDP: early double positive cells; DP: double positive cells; SP: single positive cells.

weights in patients with chronic stressful conditions. By contrast, individuals dying from cardiovascular disease or asphyxia had higher weights than those found in the normal population.

The thymus retrogresses functionally with increasing age, and these changes are paralleled by a decline of normal immune functions in older individuals.

Tissue culture studies by Oosterom and Kater have demonstrated changes in the secretory activities of thymic epithelial cells with age [128,129]. Cells from individuals older than 30 years appear to have lower hormone secretory capabilities than thymic epithelial cells from younger patients. Other studies have shown declines in the serum levels of thymopoietin and FTS with aging [80,81,99].

These hormones become non-detectable in normal serum by age 50.

Several possible mechanisms have been suggested to explain age-related thymic involution [99]. They include blockage of T-cell receptor gene rearrangements, decreased self-peptide major histocompatibility (MHC) molecules, depletion of T-cell progenitors and loss or increase of various cykokines [99]. Sex steroids probably play a role in thymic involution, providing an explanation for the acceleration of thymic decline at puberty and almost total collapse of thymopoiesis through apoptosis in patients treated with exogenous sex steroids [48,65,71]. The endocrine and neuroendocrine systems also play an important role in thymopoiesis and thymic involution [48,125].

References

1. Walter E, Wilich E, Webb WR. *The Thymus: Diagnostic Imaging, Functions and Pathologic Anatomy (Medical Radiology/Diagnostic Imaging)*. 2012; New York: Springer.

2. Marchevsky AM, Kaneko M. *Surgical Pathology of the Mediastinum*. 1991; New York: Raven Press.

3. Ugalde PA, Pereira ST, Araujo C *et al.* Correlative anatomy for the mediastinum. *Thorac Surg Clin*. 2011;21:251–72.

4. Drake RL, Vogl W. *Gray's Anatomy for Students*. 2009; New York: Churchill Livingstone.

5. Hammar JA. Zur Histogenese und Involution der Thymus-druse. *Anat Anz*. 1905;39:41–89.

6. Schambacher A. Uber die Persistenz vom DrusenKanalen in der Thymus in ihre Beziehung zur Entsehung der Hassalschen Korperchen. *Virchows Arch Pathol Anat*. 1003;172:368–94.

7. Gordon J, Manley NR. Mechanisms of thymus organogenesis and morphogenesis. *Development*. 2011;138:3865–78.

8. Shier KJ. The thymus according to Schambacher: medullary ducts and reticular epithelium of thymus and thymomas. *Cancer*. 1981;48:1183–99.

9. Lee DK, Hakim FT, Gress RE. The thymus and the immune system: layered levels of control. *J Thorac Oncol*. 2010;5:S273–S276.

10. Strutman O. *Two main features of T cell development: thymus traffic and postthymic maturation*. 1977; New York: Plenum Press.

11. Wong A, Garrett KL, Anderson JE. Myoid cell density in the thymus is reduced during mdx dystrophy and after muscle crush. *Biochem Cell Biol*. 1999;77:33–40.

12. Chan AS. Ultrastructure of myoid cells in the chick thymus. *Br Poult Sci*. 1995;36:197–203.

13. Sato T, Tamaoki N. Myoid cells in the human thymus and thymoma revealed by three different immunohistochemical markers for striated muscle. *Acta Pathol Jpn*. 1989;39:509–19.

14. Hanzlikova V. Histochemical and ultrastructural properties of myoid cells in the thymus of the frog. *Cell Tissue Res*. 1979;197:105–12.

15. Hayward AR. Myoid cells in the human foetal thymus. *J Pathol*. 1972;106:45–8.

16. Hayward A. The detection of myoid cells in the human foetal and neonatal thymus by immunofluorescence. *J Med Microbiol*. 1970;3.

17. Ito T, Hoshino T, Abe K. The fine structure of myoid cells in the human thymus. *Arch Histol Jpn*. 1969;30:207–15.

18. Bockman DE. Myoid cells in adult human thymus. *Nature*. 1968;218:286–7.

19. Drenckhahn D, von GB, Muller-Hermelink HK *et al.* Myosin and actin containing cells in the human postnatal thymus. Ultrastructural and immunohistochemical findings in normal thymus and in myasthenia gravis. *Virchows Arch B Cell Pathol Incl Mol Pathol*. 1979;32:33–45.

20. Kendall MD, Johnson HR, Singh J. The weight of the human thymus gland at necropsy. *J Anat*. 1980;131:483–97.

21. McLean G, DeSilva A, Bergman P *et al.* Solid ectopic cervical thymus in neonates with thyroid agenesis. *J Ultrasound Med*. 2012;31:1281–3.

22. Wang J, Fu H, Yang H *et al.* Clinical management of cervical ectopic thymus in children. *J Pediatr Surg*. 2011;46: e33–e36.

23. Segni M, di NR, Pucarelli I *et al.* Ectopic intrathyroidal thymus in children: a long-term follow-up study. *Horm Res Paediatr*. 2011;75:258–63.

24. Ahsan F, Allison R, White J. Ectopic cervical thymus: case report and review of pathogenesis and management. *J Laryngol Otol*. 2010;124:694–7.

25. Herman TE, Siegel MJ. Cervical ectopic thymus. *J Perinatol*. 2009;29:173–4.

26. Pai I, Hegde V, Wilson PO *et al.* Ectopic thymus presenting as a subglottic mass: diagnostic and management dilemmas. *Int J Pediatr Otorhinolaryngol*. 2005;69:573–6.

27. Kacker A, April M, Markentel CB *et al.* Ectopic thymus presenting as a solid submandibular neck mass in an infant: case report and review of literature. *Int J Pediatr Otorhinolaryngol*. 1999;49:241–5.

28. Nagoya A, Kanzaki R, Nakagiri T *et al.* Ectopic cervical thymoma accompanied by Good's Syndrome. *Ann Thorac Cardiovasc Surg*. 2013. doi: 10.5761/ atcs.cr.12.02027

29. Shien K, Shien T, Soh J *et al.* Ectopic cervical thymoma: a case report with 18F-fluorodeoxyglucose positron emission tomography findings. *Acta Med Okayama*. 2012;66:357–61.

30. Suster S, Rosai J. Histology of the normal thymus. *Am J Surg Pathol*. 1990;14:284–303.

31. Anderson G, Takahama Y. Thymic epithelial cells: working class heroes for T cell development and repertoire selection. *Trends Immunol*. 2012;33:256–63.

32. Alexandropoulos K, Danzl NM. Thymic epithelial cells: antigen presenting cells that regulate T cell repertoire and tolerance development. *Immunol Res*. 2012;54:177–90.

33. Alves NL, Huntington ND, Rodewald HR *et al.* Thymic epithelial cells: the multi-tasking framework of the T cell "cradle". *Trends Immunol*. 2009;30:468–74.

34. Rouse RV, Bolin LM, Bender JR *et al.* Monoclonal antibodies reactive with subsets of mouse and human thymic epithelial cells. *J Histochem Cytochem*. 1988;36:1511–17.

35. Schmitt D, Zambruno G, Staquet MJ *et al.* Antigenic thymus-epidermis relationships. Reactivity of a panel of anti-thymic cell monoclonal antibodies on human keratinocytes and Langerhans cells. *Dermatologica*. 1987;175:109–20.

36. von Gaudecker B. Ultrastructure of the age-involuted adult human thymus. *Cell Tissue Res*. 1978;186:507–25.

37. Pinkel D. Ultrastructure of human fetal thymus. *Am J Dis Child*. 1968;115:222–38.

38. Izon DJ, Boyd RL. The cytoarchitecture of the human thymus detected by monoclonal antibodies. *Hum Immunol*. 1990;27:16–32.

39. Kampinga J, Berges S, Boyd RL *et al.* Thymic epithelial antibodies: immunohistological analysis and introduction of nomenclature. *Thymus*. 1989;13:165–73.

40. Laster AJ, Itoh T, Palker TJ *et al.* The human thymic microenvironment: thymic epithelium contains specific keratins associated with early and late stages of epidermal keratinocyte

maturation. *Differentiation.* 1986;31:67–77.

41. Savino W, Dardenne M. Immunohistochemical studies on a human thymic epithelial cell subset defined by the anti-cytokeratin 18 monoclonal antibody. *Cell Tissue Res.* 1988;254:225–31.

42. von GB, Larche M, Schuurman HJ *et al.* Analysis of the fine distribution of thymic epithelial microenvironmental molecules by immuno-electron microscopy. *Thymus.* 1989;13:187–94.

43. Henry K. The thymus – what's new? *Histopathology.* 1989;14:537–48.

44. Janossy G, Bofill M, Trejdosiewicz LK *et al.* Cellular differentiation of lymphoid subpopulations and their microenvironments in the human thymus. *Curr Top Pathol.* 1986;75:89–125.

45. Derbinski J, Kyewski B. How thymic antigen presenting cells sample the body's self-antigens. *Curr Opin Immunol.* 2010;22:592–600.

46. Masuda K, Germeraad WT, Satoh R *et al.* Notch activation in thymic epithelial cells induces development of thymic microenvironments. *Mol Immunol.* 2009;46:1756–67.

47. Geenen V. Presentation of neuroendocrine self in the thymus: a necessity for integrated evolution of the immune and neuroendocrine systems. *Ann N Y Acad Sci.* 2012;1261:42–8.

48. Savino W, Dardenne M. Neuroendocrine interactions in the thymus: from physiology to therapy. *Neuroimmunomodulation.* 2011;18:263.

49. Moll UM. Functional histology of the neuroendocrine thymus. *Microsc Res Tech.* 1997;38:300–10.

50. Colic M, Matanovic D, Hegedis L *et al.* Immunohistochemical characterization of rat thymic non-lymphoid cells. I. Epithelial and mesenchymal components defined by monoclonal antibodies. *Immunology.* 1988;65:277–84.

51. Bearman RM, Levine GD, Bensch KG. The ultrastructure of the normal human thymus: a study of 36 cases. *Anat Rec.* 1978;190:755–81.

52. Bloodworth JM, Jr., Hiratsuka H, Hickey RC *et al.* Ultrastructure of the human thymus, thymic tumors, and myasthenia gravis. *Pathol Annu.* 1975;10:329–91.

53. Cohen-Kaminsky S, Berrih-Aknin S, Savino W *et al.* Immunodetection of the thymic epithelial P19 antigen in cultures of normal and pathological human thymic epithelium. *Thymus.* 1987;9:225–38.

54. Henry L, Anderson G. Immunoglobulins in Hassall's corpuscles of the human thymus. *J Anat.* 1990;168:185–97.

55. Esposito C, Romeo C. Surgical anatomy of the mediastinum. *Semin Pediatr Surg.* 1999;8:50–3.

56. Carter DR. The anatomy of the mediastinum. *Ear Nose Throat J.* 1981;60:153–7.

57. Kendall MD. The morphology of perivascular spaces in the thymus. *Thymus.* 1989;13:157–64.

58. Karttunen T. Basement membrane proteins and reticulin in a normal thymus and the thymus in myasthenia gravis. *Virchows Arch A Pathol Anat Histopathol.* 1987;411:245–52.

59. Bubanovic IV. Failure of blood-thymus barrier as a mechanism of tumor and trophoblast escape. *Med Hypotheses.* 2003;60:315–20.

60. Henry L, Durrant TE, Anderson G. Pericapillary collagen in the human thymus: implications for the concept of the 'blood-thymus' barrier. *J Anat.* 1992;181 (Pt 1):39–46.

61. Stet RJ, Wagenaar-Hilbers JP, Nieuwenhuis P. Thymus localization of monoclonal antibodies circumventing the blood-thymus barrier. *Scand J Immunol.* 1987;25:441–6.

62. Raviola E, Karnovsky MJ. Evidence for a blood-thymus barrier using electron-opaque tracers. *J Exp Med.* 1972;136:466–98.

63. Hofmann WJ, Momburg F, Moller P. Thymic medullary cells expressing B lymphocyte antigens. *Hum Pathol.* 1988;19:1280–7.

64. Wirt DP, Grogan TM, Nagle RB *et al.* A comprehensive immunotopographic map of human thymus. *J Histochem Cytochem.* 1988;36:1–12.

65. Geenen V. The thymus as an obligatory intersection between the immune and neuroendocrine systems: pharmacological implications. *Curr Opin Pharmacol.* 2010;10:405–7.

66. Reggiani PC, Morel GR, Console GM *et al.* The thymus-neuroendocrine axis: physiology, molecular biology, and

therapeutic potential of the thymic peptide thymulin. *Ann N Y Acad Sci.* 2009;1153:98–106.

67. Bai M, Papoudou-Bai A, Karatzias G *et al.* Immunohistochemical expression patterns of neural and neuroendocrine markers, the neural growth factor receptors and the beta-tubulin II and IV isotypes in human thymus. *Anticancer Res.* 2008;28:295–303.

68. Bodey B. Thymic reticulo-epithelial cells: key cells of neuroendocrine regulation. *Expert Opin Biol Ther.* 2007;7:939–49.

69. Geenen V. Thymus-dependent T cell tolerance of neuroendocrine functions: principles, reflections, and implications for tolerogenic/negative self-vaccination. *Ann N Y Acad Sci.* 2006;1088:284–96.

70. Geenen V, Brilot F. Role of the thymus in the development of tolerance and autoimmunity towards the neuroendocrine system. *Ann N Y Acad Sci.* 2003;992:186–95.

71. Savino W, Dardenne M. Neuroendocrine control of thymus physiology. *Endocr Rev.* 2000;21:412–43.

72. Trusen A, Beissert M, Hebestreit H *et al.* Fibrosing mediastinitis with superior vena cava obstruction as the initial presentation of Langerhans' cell histiocytosis in a young child. *Pediatr Radiol.* 2003;33:485–8.

73. Rausch E, Kaiserling E, Goos M. Langerhans cells and interdigitating reticulum cells in the thymus-dependent region in human dermatopathic lymphadenitis. *Virchows Arch B Cell Pathol.* 1977;25:327–43.

74. Hoshino T, Kukita A, Sato S. Cells containing Birbeck granules (Langerhans cell granules) in the human thymus. *J Electron Microsc (Tokyo).* 1970;19:271–6.

75. Evans VA, Lal L, Akkina R *et al.* Thymic plasmacytoid dendritic cells are susceptible to productive HIV-1 infection and efficiently transfer R5 HIV-1 to thymocytes in vitro. *Retrovirology.* 2011;8:43.

76. Vandenabeele S, Hochrein H, Mavaddat N *et al.* Human thymus contains 2 distinct dendritic cell populations. *Blood.* 2001;97:1733–41.

77. Vandenabeele S, Wu L. Dendritic cell origins: puzzles and paradoxes. *Immunol Cell Biol.* 1999;77:411–19.

78. Safar D, Aime C, Cohen-Kaminsky S *et al.* Antibodies to thymic epithelial cells in myasthenia gravis. *J Neuroimmunol.* 1991;35:101–10.

79. Hakanson R, Larsson LI, Sundler F. Peptide and amine producing endocrine-like cells in the chicken thymus. A chemical, histochemical and electron microscopic study. *Histochemistry.* 1974;39:25–34.

80. Dooley J, Liston A. Molecular control over thymic involution: from cytokines and microRNA to aging and adipose tissue. *Eur J Immunol.* 2012;42:1073–9.

81. Bach JF. Thymic hormones. *J Immunopharmacol.* 1979;1:277–310.

82. Bach JF, Bach MA, Charreire J *et al.* The mode of action of thymic hormones. *Ann N Y Acad Sci.* 1979;332:23–32.

83. Bach JF. Thymic hormones: biochemistry, and biological and clinical activities. *Annu Rev Pharmacol Toxicol.* 1977;17:281–91.

84. Trainin N. Thymic hormones and the immune response. *Physiol Rev.* 1974;54:272–315.

85. Goldstein G. Thymic hormones. *Triangle.* 1972;11:7–14.

86. Goldstein AL, Slater FD, White A. Preparation, assay, and partial purification of a thymic lymphocytopoietic factor (thymosin). *Proc Natl Acad Sci U S A.* 1966;56:1010–17.

87. Low TL, Thurman GB, Chincarini C *et al.* Current status of thymosin research: evidence for the existence of a family of thymic factors that control T-cell maturation. 1979. *Ann N Y Acad Sci.* 2012;1269:131–46.

88. Goldstein AL, Hannappel E, Sosne G *et al.* Thymosin beta4: a multifunctional regenerative peptide. Basic properties and clinical applications. *Expert Opin Biol Ther.* 2012;12:37–51.

89. Talle MA, Brown MJ, Blynn CM *et al.* Use of monoclonal antibodies to identify thymopoietin in cultured human thymic epithelial cells. *Thymus.* 1991;18:169–84.

90. Dalakas MC, Engel WK, McClure JE *et al.* Identification of human thymic epithelial cells with antibodies to thymosin alpha 1 in myasthenia gravis. *Ann N Y Acad Sci.* 1981;377:477–85.

91. Goldstein AL, Asanuma Y, White A. The thymus as an endocrine gland: properties of thymosin, a new thymus hormone. *Recent Prog Horm Res.* 1970;26:505–38.

92. Goldstein G. The isolation of thymopoietin (thymin). *Ann N Y Acad Sci.* 1975;249:177–85.

93. Goldstein G, Scheid M, Boyse EA *et al.* Thymopoietin and bursopoietin: induction signals regulating early lymphocyte differentiation. *Cold Spring Harb Symp Quant Biol.* 1977;41 Pt 1:5–8.

94. Bach JF. The mode of action of thymic hormones and its relevance to T-cell differentiation. *Transplant Proc.* 1976;8:243–8.

95. Monier JC, Dardenne M, Pleau JM *et al.* Characterization of facteur thymique serique (FTS) in the thymus. I. Fixation of anti-FTS antibodies on thymic reticulo-epithelial cells. *Clin Exp Immunol.* 1980;42:470–6.

96. Dalakas MC, Engel WK, McClure JE *et al.* Immunocytochemical localization of thymosin-alpha 1 in thymic epithelial cells of normal and myasthenia gravis patients and in thymic cultures. *J Neurol Sci.* 1981;50:239–47.

97. Monier JC, Dardenne M, Pleau JM *et al.* Characterization of facteur thymique serique (FTS) in the thymus. I. Fixation of anti-FTS antibodies on thymic reticulo-epithelial cells. *Clin Exp Immunol.* 1980;42:470–6.

98. Schmitt D, Monier JC, Dardenne M *et al.* Cytoplasmic localization of FTS (facteur thymique serique) in thymic epithelial cells. An immunoelectronmicroscopical study. *Thymus.* 1980;2:177–86.

99. Lynch HE, Goldberg GL, Chidgey A *et al.* Thymic involution and immune reconstitution. *Trends Immunol.* 2009;30:366–73.

100. Hogquist KA, Baldwin TA, Jameson SC. Central tolerance: learning self-control in the thymus. *Nat Rev Immunol.* 2005;5:772–82.

101. Miller JF. The golden anniversary of the thymus. *Nat Rev Immunol.* 2011;11:489–95.

102. Miller JF. The role of the thymus in immune processes. *Int Arch Allergy Appl Immunol.* 1965;28:61–70.

103. Miller RE, Sullivan FJ. Superior vena caval obstruction secondary to fibrosing mediastinitis. *Ann Thorac Surg.* 1973;15:483–92.

104. Miller JF. The thymus. Yesterday, today, and tomorrow. *Lancet.* 1967;2:1299–1302.

105. Miller JF, Mitchell GF. The thymus and the precursors of antigen reactive cells. *Nature.* 1967;216:659–63.

106. Miller JF, Osoba D, Dukor P. A humoral thymus mechanism responsible for immunologic maturation. *Ann N Y Acad Sci.* 1965;124:95–104.

107. Miller JF. The thymus and the development of immunologic responsiveness. *Science.* 1964;144:1544–51.

108. Miller JF. Functions of the thymus. *Sci Basis Med Annu Rev.* 1964;218–33.

109. Miller JF. The role of the thymus in immunity. *Br Med J.* 1963;2:459–64.

110. Miller JF. Immunological function of the thymus. *Lancet.* 1961;2:748–9.

111. Di George AM, Lischner HW, Dacou C *et al.* Absence of the thymus. *Lancet.* 1967;1:1387.

112. Kendall MD, van de Wijngaert FP, Schuurman HJ *et al.* Heterogeneity of the human thymus epithelial microenvironment at the ultrastructural level. *Adv Exp Med Biol.* 1985;186:289–97.

113. Hernandez JB, Newton RH, Walsh CM. Life and death in the thymus–cell death signaling during T cell development. *Curr Opin Cell Biol.* 2010;22:865–71.

114. Nakahama M, Mohri N, Mori S *et al.* Immunohistochemical and histometrical studies of the human thymus with special emphasis on age-related changes in medullary epithelial and dendritic cells. *Virchows Arch B Cell Pathol Incl Mol Pathol.* 1990;58:245–51.

115. Galy AH, Spits H. IL-1, IL-4, and IFN-gamma differentially regulate cytokine production and cell surface molecule expression in cultured human thymic epithelial cells. *J Immunol.* 1991;147:3823–30.

116. Galy AH, Dinarello CA, Kupper TS *et al.* Effects of cytokines on human thymic epithelial cells in culture. II. Recombinant IL 1 stimulates thymic epithelial cells to produce IL6 and GM-CSF. *Cell Immunol.* 1990;129:161–75.

117. Galy AH, Hadden EM, Touraine JL *et al.* Effects of cytokines on human thymic epithelial cells in culture: IL1 induces thymic epithelial cell

proliferation and change in morphology. *Cell Immunol.* 1989;124:13–27.

118. Sempowski GD, Gooding ME, Liao HX *et al.* T cell receptor excision circle assessment of thymopoiesis in aging mice. *Mol Immunol.* 2002;38:841–8.

119. Sempowski GD, Hale LP, Sundy JS *et al.* Leukemia inhibitory factor, oncostatin M, IL-6, and stem cell factor mRNA expression in human thymus increases with age and is associated with thymic atrophy. *J Immunol.* 2000;164:2180–7.

120. Carpenter AC, Bosselut R. Decision checkpoints in the thymus. *Nat Immunol.* 2010;11:666–73.

121. Griesemer AD, Sorenson EC, Hardy MA. The role of the thymus in tolerance. *Transplantation.* 2010;90:465–74.

122. Gardner JM, Fletcher AL, Anderson MS *et al.* AIRE in the thymus and beyond. *Curr Opin Immunol.* 2009;21:582–9.

123. Aw D, Palmer DB. It's not all equal: a multiphasic theory of thymic involution. *Biogerontology.* 2012;13:77–81.

124. Aw D, Palmer DB. The origin and implication of thymic involution. *Aging Dis.* 2011;2:437–43.

125. Calder AE, Hince MN, Dudakov JA *et al.* Thymic involution: where endocrinology meets immunology. *Neuroimmunomodulation.* 2011;18:281–9.

126. Hakim FT, Gress RE. Thymic involution: implications for self-tolerance. *Methods Mol Biol.* 2007;380:377–90.

127. Hsu HC, Li L, Zhang HG *et al.* Genetic regulation of thymic involution. *Mech Ageing Dev.* 2005;126:87–97.

128. Oosterom R, Kater L. The thymus in the aging individual. I. Mitogen responsiveness of human thymocytes. *Clin Immunol Immunopathol.* 1981;18:187–94.

129. Oosterom R, Kater L. The thymus in the aging individual. II. Thymic epithelial function in vitro in aging and in thymus pathology. *Clin Immunol Immunopathol.* 1981;18:195–202.

Chapter 5

Pathology of non-neoplastic conditions of the thymus

Alberto M. Marchevsky, MD, and Mark R. Wick, MD

Thymic involution

The thymus is relatively large in childhood, grows during puberty, and decreases in weight after adolescence as a result of a normal involution process that is completed by age 40 [1-6]. Abnormal acute involution with marked reduction in the weight of the gland can also occur in response to stress, as a result of a pathologic process that is mediated by endogenous corticosteroid secretion [3,4,7,8]. Acute involution can be detected on imaging studies and is associated with hyaline membrane disease in newborns, trauma, infection, radiation therapy, and other conditions [9].

Microscopically, the thymus in acute involution shows widespread lympholysis and infiltration by macrophages with large somewhat foamy cytoplasm (Fig. 5.1), giving the gland a typical "starry-sky" appearance (Fig. 5.2). These changes are most prominent in the thymic cortex. Studies using immunohistochemistry have demonstrated that the epithelial network remains unchanged in the acutely involuted thymus, while there is a progressive loss of cortical immature proliferating lymphoid cells and medullary interdigitating cells [8,10]. The degree of acute thymic involution in infancy and childhood correlates with the duration of an acute illness [10,11].

In patients with diseases resulting in chronic stress, the thymus gland undergoes complete loss of differentiation between the cortex and the medulla and remains as two involuted irregular lobes composed mostly of adipose tissue with occasional perivascular spindle epithelial cells, scanty lymphocytes, and focal elongated cystic Hassall's corpuscles lined with squamous epithelium.

Seemayer and Bolande have reported a peculiar form of involution mimicking thymic dysplasia in a premature infant with transfusion-induced graft-versus-host disease [12].

Thymic hyperplasia

The presence of a relatively large thymus in newborns and infants was identified at autopsy in the late nineteenth century and the concept of "status thymicolymphaticus" was proposed

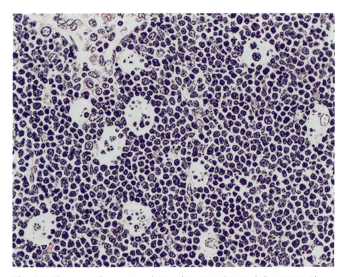

Fig. 5.1 Thymus with acute involution showing multiple histiocytes (H&E 20x).

Fig. 5.2 Thymus with acute involution showing a "starry-sky" pattern with many tangible body macrophages (H&E 40x).

Table 5.1. Thymic mean weights by age

Age range (years)	Weights (g)
0–1	24.77
1–6	23.30
6–11	28.70
11–16	33.91
16–21	20.50
21–26	18.38
26–31	14.90
31–46	13.98
46–66	12.65

Modified from Young and Turnbull (13)

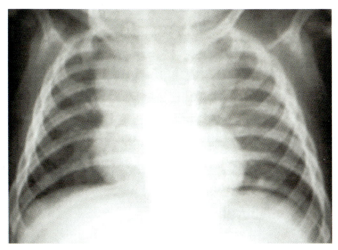

Fig. 5.3 Chest X-ray of an infant showing an enlarged thymus appearing as a prominent widening of the superior mediastinum.

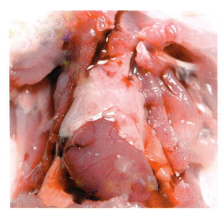

Fig. 5.4 Newborn at autopsy showing large, hyperplastic thymus compressing great vessels and other mediastinal structures.

by Paltauf in 1889 [13,14]. It was suggested that the thymus was a predisposing factor in sudden infant death but the presence of a prominent thymus in early childhood is now considered a normal finding and this theory has been discarded.

Hyperplasia of the thymus can be divided into two types based on morphologic criteria, true or simple thymic hyperplasia (TTH), and lymphoid or follicular hyperplasia (FH) [14–16].

TTH is characterized by an increase in the size and weight of a gland that retains a normal morphology for age [15]. Included in this type are two clinico-pathologic forms of TTH: (a) thymic hyperplasia with massive enlargement and (b) thymic rebound after treatment of chemotherapy [17–29].

FH is characterized by the presence of lymphoid follicles with germinal centers in the medulla of a thymus gland that is usually of normal size and weight.

Patients with combined TTH and FH have been described [30,31].

True or simple thymic hyperplasia

The diagnosis of TTH can be suspected on imaging studies (Fig. 5.3) but usually requires pathologic evaluation of the gland to determine that the glandular morphology is normal and that the size and weight of a thymus is significantly greater than the thymic age-related data published in the literature (Table 5.1) [13]. However, these tables are based on quite variable size and weight measurements obtained in autopsy studies of different patients classified as "normal". This variability should be taken into consideration in establishing the diagnosis of TTH in an individual patient, as it has been shown that the thymic weights in many apparently normal individuals can be considerably larger or smaller than those expected from the standard data of Young and Turnbull presented in Table 5.1 [32]. Judd and Welch have proposed to utilize a cutoff value of 2 standard deviations above the mean weight for age as the upper limit of normal thymus and have demonstrated

(utilizing antibodies to myoglobin and desmin) the presence of myoid cells in TTH and in LH [30,31].

True thymic hyperplasia with massive enlargement

TTH with massive enlargement of the thymus has been described in infants (Fig. 5.3), children, and young adults [17–30]. Approximately 55% of these patients present with an asymptomatic mediastinal mass that is suspicious for a thymoma or other thymic neoplasm. In the other 45% of patients, TTH with massive thymic enlargement is associated with respiratory distress, chest pain, and/or other signs secondary to compression of mediastinal structures (Fig. 5.4). Peripheral lymphocytosis is frequent. TTH with massive enlargement is not associated with autoimmune disorder or myasthenia gravis and has been described in rare patients with Grave's disease [17].

Pathologically, the massively enlarged hyperplastic thymic gland varies in size from 120 to 950 g and usually exhibits its typical bilobed shape, although in some cases the bilobation cannot be readily recognized [33]. Microscopically, the thymic architecture is well preserved, and germinal centers are absent.

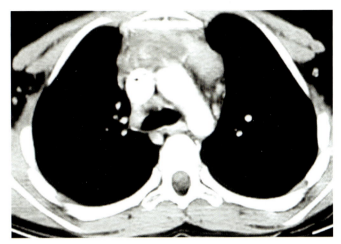

Fig. 5.5 Chest CT scan of a patient with Hodgkin's lymphoma treated with chemotherapy and showing rebound thymic hyperplasia.

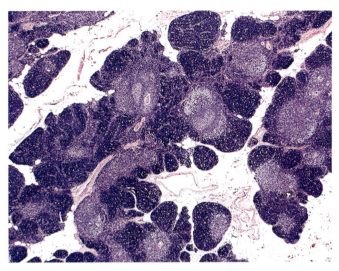

Fig. 5.6 Follicular hyperplasia. The thymus shows at low power microscopy numerous lymphoid follicles with prominent germinal centers (H&E 20x).

TTH with massive enlargement needs to be distinguished from thymomas. Grossly hyperplastic glands are usually bilobed without fibrous septa on cut section while the tumors are generally well encapsulated and have a lobulated cut surface, as discussed in the next chapter. Microscopically, the thymus in TTH with massive enlargement shows a preserved glandular architecture with distinct cortical and medullary areas; the latter with multiple Hassall's corpuscles. In contrast, thymomas exhibit a characteristic low-power-microscopy pattern of islands of lymphoepithelial tissue separated by thick, irregular fibrous trabeculae and only scanty or absent Hassall's corpuscles. In small biopsies, however, the distinction between thymoma and TTH may be difficult to make.

True thymic hyperplasia after chemotherapy and other conditions

TTH has been described as a rebound phenomenon in children and adults treated with chemotherapy for Hodgkin's disease (Fig. 5.5), germ cell tumors, breast cancer, and other malignancies [34–42]. This form of TTH probably represents an immunologic rebound phenomenon and it has been used clinically as a favorable prognostic sign of successful neoplastic control [41]. TTH after chemotherapy needs to be distinguished on chest CT and other imaging studies from tumor recurrence. The presence of an enlarged but bilobed thymus in its normal anterior mediastinal location is useful to diagnose rebound TTH.

Rare instances of TTH have also been described in children treated for hypothyroidism, in infants with Beckwith-Wiedemann syndrome and pulmonary hypoplasia and in association with sarcoidosis and Grave's disease [43,44].

Lymphoid or follicular thymic hyperplasia

FH of the thymus is characterized by the presence of germinal centers (Fig. 5.6) in the thymic medulla irrespective of the size and/or weight of the gland [45]. This definition raises the question as to whether germinal centers are normally present in the

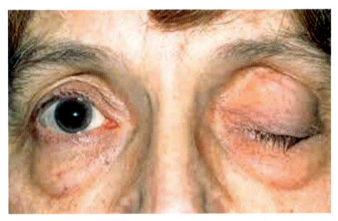

Fig. 5.7 A patient with myasthenia gravis showing characteristic ptosis of the left eye.

thymus and in what densities. Different autopsy series have reported the presence of generally small and scanty germinal centers in the thymus of 2% to 51% of "normal" individuals. These germinal centers tend to occur in the medulla and, occasionally, the fibrous septa of the normal gland [46,47].

FH has been described in association with autoimmune diseases such as myasthenia gravis (Fig. 5.7), systemic lupus erythematosus (SLE), scleroderma, and rheumatoid arthritis [48–50]. It can also be seen in patients with congenital heart disease, endocrine disorders such as hyperthyroidism, Addison's disease, acromegaly, and in liver disease [51–54].

The germinal centers in FH are generally larger than in the normal thymus (Fig. 5.8), contain immunoglobulins, and are accompanied by expansion of the thymic medulla with development of a sharp cortico-medullary junction that can be demonstrated with reticulum stains [55]. Their density, size, and configuration have been quantitated with morphometric techniques, yielding results that have varied considerably from

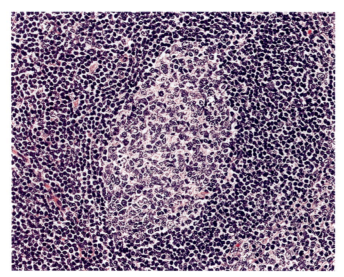

Fig. 5.8 Germinal centers in cases of follicular hyperplasia are larger than those seen in normal thymus (H&E 40x).

patient to patient and in different histologic slides from a single individual, [56,57].

The thymus in immunodeficiency syndromes

The thymus gland and the bone marrow are primary lymphoid organs that are essential for the development of a normal immune system [58-60]. Congenital absence of the thymus and congenital or acquired failure in thymic development or function is associated with the various severe immunodeficiency syndromes [61-66].

A detailed review of the pathology of immunodeficiency syndromes is beyond the scope of this volume. However, the surgical pathologist, particularly the pediatric pathologist, needs to become acquainted with the various pathologic changes present in the thymus of immunodeficiency patients, as these individuals may undergo thymic biopsy through a cervical or other approach to characterize the nature of their immunologic defect, and determine whether they will respond to immunologic reconstitution or other therapeutic modalities [64,65,67-69].

The thymus in congenital immunodeficiency syndromes

Patients with congenital immunodeficiency syndromes can exhibit complete absence of the thymus or severe hypoplasia characterized by a gland that is markedly smaller than expected for age but with a normal microscopic morphology or thymic dysplasia [70-72]. Thymic dysplasia is characterized by the presence of a small, rudimentary gland with abnormal histologic features such as the presence of only epithelial elements, scant or absent Hassall's corpuscles, and absent thymocytes [73-82].

Reticular dysgenesis is a rare and very severe congenital form of immune deficiency. Patients present with severe lymphopenia, granulocytopenia, and death *in utero* or in the newborn period [72]. This rare condition results from a failure of development of bone marrow stem cells and is characterized by the presence of a vestigial thymus.

Hypogammaglobulinemia of the Swiss type (Glanzmann–Riniker disease) is a rare autosomal recessive disease. Infants with this syndrome present clinically with manifestations of a severe combined (T- and B-cell) immunodeficiency (SCID) syndrome and usually die within a few years after birth as a result of severe bacterial, viral, fungal, and/or protozoal infections [72,83]. Glanzmann–Riniker disease is attributed to a failure in the development of lymphoid stem cells with the resulting lack of thymic lymphocytes and marked hypoplasia of peripheral lymphoid tissues [84]. A failure of thymic anlage to descend from the neck into the superoanterior mediastinum and T-cell defects resulting from the lack of inducer thymic T lymphocytes has been shown in patients with hypogammaglobulinemia of the Swiss type [72,85,86-89].

The thymus of patients with Glanzmann–Riniker disease shows severe hypoplasia or dysplasia with total absence of lymphocytes and Hassall's corpuscles [90-92].

In addition to Glanzmann–Riniker disease, there are two other forms of hypogammaglobulinemia that are not accompanied by aplasia or severe hypoplasia of the thymus: *Bruton's X-linked type of hypogammaglobulinemia* and *acquired hypogammaglobulinemia* [72]. In both syndromes, the thymus is not dysplastic or hypoplastic and exhibits changes of stress involution secondary to repeated infections.

Di George's syndrome is another rare condition characterized by the total or partial absence of the thymus and the absence or hypoplasia of the parathyroid glands resulting from a failure in the development of the third and fourth branchial pouches [93,94]. The peripheral lymphoid tissues of these patients also show severe depletion of T-cell areas. Di George's syndrome patients with thymic hypoplasia (partial Di George's syndrome) exhibit a small amount of thymic tissue with normal microscopic morphology [95].

Patients with Di George's syndrome have severe recurrent infections, various clinical problems related to hypoparathyroidism and frequent associated congenital cardiovascular defects such as truncus arteriosus [96]. Their prognosis is guarded with high mortality, although some patients have been treated successfully by thymic transplants [65,70,97-101].

Nezelof's syndrome is another rare congenital immunodeficiency disorder characterized by the absence or hypoplasia of the thymus. However, these patients exhibit normal parathyroid glands and no symptoms of hypoparathyrodism [65,102,103].

Wiscott–Aldrich syndrome is a sex-linked, recessive hereditary disease characterized by the triad of severe immunodeficiency, eczema, and thrombocytopenia [104-106]. Patients with this disorder usually have a hypoplastic thymus that is either normal histologically or exhibits changes of acute involution. They also exhibit marked depletion of parafollicular thymus-dependent areas in peripheral lymphoid tissues. Patients with Wiscott–Aldrich syndrome have a shortened life span and die of infection or malignancy (malignant lymphoma). Complete correction of the Wiscott–Aldrich syndrome by allogeneic bone transplantation has been reported [107].

Thymic dysplasia

Thymic dysplasia is characterized by absence of lymphoid tissue associated with the complete absence or presence of only very scanty Hassall's corpuscles in a thymus composed only of epithelial elements (Fig. 5.9) [108–112]. It exhibits nine morphologic patterns described in detail by Landing and associates [72].

The pinealoid pattern is the classical form of thymic dysplasia and is characterized by a gland that has only solid nests of round epithelial cells surrounded by fibro-vascular septa (Fig. 5.10). The

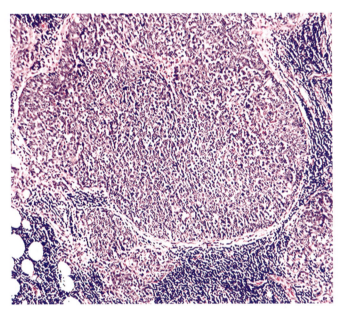

Fig. 5.9 Thymic dysplasia. The thymus shows mostly sheets of epithelial cells and scanty lymphoid cells. No distinct cortico-medullary areas or Hassall's corpuscles were present (H&E 40x).

dark spindle-cell epithelial pattern of thymic dysplasia is characterized by the presence of irregular nests of hyperchromatic spindle epithelial cells and tissue clefts ("stem cystosis"). A third variant of thymic dysplasia is the epithelial "stem-only" pattern, characterized by large aggregates of round epithelial cells surrounded by a pale myxoid stroma. The other patterns of thymic dysplasia described by Landing and associates are very rare.

The distinction among these morphologic variants of thymic dysplasia has clinical relevance. For example, patients with SCID or Nezelof's syndrome who have thymic dysplasia with the pinealoid pattern exhibit a less severe immunodeficiency that responds better to immunologic reconstitution than patients with epithelial "stem-only" features. Patients with the thymic epithelial "stem-only" pattern usually have SCID syndrome with severe immunologic deficits and associated deficiency of the enzyme adenosine deaminase (ADA) in lymphoid cells. Patients with the small dark spindle-celled pattern usually exhibit pure T-lymphocyte deficiency (so-called thymic alymphoplasia) and have a relatively better survival rate than those with the SCID syndrome.

Borzy and associates have proposed a classification of thymic dysplasia in patients with the SCID syndrome that includes five patterns: total dysplasia, partial dysplasia, partial dysplasia with phagocytosis, heterogeneous, and late fetal [113]. In their view, the thymus in total dysplasia (TDP) lacks lymphocytes, Hassall's corpuscles and distinct cortical and medullary areas, and is characterized by small lobules composed of small spindle-epithelial cells forming distinct glands (alveolar pattern) or rosettes. The thymus in partial dysplasia (PDP) has similar lobules composed of larger epithelial cells with abundant eosinophilic cytoplasm. The thymus with a heterogeneous cell population (HCP) is characterized by small distinct lobules composed of epithelial cells admixed with mononuclear cells and scanty lymphocytes. Occasional

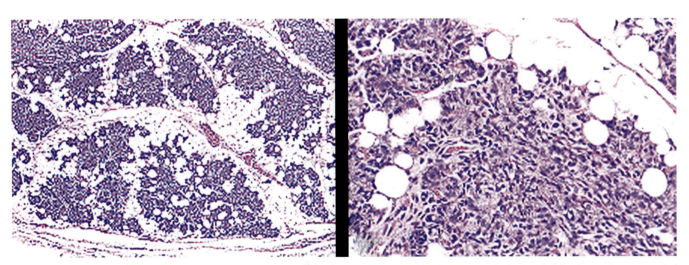

Fig. 5.10 Thymic dysplasia in an infant with severe combined immunodeficiency syndrome. The gland shows a "pinealoid pattern" of dysplasia and is composed of epithelial elements forming small cellular aggregates admixed with small blood vessels. Please note the absence of lymphoid elements, cortico-medullary differentiation, and Hassall's corpuscles (H&E 40x).

Hassall's corpuscles and a hint at corticomedullary distinction are also present. The thymus with partial dysplasia with phagocytosis (PDPP) has lobules of thymic tissue larger than those in the previous three forms, composed of epithelial cells, lymphocytes, and large numbers of phagocytic mononuclear cells. Hassall's corpuscles are absent. No cortico-medullary demarcation is present. The thymus with the late fetal pattern (LFP) resembles the fetal gland and has lobules composed of a central area of pale epithelial cells surrounded by a mantle of lymphocytes and monocytes. Focal cortico-medullary distinction is present but Hassall's corpuscles are absent.

Patients with SCID, Di George's syndrome, and other forms of immunodeficiency can exhibit low serum levels of thymopoietin and FTS [114,115]. Unfortunately, neither these abnormal hormonal levels nor other laboratory tests correlate with the thymic pathology, underscoring the value of thymic biopsy in the evaluation of patients with immune deficiency.

Serum levels of thymopoietin and FTS can return to normal values following transplants of fetal thymus in selected immunodeficiency patients [116].

Thymic abnormalities in acquired immune deficiency syndrome and other conditions

Patients with congenital diseases such as ataxia–telangiectasia, Zinsser Cole–Engman syndrome (X-linked congenital dyskeratosis with pancytopenia), and acquired conditions such as Hodgkin's lymphoma, biliary atresia, Langerhans histiocytosis, acquired immune deficiency syndrome (AIDS), SLE, and others can develop immunodeficiency associated with thymic abnormalities [65,72,117–121].

These abnormalities are seldom present at birth and usually develop progressively in a previously normal gland. For example, patients with biliary atresia develop a progressive loss of thymic epithelium over several months, and those with dysgammaglobulinemia exhibit a small thymus with cystic Hassall's corpuscles, the so-called "central Hassall's corpuscle" pattern [72]. Patients with SLE usually exhibit FH of the thymus but occasionally also show large cystic Hassall's corpuscles [122,123].

Thymic dysplasia, with absence of lymphoid cells and Hassall's corpuscles, and other pathologic abnormalities have been described in thymic biopsies and autopsies from AIDS patients [124–130,131,132]. Joshi and associates have described three histopathologic patterns in thymic biopsies from children with AIDS: precocious involution, dysinvolution mimicking dysplasia, and thymitis [133]. Biopsies with precocious involution show marked decrease in lymphocytes, microcystic Hassall's corpuscles, and an obscure cortico-medullary differentiation. Thymic dysinvolution is characterized by a decrease in thymic weight, loss of the corticomedullary differentiation, normal blood vessels, marked lymphocyte depletion, and absence of Hassall's corpuscles. Patients with thymitis have thymuses with normal location, size, weight, and vascularity that show medullary germinal centers, lymphomononuclear and/or plasma cell infiltrates that obscure the corticomedullary differentiation, and medullary giant cells.

It is controversial whether these morphologic findings are secondary to injury to the epithelial cells or other thymic structures by the Human Immunodeficiency Virus 1 (HIV-1) or the result of accelerated involution in very sick patients. Schuurman and associates have compared the thymuses at autopsy from patients who died from AIDS, congenital immunodeficiency, and after allogeneic bone marrow transplantation and detected no significant morphologic differences between the three groups [134]. In studies utilizing immunohistochemistry for HIV-1 gag and env proteins and other molecular biology techniques, the authors detected only low numbers of positive cells, disputing the theory that the thymic epithelial cells are preferentially injured by the virus. This study also confirmed the presence of epitopes of retroviral antigens in the thymic epithelium.

The thymus can so develop atrophy or hyperinvolution in bone marrow allograft recipients [97,135–138]. The glands in these patients are small and composed of subcapsular and medullary epithelium, small remnants of cortical epithelium, and only mature thymocytes. These changes may be secondary to graft-versus-host disease (GVHD), chemotherapy, and/or lethal total body irradiation. Some patients show evidence of partial reconstitution of normal thymic structures or of lymphopoiesis.

Thymus transplantation has been used to prevent graft-versus-host disease in bone marrow allograft patients [139].

The thymus in myasthenia gravis

Myasthenia gravis (MG) is a neurological disease characterized by muscular weakness and fatigability resulting from a post-synaptic defect that impairs neuromuscular transmission [140–146].

There is substantial clinical and experimental evidence indicating the autoimmune pathogenesis of the disease and the role of the thymus gland in its immunobiology, including the frequent association of MG with other autoimmune disorders and the presence in these patients of low serum levels of complement, high levels of circulating antibodies to acetylcholine receptors (AChR), and pathologic abnormalities in the thymus [147–154]. Moreover, MG can be produced experimentally by immunizing animals with purified AChR isolated from the electric organs of eels and rays.

The role of the thymus in the pathogenesis of MG has been studied in detail [155,156]. The autoantigen in MG is the nicotinic AChR encountered at the neuromuscular junction and in the myoid cells of the thymus. The number of functioning AChRs is reduced in patients with MG, as a result of circulating anti-AChR antibodies that are present in over 90% of patients with the disease. These antibodies are thought to be produced in the thymus, peripheral lymphoid organs, and the blood. The secretion of these antibodies may be modulated by AChR-specific helper T-cells. The anti-AChR autoantibodies are thought to inactivate the receptor sites at the neuromuscular junctions by

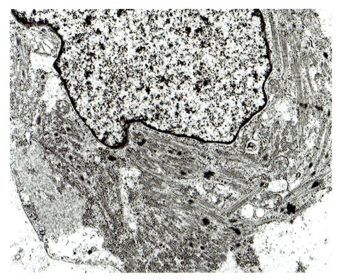

Fig. 5.11 Electron micrograph of a thymic myoid cell showing cytoplasmic myoid fibrils with focal z-bands.

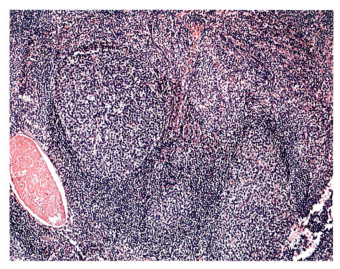

Fig. 5.12 Myasthenia gravis with follicular hyperplasia and focal microcyst (H&E 20x).

(a) activation of complement with destruction of the post-synaptic muscle cell membrane, (b) accelerated turnover and loss of the AChR, or (c) pharmacologic block of the receptor with inhibition of acetylcholine binding.

The thymus has myoid cells (Fig. 5.11), described in the human thymus by van de Velde and Friedman in 1966 [157,158]. These cells are more readily found in the medulla of the thymus of patients with MG than in controls. Myoid cells express AChR immunoreactivity and probably provide the autoantigen for intrathymic autosensitization [159–161]. In the thymus of a patient with MG, there is also an increase in the number of interdigitating cells expressing strong HLA-DR immunoreactivity [162,163]. These cells are in close contact with the myoid cells and may play an important role as antigen-presenting cells in the process of T-cell activation that takes place in the thymus of a patient with MG [164].

Wekerle and associates have proposed a three-stage model of the pathogenesis of MG based on pathological and experimental evidence. In their view, the primary event in MG is the appearance of thymic myogenic cells followed by auto-sensitization against AChR present in those cells [165,166]. In a later stage, autosensitized thymocytes interact with thymic B-cells to produce anti-AChR antibodies [97]. Several other studies support the hypothesis of the thymus as the primary site of auto-sensitization in MG [152,167–172]. The mechanisms by which the tolerance to normal antigenic epitopes is lost in patients with MG are not well known.

Heredity and certain genes appear to play a significant role in the pathogenesis of MG [173]. Cases of myasthenia gravis can be familial [174]. For example, Caucasian patients with MG have an increased incidence of the major histocompatibility complex antigens HLA-B8 and DR3, whereas their Japanese counterparts more frequently have HLA-B12. In female patients the DRw15-Dx3-positive haplotype strongly correlates with the presence of a thymoma in association with MG [175–181].

This association of HLA antigens with MG is potentially interesting because human genes in the D and DR regions are probably involved in the control of immune recognition and the generation of helper and suppressor T-cell responses [179,182–184].

Congenital myasthenia syndromes

There are several unusual forms of congenital myasthenia that have a different pathogenesis than MG [185,186]. These syndromes are usually congenital or familial and are associated with a normal thymus. They include myasthenic syndromes caused by either endplate acetylcholinesterase deficiency or a putative abnormality of the acetylcholine-induced ion channel or a postulated defect of acetylcholine resynthesis or mobilization [187].

Thymoma, follicular hyperplasia of the thymus and other abnormalities in myasthenia gravis

The thymus of myasthenia gravis (MG) patients can be normal in 10% to 25% of cases, and exhibit FH in 60% to 90% of patients (Fig. 5.12). MG is also frequently associated with other non-neoplastic changes including the presence of an increased number of medullary individual B-cells, increased densities of T-helper cells, presence of epithelial cells containing detectable intracytoplasmic thymosin, and/or an increase in visible myoid cells [188–190]. The hyperplastic follicles encountered in the thymus of MG patients with FH are located both in the interlobular/perivascular spaces and within the thymic medulla and are associated with a remodeled thymic architecture resulting from an expanded medulla, a compressed cortex, and a partial destruction of the normal network of thymic medullary epithelial cells [16,191–193]. The presence of germinal centers and the increase in individual B lymphocytes in the thymic medulla supports the theory of autoimmune activation of thymic B-cells in MG.

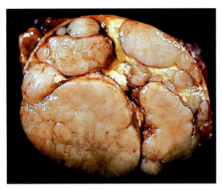

Fig. 5.13 Thymoma in a patient with myasthenia gravis. The tumor is encapsulated and shows a lobulated gray-tan surface.

MG is associated with a thymoma in 10–20% of patients (Fig. 5.13). The tumor can be diagnosed concurrently with the disease or develop metachronously [194–198].

The density of germinal centers and their significance in the thymus of MG patients with FH has been the subject of multiple studies [199–203]. The germinal centers are composed of B lymphocytes with intracytoplasmic immunoglobulins and anti-AChR antibodies, detectable with immunohistochemistry [204–206]. The density of germinal centers in the thymus of MG patients has been quantitated morphometrically in several studies, resulting in quite variable findings [207–211]. Slightly different methods have been utilized to determine (a) the presence and density of germinal centers in thymic sections (0, absent; 1 +, equivocal, rare; 2 +, present; 3 +, frequent; 4 +, numerous), (b) the degree of lymphoid cell loss and fat replacement as a measure of involution (none, less than expected, partial, complete), and (c) the number of epithelial elements present [212–215]. Penn and associates also quantitated the number of myoid cells detected in thymic sections with labeled bungarotoxin [216].

These parameters, in particular the number of germinal centers, have been correlated with the age and sex of MG patients, duration of symptoms prior to thymectomy, and response to therapy to determine their prognostic value [217]. Most studies report large numbers of germinal centers in the thymuses of MG patients and indicate that their presence is, indeed, significant [218]. Middleton, however, reported germinal centers in the thymuses of 71% of sudden death patients [219]. The density and size of thymic follicles present in their cases appear to be significantly smaller than those in MG.

Alpert and associates studied the non-neoplastic thymic tissue of MG patients at The Mount Sinai Hospital, New York, and concluded that the presence of a normal gland or a small, involuted thymus with few germinal centers correlated well with a favorable response to surgery and a rapid remission rate of the disease [220,221]. The results are controversial. For example, Mackay and associates detected a significant association between thymic germinal centers and MG but no correlation between their number and prognosis [222].

Moran and associates quantitated with morphometric techniques the germinal centers of the thymuses of patients with non-thymomatous MG and demonstrated a correlation between the size of germinal centers and clinical improvement following thymectomy [223]. Patients with germinal centers with a cross-sectional area of 0.02 mm^2, perimeter of 0.58 mm, and diameter of 0.17 mm had significantly better clinical outcomes than those with larger follicles. There was no correlation between the number of germinal centers and the clinical outcome.

References

1. Aw D, Palmer DB. The origin and implication of thymic involution. *Aging Dis.* 2011;2:437–43.

2. Aw D, Palmer DB. It's not all equal: a multiphasic theory of thymic involution. *Biogerontology.* 2012;13:77–81.

3. Calder AE, Hince MN, Dudakov JA *et al.* Thymic involution: where endocrinology meets immunology. *Neuroimmunomodulation.* 2011;18:281–9.

4. Dooley J, Liston A. Molecular control over thymic involution: from cytokines and microRNA to aging and adipose tissue. *Eur J Immunol.* 2012;42:1073–9.

5. Hakim FT, Gress RE. Thymic involution: implications for self-tolerance. *Methods Mol Biol.* 2007;380:377–90.

6. Boyd, E. The weight of the thymus gland in health and in disease. *Am J Dis Child.* 1932;43:1162–1214.

7. Hsu HC, Li L, Zhang HG *et al.* Genetic regulation of thymic involution. *Mech Ageing Dev.* 2005;126:87–97.

8. Lynch HE, Goldberg GL, Chidgey A *et al.* Thymic involution and immune reconstitution. *Trends Immunol.* 2009;30:366–73.

9. Gewolb IH, Lebowitz RL, Taeusch HW, Jr. Thymus size and its relationship to the respiratory distress syndrome. *J Pediatr.* 1979;95:108–11.

10. van Baarlen J, Schuurman HJ, Huber J. Acute thymus involution in infancy and childhood: a reliable marker for duration of acute illness. *Hum Pathol.* 1988;19:1155–60.

11. van Baarlen J, Schuurman HJ, Reitsma R *et al.* Acute thymus involution during infancy and childhood: immunohistology of the thymus and peripheral lymphoid tissues after acute illness. *Pediatr Pathol.* 1989;9:261–75.

12. Seemayer TA, Bolande RP. Thymic involution mimicking thymic dysplasia: a consequence of transfusion-induced graft versus host disease in a premature infant. *Arch Pathol Lab Med.* 1980;104:141–4.

13. Young M, Turnbull HM. An analysis of the data collected by the Status Lymphaticus Investigation Committee. *J Pathol.* 1931;34: 213–58.

14. Levine GD, Rosai J. Thymic hyperplasia and neoplasia: a review of current concepts. *Hum Pathol.* 1978;9:495–515.

15. Hofmann WJ, Moller P, Otto HF. Thymic hyperplasia. I. True thymic hyperplasia. Review of the literature. *Klin Wochenschr.* 1987;65:49–52.

16. Hofmann WJ Thymic hyperplasia. II. Lymphofollicular hyperplasia of the thymus. An immunohistologic study. *Klin Wochenschr.* 1987; 65:53–60.

17. Carvalho MR, Dias T, Baptista F et al. Graves' disease and massive thymic hyperplasia. *Thyroid*. 2010;20:227–9.

18. Gow KW, Kobrynski L, Abramowsky C et al. Massive benign thymic hyperplasia in a six-month-old girl: case report. *Am Surg*. 2003;69:717–19.

19. Green JS, Rickett AR. True massive thymic hyperplasia. *Clin Radiol*. 1996;51:598.

20. Hirasaki S, Murakami K, Kanamori T et al. Weber-Christian disease developing into mediastinitis and pleuritis with massive pleural effusion. *Intern Med*. 2012;51:943–7.

21. Lack EE. Thymic hyperplasia with massive enlargement: report of two cases with review of diagnostic criteria. *J Thorac Cardiovasc Surg*. 1981;81:741–6.

22. Lamesch AJ. Massive thymic hyperplasia in infants. *Bull Soc Sci Med Grand Duche Luxemb*. 1988;125 Spec No:20–4.

23. Hoffman W.J., Moller P, Otto H.F., Massive thymic hyperplasia in infants. *Z Kinderchir*. 1983;38:16–18.

24. McHugh K. True massive thymic hyperplasia. *Clin Radiol*. 1997;52:77–8.

25. Nezelof C, Normand C. Tumor-like massive thymic hyperplasia in childhood: a possible defect of T-cell maturation, histological and cytoenzymatic studies of three cases. *Thymus*. 1986;8:177–86.

26. Prenger KB, Poeschmann PH, Smits PH et al. Massive mediastinal hemorrhage following treatment of hyperthyroidism with radioactive iodine. *Thorac Cardiovasc Surg*. 1984;32:122–3.

27. Rice HE, Flake AW, Hori T et al. Massive thymic hyperplasia: characterization of a rare mediastinal mass. *J Pediatr Surg*. 1994;29:1561–4.

28. Szarf G, de Andrade TC, de Oliveira R, et al. Massive thymic hyperplasia presenting with respiratory insufficiency in a 2-year-old child. *Thorax*. 2010;65:555–6.

29. Woywodt A, Verhaart S, Kiss A. Massive true thymic hyperplasia. *Eur J Pediatr Surg*. 1999;9:331–3.

30. Judd RL. Massive thymic hyperplasia with myoid cell differentiation. *Hum Pathol*. 1987;18:1180–3.

31. Judd RL, Welch SL. Myoid cell differentiation in true thymic hyperplasia and lymphoid hyperplasia. *Arch Pathol Lab Med*. 1988;112:1140–4.

32. Kendall MD, Johnson HR, Singh J. The weight of the human thymus gland at necropsy. *J Anat*. 1980;131:483–97.

33. Ricci C, Pescarmona E, Rendina EA et al. True thymic hyperplasia: a clinicopathological study. *Ann Thorac Surg*. 1989;47:741–5.

34. Durkin W, Durant J. Benign mass lesions after therapy for Hodgkin's disease. *Arch Intern Med*. 1979;139:333–6.

35. Due W, Dieckmann KP, Stein H. Thymic hyperplasia following chemotherapy of a testicular germ cell tumor. Immunohistological evidence for a simple rebound phenomenon. *Cancer*. 1989;63:446–9.

36. Ford ME, Stevens R, Rosado-de-Christenson ML et al. Rebound thymic hyperplasia after pneumonectomy and chemotherapy for primary synovial sarcoma. *J Thorac Imaging*. 2008;23:178–81.

37. Hara M, McAdams HP, Vredenburgh JJ et al. Thymic hyperplasia after high-dose chemotherapy and autologous stem cell transplantation: incidence and significance in patients with breast cancer. *AJR Am J Roentgenol*. 1999;173:1341–4.

38. Hendriks JM, Van Schil PE, Schrijvers D et al. Rebound thymic hyperplasia after chemotherapy in a patient treated for pulmonary metastases. *Acta Chir Belg*. 1999;99:312–14.

39. Lin TL, Shih LY, Hung YS et al. Thymic hyperplasia following successful chemotherapy for Hodgkin's lymphoma: report of a case. *Chang Gung Med J*. 2009;32:98–103.

40. Sehbai AS, Tallaksen RJ, Bennett J et al. Thymic hyperplasia after adjuvant chemotherapy in breast cancer. *J Thorac Imaging*. 2006;21:43–6.

41. Shin MS, Ho KJ. Diffuse thymic hyperplasia following chemotherapy for nodular sclerosing Hodgkin's disease. An immunologic rebound phenomenon? *Cancer*. 1983;51:30–3.

42. Simmonds P, Silberstein M, McKendrick J. Thymic hyperplasia in adults following chemotherapy for malignancy. *Aust N Z J Med*. 1993;23:264–7.

43. Arliss J, Scholes J, Dickson PR et al. Massive thymic hyperplasia in an adolescent. *Ann Thorac Surg*. 1988;45:220–2.

44. Balcom RJ, Hakanson DO, Werner A et al. Massive thymic hyperplasia in an infant with Beckwith-Wiedemann syndrome. *Arch Pathol Lab Med*. 1985;109:153–5.

45. Mlika M, Yadi-Kaddour A, Marghli A et al. True thymic hyperplasia versus follicular thymic hyperplasia: a retrospective analysis of 13 cases. *Pathologica*. 2009;101:175–9.

46. Moran CA, Suster S, Gil J et al. Morphometric analysis of germinal centers in nonthymomatous patients with myasthenia gravis. *Arch Pathol Lab Med*. 1990;114:689–91.

47. Grody WW, Jobst S, Keesey J et al. Pathologic evaluation of thymic hyperplasia in myasthenia gravis and Lambert-Eaton myasthenic syndrome. *Arch Pathol Lab Med*. 1986;110:843–6.

48. Goldstein G, Mackay IR. The thymus in systemic lupus erythematosus: a quantitative histopathological analysis and comparison with stress involution. *Br Med J*. 1967;2:475–8.

49. Middleton G. The incidence of follicular structures in the human thymus at autopsy. *Aust J Exp Biol Med Sci*. 1967;45:189–99.

50. Biggart JD, Nevin NC. Hyperplasia of the thymus in progressive systemic sclerosis. *J Pathol Bacteriol*. 1967;93:334–7.

51. Vetters M, Barclay RS. The incidence of germinal centres in thymus glands of patients with congenital heart disease. *J Clin Pathol*. 1973;26:583–91.

52. Mackay IR, Degail P. Thymic "germinal centres" and plasma cells in systemic lupus erythematosus. *Lancet*. 1963;2:667.

53. Corridan M. The thymus in hepatic cirrhosis. *J Clin Pathol*. 1963;16:445–7.

54. Kamegaya K, Tsuchiya M, Sambe K. Thymic abnormalities and the chronicity of liver disease–report of 10 cases and follow-up study. *Keio J Med*. 1971;20:77–90.

55. Rosai J, Levine GD. *Tumors of the thymus*. 1976; Washington: Armed Forces Institute of Pathology.

56. Alpert LI, Papatestas A, Kark A et al. A histologic reappraisal of the thymus in myasthenia gravis. A correlative study of thymic pathology and response

to thymectomy. *Arch Pathol.* 1971;91:55–61.

57. Moran CA, Suster S, Gil J *et al.* Morphometric analysis of germinal centers in nonthymomatous patients with myasthenia gravis. *Arch Pathol Lab Med.* 1990; 114:689–91.

58. Amariglio N, Lev A, Simon A *et al.* Molecular assessment of thymus capabilities in the evaluation of T-cell immunodeficiency. *Pediatr Res.* 2010;67:211–16.

59. Poliani PL, Vermi W, Facchetti F. Thymus microenvironment in human primary immunodeficiency diseases. *Curr Opin Allergy Clin Immunol.* 2009;9:489–95.

60. Linder J. The thymus gland in secondary immunodeficiency. *Arch Pathol Lab Med.* 1987;111:1118–22.

61. Scinicariello F, Kourtis AP, Nesheim S *et al.* Limited evolution of human immunodeficiency virus type 1 in the thymus of a perinatally infected child. *Clin Infect Dis.* 2010;50:726–32.

62. D'Andrea V, Ambrogi V. Thymus biopsy in patients with AIDS and ARC. *Thymus.* 1991;18:61–2.

63. Schuurman HJ, Krone WJ, Broekhuizen R *et al.* The thymus in acquired immune deficiency syndrome. Comparison with other types of immunodeficiency diseases, and presence of components of human immunodeficiency virus type 1. *Am J Pathol.* 1989;134:1329–38.

64. D'Andrea V, Naso G, Loreto CG *et al.* Biopsy of the thymus in patients with acquired immunodeficiency syndrome. *Thymus.* 1989;14:261–3.

65. Nezelof C. Pathology of the thymus in immunodeficiency states. *Curr Top Pathol.* 1986;75:151–77.

66. Grody WW, Fligiel S, Naeim F. Thymus involution in the acquired immunodeficiency syndrome. *Am J Clin Pathol.* 1985;84:85–95.

67. Borzy MS, Schulte-Wissermann H, Gilbert E *et al.* Thymic morphology in immunodeficiency diseases: results of thymic biopsies. *Clin Immunol Immunopathol.* 1979;12:31–51.

68. D'Andrea V, Ambrogi V. Thymus biopsy in patients with AIDS and ARC. *Thymus.* 1991;18:61–2.

69. Joshi VV, Oleske JM, Saad S *et al.* Thymus biopsy in children with

acquired immunodeficiency syndrome. *Arch Pathol Lab Med.* 1986;110:837–42.

70. Taylor MJ, Josifek K. Multiple congenital anomalies, thymic dysplasia, severe congenital heart disease, and oligosyndactyly with a deletion of the short arm of chromosome 5. *Am J Med Genet.* 1981;9:5–11.

71. Lewis JF, Matthews WP. Thymic dysplasia associated with lymphopenia. *South Med J.* 1972;65:998–1000.

72. Landing BH, Yutuc I.L., Swanson VL. Cinicopathologic correlations in immunologic deficiency diseases of children, with emphasis on thymic histologic patterns. In: *Proceedings of the International Symposium on Immunodeficiency.*1976. Tokyo: Tokyo University Press.

73. Elie R, Laroche AC, Arnoux E *et al.* Thymic dysplasia in acquired immunodeficiency syndrome. *N Engl J Med.* 1983;308:841–2.

74. Sutton AL, Smithwick EM, Seligman SJ *et al.* Fatal disseminated herpesvirus hominis type 2 infection in an adult with associated thymic dysplasia. *Am J Med.* 1974;56:545–53.

75. Lewis JF, Matthews WP. Thymic dysplasia associated with lymphopenia. *South Med J.* 1972;65:998–1000.

76. Say B, Tinaztepe B, Tinaztepe K *et al.* Thymic dysplasia associated with dyschondroplasia in an infant. *Am J Dis Child.* 1972;123:240–4.

77. Leikin S, Purugganan G, Chandra R. Thymic dysplasia. *J Pediatr.* 1969;75:229–35.

78. Lamvik J, Moe PJ. Thymic dysplasia with immunological deficiency. Report of two unusual cases. *Acta Pathol Microbiol Scand.* 1969;76:349–60.

79. Berry CL, Thompson EN. Clinico-pathological study of thymic dysplasia. *Arch Dis Child.* 1968;43:579–84.

80. Miller ME, Schieken RM. Thymic dysplasia. A separable entity from "swiss agammaglobulinemia". *Am J Med Sci.* 1967;253:741–50.

81. Miller ME, Hummeler K. Thymic dysplasia ("Swiss agammaglobulinemia"). II. Morphologic and functional observations. *J Pediatr.* 1967;70:737–44.

82. Miller ME. Thymic dysplasia ("Swiss agammaglobulinemia"). I. Graft versus host reaction following bone-marrow transfusion. *J Pediatr.* 1967;70:730–6.

83. Pahwa RN, Pahwa SG, Good RA. T-lymphocyte differentiation in severe combined immunodeficiency: defects of the thymus. *Clin Immunol Immunopathol.* 1978;11:437–44.

84. Miller ME, Schieken RM. Thymic dysplasia. A separable entity from "swiss agammaglobulinemia". *Am J Med Sci.* 1967;253:741–50.

85. Borzy MS, Schulte-Wissermann H, Gilbert E *et al.* Thymic morphology in immunodeficiency diseases: results of thymic biopsies. *Clin Immunol Immunopathol.* 1979;12:31–51.

86. Ratech H, Lett J, Hong R. Thymic morphology in immunodeficiency diseases: results of thymic biopsies. *Clin Immunol Immunopathol.* 1979;12:31–51.

87. Poliani PL, Vermi W, Facchetti F. Thymus microenvironment in human primary immunodeficiency diseases. *Curr Opin Allergy Clin Immunol.* 2009;9:489–95.

88. Linder J. The thymus gland in secondary immunodeficiency. *Arch Pathol Lab Med.* 1987;111:1118–22.

89. Pahwa RN, Pahwa SG, Good RA. T-lymphocyte differentiation in severe combined immunodeficiency: defects of the thymus. *Clin Immunol Immunopathol.* 1978;11:437–44.

90. Miller ME, Schieken RM. Thymic dysplasia. A separable entity from "swiss agammaglobulinemia". *Am J Med Sci.* 1967;253:741–50.

91. Miller ME. Thymic dysplasia ("Swiss agammaglobulinemia"). I. Graft versus host reaction following bone-marrow transfusion. *J Pediatr.* 1967;70:730–6.

92. Miller ME, Hummeler K. Thymic dysplasia ("Swiss agammaglobulinemia"). II. Morphologic and functional observations. *J Pediatr.* 1967;70:737–44.

93. Joshi VV, Oleske JM, Saad S *et al.* Thymus biopsy in children with acquired immunodeficiency syndrome. *Arch Pathol Lab Med.* 1986;110:837–42.

94. Di George AM, Lischner HW, Dacou C *et al.* Absence of the thymus. *Lancet.* 1967;1:1387.

95. Pahwa RN, Pahwa SG, Good RA. T-lymphocyte differentiation in severe combined immunodeficiency: defects of the thymus. *Clin Immunol Immunopathol.* 1978;11:437–44.

96. Jung LKL. T-lymphocyte differentiation in severe combined immunodeficiency: defects of the thymus. *Clin Immunol Immunopathol.* 1978;11:437–44.

97. Haynes BF, Markert ML, Sempowski GD *et al.* The role of the thymus in immune reconstitution in aging, bone marrow transplantation, and HIV-1 infection. *Annu Rev Immunol.* 2000;18:529–60.

98. Joshi VV, Oleske JM, Saad S *et al.* Thymus biopsy in children with acquired immunodeficiency syndrome. *Arch Pathol Lab Med.* 1986;110:837–42.

99. Bach JF. The thymus in immunodeficiency diseases: new therapeutic approaches. *Birth Defects Orig Artic Ser.* 1983;19:245–53.

100. Kirkpatrick JA, Jr., Di George AM. Congenital absence of the thymus. *Am J Roentgenol Radium Ther Nucl Med.* 1968;103:32–7.

101. Lischner HW, Dacou C, Di George AM. Normal lymphocyte transfer (NLT) test: negative response in a patient with congenital absence of the thymus. *Transplantation.* 1967;5:555–7.

102. Suvatte V, Tuchinda M, Bukkavesa S *et al.* Thymic dysplasia with normal immunoglobulins (Nezelof syndrome): a case report. *J Med Assoc Thai.* 1976;59:224–33.

103. Berkel AI, Caglar M, Tinatepe K *et al.* Thymic dysplasia with normal immunoglobulins (the Nezelof syndrome). (A case report). *Turk J Pediatr.* 1976;18:45–52.

104. Chellaiah MA, Kuppuswamy D, Lasky L *et al.* Phosphorylation of a Wiscott–Aldrich syndrome protein-associated signal complex is critical in osteoclast bone resorption. *J Biol Chem.* 2007;282:10104–16.

105. Li R. Bee1, a yeast protein with homology to Wiscott–Aldrich syndrome protein, is critical for the assembly of cortical actin cytoskeleton. *J Cell Biol.* 1997;136:649–58.

106. Shapiro RS, Gerrard JM, Perry GS, *et al.* Wiskott–Aldrich syndrome: detection of carrier state by metabolic stress of platelets. *Lancet.* 1978;1:121–3.

107. Parkman R, Rappeport J, Geha R *et al.* Complete correction of the Wiskott–Aldrich syndrome by allogeneic bone-marrow transplantation. *N Engl J Med.* 1978;298:921–7.

108. Andronikou S, Kollios K, Dimou S *et al.* Hemolytic uremic syndrome and thymic dysplasia in an infant. *Pediatr Nephrol.* 1998;12:231–3.

109. Elie R, Laroche AC, Arnoux E *et al.* Thymic dysplasia in acquired immunodeficiency syndrome. *N Engl J Med.* 1983;308:841–2.

110. Suvatte V, Tuchinda M, Bukkavesa S *et al.* Thymic dysplasia with normal immunoglobulins (Nezelof syndrome): a case report. *J Med Assoc Thai.* 1976;59:224–33.

111. Roberts PF. Thymic dysplasia, persistence of measles virus, and unexpected infant death. *Arch Dis Child.* 1975;50:401–3.

112. Lewis JF, Matthews WP. Thymic dysplasia associated with lymphopenia. *South Med J.* 1972;65:998–1000.

113. Borzy MS, Schulte-Wissermann H, Gilbert E *et al.* Thymic morphology in immunodeficiency diseases: results of thymic biopsies. *Clin Immunol Immunopathol.* 1979;12:31–51.

114. Pahwa R, Ikehara S, Pahwa SG *et al.* Thymic function in man. *Thymus.* 1979;1:27–58.

115. Pahwa RN, Pahwa SG, Good RA. T-lymphocyte differentiation in severe combined immunodeficiency: defects of the thymus. *Clin Immunol Immunopathol.* 1978;11:437–44.

116. Atkinson K, Storb R, Ochs HD *et al.* Thymus transplantation after allogeneic bone marrow graft to prevent chronic graft-versus-host disease in humans. *Transplantation.* 1982;33:168–73.

117. D'Andrea V, Ambrogi V. Thymus biopsy in patients with AIDS and ARC. *Thymus.* 1991;18:61–2.

118. Linder J. The thymus gland in secondary immunodeficiency. *Arch Pathol Lab Med.* 1987;111:1118–22.

119. Welch K. The thymus in AIDS. *Am J Clin Pathol.* 1986;85:531.

120. Perreault S, Bernard G, Lortie A *et al.* Ataxia-telangiectasia presenting with a novel immunodeficiency. *Pediatr Neurol.* 2012;46:322–4.

121. Ortega JA, Swanson VL, Landing BH *et al.* Congenital dyskeratosis. Zinsser-Engman-Cole syndrome with thymic dysplasia and aplastic anemia. *Am J Dis Child.* 1972;124:701–4.

122. Pasqualoni E, Aubart F, Brihaye B *et al.* Lambert-Eaton myasthenic syndrome and follicular thymic hyperplasia in systemic lupus erythematosus. *Lupus.* 2011;20:745–8.

123. Goldstein G, Mackay IR. The thymus in systemic lupus erythematosus: a quantitative histopathological analysis and comparison with stress involution. *Br Med J.* 1967;2:475–8.

124. Alves K, Canzian M, Delwart EL. HIV type 1 envelope quasispecies in the thymus and lymph nodes of AIDS patients. *AIDS Res Hum Retroviruses.* 2002;18:161–5.

125. Chhieng DC, Demaria S, Yee HT *et al.* Multilocular thymic cyst with follicular lymphoid hyperplasia in a male infected with HIV. A case report with fine needle aspiration cytology. *Acta Cytol.* 1999;43:1119–23.

126. Markert ML. Perspective: research highlights at the Duke University center for AIDS research. Immunoreconstitution in HIV infection: the role of the thymus. *AIDS Res Hum Retroviruses.* 1996;12:751–5.

127. Harris PJ, Candeloro PD, Bunn JE. HIV infection of the adult thymus: an even more conventional theory explaining CD4 cell decrease and CD8 cell increase in AIDS. *Med Hypotheses.* 1991;36: 379–80.

128. D'Andrea V, Ambrogi V. Thymus biopsy in patients with AIDS and ARC. *Thymus.* 1991;18:61–2.

129. Hermans P, Clumeck N. Preliminary results on clinical and immunological effects of thymus hormone preparations in AIDS. *Med Oncol Tumor Pharmacother.* 1989;6:55–8.

130. Welch K. The thymus in AIDS. *Am J Clin Pathol.* 1986;85:531.

131. Elie R, Laroche AC, Arnoux E *et al.* Thymic dysplasia in acquired immunodeficiency syndrome. *N Engl J Med.* 1983;308:841–2.

132. Joshi VV, Oleske JM. Pathologic appraisal of the thymus gland in acquired immunodeficiency syndrome in children. A study of four cases and a review of the literature. *Arch Pathol Lab Med.* 1985;109:142–6.

133. Joshi VV, Oleske JM, Saad S *et al.* Thymus biopsy in children with acquired immunodeficiency syndrome. *Arch Pathol Lab Med.* 1986;110:837–42.

134. Schuurman HJ, Krone WJ, Broekhuizen R *et al.* The thymus in acquired immune deficiency syndrome. Comparison with other types of immunodeficiency diseases, and

presence of components of human immunodeficiency virus type 1. *Am J Pathol.* 1989;134:1329–38.

135. Honda K, Takada H, Nagatoshi Y *et al.* Thymus-independent expansion of T lymphocytes in children after allogeneic bone marrow transplantation. *Bone Marrow Transplant.* 2000;25:647–52.

136. McBride WH, Vegesna V. Role of the thymus in radiation-induced lung damage after bone marrow transplantation. *Radiat Res.* 1997;147:501–5.

137. Parkman R, Rappeport J, Geha R *et al.* Complete correction of the Wiskott–Aldrich syndrome by allogeneic bone-marrow transplantation. *N Engl J Med.* 1978;298:921–7.

138. Thomas JA, Sloane JP, Imrie SF *et al.* Immunohistology of the thymus in bone marrow transplant recipients. *Am J Pathol.* 1986;122:531–40.

139. Atkinson K, Storb R, Ochs HD *et al.* Thymus transplantation after allogeneic bone marrow graft to prevent chronic graft-versus-host disease in humans. *Transplantation.* 1982;33:168–73.

140. Beeson D, Bond AP, Corlett L *et al.* Thymus, thymoma, and specific T cells in myasthenia gravis. *Ann N Y Acad Sci.* 1998;841:371–87.

141. Carrieri PB, Marano E, Perretti A *et al.* The thymus and myasthenia gravis: immunological and neurophysiological aspects. *Ann Med.* 1999;31 Suppl 2:52–6.

142. Castleman B. The pathology of the thymus gland in myasthenia gravis. *Ann N Y Acad Sci.* 1966;135:496–505.

143. Cavalcante P, Le Panse R, Berrih-Aknin S *et al.* The thymus in myasthenia gravis: Site of "innate autoimmunity"? *Muscle Nerve.* 2011;44:467–84.

144. Cizeron-Clairac G, Le Panse R, Frenkian-Cuvelier M *et al.* Thymus and Myasthenia Gravis: what can we learn from DNA microarrays? *J Neuroimmunol.* 2008;201–2:57–63.

145. Fraser K. The thymus and myasthenia gravis. *Scott Med J.* 1966;11:203–7.

146. Hohlfeld R, Wekerle H. The thymus in myasthenia gravis. *Neurol Clin.* 1994;12:331–42.

147. Alpert LI, Rule A, Norio M *et al.* Studies in myasthenia gravis: cellular hypersensitivity to skeletal muscle. *Am J Clin Pathol.* 1972;58:647–53.

148. Hohlfeld R, Wekerle H. The role of the thymus in myasthenia gravis. *Adv Neuroimmunol.* 1994;4:373–86.

149. Keesey JC. Thymus, antibodies, and myasthenia. *Neurology.* 1992;42:2227.

150. Leite MI, Jones M, Strobel P *et al.* Myasthenia gravis thymus: complement vulnerability of epithelial and myoid cells, complement attack on them, and correlations with autoantibody status. *Am J Pathol.* 2007;171:893–905.

151. Levinson AI, Wheatley LM. The thymus and the pathogenesis of myasthenia gravis. *Clin Immunol Immunopathol.* 1996;78:1–5.

152. Melms A, Luther C, Stoeckle C *et al.* Thymus and myasthenia gravis: antigen processing in the human thymus and the consequences for the generation of autoreactive T cells. *Acta Neurol Scand Suppl.* 2006;183:12–13.

153. Moulian N, Wakkach A, Guyon T *et al.* Respective role of thymus and muscle in autoimmune myasthenia gravis. *Ann N Y Acad Sci.* 1998;841:397–406.

154. Onodera H. The role of the thymus in the pathogenesis of myasthenia gravis. *Tohoku J Exp Med.* 2005;207:87–98.

155. Levinson AI, Wheatley LM. The thymus and the pathogenesis of myasthenia gravis. *Clin Immunol Immunopathol.* 1996;78:1–5.

156. Onodera H. The role of the thymus in the pathogenesis of myasthenia gravis. *Tohoku J Exp Med.* 2005;207:87–98.

157. van de Velde R, Friedman NB. Thymic myoid cells and myasthenia gravis. *Am J Pathol.* 1970;59:347–68.

158. van de Velde R, Friedman NB. The thymic "myoidzellen" and myasthenia gravis. *JAMA.* 1966;198:287–8.

159. Scadding GK, Calder L, Vincent A *et al.* Anti-acetylcholine receptor antibodies induced in mice by syngeneic receptor without adjuvants. *Immunology.* 1986;58:151–5.

160. Scadding GK, Vincent A, Newsom-Davis J *et al.* Acetylcholine receptor antibody synthesis by thymic lymphocytes: correlation with thymic histology. *Neurology.* 1981;31:935–43.

161. Scadding GK, Thomas HC, Havard CW. Myasthenia gravis: acetylcholine-receptor antibody titres after thymectomy. *Br Med J.* 1977;1:1512.

162. Kirchner T, Schalke B, Melms A *et al.* Immunohistological patterns of non-neoplastic changes in the thymus in myasthenia gravis. *Virchows Arch B Cell Pathol Incl Mol Pathol.* 1986;52:237–57.

163. Kornstein MJ, Brooks JJ, Anderson AO *et al.* The immunohistology of the thymus in myasthenia gravis. *Am J Pathol.* 1984;117:184–94.

164. Kirchner T, Hoppe F, Schalke B *et al.* Microenvironment of thymic myoid cells in myasthenia gravis. *Virchows Arch B Cell Pathol Incl Mol Pathol.* 1988;54:295–302.

165. Hohlfeld R, Wekerle H. The thymus in myasthenia gravis. *Neurol Clin.* 1994;12:331–42.

166. Wekerle H. The thymus in myasthenia gravis. *Ann N Y Acad Sci.* 1993;681:47–55.

167. Hohlfeld R, Wekerle H. The thymus in myasthenia gravis. *Neurol Clin.* 1994;12:331–42.

168. Carrieri PB, Marano E, Perretti A *et al.* The thymus and myasthenia gravis: immunological and neurophysiological aspects. *Ann Med.* 1999;31 Suppl 2:52–6.

169. Cizeron-Clairac G, Le Panse R, Frenkian-Cuvelier M *et al.* Thymus and myasthenia gravis: what can we learn from DNA microarrays? *J Neuroimmunol.* 2008;201–2:57–63.

170. Fraser K. The thymus and myasthenia gravis. *Scott Med J.* 1966;11:203–7.

171. Keesey JC. Thymus, antibodies, and myasthenia. *Neurology.* 1992;42:2227.

172. Onodera H. The role of the thymus in the pathogenesis of myasthenia gravis. *Tohoku J Exp Med.* 2005;207:87–98.

173. Landoure G, Knight MA, Stanescu H *et al.* A candidate gene for autoimmune myasthenia gravis. *Neurology.* 2012;79:342–7.

174. Feng HY, Liu WB, Luo CM *et al.* A retrospective review of 15 patients with familial myasthenia gravis over a period of 25 years. *Neurol Sci.* 2012;33:771–7.

175. Pahwa RN, Pahwa SG, Good RA. T-lymphocyte differentiation in severe combined immunodeficiency: defects of the thymus. *Clin Immunol Immunopathol.* 1978;11:437–44.

176. Deitiker PR, Oshima M, Smith RG *et al.* Association with HLA DQ of early onset myasthenia gravis in Southeast Texas region of the United States. *Int J Immunogenet.* 2011;38:55–62.

177. Fekih-Mrissa N, Klai S, Zaouali J et al. Association of HLA-DR/DQ polymorphism with myasthenia gravis in Tunisian patients. *Clin Neurol Neurosurg.* 2013;115:32–6.

178. Shinomiya N, Nomura Y, Segawa M. A variant of childhood-onset myasthenia gravis: HLA typing and clinical characteristics in Japan. *Clin Immunol.* 2004;110:154–8.

179. Testi M, Terracciano C, Guagnano A et al. Association of HLA-DQB1 *05:02 and DRB1 *16 Alleles with late-onset, nonthymomatous, AChR-Ab-positive myasthenia gravis. *Autoimmune Dis.* 2012;541760.

180. Vandiedonck C, Raffoux C, Eymard B et al. Association of HLA-A in autoimmune myasthenia gravis with thymoma. *J Neuroimmunol.* 2009;210:120–3.

181. Zhu WH, Lu JH, Lin J et al. HLA-DQA1*03:02/DQB1*03:03:02 is strongly associated with susceptibility to childhood-onset ocular myasthenia gravis in Southern Han Chinese. *J Neuroimmunol.* 2012;247:81–5.

182. Deitiker PR, Oshima M, Smith RG et al. Association with HLA-DQ of early onset myasthenia gravis in Southeast Texas region of the United States. *Int J Immunogenet.* 2011;38:55–62.

183. Fekih-Mrissa N, Klai S, Zaouali J et al. Association of HLA-DR/DQ polymorphism with myasthenia gravis in Tunisian patients. *Clin Neurol Neurosurg.* 2013;115:32–6.

184. Vandiedonck C, Raffoux C, Eymard B et al. Association of HLA-A in autoimmune myasthenia gravis with thymoma. *J Neuroimmunol.* 2009;210:120–3.

185. Engel AG. Morphologic and immunopathologic findings in myasthenia gravis and in congenital myasthenic syndromes. *J Neurol Neurosurg Psychiatry.* 1980;43:577–89.

186. Shen XM, Fukuda T, Ohno K et al. Congenital myasthenia-related AChR delta subunit mutation interferes with intersubunit communication essential for channel gating. *J Clin Invest.* 2008;118:1867–76.

187. Engel AG. Morphologic and immunopathologic findings in myasthenia gravis and in congenital myasthenic syndromes. *J Neurol Neurosurg Psychiatry.* 1980;43:577–89.

188. Cossins J, Belaya K, Zoltowska K et al. The search for new antigenic targets in myasthenia gravis. *Ann N Y Acad Sci.* 2012;1275:123–8.

189. Gilhus NE. Myasthenia and the neuromuscular junction. *Curr Opin Neurol.* 2012;25:523–9.

190. Pal J, Rozsa C, Komoly S et al. Clinical and biological heterogeneity of autoimmune myasthenia gravis. *J Neuroimmunol.* 2011;231:43–54.

191. Marx A, Pfister F, Schalke B et al. Thymus pathology observed in the MGTX trial. *Ann N Y Acad Sci.* 2012;1275:92–100.

192. Mlika M, yadi-Kaddour A, Marghli A et al. True thymic hyperplasia versus follicular thymic hyperplasia: a retrospective analysis of 13 cases. *Pathologica.* 2009;101:175–9.

193. Middleton G. The incidence of follicular structures in the human thymus at autopsy. *Aust J Exp Biol Med Sci.* 1967;45:189–99.

194. Marx A, Pfister F, Schalke B et al. Thymus pathology observed in the MGTX trial. *Ann N Y Acad Sci.* 2012;1275:92–100.

195. Cavalcante P, Le PR, Berrih-Aknin S et al. The thymus in myasthenia gravis: Site of "innate autoimmunity"? *Muscle Nerve.* 2011;44:467–84.

196. Ragheb S, Lisak RP. The thymus and myasthenia gravis. *Chest Surg Clin N Am.* 2001;11:311–27.

197. Butcovan D, Tinica G, Stefanescu C et al. Pathological comparative assessment of two cases of thymic cyst and cystic thymoma and review of the literature. *Rev Med Chir Soc Med Nat Iasi.* 2012;116:812–16.

198. Marchevsky AM, McKenna RJ, Jr., Gupta R. Thymic epithelial neoplasms: a review of current concepts using an evidence-based pathology approach. *Hematol Oncol Clin North Am.* 2008;22:543–62.

199. Mackay IR, Whittingham S, Goldstein G et al. Myasthenia gravis: clinical, serological and histological studies in relation to thymectomy. *Australas Ann Med.* 1968;17:1–11.

200. Goldstein G. Thymic germinal centres in myasthenia gravis: a correlative study. *Clin Exp Immunol.* 1967;2:103–7.

201. Osserman KE, Genkins G. Studies in myasthenia gravis: review of a twenty-year experience in over 1200 patients. *Mt Sinai J Med.* 1971;38:497–537.

202. Papatestas AE, Alpert LI, Osserman KE et al. Studies in myasthenia gravis: effects of thymectomy. Results on 185 patients with nonthymomatous and thymomatous myasthenia gravis, 1941–1969. *Am J Med.* 1971;50:465–74.

203. Alpert LI, Papatestas A, Kark A et al. A histologic reappraisal of the thymus in myasthenia gravis. A correlative study of thymic pathology and response to thymectomy. *Arch Pathol.* 1971;91:55–61.

204. Cossins J, Belaya K, Zoltowska K et al. The search for new antigenic targets in myasthenia gravis. *Ann N Y Acad Sci.* 2012;1275:123–8.

205. Ragheb S, Lisak RP. The thymus and myasthenia gravis. *Chest Surg Clin N Am.* 2001;11:311–27.

206. Oger JJ. Thymus histology and acetylcholine receptor antibodies in generalized myasthenia gravis. *Ann N Y Acad Sci.* 1993;681:110–12.

207. Alpert LI, Rule A, Norio M et al. Studies in myasthenia gravis: cellular hypersensitivity to skeletal muscle. *Am J Clin Pathol.* 1972;58:647–53.

208. Perlo VP, Arnason B, Poskanzer D et al. The role of thymectomy in the treatment of myasthenia gravis. *Ann N Y Acad Sci.* 1971;183:308–15.

209. Papatestas AE, Alpert LI, Osserman KE et al. Studies in myasthenia gravis: effects of thymectomy. Results on 185 patients with nonthymomatous and thymomatous myasthenia gravis, 1941–1969. *Am J Med.* 1971;50:465–74.

210. Alpert LI, Papatestas A, Kark A et al. A histologic reappraisal of the thymus in myasthenia gravis. A correlative study of thymic pathology and response to thymectomy. *Arch Pathol.* 1971;91:55–61.

211. Osserman KE, Genkins G. Studies in myasthenia gravis: review of a twenty-year experience in over 1200 patients. *Mt Sinai J Med.* 1971;38:497–537.

212. Alpert LI, Rule A, Norio M et al. Studies in myasthenia gravis: cellular hypersensitivity to skeletal muscle. *Am J Clin Pathol.* 1972;58:647–53.

213. Perlo VP, Arnason B, Poskanzer D et al. The role of thymectomy in the treatment of myasthenia gravis. *Ann N Y Acad Sci.* 1971;183:308–15.

214. Papatestas AE, Alpert LI, Osserman KE *et al.* Studies in myasthenia gravis: effects of thymectomy. Results on 185 patients with nonthymomatous and thymomatous myasthenia gravis, 1941–1969. *Am J Med.* 1971;50:465–74.

215. Alpert LI, Papatestas A, Kark A *et al.* A histologic reappraisal of the thymus in myasthenia gravis. A correlative study of thymic pathology and response to thymectomy. *Arch Pathol.* 1971;91:55–61.

216. Penn AS, Jaretzki A, Wolff M *et al.* Thymic abnormalities: antigen or antibody? Response to thymectomy in myasthenia gravis. *Ann N Y Acad Sci.* 1981;377:786–804.

217. Maggi G, Casadio C, Cavallo A *et al.* Thymectomy in myasthenia gravis. Results of 662 cases operated upon in 15 years. *Eur J Cardiothorac Surg.* 1989;3:504–9.

218. Zeldowicz LR, Saxton GD. Myasthenia gravis: comparative evaluation of medical and surgical treatment. *Can Med Assoc J.* 1969;101:88–93.

219. Middleton G. The incidence of follicular structures in the human thymus at autopsy. *Aust J Exp Biol Med Sci.* 1967;45:189–99.

220. Alpert LI, Rule A, Norio M *et al.* Studies in myasthenia gravis: cellular hypersensitivity to skeletal muscle. *Am J Clin Pathol.* 1972;58:647–53.

221. Alpert LI, Papatestas A, Kark A *et al.* A histologic reappraisal of the thymus in myasthenia gravis. A correlative study of thymic pathology and response to thymectomy. *Arch Pathol.* 1971;91:55–61.

222. Mackay IR, Whittingham S, Goldstein G *et al.* Myasthenia gravis: clinical, serological and histological studies in relation to thymectomy. *Australas Ann Med.* 1968;17:1–11.

223. Moran CA, Suster S, Gil J *et al.* Morphometric analysis of germinal centers in nonthymomatous patients with myasthenia gravis. *Arch Pathol Lab Med.* 1990;114:689–91.

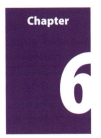

Chapter

6

Low-grade and intermediate-grade malignant epithelial tumors of the thymus: thymomas

Alberto M. Marchevsky, MD, Saul Suster, MD, and Mark R. Wick, MD

The thymus gland can be the site of origin of a wide variety of benign, low-grade malignant, and malignant neoplasms [1,2]. Although these tumors are relatively infrequent in the general population, they have elicited a great deal of interest in the medical literature because of their association with myasthenia gravis and other neurological diseases, red cell aplasia, extrathymic malignancies, and other diseases [3–5] (Table 6.1).

The term thymoma has been applied in the literature to indicate any type of tumor that originates in the thymus, but it is currently restricted to neoplasms other than thymic carcinomas originating from thymic epithelial cells [6–8]. The presence of benign neoplasms derived from thymic epithelial cells is currently not accepted in the literature, although some histopathological variants of thymomas have been considered in the past literature as "benign thymomas" [6,9,10]. The concept of "benign thymomas" has been advocated because spindle cell thymomas or "thymomas A", described later on in this chapter, seldom recur or metastasize [10,11]. However, thymomas are currently considered as low-grade and intermediate-grade malignancies of thymic epithelial cell origin as they have the potential to invade extra-thymic mediastinal structures, recur intrathoracically, and/or metastasize to bone and other distant sites [12–14]. Higher grade malignant tumors of thymic epithelial cell origin are currently classified as thymic carcinomas and are discussed in the next chapter [15,16]. The thymus can also be the site of origin of various benign and malignant mesenchymal tumors and many other neoplasms of lymphoid and germ cell origin, described in other chapters of this volume.

Epidemiology

Thymomas have no predilection for any particular age group, sex, race, or geographic area and can affect patients of all ages, including, in rare cases, children [17–19]. Most cases are diagnosed in patients older than 40 years of age and as many as 70% of thymoma patients are detected in the fifth and sixth decades of life [2]. Thymomas can rarely present as a familial disease, sometimes associated with autoimmune myasthenia gravis (MG) [20,21].

Location

Approximately 95% of thymomas occur in the anterosuperior compartment of the mediastinum but can occur in the middle and posterior mediastinum [22,23]. Less frequently, they can occur as a mass in the neck, pulmonary hilus, and supradiaphragmatic area. Thymomas have rarely been found as an endotracheal polypoidal mass [24].

Clinical features

Thymoma patients are asymptomatic in approximately one-third of instances, and the tumor is found as an incidental mediastinal mass in chest roentgenograms (Fig. 6.1 and Fig. 6.2), computerized tomograms (Fig. 6.3) or other imaging studies [18,22]. Other patients present with a variety of clinical manifestations. Twenty-five to 30% of patients present with local signs or symptoms secondary to compression of intrathoracic structures, such as cough, chest pain, dysphagia, dyspnea, hoarseness, and/or respiratory infections [25]. Dyspnea and other respiratory symptoms can also result from seeding by multiple pleural nodules with pleural effusion or bronchial obstruction resulting from polypoid endobronchial extension of an invasive mediastinal tumor [26–28]. Thymomas can also present as a neck mass, or as a lesion that simulates cardiomegaly, pulmonary stenosis or constrictive pericarditis, with manifestations of the superior vena cava syndrome or, infrequently, sudden death following compression of the right atrium [27,29,30]. As many as half of thymoma patients are associated with MG or one of the other systemic disorders listed in Table 6.1 [5,31].

Thymoma and other diseases

The association between MG and thymic neoplasms was first established by Weigert in 1901 [32]. It has been estimated that 8% to 15% of patients with MG have a thymoma, and that approximately 30% to 50% of thymomas are associated with MG [3,5,31,33–37]. The neuromuscular syndrome usually becomes clinically evident prior to the discovery of the thymic tumor,

---

Table 6.1. Clinical disorders associated with thymomas

Neuromuscular syndromes
  Myasthenia gravis
  Myotonic dystrophy
  Lambert–Eaton syndrome
  Myositis
  Subacute motor neuronopathy
  Progressive systemic sclerosis
  Limbic encephalitis
  Neuromyotonia (Morvan disease)

Hematologic syndromes
  Pure red cell aplasia
  Erythrocytosis
  Pancytopenia
  Megakaryocytopenia
  T-cell lymphocytosis
  Acute leukemia
  Multiple myeloma
  Others

Immune deficiency syndromes
  Hypogammaglobulinemia
  T-cell deficiency syndrome
  Epstein–Barr virus infections

Collagen diseases and autoimmune disorders
  Systemic lupus erythematosus
  Rheumatoid arthritis
  Polymyositis
  Myocarditis
  Sjögren's syndrome
  Scleroderma

Dermatologic diseases
  Pemphigus (vulgaris, erythematosus)
  Chronic muco-cutaneous candidiasis

Endocrine disorders
  Hyperparathyroidism
  Hashimoto's thyroiditis
  Addison's disease

Renal diseases
  Nephrotic syndrome
  Minimal-change nephropathy

Bone disorders
  Hypertrophic osteoarthropathy

Malignancy
  Malignant lymphoma (Hodgkin's disease, non-Hodgkin's lymphomas)
  Carcinomas (lung, colon, others)
  Kaposi's sarcoma

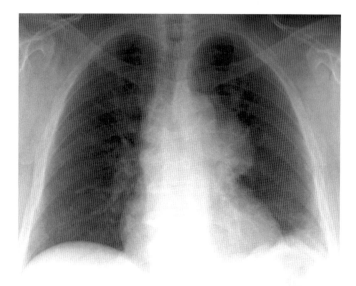

Fig. 6.1 Thymoma presenting as an asymptomatic mass in a routine posteroanterior chest film.

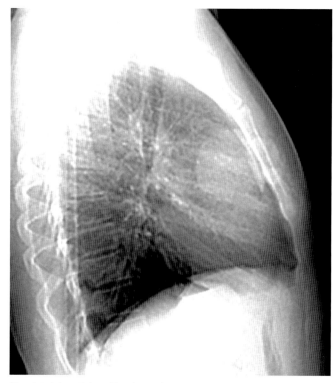

Fig. 6.2 A lateral chest film shows that the thymoma is in the anterior mediastinum.

relapsing polychondritis, and demyelinating neuropathy synchronously or metachronously [38–45].

Thymoma and myasthenia gravis

Although MG is more likely to be diagnosed in thymoma patients in their fourth to sixth decades of life because of the higher prevalence of the tumor in this age group, an

but it can occur after the diagnosis of the lesion and even after thymectomy for removal of a thymoma.

Thymoma patients can also develop one of the other associated conditions listed in Table 6.1 such as aplastic anemia, stiff-man syndrome, multiple schwannomas, gammopathies,

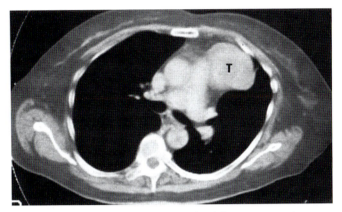

Fig. 6.3 Chest CT scan showing an encapsulated thymoma presenting as an anterior mediastinal mass (T).

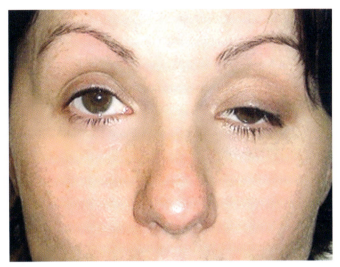

Fig. 6.4 A patient with myasthenia gravis associated with thymoma, showing characteristic ptosis of the left eye.

association between the two conditions is more frequent in younger thymoma patients [37,46]. This may be related to the earlier detection of the thymic tumors in symptomatic patients.

The prognostic significance of the presence of thymomas in patients with MG has been the subject of controversy. Older studies such as those of Wilkins and Castleman have suggested that the presence of MG is a bad prognostic sign in thymoma patients but, perhaps as a result of improvements in the clinical management of MG, the neuromuscular disease is no longer considered to have a significant effect on the long-term survival of patients with a mediastinal tumor [46–48].

Patients develop muscle weakness that worsens after the muscle is used repeatedly and affects the eye muscles causing unilateral or bilateral ptosis (Fig. 6.4), and/or diplopia. Involvement of other muscles results in altered speaking, difficulty swallowing, limited facial expressions, and weakness in the neck, arms, and legs.

The value of thymectomy for the treatment of MG in patients with thymomas is controversial [9,46,49]. For example, Wilkins and Castleman have reported beneficial clinical effects with remission of the neuromuscular symptoms in about 25% of MG patients undergoing thymectomy for removal of a thymoma, while other studies have shown no clear improvement post-thymectomy [47,48]. The clinical improvement in MG symptoms can be delayed for periods of up to two years following surgery.

Pathogenesis of myasthenia gravis in thymoma patients

MG is an autoimmune disease characterized by the presence of circulating anti-acetylcholine receptor (AChR) antibodies [50–55] in over 90% of patients [3,52,56,57]. The receptor has four subunits (alpha, beta, gamma, and delta), and its tridimensional structure is known. The antibodies to AChR are thought to play a role in the pathogenesis of the disease by various mechanisms, including activation of complement with destruction of the postsynaptic muscle membrane, antigenic modulation resulting in

increased degradation of the receptor, and pharmacologic block of the receptor. As the thymus has rare myoid cells, it has been postulated that autoantibodies develop in response to the intrathymic release of AChR antigens by degenerating myoid cells (see Chapter 5) [58–61]. Indeed, the number of myoid cells is smaller in the thymus of patients with MG.

The pathogenesis of MG may be heterogeneous, and patients with thymoma may develop the disease as a result of different mechanisms than those activated in individuals with thymic hyperplasia [62,63]. Experiments with monoclonal antibodies have indicated that the spectrum of anti-AChR antibodies is different in both patient populations. There is no predisposition regarding gender or human leukocyte antigen (HLA) for patients with MG associated with thymoma [64–73]. However, female patients with the HLA-B8/DR3 haplotype are more likely to develop thymic hyperplasia associated with MG [64–70]. Furthermore, thymoma patients with MG very frequently have antistriated muscle autoantibodies that are only seldom seen in patients with thymic hyperplasia [74]. These antibodies are thought to develop as the result of autosensitization to cytoskeletal contractile proteins such as myosin, alpha actinin, or actin. These epitopes have been detected on epithelial cells from thymomas that share a common epitope, defined by monoclonal antibodies, with skeletal muscle. These antibodies do not cross-react with the normal thymus, except for rare Hassall's corpuscles, label a large number of cells in thymomas, and recognize cross-striations from skeletal muscle cells.

Thymomas and other neurologic disorders

Thymoma has been encountered in patients with myotonic dystrophy, Lambert–Eaton syndrome, myositis, subacute motor neuronopathy, progressive systemic sclerosis, limbic encephalitis, and myasthenia gravis–Lambert–Eaton syndrome [43,45,75]. The role played by the thymic neoplasm in the pathogenesis of these disorders is unknown.

Thymoma and hematologic disorders

Red cell aplasia is a rare hematologic disorder characterized by the almost total absence of bone marrow erythroblasts and blood reticulocytes [39–41,76]. Thymomas have been described in 50% of these patients. However, only 5% of patients with thymoma exhibit this hematologic disorder. Pure red cell aplasia has also been described in association with other thymic neoplasms such as thymolipomas and Hodgkin's disease.

Pure red cell aplasia is associated with spindle cell thymomas (see below) in 70% of cases [11]. Anemia is usually diagnosed when the mediastinal mass is being clinically evaluated, but occasionally the tumor is unexpectedly encountered in a patient being studied for the hematologic disorder [77]. There are also a few instances of pure red cell aplasia developing after thymectomy or radiation therapy for a thymoma [76,78].

The role of either the thymus gland or thymomas in the pathogenesis of red cell aplasia is unclear. Several autoantibodies have been described in patients with pure red cell aplasia including antierythroblast antibody, and antierythropoietin antibody [76,79–82]. They can also exhibit an altered cellular immune system with increase of suppressor T-cells against the erythrocyte maturation cycle, increase of gamma interferon, and decrease in interleukin-3.

Masaoka and associates reported that the non-neoplastic thymus adjacent to thymomas associated with pure red cell aplasia is involuted with no germinal centers present. They suggested that thymomas may produce suppressor T-cells that inhibit erythrocyte maturation [83]. Approximately a third of patients have remission of their symptoms following thymectomy.

Thymomas have also been described with other hematologic disorders including leukopenia, thrombocytopenia, pancytopenia, T-cell lymphocytosis, megakaryocytopenia, lymphocytic leukemias, multiple myeloma, bone marrow eosinophilia, agranulocytosis, chronic lymphocytic leukemia, pure white blood cell aplasia, pernicious anemia, and polycythemia vera [84–90].

Thymoma and immune deficiency syndromes

Thymoma has been described in association with Good's syndrome, a form of hypogammaglobulinemia that usually affects elderly people and rarely involves children [91]. Patients present with repeated episodes of severe bacterial infections and opportunistic viral infections by cytomegalovirus, herpes virus, and/or muco-cutaneous candidiasis. Hypogammaglobulinemia is usually apparent when the thymoma is discovered, but it may develop following thymectomy. In most instances, the removal of the thymic neoplasm does not have a beneficial effect on the immunoglobulins.

A few of these patients have been shown to lack surface immunoglobulin-bearing cells in their peripheral blood. Waldmann and associates also demonstrated a population of suppressor T-cells inhibiting immunoglobulin synthesis in two out of three patients with thymoma and hypogammaglobulinemia [92].

However, most patients with the syndrome have normal numbers of circulating T-cells, normal *in vitro* immunologic tests (mitogenic responsiveness, antigen-stimulated lymphocyte transformation), and normal skin reactivity to common antigens.

A few patients with thymomas have had severe opportunistic skin infections such as herpes simplex and muco-cutaneous candidiasis with increased numbers of T suppressor lymphocytes and decreased numbers of circulating B-cells [93–95]. More recently, Kisand *et al.* have proposed that muco-cutaneous candidiasis and the rare automosomal recessive disease autoimmune polyendocrinopathy candidiasis ectodermal dystrophy (APECED) develop as a result of autoimmune mechanisms with mutation in the autoimmune regulator (AIRE) protein [96].

Epstein–Barr virus infection and thymoma

The incidence of thymoma associated with MG appears to be considerably higher in patients from China, where the incidence of Epstein–Barr virus (EBV) is more prevalent than in Western countries [97–100]. Antibodies of EBV have been detected in patients with thymic tumors, and the viral genome has been demonstrated by Southern blot hybridization analysis in thymomas studied in Hong Kong. Western thymomas studied with Southern blot hybridization and polymerase chain reaction for EBV genome have been negative.

Thymomas associated with skin diseases and autoimmune disorders

Pemphigus vulgaris and pemphigus erythematosus have been described in patients with thymoma [101–104]. These autoimmune bullous diseases are usually present at the time of diagnosis of a mediastinal mass but may develop after thymectomy for removal of a thymoma. Patients with these diseases have elevated serum levels of antibodies to striated muscle, skin, and DNA antigens. Gibson and Muller have reported cutaneous fungal diseases, lichen planus, pemphigus, myositis, and lupus-like disease in a review of 172 patients with thymoma [105].

Thymomas have also been described in patients with other autoimmune diseases such as systemic lupus erythematosus, rheumatoid arthritis, polymyositis, scleroderma, Sjögren's syndrome, and Hashimoto's thyroiditis [106–109].

The role of the thymic neoplasm in the pathogenesis of these diseases is unclear, but it has been postulated that the autoimmune disorder may be the result of a lack of immunologic surveillance by thymic T-cells. Thymus-derived lymphocytes are thought to prevent autoimmunity in normal individuals, and their derangement could be "permissive", resulting in the formation of clones of lymphocytes that produce autoantibodies. Excess numbers of helper T-cells could also result in increased production of autoantibodies.

Thymoma and renal disorders

Nephrotic syndrome related to membranous glomerulonephritis or minimal-change "lipoid" nephropathy has been described in a few patients with thymomas and is a well-recognized systemic manifestation of other neoplasms such as Hodgkin's disease [110,111]. It may be related to the formation of antigen–antibody complexes that cross react with the patients' neoplasm and glomeruli.

Glomerular injury in minimal-change nephropathy may also represent a T-cell-mediated abnormality secondary to the production of abnormal lymphokines by thymocytes or to the abnormal production of a normal lymphokine by T lymphocytes.

Thymoma and other neoplasms

Thymomas have been reported in association with extrathymic malignancies including non-Hodgkin's lymphomas, Hodgkin's disease, carcinomas of the gastrointestinal tract, genitourinary system, lung, breast, and thyroid, brain tumors, leukemia, multiple myeloma, and Kaposi's sarcoma [112,113]. Souadjian and associates encountered second neoplasms in 21% of 146 patients with thymomas [114]. These second malignancies may develop as a consequence of defective immunologic surveillance mechanisms in these patients with immune deficiency.

Thymoma and bone disorders

Hypertrophic osteoarthropathy has been reported in two patients with malignant thymomas [115]. In one patient reported by Lesser and associates, the subjective and objective findings of the osteoarticular disease disappeared following the surgical resection and postoperative radiotherapy of the thymoma [115].

Thymoma and endocrine disorders

Palmer and Sawyers reported patients with thymoma and hyperparathyroidism [116]. There is no evidence of a causal relationship. Hashimoto's thyroiditis and Addison's disease have also been associated with thymomas [109].

Diagnosis of thymomas using imaging techniques

Thymomas can be detected with chest X-rays, chest CT, and other imaging modalities discussed in more detail in Chapter 2 [22]. They usually appear as round or oval well-circumscribed, coarsely lobulated masses in the anterior and superior mediastinum or in any of the other locations discussed previously (Figs. 6.1 to 6.3) [23]. In 6% to 20% of instances, the tumors have coarse, dense, irregular or ring-like calcifications that may be confused with those seen in mediastinal teratomas or aortic aneurysms. Cystic degeneration is seen in a small number of thymomas.

More advanced thymomas can present with invasive lesions that compress mediastinal vascular and other structures, invade the pleura with multiple pleural nodules, pericardium, diaphragm and other intrathoracic structures visible on chest CT and other modalities [22,23].

Detection of serum autoantibodies in thymoma patients with myasthenia gravis

Thymomas are associated with MG in up to 50% of patients and detection of various serum autoantibodies present in patients with this disease can sometimes suggest the possibility that the patient has a thymic neoplasm that may be difficult to visualize on imaging studies due to small size [74,117]. MG is a disorder of neuromuscular transmission associated with auto-antibodies against the nicotinic acethylcholine receptor (AChR antibodies) [118]. These antibodies can be detected in the serum of 80–90% of patients with generalized MG. Other autoantibodies have been described in patients with the disease, including against myosin, filamin, vinculin, tropomyosin, rapsyn and, exceptionally, muscle specific kinase (MuSK). MG patients can also have elevated serum levels of non-AChR antibodies, particularly when the disease is associated with a thymoma, such as antibodies to alfa-actinin, actin, IFN-alpha, interleukin (IL)-12 and others.

Pathologic features of thymomas: gross pathology

Thymomas are usually well encapsulated tumors that vary in size from microscopic to giant lesions (Fig. 6.5) [1]. The thymoma reported by Smith and associates in a 15-year-old boy is one of the largest on record and weighed 5,700 g [119]. Thymomas usually present as single lesions but can also be multiple (Fig. 6.6), as a result of multicentric development [2]. However,

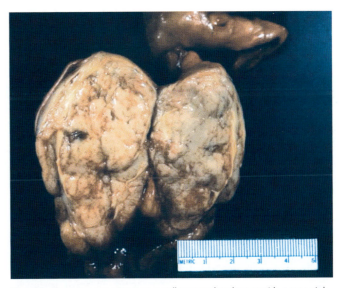

Fig. 6.5 Thymoma presenting as a well encapsulated mass with a gray-pink lobulated surface. Note the presence of the residual normal thymic tissue in the right upper portion of the photograph.

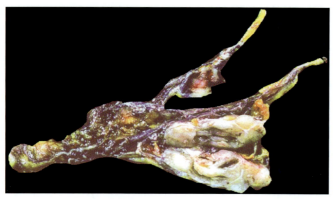

Fig. 6.6 Thymus gland containing multiple small thymomas, represented by well circumscribed gray-tan lesions with a characteristic lobulated cut surface.

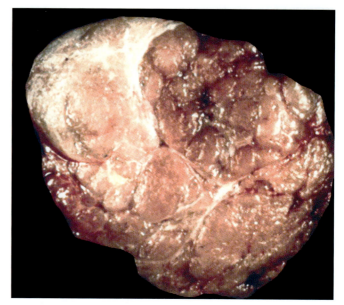

Fig. 6.7 Thymoma with a somewhat bosselated surface. The entire lesion is surrounded by a thin fibrous capsule.

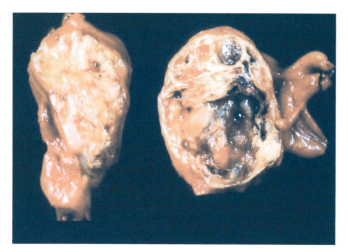

Fig. 6.8 Thymoma with cystic change. Cystic degeneration of a thymoma occurs in up to 40% of cases.

they can be locally invasive, with partial encapsulation, extending into peri-thymic adipose tissue, pleura, pericardium, intrathoracic nerves, vascular structures, and other intrathoracic areas.

The term microscopic thymoma has been proposed by the World Health Organization (WHO) classification of thymomas to define lesions smaller than 1 mm in greatest dimension [17]. However, it is unclear how to distinguish these "tumors" from focally hyperplastic thymic tissue, particularly as so-called microscopic thymomas have been described in MG patients with follicular hyperplasia.

Thymomas usually have a bosselated outer surface (Fig. 6.7) [17]. They occasionally appear as flattened masses adherent to the chest wall, simulating a fibrotic plaque [1]. The parenchyma of thymomas is usually solid, with a soft, tan or gray–pink "fish flesh" surface that grossly resembles lymphoid tissue and can exhibit variable cystic change. This "fish flesh" tissue is usually separated into visible lobules by generally uniform white–gray fibrous tissue septa. In most instances, the tumor is contiguous with a portion of visible thymic tissue. Although other tumors may occasionally simulate a thymoma,

these features in a mediastinal mass are almost pathognomonic of a thymoma. The nodular sclerosis variant of Hodgkin's disease can present as a lobulated lymphoid mass of the thymus but is usually firmer, less well circumscribed, and composed of smaller nodules than a thymoma, with considerable irregularity of the fibrous tissue component. Other thymic tumors such as B large cell lymphoma and seminoma with abundant lymphoid stroma also have a soft, tan, "fish flesh" gross appearance. These tumors, however, are usually not lobulated.

Grossly visible cysts are seen in as many as 40% of thymomas and are more frequent in large lesions (Fig. 6.8) [1,120]. The cystic spaces probably follow liquefactive necrosis of tumor cells, fluid accumulation in perivascular spaces, and/or hemorrhage [121]. Cysts vary in size from a few millimeters to several centimeters in diameter and contain serous or pasty brown hemorrhagic material in their lumen. Rarely, the tumor becomes almost completely cystic (Fig. 6.9), and multiple histologic sections taken from focal solid areas in the cyst wall are necessary to distinguish a cystic thymoma from a benign thymic cyst [120,121].

Thymomas can become quite large and invade the lung (Fig. 6.10) or compress mediastinal structures such as the heart and great vessels. In these instances, they can clinically simulate syndromes of constrictive pericarditis or pulmonary stenosis.

Complete cystic degeneration of an invasive thymoma offers no guarantee of a good prognosis. For example, Effler and McCormack described a patient with a thymic cyst from which a definitive histological diagnosis of thymoma could not be established but the lesion recurred three years later [122]. The recurrent local and pericardial nodules had histologic features of an invasive thymoma.

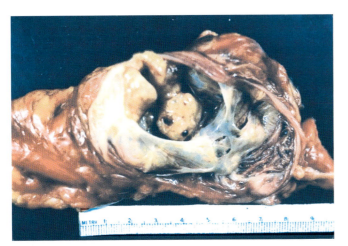

Fig. 6.9 Cystic thymoma. Rarely, thymomas can be predominantly cystic and can be confused with a benign thymic cyst. Note the presence of a small, gray nodular area on the left side of the cyst that represents residual solid tumor. Areas such as this need to be sampled histologically to identify the neoplasm.

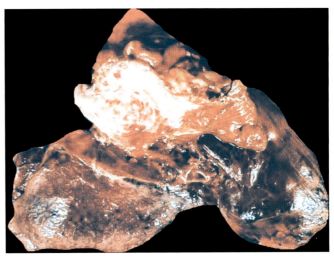

Fig. 6.10 Invasive thymoma infiltrating the lung. Thymomas can infiltrate into other various mediastinal structures as well.

Thymomas also frequently exhibit areas of calcification of the capsule or the tumor stroma. Foci of hemorrhage and necrosis are not infrequent and may be seen in up to a third of cases.

Clinico-pathological classification of thymomas and other malignant epithelial neoplasms of the thymus

The histopathological classification of thymomas has been the subject of longstanding and at times heated debate. Bernatz *et al.* proposed in 1961 a classification schema of thymomas into four histopathological variants: lymphocytic-predominant, epithelial-predominant, mixed (lymphoepithelial), and spindle cell thymomas [123]. Levine and Rosai extended this classification schema with the general concept that encapsulated thymomas, as classified above, are benign neoplasms whereas invasive lesions are malignant [6]. This classification was widely used in the United States until the late 1990s.

Thymic carcinomas were recognized as a distinct category of malignant thymic epithelial neoplasms, raising some confusion amongst practicing pathologists, thoracic surgeons, and oncologists regarding which thymic epithelial neoplasms were indeed malignant [124]. Marino and Mueller-Hermelink proposed in 1985 a "histogenetic" classification of thymomas that classified these lesions, based on the presumed cell of origin as suggested by their immunophenotype, into cortical and medullary thymomas and their variants [125,126]. They also advocated the concept that this classification had prognostic value. However, other studies have questioned the interobserver reproducibility of the Marino and Mueller-Hermelink classification, its "histogenetic" accuracy, and its prognostic value [127].

An international panel of pathology experts sponsored by the World Health Organization (WHO) proposed a grouping of thymic epithelial tumors into thymomas A, B1-B3, AB, and C in 1999 that was intended to translate the nomenclatures proposed by Rosai and Levine, and Marino and Muller-Hermelink [17,128]. Although this publication explicitly stated that this "grouping of thymomas" was not intended as a formal clinico-pathologic classification, it became de-facto the most widely used classification schema for thymomas. The WHO classification of thymomas was revised by another panel of experts in 2004 and the category of thymomas C was changed to thymic carcinomas [17]. Multiple international publications have evaluated the reproducibility and prognostic value of the 1999 and 2004 WHO classification of thymomas, with variable results [129–135].

The WHO classification scheme for classification of thymomas was criticized almost from its outset by several prominent American pathologists because of inter-observer variability problems in classification and variable correlation between certain WHO types and prognosis [12–14,136]. For example, it was noted that the system does not provide specific criteria to classify heterogeneous tumors that exhibit different "types" in separate tissue samples from a single neoplasm, distinguish thymomas A or B1 from AB lesions, or stratify thymomas B1-B3 in a reproducible manner. Clinical studies also raised questions about the practical value of the WHO classification scheme of thymomas for the management of patients with these neoplasms, as most thymoma patients are treated with thymectomy regardless of WHO histologic type [131].

Suster and Moran have proposed a clinico-pathologic classification of thymomas into simply "thymomas" and "atypical thymomas" and have stressed the concept that a morphologic classification of thymoma in the absence of correlation with the clinical staging is meaningless from a clinical standpoint [137]. Their classification is based on the premise that subclassifying tumors that are highly heterogeneous, such as thymoma, into multiple histologic subtypes does not make practical sense unless the stratification shows significant correlation with prognosis [136,138,139].

Table 6.2. Comparison of different thymoma classification schema

Traditional (Beratz et al., 1961)	Kirchner and Muller-Hermelink (1989)	WHO (1999)	Suster and Moran (1999)
Spindle cell	Medullary	Type A	Thymoma, well differentiated
–	Mixed	Type AB	Thymoma, well differentiated
–	Predominantly cortical	Type B1	Thymoma, well differentiated
Lymphocyte-rich	Cortical	Type B2	Thymoma, well differentiated
Lymphoepithelial	Cortical	Type B2	Thymoma, well differentiated
Epithelial-rich	Well-differentiated thymic carcinoma	Type B3	Atypical thymoma
–	High-grade thymic carcinoma	Type C	Thymic carcinoma

WHO, World Health Organization

Table 6.3. Clinico-pathological classification of thymic malignant epithelial neoplasms

Low-grade thymic malignant epithelial neoplasms
- Spindle cell thymoma (WHO A)
- Lymphocyte-rich thymoma (WHO B1)
- Lymphocyte-rich with variable number of spindle cells thymoma (WHO AB)
- Lymphocyte-rich with atypia thymoma (WHO B2)*

Unusual thymomas**
- Metaplastic thymoma (same as WHO)
- Micronodular thymoma (same as WHO)
- Plasma-rich thymoma (not in WHO)
- Rhabdomyomatous thymoma (not in WHO)
- Sclerosing thymoma (same as WHO)
- Thymoma with prominent glandular differentiation (not in WHO)
- Spindle cell thymoma with prominent papillary and pseudo-papillary features (not in WHO)
- Lipofibroadenoma (same as WHO)

Intermediate-grade thymic malignant epithelial neoplasms
- Spindle cell with atypia thymoma (WHO A, atypical variant)
- Lymphocyte-depleted with atypia thymoma (WHO B3)
- Well-differentiated squamous cell carcinoma
- Well-differentiated mucoepidermoid carcinoma

High-grade thymic malignant epithelial neoplasms**
- Moderately and poorly differentiated squamous cell carcinoma
- Lymphoepithelioma-like thymic carcinoma
- Adenosquamous carcinoma
- Papillary adenocarcinoma
- Basaloid squamous cell carcinoma
- Sarcomatoid carcinoma
- Anaplastic carcinoma
- Rhabdoid carcinoma
- Mucinous carcinoma

Uncertain-grade thymic malignant epithelial neoplasms
- Clear cell carcinoma
- Micronodular lymphoid-rich carcinoma

Heterologous thymomas (grade depends on components)

* The prognosis of this lesion is disputed, as it has probably been diagnosed variably in the past.
** The prognosis of unusual thymomas and several variants of thymic carcinoma is uncertain, as only a small number of cases have been reported. The table provides a tentative prognostic stratification for these neoplasms that needs to be investigated in future studies.

The main difference between the classification schema proposed by WHO experts and by Suster and Moran is that the former emphasizes a "morphological approach" that classifies thymomas into as many recognizable histopathological variants as possible, albeit using simply letters and numbers to designate them, while the latter approaches the problem from a "managerial approach" that emphasizes prognostic value. Table 6.2 compares the nomenclature used in the various classification schemas proposed for thymomas.

"Morphological", "managerial" and other classification paradigms have pros and cons that have been discussed in detail in a recent volume on Evidence-Based Pathology [140].

In our current view, the stratification of thymomas proposed by WHO uses a somewhat unorthodox and arbitrary terminology that does not help pathologists intuitively appreciate how these neoplasms appear under the microscope, and does not provide "at a glance" information to thoracic surgeons and oncologists about the prognostic significance of a particular diagnosis. Indeed, in our daily experience it is not infrequent to listen to inexperienced thoracic surgeons and oncologists discuss patients with "benign thymomas". In addition, there appears to be genuine confusion amongst clinical colleagues between thymomas, touted by pathologists as malignant neoplasms and thymic carcinomas (? "Malignant ++"). Unfortunately, even some recent publications still stratify thymomas into benign and malignant lesions [28].

The discussion as to whether there are benign and malignant thymomas is not merely academic. It has been shown that all thymoma variants, described below, can recur and/or metastasize. However, as some encapsulated thymomas have been considered benign lesions in the past, patients have been treated with incomplete resection, resulting in recurrences or other preventable clinical problems.

A clinico-pathological classification of thymic epithelial lesions that emphasizes that all of them are malignant and stratifies thymomas and thymic carcinomas according to their prognosis, expressed as tumor grade, and most prominent histopathological features is shown in Table 6.3. The grading

(a)

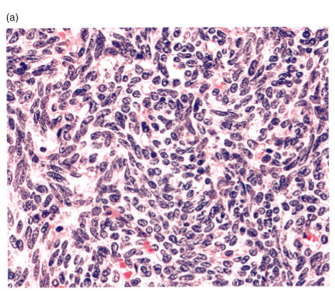

(b)

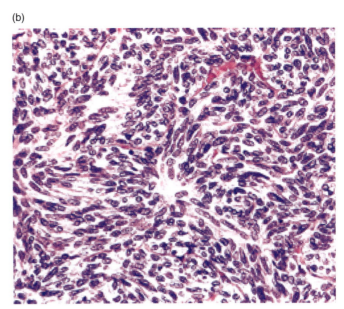

Fig. 6.11 (a) Spindle cell thymoma composed of solid sheets of fusiform epithelial cells with few lymphocytes (H&E 200x). **(b)** Spindle cell thymoma composed of cells with fusiform nuclei showing minimal anisocytosis. No cytologic atypia, mitoses, or necrosis are seen (H&E 200x).

system is somewhat arbitrary, particularly for thymic carcinomas, and was derived from limited level II evidence provided by two studies with meta-analysis of approximately 1,000 thymomas from the literature and our own experience [141,142]. The table also lists in parenthesis the corresponding WHO cell type. Low-grade malignant thymic epithelial neoplasms most frequently present as encapsulated thymic lesions, but can be locally invasive, recur in the thorax, and rarely metastasize systemically many years after initial diagnosis. They usually do not respond to platinum-based chemotherapy or other cytotoxic drugs used for carcinomas of the lung and other origin. Intermediate-grade malignant thymic epithelial neoplasms present more frequently as locally invasive mediastinal tumors, but also have a somewhat indolent clinical behavior, with local recurrences, pleural metastasis, and late pulmonary or extrathoracic metastasis. High-grade thymic epithelial neoplasms usually behave as systemic malignancies that frequently metastasize to the lung and other organs and are treated with chemotherapy.

Low-grade malignant thymic epithelial neoplasms

Low-grade malignant thymic epithelial neoplasms include several histopathological variants of thymomas that are usually diagnosed at Masaoka-Koga stages I and II of the disease and have an excellent prognosis [143]. However, a small proportion of them can infiltrate mediastinal structures, recur as multiple pleural nodules, and/or metastasize. Indeed, any individual case of thymoma can be initially diagnosed at Masaoka-Koga stages I–IV.

Spindle cell thymoma (WHO A)

Spindle cell thymomas are usually encapsulated lesions that only occasionally present with capsular invasion [11,17,144]. Most but not all cases exhibit a solid, diffuse gray surface without the distinct lobulation that is characteristic of other thymoma variants. The tumor capsule and surface can be partially cystic and/or calcified but areas of necrosis are unusual.

Microscopically, spindle cell thymomas are composed almost exclusively of spindle epithelial cells with few or absent lymphocytes (Fig. 6.11a). The epithelial cells exhibit spindle- or oval-shaped nuclei showing minimal anisocytosis, dispersed chromatin, and inconspicuous nucleoli and scanty amphophilic cytoplasm with indistinct cellular borders (Fig. 6.11b). The neoplastic cells are arranged in solid sheets without any particular growth pattern, although in some cases they can be arranged in a perivascular distribution simulating the appearance of a hemangiopericytoma (Fig. 6.12). Mitoses are infrequent and necrosis is usually absent.

Spindle cell thymomas usually exhibit no significant cytological atypia, mitoses, or necrosis. The presence of any of these features should raise the suspicion that the lesion is a spindle cell thymoma with atypia, a form of grade III malignant thymic epithelial tumor that is more likely to behave in a more aggressive manner [137]. It should also prompt the pathologist to examine additional sections to exclude the possibility of other thymoma variants or of an associated thymic carcinoma, as thymomas are often heterogeneous. Reticulin stains can be helpful to demonstrate the presence of reticulin around each individual tumor cell.

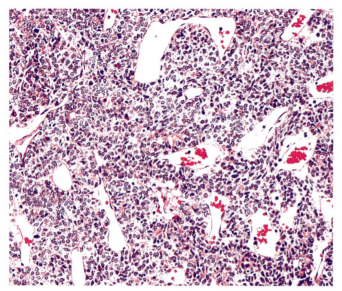

Fig. 6.12 Spindle cell thymoma showing epithelial cells arranged in a distinctive perivascular pattern that simulates the appearance of a hemangiopericytoma (H&E 40x).

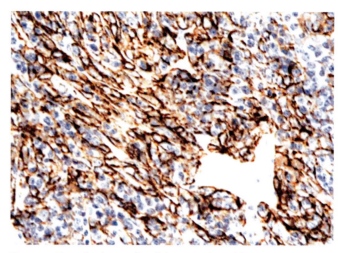

Fig. 6.13 The cells of a spindle cell thymoma show diffuse cytoplasmic immunoreactivity for keratin (PAP 200x).

(a)

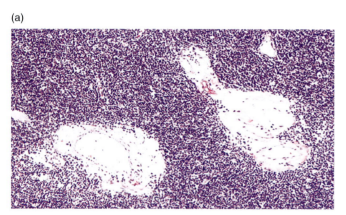

(b)

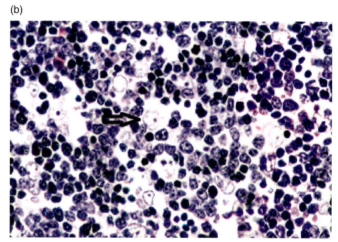

Fig. 6.14 (a) Lymphocyte-rich thymoma showing solid sheets of lymphoid cells admixed with dispersed epithelial cells. On low-power microscopy the latter may simulate histiocytes. Note the presence of two perivascular spaces around central venules surrounded by serum pools that contain a number of lymphocytes. These structures are not seen in malignant lymphomas and are characteristic of thymomas. However, they may be only focally present in lymphocyte-rich thymomas (H&E 20x). (b) Lymphocyte-rich thymoma showing epithelial cells (arrow) with round, hypochromatic nuclei and indistinct clear cytoplasm admixed with immature lymphoid cells (H&E 400x).

The spindle cells exhibit cytoplasmic immunoreactivity for cytokeratin AE1/AE3 (Fig. 6.13), a useful feature to distinguish these neoplasms from solitary fibrous tumors and other mediastinal mesenchymal tumors composed of spindle cells [1,145]. Various cytokeratins other than CK20 as well as epithelial membrane antigen (EMA) can be positive in some of these tumors. The tumor cells also exhibit immunoreactivity for thymic specific antigens such as metallothionein and PE-35 but antibodies to these epitopes are not available for routine diagnostic use [146]. The scanty lymphocytes present in the tumor are CD3+ and CD5+ lymphocytes. CD1a+ and CD99+ cells can also be focally present. More recently the presence of PAX-8 was noted in thymomas. [147]

Lymphocyte-rich thymoma (WHO B1)

Lymphocyte-rich thymoma is a relatively infrequent variant of the neoplasm that shows similar gross features to those described for spindle cell thymomas and also tends to lack the typical lobulation seen in the more frequent variants of the thymic epithelial neoplasm [17,148]. It can exhibit cystic degeneration, fibrosis, and focal necrosis. The latter feature is very unusual in our personal experience.

Microscopically, lymphocyte-rich thymomas show an architecture that resembles an expanded thymic cortex, with only focal fibrous, usually thin, septa intersecting sheets of immature T-lymphocytes and dividing the tumor into incomplete lobules (Fig. 6.14a–b) [1]. The immature lymphocytes are less dense in focal areas, forming areas that simulate medullary differentiation (Fig. 6.15) or lymphoid follicles at low-power microscopy. However, unlike lymphoid follicles they are composed of only some immature T-cells. Lymphocyte-rich thymoma has been described as predominantly cortical or organoid thymoma because of its resemblance to the thymic cortex (Fig. 6.16a–b). Epithelial cells are inconspicuous and have round to oval hypochromatic nuclei with absent or inconspicuous nucleoli (Fig. 6.14b). The epithelial cells resemble histiocytes, as they are dispersed without forming cellular aggregates. Macrophages in the form of tingible-body macrophages are also present,

imparting to some lesions a "starry-sky" appearance at low-power microscopy. Perivascular spaces, a useful diagnostic finding in other variants of thymoma, are usually absent or inconspicuous. Hassall's corpuscles can be focally present.

Immunostains for keratin A1/AE3 (Fig. 6.17) are very helpful to diagnose lymphocyte-rich thymoma, as they allow for the clear distinction between the neoplastic epithelial cells and lymphoid cells [149–151]. The tumor cells also exhibit cytoplasmic immunoreactivity for CK7, CK18, CD19 and other cytokeratins, and for PAX-8 (Fig. 6.18) but these findings are of limited value in daily clinical practice [1]. The immature lymphoid cells of lymphocyte-rich thymomas (WHO B1) exhibit immunoreactivity for TdT and cytoplasmic immunoreactivity for CD3, CD4, and CD8 (double positive cells), and other lymphoid markers. CD1a positive antigen presenting cells are also present, interspersed amongst the immature lymphocytes. The medullary areas of lymphocyte-rich thymomas exhibit mature CD3+, CD1a negative and TdT negative lymphoid cells.

Lymphocyte-rich thymomas are difficult to diagnose on frozen section and small biopsies because they closely resemble a malignant lymphoma in some cases and hyperplastic thymic tissue in others. Immunostains for TdT can be particularly misleading as they could be misinterpreted as evidence for a lymphoblastic lymphoma (Fig. 6.19). Recognition of a meshwork composed of keratin positive dispersed throughout the lesion helps formulate the correct diagnosis (Fig. 6.17). Lymphocyte-rich thymomas can also be difficult to distinguish from hyperplastic thymic tissue, particularly if areas of medullary differentiation are mistaken for lymphoid follicles diagnostic of follicular hyperplasia. Recognition that these structures lack the various lymphoid cells usually present in lymphoid follicles and detection of fibrous septa dividing the

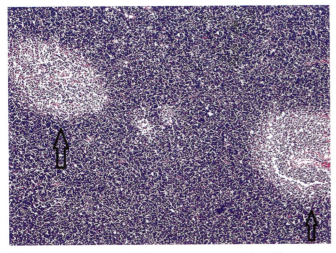

Fig. 6.15 Lymphocyte-rich thymoma with areas of medullary differentiation (arrows). They consist of round aggregates of lymphoid cells that are less dense than the remainder of the tumor, simulating the distinction between cortex and medulla seen in the normal thymus (H&E 20x).

(a)

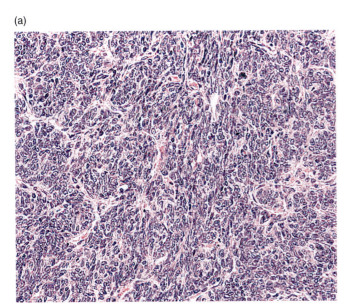

(b)

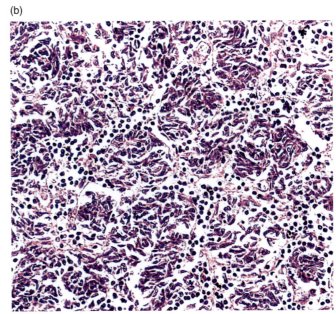

Fig. 6.16 (a) Thymoma with an organoid pattern, resembling the appearance of the thymic cortex (H&E 40x). **(b)** Thymoma with an organoid growth pattern (H&E 100x).

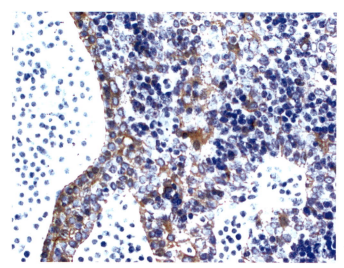

Fig. 6.17 The cells of a lymphocyte-rich thymoma show membrane immunoreactivity for keratin. Note that the tumor cells are admixed with many lymphoid cells that are keratin-negative. This feature is helpful in distinguishing this variant of thymoma from malignant lymphomas (PAP 40 X).

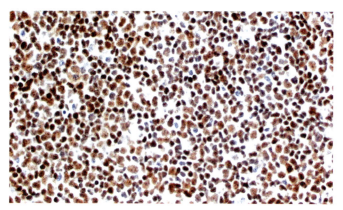

Fig. 6.19 The immature lymphoid cells of lymphocyte-rich thymomas exhibit nuclear immunoreactivity for terminal deoxynucleotidyl transferase (TdT). This finding can result in a misdiagnosis of lymphoblastic lymphoma (LBL). However, the latter tumor is most frequently seen in children, rather than in middle-aged adults, as true of thymomas. LBL is composed of more atypical lymphoid cells without interspersed epithelial cells. Attention to the cytological features of the lesion and immunostaining for keratin can avoid confusion between LBL and thymoma (PAP 200 X).

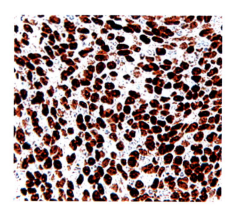

Fig. 6.18 Thymoma showing immunoreactivity for PAX-8. This marker can be seen in virtually all variants of thymoma and thymic carcinoma (PAP 400 X).

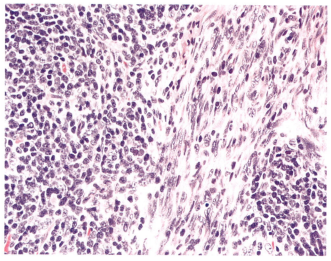

Fig. 6.20 Lymphocyte-rich thymoma with spindle cells. The neoplastic spindle cells are seen in the center of the photograph while other areas show a lymphocyte-rich image. The lesion also contains some plasma cells (H&E 200 X).

lesion into incomplete lobules can be helpful features in the differential diagnosis.

Lymphocyte-rich thymomas can also be difficult to distinguish from lymphocyte-rich thymoma with atypia (WHO B2) in cases that exhibit a small number of large epithelial cells with slightly prominent nucleoli [137,152–159]. The presence of distinct lobulation and perivascular spaces favors the latter diagnoses.

Lymphocyte-rich thymoma with spindle cells (WHO AB)

Lymphocyte-rich thymoma with spindle cells is characterized by the presence of lymphocyte-rich areas with or without atypia admixed with variable numbers of spindle epithelial cells (WHO A) (Fig. 6.20) [17]. In contrast to spindle cell thymomas (WHO A) and lymphocyte-rich thymomas (WHO B1), lymphocyte-rich thymoma with spindle cells tend to show better defined fibrous septa dividing the neoplastic cells into multiple tan-gray nodules [1].

Lymphocyte-rich thymoma with spindle cells is probably the most frequent variant of thymoma. The spindle cells vary in frequency and can appear as individual epithelial cells or in aggregates. They show similar histopathologic features to fibroblasts and endothelial cells, but the mesenchymal cells usually have more elongated, more spindly nuclei (Fig. 6.21). Immunostains for keratin A1/AE3 (Fig. 6.22) are helpful for the identification of neoplastic epithelial cells. Mesenchymal cells exhibit immunoreactivity for vimentin and endothelial cells for CD31, CD34, and other endothelial markers.

This variant of thymoma is probably one that has been diagnosed quite variably by different pathologies, as the minimum number of spindle epithelial cells required for diagnoses has not been explained explicitly in the pathology literature and mesenchymal cells can be mistaken for neoplastic cells in some cases [160,161].

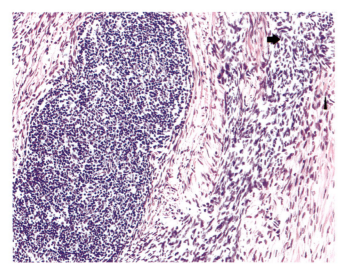

Fig. 6.21 Lymphocyte-rich thymoma with spindle cells. The neoplastic cells (arrow) contain fusiform nuclei and indistinct cytoplasm. Stromal cells (arrowhead) show more elongated nuclei and amphophilic cytoplasm (H&E 100x).

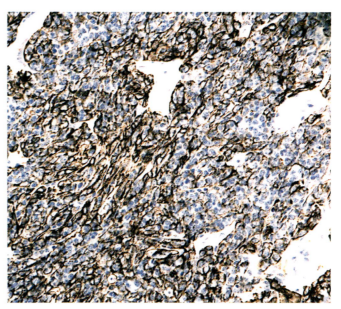

Fig. 6.22 Keratin imunostaining shows reactivity in the cytoplasm of spindled neoplastic cells, a feature that distinguishes them from fibroblasts (PAP 200x).

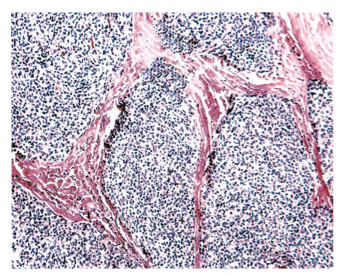

Fig. 6.23 Lymphocyte-rich thymoma with atypia. The lesion shows multiple thin fibrous septa and typical lobulation at low-power microscopy (H&E 20x).

The immunophenotype of lymphocyte-rich thymoma with spindle cells is similar to that of spindle cell thymomas [1]. Round to polygonal epithelial cells can also exhibit cytokeratin CK14 immunoreactivity.

Lymphocyte-rich thymoma with atypia (WHO B2)

Lymphocyte-rich thymoma with atypia (WHO B2) is one of the more frequent variants of thymoma [17]. It is tentatively included in Table 6.3 as a low-grade malignant thymic epithelial lesion, although its prognosis remains controversial, perhaps as a result of inter-observer diagnostic problems between different investigators. Indeed, even two of the authors of this chapter have reported conflicting data (AM and SS).

A meta-analysis performed by Marchevsky *et al.* demonstrated that patients with this thymoma variant have a less favorable prognosis than those with WHO thymomas A, AB, and B1, supporting the classification of this lesion as a higher than low-grade thymic malignant epithelial lesion [141,142]. In contrast, Moran and Suster have argued that these neoplasms have similar prognosis to most other thymomas and have classified lymphocyte-rich thymoma with atypia (WHO B2) under their generic "thymoma" category rather than as "atypical thymomas" [14,138,139]. There is a need for a more detailed description of the diagnostic features of lymphocyte-rich thymoma with atypia (WHO B2) and prospective studies of their prognosis.

Lymphocyte-rich thymoma with atypia (WHO B2) shows similar gross pathologic features to those described for lymphocyte-rich thymoma with spindle cells and presents as encapsulated lesions with a lobulated cut surface [136,138].

Microscopically the lesions exhibit multiple lobules separated by thin fibrous septa (Fig. 6.23). The lobules are composed of numerous lymphocytes admixed with variable numbers of round to slightly oval epithelial cells (Fig. 6.24a). The latter can appear singly or in small aggregates, and have round nuclei that are larger than those seen in the epithelial cells of lymphocyte-rich thymomas and usually exhibit somewhat prominent central nucleoli (Fig. 6.24b). Perivascular spaces showing a central venule surrounded by a clear space are present in variable numbers (Fig. 6.25). They can blend into microscopic cysts due to edema (Fig. 6.26) [162]. Medullary islands, as seen in lymphocyte-rich thymomas, are usually absent. Small Hassall's corpuscles and epithelial rosettes or pseudorosettes can be present (Fig. 6.27).

Lymphocyte-rich thymomas with atypia can be difficult to distinguish from lymphocyte-rich thymomas. The presence of

(a)

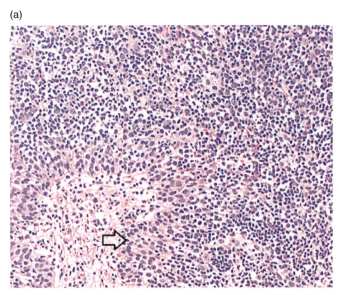

(b)

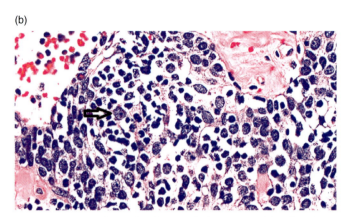

Fig. 6.24 (a) Lymphocyte-rich with atypia thymoma. The epithelial cells (arrow) are more conspicuous than in lymphocyte-rich thymomas and they form loose aggregates admixed with lymphoid cells. Mild anisocytosis is present but no significant cytologic atypia is seen in this microscopic field (H&E 100x). **(b)** Lymphocyte-rich with atypia thymoma. The epithelial cells are slightly anisocytotic and they contain focal small nucleoli (arrow) (H&E 400x).

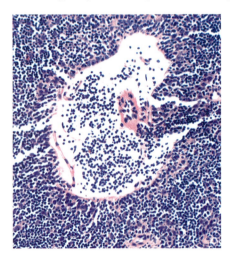

Fig. 6.25 Lymphocyte-rich with atypia thymoma showing a characteristic perivascular space. It contains a central venule surrounded by edema fluid and suspended lymphoid cells (H&E 40x).

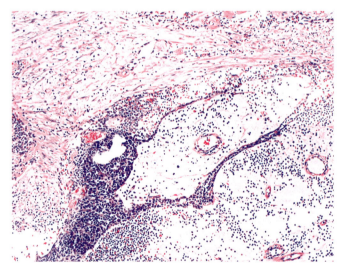

Fig. 6.26 Lymphocyte-rich with atypia thymoma showing prominent perivascular spaces with extensive edema and microcystic change (H&E 40x).

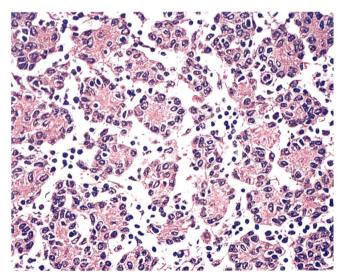

Fig. 6.27 Lymphocyte-rich with atypia thymoma showing epithelial rosettes (H&E 100x).

lobulation and perivascular spaces and the presence of polygonal epithelial cells with conspicuous nucleoli are helpful features for the diagnosis. As recognition of cellular atypia and lymphoid cell density can be subjective (Fig. 6.28), lymphocyte-rich thymomas with atypia (WHO B2) (Fig. 6.29a) can also be difficult to distinguish from lymphocyte-depleted thymoma with atypia (WHO B3) (Fig. 6.29b). We favor the latter diagnoses in lesions that exhibit only a relatively small number of lymphocytes and are composed mostly of round to oval epithelial cells exhibiting modest cytologic atypia and/or only focal severe atypia (Fig. 6.29b).

Malignant lymphomas can usually be readily distinguished from lymphocyte-rich thymomas with atypia as

the majority of mediastinal lymphoid lesions are composed of larger and more atypical lymphocytes than seen in thymomas. The differential diagnosis from Hodgkin's lymphoma can be more difficult, as this lesion shows small lymphocytes and lobulation in the nodular sclerosing variant and can be associated with thymic cysts. The presence of "popcorn", Reed-Sternberg, and other atypical lymphoid cells and/or eosinophils in Hodgkin's lymphoma are helpful features for the differential diagnoses. In addition, the fibrous septa in Hodgkin's lymphoma are thicker and more irregular than those seen in thymomas.

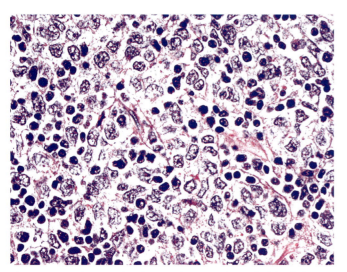

Fig. 6.28 Lymphocyte-rich with atypia thymoma. The epithelial cells show more prominent anisocytosis and nucleolar prominence than the examples in previous figures. Some observers may prefer to categorize such a tumor as a WHO B3 thymoma. The lesion contains lymphoid cells admixed with epithelial cells that do not form solid sheets, and therefore a WHO B2 lesion seems to be a better classification (H&E 400x).

Intermediate-grade malignant thymic epithelial lesions

Two overlapping histopathological variants of thymomas and two variants of thymic carcinomas are usually associated with higher stage at diagnosis and less favorable prognosis than the previously described low-grade malignant thymic epithelial lesions. The thymomas are classified by the current WHO expert panel as two specific variants and were both included in the classification scheme by Suster and Moran as atypical thymomas [137]. In practice atypical thymomas usually show an admixture of epithelial cells with round, oval, or spindle shaped nuclei, although some lesions are composed predominantly of spindle cells and others of round/oval cells. Spindle cell thymomas with atypia were not explicitly included under the category WHO B3 in the past and are described separately from other atypical thymomas to emphasize that not all spindle cell thymomas are low-grade lesions.

The pathology of well-differentiated squamous cell carcinoma and mucoepidermoid carcinoma of the thymus is discussed in the next chapter.

Spindle cell thymoma with atypia (not in 2004 WHO classification)

Spindle cell thymoma with atypia is an incompletely characterized lesion composed of spindle epithelial cells with moderate and perhaps focally severe nuclear atypia and focal necrosis. Some cases have probably been classified in the past as either WHO A or WHO B3 thymomas [17]. Recently, Nonaka and Rosai reported a pilot study of 13 WHO type A thymomas displaying increased mitotic activity, mild to moderate nuclear atypia, and focal areas of necrosis; no correlation with prognosis was provided [163]. Vladislav *et al.* reported that 43% of 23 thymomas classified in their database as WHO type A had recurrence or

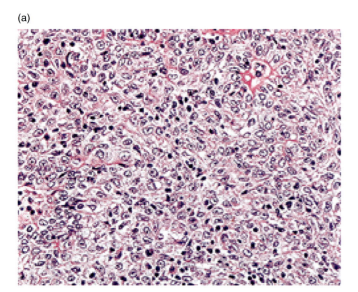

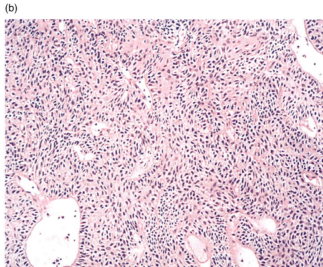

(a)

(b)

Fig. 6.29 (a) Lymphocyte-rich with atypia thymoma. The tumor cells exhibit mild anisocytosis and small nucleoli. They are admixed with a modest number of mature lymphocytes (H&E 200x). **(b)** Lymphocyte-depleted with atypia thymoma. The tumor cells exhibit greater anisocytosis and cytologic atypia than seen in the previous figure and they form solid sheets with few lymphocytes (H&E 100x).

(a) (b)

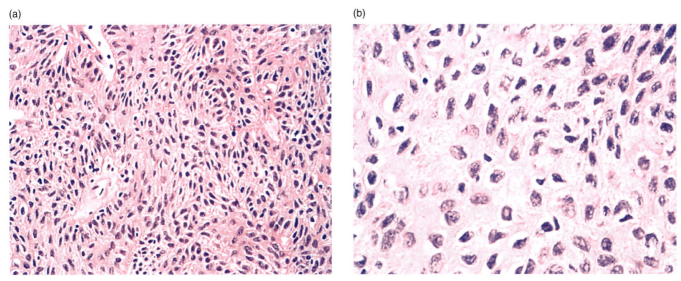

Fig. 6.30 (a) Spindle cell thymoma with atypia. The epithelial cells are atypical and form solid sheets admixed with relatively few lymphocytes (H&E 200x). **(b)** Spindle cell thymoma with atypia. The atypical epithelial cells show irregular rounded or spindled nuclei with considerable anisocytosis and somewhat irregular nuclear membranes. This lesion can be difficult to distinguish from a well-differentiated squamous cell carcinoma. However, the thymoma lacks the presence of intercellular bridges, keratinization, necrosis, and prominent nucleolation (H&E 400x).

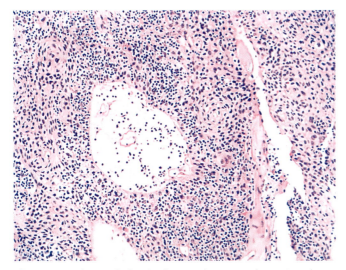

Fig. 6.31 Lymphocyte-depleted with atypia thymoma with a perivascular space (H&E 100x).

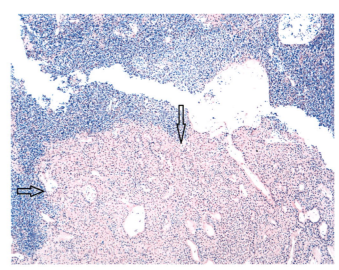

Fig. 6.32 The same tumor shown in the previous figure contains other areas comprising solid sheets of epithelial cells (arrows) that form focal glandular spaces (H&E 40x).

metastases. The presence of necrosis correlated with recurrence and metastases but not with Masaoka stage. No clinical or histological features correlated with aggressive behavior [164].

In contrast to spindle cell thymomas (WHO A), these lesions exhibit variable anisocytosis, mitoses in variable numbers, rare atypical mitoses, and focal necrosis (Fig. 6.30a and b). Reticulin stains usually fail to show staining around each of the epithelial neoplastic cells, a pattern characteristic of spindle cell thymomas.

Lymphocyte-depleted thymoma with atypia (WHO B3)

Lymphocyte-depleted thymoma with atypia (WHO B3) accounts for 7–25% of thymic epithelial lesions [17,152,153,157]. They are usually not encapsulated or are poorly encapsulated

and exhibit a gray, irregularly lobulated surface. Microscopically, they are composed of diffuse sheets or vaguely nodular areas of polygonal epithelial cells admixed with relatively few lymphoid cells. Variable numbers of perivascular spaces are usually present (Fig. 6.31).The epithelial cells can show considerable nuclear atypia with anisocytosis, prominent nucleoli, and high N:C ratio in focal areas (Fig. 6.32).

Spindle cell thymoma with atypia and lymphocyte depleted thymoma with atypia need to be distinguished from well differentiated thymic carcinomas, particularly non-keratinizing squamous cell carcinoma [165]. The latter exhibit more prominent cytologic atypia, focal dyskeratosis, and/or intercellular bridges (Figs. 6.33a and b). Both lesions can

(a)

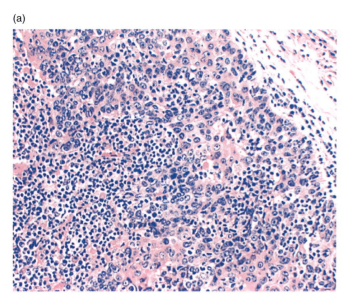

(b)

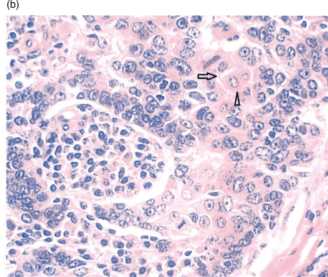

Fig. 6.33 (a) Lymphocyte-depleted with atypia thymoma. This tumor comprises epithelial cells with prominent nucleoli and focal cytoplasmic eosinophilia. This type of lesion can be difficult to distinguish with certainty from well differentiated squamous cell carcinoma (H&E 200x). **(b)** Other areas of the same tumor indeed did show foci of well-differentiated squamous cell carcinoma with a greater degree of cytologic atypia than seen in Fig. 6.33a. In addition, the tumor cells exhibited focal intercellular bridges (arrow) and prominent cytoplasmic eosinophilia (arrowhead) suggestive of dyskeratosis (H&E 400x).

exhibit cytoplasmic immunoreactivity for CK5/6. To our knowledge, the use of antibodies such as p40, desmoglein, p63, and others being currently utilized for the diagnosis of squamous cell carcinoma of the lung and other sites has not been evaluated in spindle cell thymomas with atypia [166].

Lymphocyte-depleted thymoma with atypia exhibits a similar immunophenotype to other thymomas other than lymphocyte-rich thymoma. The epithelial cells can also exhibit cytoplasmic immunoreactivity for CD5 and EMA, findings usually associated with a thymic carcinoma.

Lymphocyte-depleted thymoma with atypia (WHO B3) also needs to be distinguished from well-differentiated carcinomas based on the features described above.

Heterologous thymomas

Thymomas are often heterologous neoplasms that exhibit different morphological features in different samples examined from the same tumor. Moran *et al.* have elegantly demonstrated that the greater the number of histologic sections collected from a thymoma, the higher the probability that more than a single WHO histologic type will be encountered [167]. In their view, this finding supports their concept that a subclassification based on histopathology of these lesions is unnecessary. In a recent study of 250 thymomas evaluated at the M.D. Anderson Cancer Center, 53% of the lesions were of mixed histologic types [168].

There are no consensus criteria or evidence-based criteria regarding the minimum thresholds necessary to classify a lesion as heterologous thymoma [169,170]. Previous WHO classification of thoracic neoplasms has proposed the use of an arbitrary 10% cut-off to label tumors with mixed histopathologic features as a separate category [17]. For example a

squamous cell carcinoma (SCC) of the lung with less than 10% glandular features would be diagnosed as SCC with focal glandular features, while another with 10% or greater adeno-carcinoma component would be labeled as adeno-squamous carcinoma. Readers may elect to use this arbitrary nomenclature in the diagnoses of heterologous thymoma. We prefer to label as such all lesions as heterologous thymomas without using an arbitrary minimum cut-off value, listing the different components, according to their relative density within a lesion.

To our knowledge, there is no high-level evidence evaluating the prognosis of patients with heterologous thymomas, particularly as there is no consensus on how to classify them.

Combined thymoma–thymic carcinoma

Thymic neoplasms can also exhibit distinct areas of thymoma combined with other areas of thymic carcinoma or other thymic neoplasms (Figs. 6.33a and b) [171–173]. The carcinoma component of the neoplasm is the one that usually recurs and/or metastasizes [1]. In cases exhibiting spindle cell thymoma with atypia (WHO A, atypical) or lymphocyte-depleted thymoma with atypia (WHO B3) and carcinoma areas, it is often difficult to determine with certainty which areas belong to each of the neoplastic components.

Unusual thymoma variants

Thymoma with pseudosarcomatous stroma (WHO metaplastic thymoma)

This unusual thymic neoplasm has been reported under various designations, including thymoma with pseudosarcomatous stroma, low-grade metaplastic carcinoma, biphasic

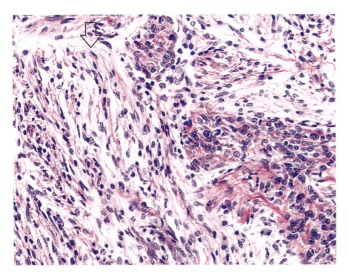

Fig. 6.34 Thymoma with pseudosarcomatous stroma. Note the presence of the cellular stroma (arrow) with a resemblance to spindle cell thymoma. However the mesenchymal cells in that portion of the tumor showed no keratin immunoreactivity (H&E 100x).

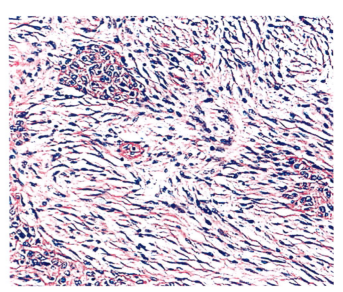

Fig. 6.35 Thymoma with pseudosarcomatous stroma. The lesion lacks lobulation and prominent lymphoid infiltrates as seen in other thymomas (H&E 100x).

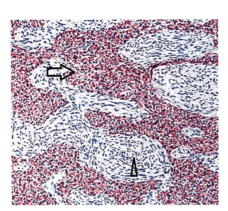

Fig. 6.36 Thymoma with pseudosarcomatous stroma. The epithelial tumor cells show cytoplasmic reactivity for keratin (arrow) whereas the stromal cells are negative (arrowhead) (PAP 40x).

thymoma, and mixed polygonal and spindle cell type thymoma [174–180]. It occurs in adult patients, usually in the sixth decade of life, and appears to be more frequent in men than in women.

Thymomas with pseudosarcomatous stroma have been described only in the mediastinum in patients without MG or other paraneoplastic syndromes [1]. They can have variable size, and lesions measuring up to 16 cm have been described. They are usually well-encapsulated tumors, but can appear as locally invasive lesions in less than 10% of cases.

Microscopically, they are lymphocyte-depleted lesions composed of anastomosing round and irregular islands of polygonal, ovoid, or spindle epithelial cells, admixed with sheets and narrow zones of spindle cells that can exhibit focal storiform growth pattern (Fig. 6.34). In contrast with lymphocyte-rich thymomas with spindle cells, the lesions lack prominent lymphoid component and lobulation (Fig. 6.35). The epithelial cells can exhibit variable degrees of cytologic atypia, with enlarged hypochromatic or hyperchromatic nuclei, and high N:C ratio. However, in spite of the cytological atypia, the epithelial cells exhibit only infrequent mitoses and no significant necrosis, in contrast to carcinomas. The spindle cells of metaplastic thymomas have bland nuclei and are organized in solid sheets, fascicles, or storiform areas. Mitoses are rare in spindle cell areas.

Immunostains can be helpful for the diagnosis of thymomas with pseudosarcomatous stroma. The epithelial cells exhibit cytoplasmic keratin AE1/AE3 immunoreactivity but the spindle cells are usually negative (Fig. 6.36), with only rare positive cells [1]. Proliferative activity, as measured by Ki-67, is usually lower than 5%. Immunostain for CD5, a frequent finding in thymic carcinomas, is negative. The spindle cells lack keratin immunoreactivity. This finding is different than usually seen in metaplastic carcinomas of breast and other origin and favors the concept that the spindle cells are stromal in origin, rather than metaplastic. Cytogenetic abnormalities have been reported in rare cases of thymoma with pseudosarcomatous stroma, a finding that was interpreted by the authors of the WHO classification of thymomas as supportive of a metaplastic origin.

Thymomas with pseudosarcomatous stroma behave in a similar manner to other low-grade thymomas. Most patients are diagnosed in Masaoka stage I, although stage II and III patients have been described [175–180]. They can recur intrathoracically following thymectomy and can rarely be fatal.

The differential diagnosis usually includes sarcomatoid carcinoma of the thymus, a lesion that usually exhibits greater mitotic activity, atypical mitoses, and multifocal areas of necrosis (see Chapter 7). There have been a few reports of thymic sarcomatoid carcinoma arising from a metaplastic thymoma [177,178].

(a)

(b)

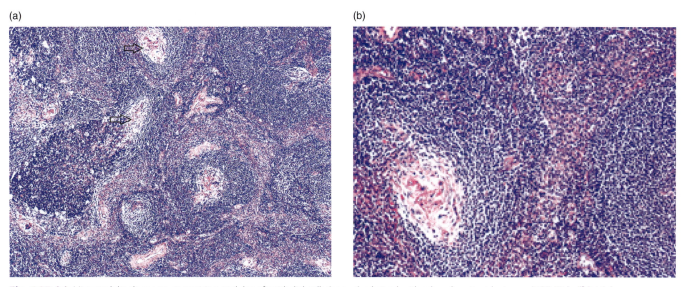

Fig. 6.37 (a) Micronodular thymoma comprising nodules of epithelial cells (arrows) admixed with a lymphocyte-rich stroma (H&E 40x). **(b)** Higher power of the same lesion (H&E 100x).

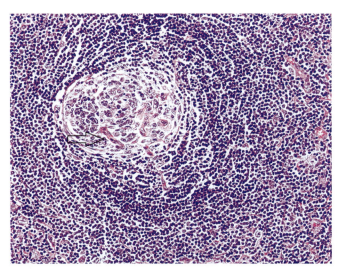

Fig. 6.38 Micronodular thymoma showing focal neovascularization in an epithelial focus (arrow) that resembles the image of Castleman disease (H&E 40x).

Fig. 6.39 Keratin immunostain highlights the presence of epithelial foci surrounded by dense lymphoid infiltrate in a micronodular thymoma (PAP 20x).

Micronodular thymoma (WHO micronodular thymoma)

This is an unusual variant of thymoma that occurs almost exclusively in the mediastinum, with only rare cases reported in the neck [179–182]. It involves adults in their fifth to ninth decade of life, with no sex predilection. They are not associated with MG or other systemic conditions. Micronodular thymomas appear grossly as encapsulated nodules of variable size that can be as large as 15 cm, with infrequent local invasion. They frequently show cystic areas. Microscopically, micronodular thymomas are characterized by the presence of multiple microscopic nodules of polygonal or spindle epithelial cells admixed with a lymphocyte-rich stroma that can contain germinal centers and plasma cells (Fig. 6.37a and b). Focal areas of neovascularization resembling Castleman disease can be present (Fig. 6.38). Interestingly, the micronodules of epithelial

cells are devoid of lymphocytes. Rosettes can be found in micronodular thymomas, but Hassall's corpuscles, mitoses, and areas or necrosis are absent.

The epithelial cells of micronodular thymomas exhibit cytoplasmic immunoreactivity for cytokeratins AE1/AE3 (Fig. 6.39), CK5/6, and CAM5.2 [181,183]. Epithelial cells lining cystic areas also show EMA cytoplasmic immunoreactivity. In contrast with other variants of thymomas, the majority of the lymphocytes in micronodular thymomas are CD20+ B-cells, although variable numbers of CD3+, CD5+ T-cells are also present. Scanty immature TdT+, CD99+ thymocytes can be seen in areas surrounding the epithelial micronodules. Usually plasma cells do not exhibit light-chain restriction [181].

Patients with micronodular thymomas have an excellent prognosis, with no reported recurrences, metastases, or fatalities.

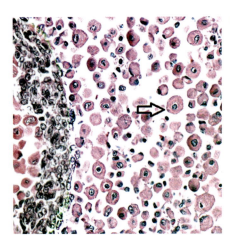

Fig. 6.40 Rhabdomyomatous thymoma showing stromal cells with characteristically eosinophilic cytoplasm (arrow) (H&E 200x).

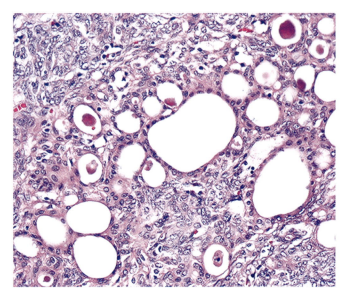

Fig. 6.41 Thymoma with prominent glandular differentiation (H&E 100x).

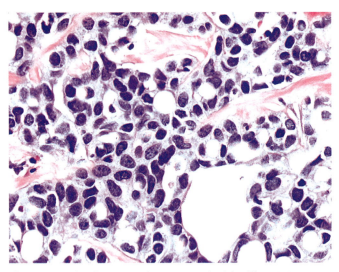

Fig. 6.42 Another thymoma with prominent glandular differentiation (H&E 200x).

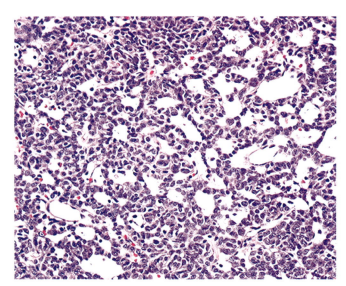

Fig. 6.43 Thymoma with prominent glandular differentiation and adenomatoid features (H&E 100x).

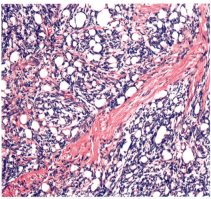
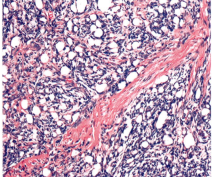

Fig. 6.44 Thymoma containing pseudoglands (H&E 100x).

Rhabdomyomatous thymoma (not included in WHO)

Moran and Koss reported an encapsulated thymic neoplasm composed of epithelial and myoid cells (Fig. 6.40) that they classified as rhabdomyomatous thymoma [184,185]. The myoid cells exhibited immunoreactivity for myoglobin and desmin [186]. More recently, a rhabdomyomatous spindle cell thymoma with mucinous cystic degeneration has been reported in a pericardial location [187].

Sclerosing thymoma (WHO sclerosing thymoma)

Sclerosing thymoma is a very unusual tumor characterized by the presence of morphological features of a thymoma but with prominent areas of stromal fibrosis and hyalinization [188]. It remains controversial whether, in the absence of necrosis the fibroblastic response is secondary to epithelial cell stimulation or a regressive change [189].

Thymoma with prominent glandular differentiation (not included in WHO)

Different variants of thymomas can show focal mucinous and non-mucinous glandular structures (Figs. 6.41 and 6.42) [1]. Foci with adenomatoid features (Fig. 6.43), pseudoglands (Fig. 6.44), and signet-ring cells (Fig. 6.45) can also be present. Recently, Weissferdt and Moran reported 12 thymomas with prominent glandular differentiation in patients without a history of MG or other autoimmune disorders [190]. Tumor epithelial cells showed immunoreactivity for CAM 5.2 and CK 5/6.

Spindle cell thymoma with prominent papillary and pseudo-papillary features (not in WHO)

Kalhor et al. recently described ten cases of spindle cell thymoma with prominent papillary and pseudo-papillary features (Fig. 6.46a and b) and emphasized the recognition of these unusual neoplasms to avoid misdiagnosis with other mediastinal neoplasms [191].

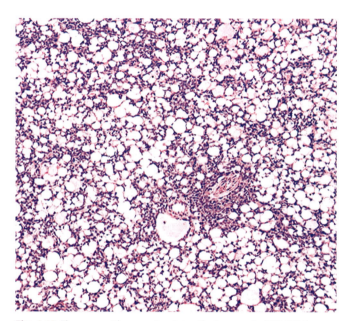

Fig. 6.45 Thymoma with many signet-ring-like tumor cells (H&E 100x).

Other thymic lesions

Lipofibroadenoma (WHO lipofibroadenoma)

So-called lipofibroadenoma is a rare thymic lesion that exhibits a sparse lymphoid component and is composed of epithelial and stromal elements arranging a matter that resembles a fibroadenoma of breast origin [1,192]. It is unclear whether the epithelial cells present in this lesion are neoplastic or reactive thymic epithelial cells.

Thymomas with "monster" atypical cells (not in WHO)

Rarely, thymomas exhibit very large and atypical "monster" cells (Fig. 6.47a and b). These lesions could probably be classified as "simplastic thymoma" but to our knowledge such an entity has yet to be defined in the literature.

Thymomas in myasthenia gravis patients

There is no single morphological feature of a thymoma that is specifically associated with MG, although the neoplasms in these patients are probably more likely to have germinal centers and Hassall's corpuscles (Fig. 6.48) than tumors in non-MG patients [5,35–37,46,193–195]. In contrast, thymomas in non-MG patients are more likely to exhibit rosettes, a spindle cell morphology, and pseudoglandular formation [2].

Follicular hyperplasia of the thymus is the most significant pathology detected in the non-neoplastic thymic tissue adjacent to a thymoma in MG patients [196–198]. Alpert and associates have reported that 53% of patients with both thymoma and MG have follicular hyperplasia of the thymus whereas none of the non-myasthenic patients with thymoma exhibited that finding [197]. However, the significance of thymic follicular hyperplasia in an individual patient with thymoma is not diagnostic of the presence of MG, as this finding can be seen in patients without the neuromuscular disease.

(a)

(b)

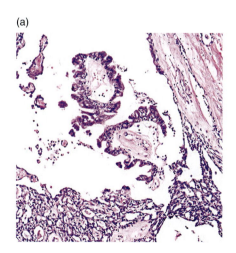
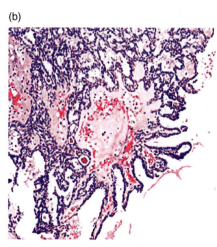

Fig. 6.46 (a) Spindle cell thymoma with focally prominent papillary features (H&E 100x).
(b) Higher power of the same lesion demonstrating papillary and pseudo-papillary structures (H&E 200x).

(a) (b)

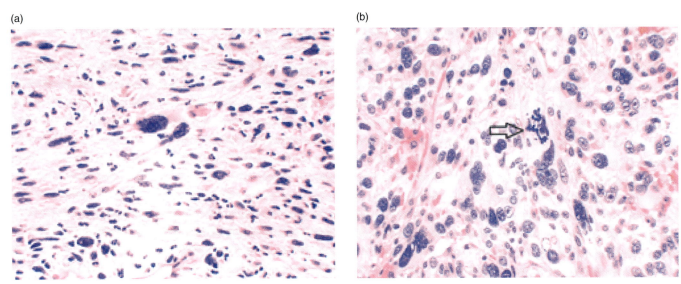

Fig. 6.47 **(a)** Spindle cell thymoma with cytologic atypia, showing a few markedly pleomorphic (monster) cells. This finding was present only in a small area of a tumor that otherwise lacked significant cellular pleomorphism, necrosis, and mitotic activity (H&E 400x). **(b)** The same lesion shows a rare atypical mitotic figure in an area adjacent to that shown in Fig. 6.47a (arrow) (H&E 400x). Does this represent a microscopic focus of carcinoma arising in a thymoma? The prognosis of these tumors is uncertain because this entity has not been well characterized to date.

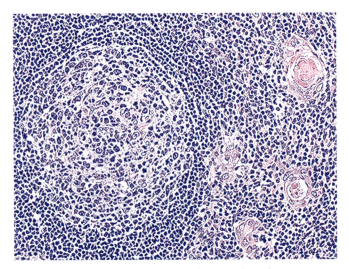

Fig. 6.48 Follicular lymphoid hyperplasia of non-neoplastic thymic tissue, a common finding in patients with myasthenia gravis (H&E 40x).

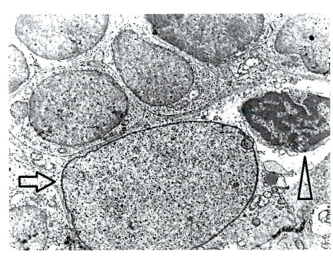

Fig. 6.49 Electron micrograph of thymoma showing cohesive epithelial cells (arrow) forming a space that contains a mature lymphocyte (arrowhead).

Degenerative changes in thymomas

All thymoma variants can exhibit a variety of degenerative microscopic changes, including "starry-sky" pattern, collections of "foamy histiocytes", microcystic degeneration, areas of old and recent hemorrhage, granulomas, and calcification with occasional formation of "sclerosiderotic nodules" [1].

The "starry-sky" pattern is characterized by the presence of large numbers of phagocytic histiocytes among the lymphocytic component of thymomas. They may represent a response to cellular destruction. Foamy histiocytes are found in clusters admixed with tumor cells or in perivascular spaces in 15% to 27% of thymomas.

Microcysts are present in 16% to 41% of thymomas and appear as round, empty holes containing either degenerated or viable cells in their lumina. They are found most frequently in lymphoid areas of the tumor and have no cyst lining [120].

Hemorrhagic foci are not infrequent in thymomas. They may become calcified. Sclerosiderotic nodules similar to Gamna–Gandy nodules can occur. Epithelioid granulomas are infrequent in thymomas [2].

Ultrastructural features of thymomas

Thymomas mimic, at the ultrastructural level, the structure of the normal thymus gland (Fig. 6.49) [146,199–201]. Epithelial-reticular cells have characteristic long cytoplasmic processes connected by desmosomal attachments and form irregular

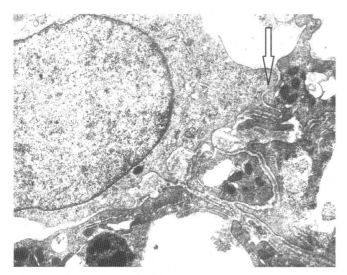

Fig. 6.50 Electron micrograph of thymoma showing epithelial cells with interdigitating cellular processes (arrow).

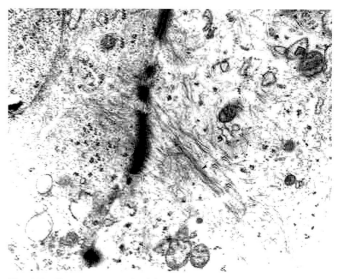

Fig. 6.51 Electron micrograph of thymoma showing intracytoplasmic tonofilaments in the cytoplasm of the epithelial tumor cells.

sheets with multiple spaces in which lymphocytes lay. The epithelial cells of thymomas are oval, polyhedral, spindle, or irregular in shape and have multiple elongated cell processes measuring up to 20 μm in length (Figs. 6.50 and 6.51). These cord-like processes can be best seen with scanning electron microscopy and give the epithelial cells a markedly irregular cell contour. The elongated cell processes of epithelial cells are in close contact with basement membrane material and become attached to adjacent epithelial cells by well-formed macula-adherens-type junctions (desmosomes). In this way, the tumor cells become interlocked in a complex pattern of cell-to-cell relationships. The cytoplasm of epithelial cells of thymomas has characteristic prominent tonofilaments, which form branching and interconnecting bundles measuring about 70 nm in thickness and up to 2 μm in length. These tonofilaments frequently extend into the cellular membrane and establish contact with desmosomes through thickenings of the subplasmalemmal regions. They become particularly prominent in epithelial cells exhibiting keratinization. In addition, epithelial cells of thymomas have other cytoplasmic organelles, including large numbers of mitochondria, moderately well-developed Golgi apparatus, centriole, pinocytotic vesicles, scanty rough endoplasmic reticulum, lysosomes, occasional lipid droplets, and rare cilia. In some instances, they also have prominent cytoplasmic vacuoles lined by a smooth membrane. These probably represent a degenerative phenomenon and are present in thymomas that exhibit clear cells with light microscopy. The nucleus of the epithelial cells of thymomas is round or oval and has a smooth or indented contour. Heterochromatin is condensed beneath the nuclear membrane, and there are well-formed nucleoli with moderately developed nucleololemmas.

The epithelial cells of thymomas may become organized in structures already described at the light microscopic level. They can form gland-like spaces lined by cuboidal or flattened cells connected by desmosomes and arranged around a space filled with electron-dense amorphous material. These epithelial cells have prominent microvilli, which project into the lumen. Occasionally, epithelial cells become concentrically arranged around a central area composed of degenerating and necrotic cells (Hassall's corpuscles). The epithelial cells of thymomas can also grow around vascular structures and establish a close relationship with capillaries, forming perivascular spaces characteristic of thymomas. These dilated spaces are present between the basal lamina of endothelial cells of capillaries and those of epithelial cells growing around the vessel. The central vessel is composed of endothelial cells with abundant cytoplasm. The epithelial cells are flattened or columnar and have basal nuclei and desmosomal attachments. The perivascular spaces contain fibrous long-spacing collagen, plasma, a variable number of lymphocytes, occasional red blood cells, macrophages, and/or mesenchymal cells. Lymphocytes can occasionally be seen migrating across the epithelial basal lamina into the epithelial site and can probably cross the endothelial basement membrane, as demonstrated in the animal thymus.

Secretory activities of thymomas

Patients with thymomas showing elevated serum levels of thymopoietin, serum thymic factor (FTS), and other thymic hormones have been reported in patients with immune disorders[202–204].

Hormone receptors in thymomas

Estrogen receptors and other hormone receptors have been described in thymomas and in thymic hyperplasia, suggesting the potential for hormonal treatment of these conditions[205,206].

Analysis of nuclear DNA content in thymomas

DNA cytofluorometry and morphometry is not useful for the classification of malignant thymic epithelial neoplasms as all variants can exhibit aneuploidy or abnormal S-fractions[85,207].

(a)

(b)

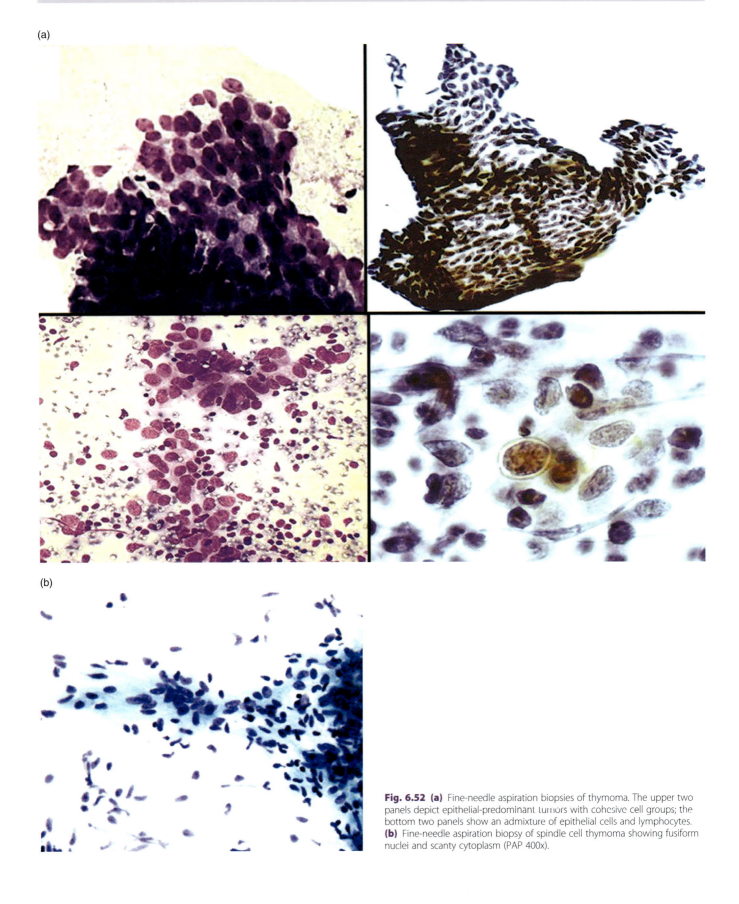

Fig. 6.52 (a) Fine-needle aspiration biopsies of thymoma. The upper two panels depict epithelial-predominant tumors with cohesive cell groups; the bottom two panels show an admixture of epithelial cells and lymphocytes. **(b)** Fine-needle aspiration biopsy of spindle cell thymoma showing fusiform nuclei and scanty cytoplasm (PAP 400x).

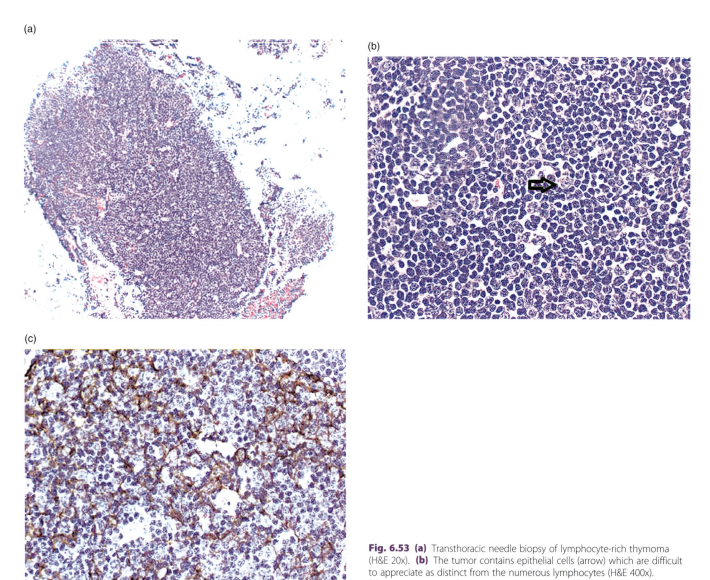

(a)

(b)

(c)

Fig. 6.53 (a) Transthoracic needle biopsy of lymphocyte-rich thymoma (H&E 20x). (b) The tumor contains epithelial cells (arrow) which are difficult to appreciate as distinct from the numerous lymphocytes (H&E 400x). (c) Immunostaining for keratin shows reactivity in the cytoplasm of the epithelial cells (PAP 400x). This is a helpful feature in distinguishing lymphocyte-rich thymoma from malignant lymphoma.

Cytogenetic and molecular studies in thymomas

Multiple cytogenetic and molecular abnormalities have been described in thymomas [16,85,208–215]. They include the presence of ras oncogene p21, various translocations such as t(15:22)(p11;q11), t(1:8)(p13;p11), deletion of chromosome 6, formation of ring chromosome, abnormalities in p53 gene, and others. A comprehensive review of these abnormalities is beyond the scope of this volume.

Diagnosis of malignant thymic epithelial lesions on small biopsy specimens

The diagnosis of a thymoma can be established preoperatively by transthoracic CT-guided fine-needle aspiration biopsy (FNA) (Fig. 6.52a–b), percutaneous needle core biopsies (Fig. 6.53a–c), and incisional biopsies by mediastinoscopy, video-assisted thoracoscopic surgery (VATS), minithoracotomy/Chamberlain procedure, and other biopsy techniques [22,131,216–218]. Biopsies of cystic lesions are generally approached cautiously as they can seed malignant cells or infection, but in general there is little evidence that biopsies of thymic lesions contribute to the spread of the disease.

The use of biopsies and FNA for the diagnosis of malignant thymic epithelial lesions was recently reviewed by a workgroup sponsored by the International Thymic Malignancy Interest Group (ITMIG). Transthoracic FNA yields sensitivity of 71–100%, specificity of 77–100%, and positive predictive value of 69–100% [170]. Percutaneous core biopsy yields sensitivity of 40–93%, specificity of 76–100%, and positive predictive value of 83–91%. Interpretation should be correlated with the clinical and imaging findings. Consultation with an experienced

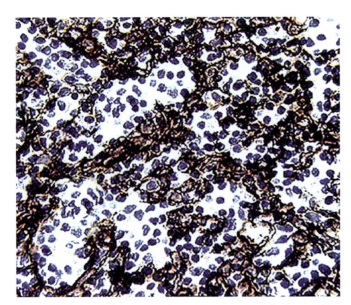

Fig. 6.54 Thymoma showing cytoplasmic immunoreactivity for keratin 5/6 (PAP 400x).

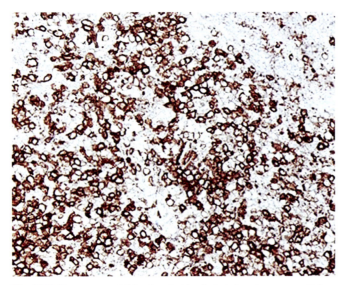

Fig. 6.56 Thymoma containing lymphoid cells that show immunoreactivity for CD 99 (PAP 200x).

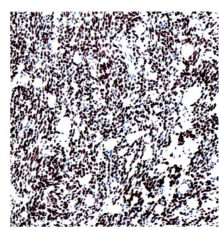

Fig. 6.55 Lymphocyte-rich thymoma showing numerous lymphoid cells with nuclear labeling for terminal deoxynucleotidyl transfersase (TdT) (PAP 400x).

EMA. Neuroendocrine markers such as synaptophysin, chromogranin, and CD56, and germ cell markers such as OCT ¾, SALL4, alpha-fetoprotein, PLAP, and hCG are helpful to diagnose neuroendocrine neoplasms and germ cell tumors, respectively.

Thymomas may be very difficult to distinguish from thymic hyperplasia on smears of aspirated material or small biopsies, but their cytological and histopathological features are generally distinct from those seen in other mediastinal lesions[219,220]. For example, metastatic small-cell carcinomas of the lung exhibit dispersed small round, ovoid, or spindle cells with scanty cytoplasm and hyperchromatic nuclei. Lymphomas usually exhibit large, irregular lymphoid cells with obvious cytologic atypia. Lymphoblastic lymphomas, frequent in the mediastinum, show convoluted lymphoid cells. Low-grade lymphomas, however, may pose diagnostic problems. They exhibit small, round lymphocytes with minimal nuclear atypia, as seen in thymomas. They lack, however, the presence of clusters of epithelial cells seen in thymic neoplasms. Other mediastinal lesions such as teratomas exhibit cytologic features that are distinct from those seen in thymomas.

second pathologist is recommended whenever there is any diagnostic difficulty.

Selected immunohistochemical markers are very helpful to diagnose malignant thymic epithelial lesions on small biopsy samples and distinguish them from other mediastinal neoplasms. Thymomas and thymic carcinomas exhibit immunoreactivity for cytokeratins such as AE1/AE3 (Fig. 6.53c) and CK5/6 (Fig. 6.54), PAX-8 (Fig. 6.18) and other markers. Lymphoid cells exhibit immunoreactivity for various T-cell and other markers such as TdT (Fig. 6.55) and CD99 (Fig. 6.56). Thymic carcinomas but usually not thymomas can exhibit immunoreactivity for CD117, CD5, CD70, and

Clinico-pathological staging of patients with malignant thymic epithelial lesions

The American Joint Commission on Cancer (AJCC) has not developed a staging system for thymomas and thymic carcinomas, perhaps because of past controversies regarding whether there are benign and malignant thymomas. Bergh *et al.* and Wilkins *et al.* proposed systems for the staging of thymoma patients but the most widely used system for staging of these lesions is the Masaoka-Koga stage classification system shown in Table 6.4[47,143,221,222].

Stage I lesions are grossly and microscopically completely encapsulated. Stage IIa show microscopic transcapsular invasion while Stage IIb exhibit macroscopic invasion into surrounding tissues. Stage III lesions show macroscopic invasion into adjacent organs such as the pericardium, lung, and others.

Table 6.4. Masaoka-Koga staging system for thymic malignant epithelial tumors

Stage	Definitions
I	Grossly and microscopically completely encapsulated tumors.
IIa	Microscopic transcapsular invasion.
IIb	Macroscopic invasion into perithymic or surrounding fatty tissue or grossly adherent to but not breaking through mediastinal pleura or pericardium.
III	Macroscopic invasion into neighboring organs (lung, pericardium, or great vessels).
IVa	Pleural or pericardial metastases.
IVb	Distant metastases.

Table 6.5. Moran *et al.*, clinico-pathologic staging of thymomas

Stage 0: encapsulated thymomas.

Stage I: invasive thymoma, with histologically proven invasion into peri-thymic adipose tissue.

Stage II: a; invasive thymoma with direct invasion into innominate vein, mediastinal pleura, and/or lung.

b; invasive thymoma with extension into the pericardium.

c; invasive thymoma with extension into the great vessels and/or heart.

Stage III: a; metastatic disease to intrathoracic structures and lymph nodes.

b; metastatic disease to extrathoracic sites.

(a)

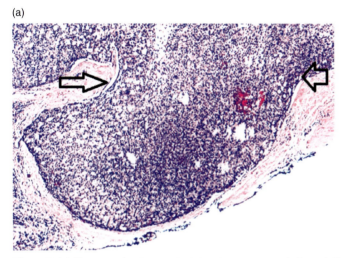

(b)

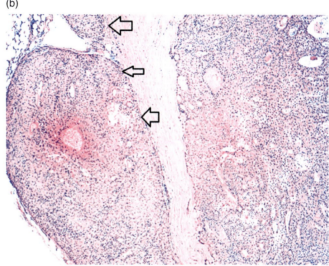

Fig. 6.57 (a) Thymoma showing neoplastic invasion into its capsule (arrows). The tumor has not infiltrated into the adjacent soft tissues and this finding is therefore insufficient to classify the lesion as an invasive Masaoka-Koga stage IIa thymoma (H&E 40x). **(b)** Thymoma with transcapsular invasion. The tumor has grown through its capsule, indicated by arrows, into adjacent soft tissues shown at the left of the photograph (H&E 40x).

Stage IVa malignant thymic epithelial lesions show pleural or pericardial metastases while Stage IVb tumors show lymphatic or hematogenous metastasis. Detterbeck *et al.* have recently published guidelines for clarification and definition of terms in the use of the Masaoka-Koga stage classification system for thymic malignancies [143].

The presence of microscopic transcapsular invasion in thymomas allows for the distinction between stages I and IIa of disease (Fig. 6.57a and b). A thymoma is staged as IIa when it grows through the capsule (transcapsular), as shown in Fig. 6.57b but not Fig. 6.57a. The presence of transcapsular invasion has been emphasized as a very important feature to evaluate during the pathological work-up of a thymoma [1,6,17]. However, review of the literature with meta-analysis demonstrated that this feature is not associated with significant prognostic differences [223]. In daily practice, it is more important to evaluate resection margins to inform the surgeon whether the entire lesion has been resected.

Moran *et al.* recently proposed a somewhat different clinico-pathologic staging system shown in Table 6.5 and Fig. 6.58a–f, based on their experience with 250 thymoma cases treated at M.D. Anderson Cancer Center [168]. The number of recurrences were 0%, 6.1%, 22.7%, and 20% by stages 0, I, II, and III respectively. Nine of 20 patients in stage III were dead, while patients in lower stages were alive with or without recurrence [168].

Treatment and prognosis of thymoma patients

The treatment of thymoma patients is generally selected on the basis of Masaoka-Koga stage or stage determined by another system [30,131,143]. The clinical value of the WHO classification of thymomas, by stage, is controversial, although recent studies suggest that WHO B3 thymomas may benefit more from neoadjuvant chemotherapy than patients with other variants of the disease [49,141,211,224,225].

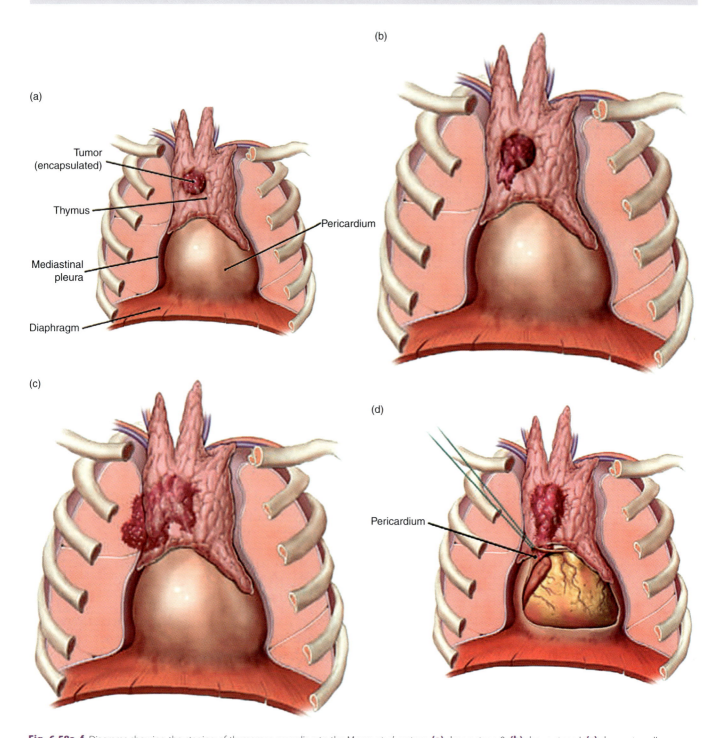

Fig. 6.58a–f Diagrams showing the staging of thymomas according to the Moran *et al.* system. **(a)** shows stage 0, **(b)** shows stage I, **(c)** shows stage IIa, **(d)** shows stage IIb, **(e)** shows stage IIc, and **(f)** shows stage IIIa (please see Table 6.5).

Surgical resection is the mainstay of treatment for thymoma patients [226,227]. Patients with stage I and II undergo thymectomy with excision not only of the neoplasm but of all visible thymic tissues [227]. The thymectomy specimen needs to be oriented properly by the surgeon in the operating room to allow for accurate pathological evaluation of resection margins. Detterbeck *et al.* recently published ITMIG policies and procedures for surgeons and pathologists regarding resection of thymic malignancies [169]. They recommended that the areas such as those immediate to the pericardium, pleura, or other structures of interest be identified by the surgeon and that the surgeon should help orient the specimen to the pathologist before placing it in formalin. Removal of lymph nodes adjacent to the thymus was encouraged. Pathologists should examine resection margins carefully, as incompletely excised thymomas have a higher incidence of recurrences.

(f)

(e)

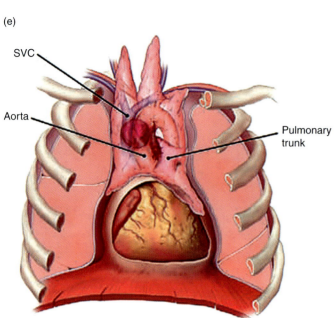

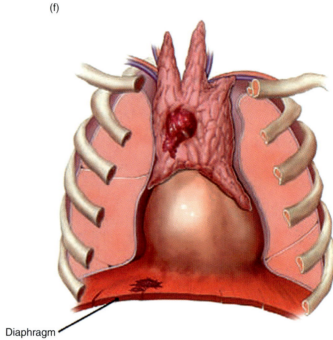

Fig. 6.58a–f (cont.)

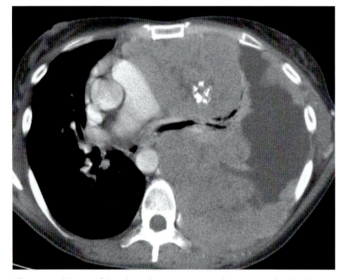

Fig. 6.59 CT scan of the chest showing invasive thymoma with pleural implants and a pleural effusion.

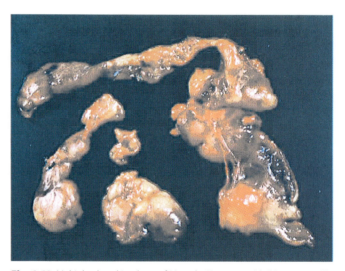

Fig. 6.60 Multiple pleural implants of Masaoka-Koga stage IVa/Moran stage IIIa thymoma, resected at thoracotomy.

The use of post-operative radiation therapy for the treatment of stage I and II thymoma patients has been controversial but there is no evidence demonstrating survival advantages, particularly as the neoplasms tend to recur as pleural or mediastinal nodules separate from the original tumor site [228–231].

Patients with stage III thymomas are treated with radical thymectomy and procedures that sometimes involve vascular grafts [226]. The value of neo-adjuvant and adjuvant chemotherapy is being investigated [230,232]. Most patients are treated with post-operative radiation therapy, with variable results.

Patients with stage IVa thymomas (Fig. 6.59) undergo surgical resection of their pleural nodules and tumor debulking (Fig. 6.60), followed in selected patients by radiation therapy and chemotherapy [49,211,225,228,233–239]. Patients with stage IVb disease (Fig. 6.61) are treated with chemotherapy.

Patients with thymomas need to be followed clinically for long periods of time, as the neoplasms can recur up to 20 years following initial diagnosis.

Table 6.6 summarizes the results of various cohorts of thymoma patients. Fig. 6.62 shows survival statistics of a group of thymomas staged by Masaoka-Koga, as recently reported by

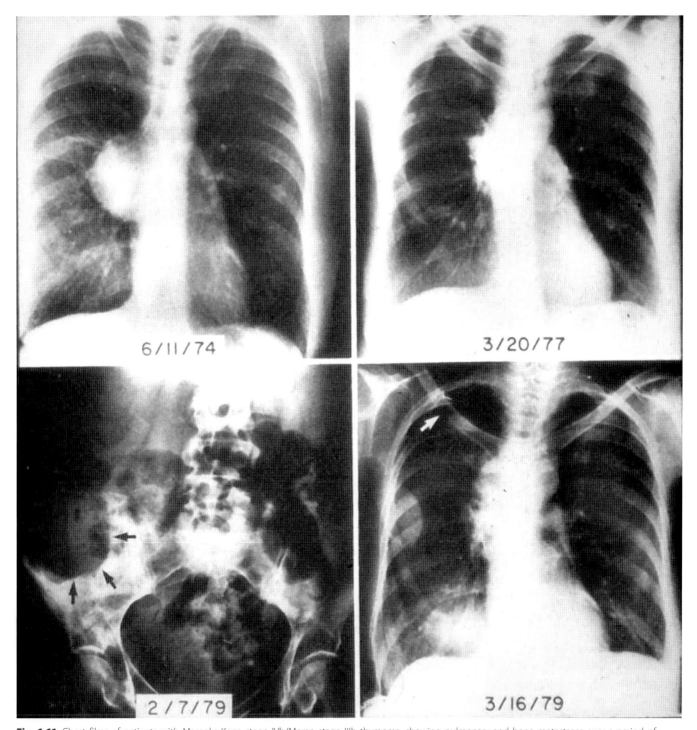

Fig. 6.61 Chest films of patients with Masaoka-Koga stage IVb/Moran stage IIIb thymoma, showing pulmonary and bone metastases over a period of five years.

Masaoka [222]. Figs. 6.63 and 6.64 show the experience at M.D. Anderson Cancer Center, reported by Moran *et al.* [168].

Thymomas in children

Thymomas have been reported in children as young as eight months of age and present several distinct clinical features in patients younger than 15 years of age [28,240,241].

Thymomas are infrequent in children. They account for 12% to 20% of all mediastinal tumors in adults but only 5% of mediastinal neoplasms in children. Most mediastinal tumors in patients younger than 15 years of age are teratomas or lymphoid tumors.

The clinical presentation of the thymic neoplasm may also be different in young patients. Thymomas are

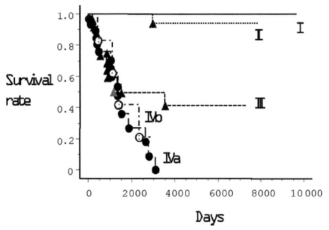

Masaoka stages and progression-free survival.
Those of stage IVa and IVb become nearly superimposed. I versus any stage: not available; II versus III: $p < 0.0001$; II versus IVa: $p < 0.0001$; II versus IVb: $p < 0.0001$; III versus IVa: $p = 0.1028$; III versus IVb: $p = 0.7426$; IVa versus IVb: $p = 0.6021$.

Fig. 6.62 Progression-free survival of thymoma patients staged by the Masaoka-Koga system [220].

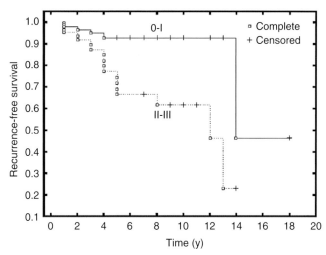

Recurrence-free survival curve showing a statistically significant difference ($P = 0.016$). Kaplan-Meier analysis; cumulative proportion surviving, n = 231.

Fig. 6.63 Recurrence-free survival of thymoma patients staged by the system of Moran et al. [166].

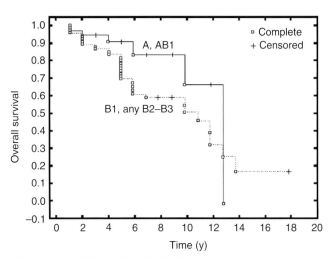

Comparison of histologic subtyping for types A and AB1 vs B1, B2, and B3 and overall survival (Kaplan–Meier analysis; comulative proportion surviving, n = 231). $P = 0.226$ (statistically not significant).

Fig. 6.64 Overall survival of thymoma cases as categorized by WHO tumor type, as reviewed at the MD Anderson Cancer Center [169].

frequently symptomatic, and patients present with signs and symptoms of respiratory and/or vascular compression including cough, dyspnea, cyanosis, wheezing, and superior vena cava syndrome. Except for a few isolated reports of MG, aplastic anemia, or leukemia, most children with the tumor have had no associated systemic disease.

The pathologic features of childhood thymomas are somewhat different from those of adults. Dehner and associates suggest that these tumors in young patients lack the typical features of thymomas in adults, such as the distinct

lobulation, and that they are usually composed of proliferating bands of epithelium containing numerous Hassall's corpuscles, lymphocytes, and connective tissue septa [242]. These differences probably fall, however, within the wide spectrum of morphologic features that can be found in thymomas.

Thymomas in children have a higher incidence of invasiveness than their counterparts in adult patients. For example, of 12 patients with thymoma reviewed at Children's Hospital Medical Center in Boston, 43% had invasive features [243]. This incidence of invasiveness is higher than the 7% to 33% encountered in adults. Indeed, childhood thymomas may be more aggressive than their adult counterparts. Most lesions reported have followed a rapid clinical course with progression to death within six months of onset of symptoms. Bowie and associates, for example, in a review of 20 patients from the literature and their own experience, reported a 78% mortality in children with thymoma [244]. This survival rate compares with an overall 65% five-year survival rate of adult patients with thymoma.

Other authors have had much better therapeutic results and have indicated that the prognosis of thymomas in children is not necessarily dismal if patients are treated with aggressive surgical excision and adjuvant radiotherapy and chemotherapy. The Boston Children's Hospital patients were staged clinically according to the scheme of Bergh and associates. All patients underwent excision of their primary lesions and satellite nodules [243]. Patients at stages II and III received adjuvant radiotherapy and/or chemotherapy. Four of these patients with more advanced disease survived 15 months to nine years following onset of symptoms. The approximate long-term survival in this series is 60%, similar to that reported in adults with thymomas.

Table 6.6. Overall survival rates of thymoma patients (with permission from Detterbeck *et al.*)

Overall survival references	n	Years included	Treatment (%) R₀	Ch	RT	5–yr suvival (%) I	II	III	IVa	10-yr survival (%) I	II	III	IVa
Regnard *et al.*	307	55–93	85	6	52	89	87	68	66	80	78	47	30
Maggi *et al.*	241	59–88	88	–	–	89	71	72	59	87	60	64	40
de Jong.	232	94–03	41	10^a	33^a	83	89	58	56	–	–	–	–
Verley and Hollmann	200	55–82	–	Few	Most	85	60	––33––		80	42	––23––	
Chen *et al.*	200	69–96	–	4	28	97	94	53	24	90	82	37	_
Ströbel *et al.*	179	–	77^a	12	25	100	100	87	66	100	91	84	47
Park *et al.*	150	92–02	69	–	–	100	88	63	23	–	–	–	–
Nakahara *et al.*^{b}	141	57–85	80	Few	84	100	92	88	47^c	100	84	77	47^c
Wilkins *et al.*	136	57–97	68	7	37	84	66	63	40	75	50	44	40
Blumberg *et al.*	118	49–93	73	32	58	95	70	50	100	86	54	26^d	–
Quintanilla-Martinez *et al.*	116	39–90	94	1	26	100	100	70	(70)^e	100	100	60	(0)^e
Pan *et al.*^{b}	112	61–91	80	–	–	94	85	63	41	87	69	58	22
Ogawa^b	103	79–98	100	–	100	100	90	56	–	100	90	48	–
Elert *et al.*	102	57–87	–	–	–	83	90	46	–^{e}	–	–	–	–
Kondo *et al.*	100	73–01	84	28	37	100	100	69	57^c	100	100	69	–
Average^f	**2437**					**93**	**85**	**65**	**53**	**90**	**75**	**56**	**38**

Inclusion criteria: results of ≥100 patients, with results by Masaoka stage.
^{a} Estimated from data provided.
^{b} Thymic carcinoma excluded.
^{c} Stage IVa, b.
^{d} 9-yr survival data
^{e} <5 patients.
^{f} Excluding values in parentheses.
Ch, chemotheraphy; R₀, complete resection; RT, radiotherapy.

References

1. Shimosato Y, Mukai K, Matsuno Y. *Tumors of the Mediastinum.* 2010; Washington: American Registry of Pathology.

2. Marchevsky AM, Kaneko M. *Surgical Pathology of the Mediastinum.* 1991; New York: Raven Press.

3. Marx A, Muller-Hermelink HK, Strobel P. The role of thymomas in the development of myasthenia gravis. *Ann N Y Acad Sci.* 2003;998:223–36.

4. Marx A, Schultz A, Wilisch A *et al.* Paraneoplastic autoimmunity in thymus tumors. *Dev Immunol.* 1998;6:129–40.

5. Marx A, Willcox N, Leite MI *et al.* Thymoma and paraneoplastic myasthenia gravis. *Autoimmunity.* 2010;43:413–27.

6. Levine GD, Rosai J. Thymic hyperplasia and neoplasia: a review of current concepts. *Hum Pathol.* 1978;9:495–515.

7. Rosai J. Thymomas, committees, and memory lapses. *Am J Clin Pathol.* 2011;135:648.

8. Rosai J. The pathology of thymic neoplasia. *Monogr Pathol.* 1987;161–83.

9. Finsterer J, Mullauer L. Is resection of a thymoma WHO A indicated in the absence of myasthenia gravis? *Clin Ter.* 2011;162:37–9.

10. Jain RK, Mehta RJ, Henley JD *et al.* WHO types A and AB thymomas: not always benign. *Mod Pathol.* 2010;23:1641–9.

11. Moran CA, Kalhor N, Suster S. Invasive spindle cell thymomas (WHO Type A): a clinicopathologic correlation of 41 cases. *Am J Clin Pathol.* 2010;134:793–8.

12. Suster S, Moran CA. Histologic classification of thymoma: the World Health Organization and beyond. *Hematol Oncol Clin North Am.* 2008;22:381–92.

13. Suster S. Problem areas and inconsistencies in the WHO classification of thymoma. *Semin Diagn Pathol.* 2005;22:188–97.

14. Suster S. Thymoma classification: current status and future trends. *Am J Clin Pathol.* 2006;125:542–54.

15. Koksal D, Bayiz H, Mutluay N *et al.* Fibrosing mediastinitis mimicking

bronchogenic carcinoma. *J Thorac Dis.* 2013;5:E5–E7.

16. Strobel P, Hohenberger P, Marx A. Thymoma and thymic carcinoma: molecular pathology and targeted therapy. *J Thorac Oncol.* 2010;5: S286–S290.

17. Travis WD, Brambilla E, Muller-Hermelink HK *et al. Tumours of the Lung, Pleura, Thymus and Heart.* 2004; Lyon: IARC Press.

18. LeGolvan DP, Abell MR. Thymomas. *Cancer.* 1977;39:2142–57.

19. Engels EA. Epidemiology of thymoma and associated malignancies. *J Thorac Oncol.* 2010;5:S260–S265.

20. Wick MR, Scheithauer BW, Dines DE. Thymic neoplasia in two male siblings. *Mayo Clin Proc.* 1982;57:653–6.

21. Pascuzzi RM, Sermas A, Phillips LH *et al.* Familial autoimmune myasthenia gravis and thymoma: occurrence in two brothers. *Neurology.* 1986;36:423–7.

22. Walter E, Wilich E, Webb WR. *The Thymus: Diagnostic Imaging, Functions and Pathologic Anatomy (Medical Radiology/Diagnostic Imaging).* 2012; New York: Springer.

23. Heitzman ER. *The Mediastinum: Radiologic Correlations with Pathology.* 2012; New York: Springer.

24. Hwang JT, Kim MH, Chang KJ *et al.* A case of invasive thymoma with endotracheal polypoid growth. *Tuberc Respir Dis (Seoul).* 2012;73:331–5.

25. Lavini C, Moran CA, Morandi U *et al. Thymus Gland Pathology: Clinical, Diagnostic and Therapeutic.* 2008; New York: Springer.

26. Lewis JE, Wick MR, Scheithauer BW *et al.* Thymoma. A clinicopathologic review. *Cancer.* 1987;60:2727–43.

27. Kurata A, Saji H, Ikeda N *et al.* Intracaval and intracardiac extension of invasive thymoma complicated by superior and inferior vena cava syndrome. *Pathol Int.* 2013;63:56–62.

28. Yalcin B, Demir HA, Ciftci AO *et al.* Thymomas in childhood: 11 cases from a single institution. *J Pediatr Hematol Oncol.* 2012;34:601–5.

29. Toker A, Tireli E, Tanju S *et al.* Transcaval invasion of right atrium by thymoma: resection via transient cava-pulmonary shunt. *Eur J Cardiothorac Surg.* 2012;41:1175–7.

30. Rosa GR, Takizawa N, Schimidt D *et al.* Surgical treatment of superior vena cava syndrome caused by invasive thymoma. *Rev Bras Cir Cardiovasc.* 2010;25:257–60.

31. Tormoehlen LM, Pascuzzi RM. Thymoma, myasthenia gravis, and other paraneoplastic syndromes. *Hematol Oncol Clin North Am.* 2008;22:509–26.

32. Weigert C. Pathogisch-Anatomischer Beirtrag zur Erbschen Krankhei. *Neurol Zentralbl.* 1901;597.

33. Strobel P, Preisshofen T, Helmreich M *et al.* Pathomechanisms of paraneoplastic myasthenia gravis. *Clin Dev Immunol.* 2003;10:7–12.

34. Strobel P, Helmreich M, Menioudakis G *et al.* Paraneoplastic myasthenia gravis correlates with generation of mature naive CD4(+) T cells in thymomas. *Blood.* 2002;100:159–66.

35. Spuler S, Sarropoulos A, Marx A *et al.* Thymoma-associated myasthenia gravis. Transplantation of thymoma and extrathymomal thymic tissue into SCID mice. *Am J Pathol.* 1996;148:1359–65.

36. Muller-Hermelink HK, Marx A, Geuder K *et al.* The pathological basis of thymoma-associated myasthenia gravis. *Ann N Y Acad Sci.* 1993;681:56–65.

37. Mao ZF, Mo XA, Qin C *et al.* Incidence of thymoma in myasthenia gravis: a systematic review. *J Clin Neurol.* 2012;8:161–9.

38. Piccolo G, Martino G, Moglia A *et al.* Autoimmune myasthenia gravis with thymoma following the spontaneous remission of stiff-man syndrome. *Ital J Neurol Sci.* 1990;11:177–80.

39. de Castro MA, de Castro MA, Arantes AM *et al.* Thymoma followed by aplastic anemia – two different responses to immunosuppressive therapy. *Rev Bras Hematol Hemoter.* 2011;33:476–7.

40. Bajel A, Ryan A, Roy S *et al.* Aplastic anaemia: autoimmune sequel of thymoma. *Br J Haematol.* 2009;147:591.

41. Gaglia A, Bobota A, Pectasides E *et al.* Successful treatment with cyclosporine of thymoma-related aplastic anemia. *Anticancer Res.* 2007;27:3025–8.

42. Coplu L, Selcuk ZT, Haznedaroglu IC *et al.* Aplastic pancytopenia associated with thymoma. *Ann Hematol.* 2000;79:648–50.

43. van SA, Wirtz PW, Verschuuren JJ *et al.* Paraneoplastic syndromes of the neuromuscular junction: therapeutic options in myasthenia gravis, lambert-eaton myasthenic syndrome, and neuromyotonia. *Curr Treat Options Neurol.* 2013;15:224–39.

44. Kon T, Mori F, Tanji K *et al.* Giant cell polymyositis and myocarditis associated with myasthenia gravis and thymoma. *Neuropathology.* 2013 Jun;33 (3):281–7. doi: 10.1111/j.1440-1789.2012.01345.x. E-pub 2012 Sep 19.

45. Miyazaki Y, Hirayama M, Watanabe H *et al.* Paraneoplastic encephalitis associated with myasthenia gravis and malignant thymoma. *J Clin Neurosci.* 2012;19:336–8.

46. Silvestri NJ, Wolfe GI. Myasthenia gravis. *Semin Neurol.* 2012;32:215–26.

47. Wilkins EW, Jr., Castleman B. Thymoma: a continuing survey at the Massachusetts General Hospital. *Ann Thorac Surg.* 1979;28:252–6.

48. az-Manera J, Rojas GR, Illa I. Treatment strategies for myasthenia gravis: an update. *Expert Opin Pharmacother.* 2012;13:1873–83.

49. Spaggiari L, Casiraghi M, Guarize J. Multidisciplinary treatment of malignant thymoma. *Curr Opin Oncol.* 2012;24:117–22.

50. Maclennan CA, Vincent A, Marx A *et al.* Preferential expression of AChR epsilon-subunit in thymomas from patients with myasthenia gravis. *J Neuroimmunol.* 2008;201–2:28–32.

51. Gattenlohner S, Brabletz T, Schultz A *et al.* Cloning of a cDNA coding for the acetylcholine receptor alpha-subunit from a thymoma associated with myasthenia gravis. *Thymus.* 1994;23:103–13.

52. Siara J, Rudel R, Marx A. Absence of acetylcholine-induced current in epithelial cells from thymus glands and thymomas of myasthenia gravis patients. *Neurology.* 1991;41:128–31.

53. Marx A, O'Connor R, Geuder KI *et al.* Characterization of a protein with an acetylcholine receptor epitope from myasthenia gravis-associated thymomas. *Lab Invest.* 1990;62:279–86.

54. Geuder KI, Schoepfer R, Kirchner T *et al.* The gene of the alpha-subunit of the acetylcholine receptor: molecular organisation and transcription in myasthenia-associated thymomas. *Thymus.* 1989;14:179–86.

55. Marx A, O'Connor R, Tzartos S *et al.* Acetylcholine receptor epitope in

proteins of myasthenia gravis-associated thymomas and non-thymic tissues. *Thymus.* 1989;14:171–8.

56. Wilisch A, Gutsche S, Hoffacker V *et al.* Association of acetylcholine receptor alpha-subunit gene expression in mixed thymoma with myasthenia gravis. *Neurology.* 1999;52:1460–6.

57. Marx A, Wilisch A, Schultz A *et al.* Pathogenesis of myasthenia gravis. *Virchows Arch.* 1997;430:355–64.

58. Judd RL, Welch SL. Myoid cell differentiation in true thymic hyperplasia and lymphoid hyperplasia. *Arch Pathol Lab Med.* 1988;112:1140–4.

59. Hayward AR. Myoid cells in the human foetal thymus. *J Pathol.* 1972;106:45–8.

60. Hayward A. The detection of myoid cells in the human foetal and neonatal thymus by immunofluorescence. *J Med Microbiol.* 1970;3:v.

61. Ito T, Hoshino T, Abe K. The fine structure of myoid cells in the human thymus. *Arch Histol Jpn.* 1969;30:207–15.

62. Marx A, Pfister F, Schalke B *et al.* The different roles of the thymus in the pathogenesis of the various myasthenia gravis subtypes. *Autoimmun Rev.* 2013.

63. Kirchner T, Tzartos S, Hoppe F *et al.* Pathogenesis of myasthenia gravis. Acetylcholine receptor-related antigenic determinants in tumor-free thymuses and thymic epithelial tumors. *Am J Pathol.* 1988;130:268–80.

64. Yang H, Hao J, Peng X *et al.* The association of HLA-DQA1*0401 and DQB1*0604 with thymomatous myasthenia gravis in northern Chinese patients. *J Neurol Sci.* 2012;312:57–61.

65. Kont V, Murumagi A, Tykocinski LO *et al.* DNA methylation signatures of the AIRE promoter in thymic epithelial cells, thymomas and normal tissues. *Mol Immunol.* 2011;49:518–26.

66. Deitiker PR, Oshima M, Smith RG *et al.* Association with HLA DQ of early onset myasthenia gravis in Southeast Texas region of the United States. *Int J Immunogenet.* 2011;38:55–62.

67. Vandiedonck C, Raffoux C, Eymard B *et al.* Association of HLA-A in autoimmune myasthenia gravis with thymoma. *J Neuroimmunol.* 2009;210:120–23.

68. Santos SG, Antoniou AN, Sampaio P *et al.* Lack of tyrosine 320 impairs spontaneous endocytosis and enhances

69. Donmez B, Ozakbas S, Oktem MA *et al.* HLA genotypes in Turkish patients with myasthenia gravis: comparison with multiple sclerosis patients on the basis of clinical subtypes and demographic features. *Hum Immunol.* 2004;65:752–7.

70. Antoniou AN, Ford S, Taurog JD *et al.* Formation of HLA-B27 homodimers and their relationship to assembly kinetics. *J Biol Chem.* 2004;279:8895–902.

71. Garcia-Ramos G, Tellez-Zenteno JF, Zapata-Zuniga M *et al.* HLA class II genotypes in Mexican Mestizo patients with myasthenia gravis. *Eur J Neurol.* 2003;10:707–10.

72. Machens A, Loliger C, Pichlmeier U *et al.* Correlation of thymic pathology with HLA in myasthenia gravis. *Clin Immunol.* 1999;91:296–301.

73. Vieira ML, Caillat-Zucman S, Gajdos P *et al.* Identification by genomic typing of non-DR3 HLA class II genes associated with myasthenia gravis. *J Neuroimmunol.* 1993;47:115–22.

74. Zisimopoulou P, Brenner T, Trakas N *et al.* Serological diagnostics in myasthenia gravis based on novel assays and recently identified antigens. *Autoimmun Rev.* 2013; 12:924–30.

75. Aysal F, Baybas S, Selcuk HH *et al.* Paraneoplastic extralimbic encephalitis associated with thymoma and myasthenia gravis: Three years follow up. *Clin Neurol Neurosurg.* 2013;115:628–31.

76. Beard ME, Krantz SB, Johnson SA *et al.* Pure red cell aplasia. *Q J Med.* 1978;47:339–48.

77. Korn D, Gelderman A, Cage G *et al.* Immune deficiencies, aplastic anemia and abnormalities of lymphoid tissue in thymoma. *N Engl J Med.* 1967;276:1333–9.

78. Shibata K, Masaoka A, Mizuno T *et al.* Pure red cell aplasia following irradiation of an asymptomatic thymoma. *Jpn J Surg.* 1982;12:419–23.

79. Saha M, Ray S, Kundu S *et al.* Pure red cell aplasia following autoimmune hemolytic anemia: An enigma. *J Postgrad Med.* 2013;59:51–3.

80. Balikar R, Redkar NN, Patil MA *et al.* Myasthenia gravis and pure red cell aplasia: a rare association. *BMJ Case*

Rep. 2013. doi:pii: bcr2012008224. 10.1136/bcr-2012-008224.

81. Baral A, Poudel B, Agrawal RK *et al.* Pure red cell aplasia caused by Parvo B19 virus in a kidney transplant recipient. *JNMA J Nepal Med Assoc.* 2012;52:75–8.

82. Sreenivasan P, Mani NS. Pure red cell aplasia in systemic onset juvenile idiopathic arthritis. *Indian J Hematol Blood Transfus.* 2012;28:42–3.

83. Masaoka A, Hashimoto T, Shibata K *et al.* Thymomas associated with pure red cell aplasia. Histologic and follow-up studies. *Cancer.* 1989;64:1872–8.

84. Voigt S. Polycytaemia vera associated with thymoma. Case report. *Acta Pathol Microbiol Immunol Scand A.* 1986;94:351–2.

85. Ertel V, Fruh M, Guenther A *et al.* Thymoma with molecularly verified "conversion" into T lymphoblastic leukemia/lymphoma over nine years. *Leuk Lymphoma.* 2013.

86. Sichere P, Galimard E, Fromaget M *et al.* Myeloma and thymoma: an as yet unreported association. *Rev Rhum Engl Ed.* 1997;64:518–19.

87. Weir AB, Dow LW. Response of agranulocytosis to thymectomy in a patient with thymoma and chronic lymphocytic leukemia. *Med Pediatr Oncol.* 1989;17:58–61.

88. Davila DG, Ryan DH. Thymoma, hypogammaglobulinemia, and pernicious anemia. *South Med J.* 1986;79:904–6.

89. Lyonnais J. Thymoma and pancytopenia. *Am J Hematol.* 1988;28:195–6.

90. Fitzmaurice RJ, Gardner DL. Thymoma with bone marrow eosinophilia. *J R Soc Med.* 1990;83:270–1.

91. Kikuchi R, Mino N, Okamoto T *et al.* A case of Good's syndrome: a rare acquired immunodeficiency associated with thymoma. *Ann Thorac Cardiovasc Surg.* 2011;17:74–6.

92. Waldmann TA, Broder S, Durm M *et al.* Suppressor T cells in the pathogenesis of hypogammaglobulinemia associated with a thymoma. *Trans Assoc Am Physicians.* 1975;88:120–34.

93. Habbe N, Waldmann J, Bartsch DK *et al.* Multimodal treatment of sporadic and inherited neuroendocrine tumors of the thymus. *Surgery.* 2008;144:780–5.

94. Montes LF, Ceballos R, Cooper MD et al. Chronic mucocutaneous candidiasis, myositis, and thymoma. A new triad. JAMA. 1972;222:1619–23.

95. Kauffman CA, Linnemann CC, Jr., Alvira MM. Cytomegalovirus encephalitis associated with thymoma and immunoglobulin deficiency. Am J Med. 1979;67:724–8.

96. Kisand K, Lilic D, Casanova JL, et al. Mucocutaneous candidiasis and autoimmunity against cytokines in APECED and thymoma patients: clinical and pathogenetic implications. Eur J Immunol 2011;41(6):1517–727.

97. Chen PC, Pan CC, Yang AH et al. Detection of Epstein-Barr virus genome within thymic epithelial tumours in Taiwanese patients by nested PCR, PCR in situ hybridization, and RNA in situ hybridization. J Pathol. 2002;197:684–8.

98. Borisch B, Kirchner T, Marx A et al. Absence of the Epstein-Barr virus genome in the normal thymus, thymic epithelial tumors, thymic lymphoid hyperplasia in a European population. Virchows Arch B Cell Pathol Incl Mol Pathol. 1990;59:359–65.

99. Inghirami G, Chilosi M, Knowles DM. Western thymomas lack Epstein-Barr virus by Southern blotting analysis and by polymerase chain reaction. Am J Pathol. 1990;136:1429–36.

100. McGuire LJ, Huang DP, Teoh R et al. Epstein-Barr virus genome in thymoma and thymic lymphoid hyperplasia. Am J Pathol. 1988;131:385–90.

101. Yoshida M, Miyoshi T, Sakiyama S et al. Pemphigus with thymoma improved by thymectomy: report of a case. Surg Today. 2012; 20:479–81.

102. Rota C, Lupi F, De PO et al. Pemphigus foliaceous with thymoma and multiple comorbidities: a fatal case. Eur J Dermatol. 2011;21:424–5.

103. Barbetakis N, Samanidis G, Paliouras D et al. Paraneoplastic pemphigus regression after thymoma resection. World J Surg Oncol. 2008;6:83.

104. Winkler DT, Strnad P, Meier ML et al. Myasthenia gravis, paraneoplastic pemphigus and thymoma, a rare triade. J Neurol. 2007;254:1601–3.

105. Gibson LE, Muller SA. Dermatologic disorders in patients with thymoma. Acta Derm Venereol. 1987;67:351–6.

106. Holbro A, Jauch A, Lardinois D et al. High prevalence of infections and autoimmunity in patients with thymoma. Hum Immunol. 2012;73:287–90.

107. Shelly S, gmon-Levin N, Altman A et al. Thymoma and autoimmunity. Cell Mol Immunol. 2011;8:199–202.

108. Sherer Y, Bardayan Y, Shoenfeld Y. Thymoma, thymic hyperplasia, thymectomy and autoimmune diseases (Review). Int J Oncol. 1997;10:939–43.

109. Yapali S, Oruc N, Ilgun S et al. Acute presentation of autoimmune hepatitis in a patient with myasthenia gravis, thymoma, Hashimoto thyroiditis and connective tissue disorder. Hepatol Res. 2012;42:835–39.

110. Karras A, de Montpreville V, Fakhouri F et al. Renal and thymic pathology in thymoma-associated nephropathy: report of 21 cases and review of the literature. Nephrol Dial Transplant. 2005;20:1075–82.

111. Varsano S, Bruderman I, Bernheim JL et al. Minimal-change nephropathy and malignant thymoma. Chest. 1980;77:695–7.

112. Skinnider LF, Alexander S, Horsman D. Concurrent thymoma and lymphoma: a report of two cases. Hum Pathol. 1982;13:163–6.

113. Ridell B, Larsson S. Coexistence of a thymoma and Hodgkin's disease of the thymus. A case report. Acta Pathol Microbiol Scand A. 1980;88:1–4.

114. Souadjian JV, Silverstein MN, Titus JL. Thymoma and cancer. Cancer. 1968;22:1221–5.

115. Lesser M, Mouli CC, Jothikumar T. Hypertrophic osteoarthropathy associated with a malignant thymoma. Mt Sinai J Med. 1980;47:24–30.

116. Palmer FJ, Sawyers TM. Hyperparathyroidism, chemodectoma, thymoma, and myasthenia gravis. Arch Intern Med. 1978;138:1402–3.

117. Vincent A, Waters P, Leite MI et al. Antibodies identified by cell-based assays in myasthenia gravis and associated diseases. Ann N Y Acad Sci. 2012;1274:92–8.

118. Vernino S, Lennon VA. Autoantibody profiles and neurological correlations of thymoma. Clin Cancer Res. 2004;10:7270–5.

119. Smith WF, DeWall RA, Krumholz RA. Giant thymoma. Chest. 1970;58:383–4.

120. Rieker RJ, Aulmann S, Schnabel PA et al. Cystic thymoma. Pathol Oncol Res. 2005;11:57–60.

121. Moran CA, Suster S. Thymoma with prominent cystic and hemorrhagic changes and areas of necrosis and infarction: a clinicopathologic study of 25 cases. Am J Surg Pathol. 2001;25:1086–90.

122. Effler DB, McCormack LJ. Thymic neoplasms. J Thorac Surg. 1956;31:60–77.

123. Bernatz PE, Harrison EG, Clagett OT. Thymoma: a clinicopathologic study. J Thorac Cardiovasc Surg. 1961;42:424–44.

124. Snover DC, Levine GD, Rosai J. Thymic carcinoma. Five distinctive histological variants. Am J Surg Pathol. 1982;6:451–70.

125. Muller-Hermelink HK, Marino M, Palestro G. Pathology of thymic epithelial tumors. Curr Top Pathol. 1986;75:207–68.

126. Muller-Hermelink HK, Marx A. Towards a histogenetic classification of thymic epithelial tumours? Histopathology. 2000;36:466–9.

127. Suster S, Moran CA. Thymoma classification. The ride of the valkyries? Am J Clin Pathol. 1999;112:308–10.

128. Dadmanesh F, Sekihara T, Rosai J. Histologic typing of thymoma according to the new World Health Organization classification. Chest Surg Clin N Am. 2001;11:407–20.

129. Chalabreysse L, Roy P, Cordier JF et al. Correlation of the WHO schema for the classification of thymic epithelial neoplasms with prognosis: a retrospective study of 90 tumors. Am J Surg Pathol. 2002;26:1605–11.

130. Chen G, Marx A, Chen WH et al. New WHO histologic classification predicts prognosis of thymic epithelial tumors: a clinicopathologic study of 200 thymoma cases from China. Cancer. 2002;95:420–9.

131. Detterbeck FC. Clinical value of the WHO classification system of thymoma. Ann Thorac Surg. 2006;81:2328–34.

132. Kondo K, Yoshizawa K, Tsuyuguchi M et al. WHO histologic classification is a prognostic indicator in thymoma. Ann Thorac Surg. 2004;77:1183–8.

133. Okumura M, Ohta M, Miyoshi S et al. Oncological significance of WHO histological thymoma classification. A clinical study based on 286 patients.

Jpn J Thorac Cardiovasc Surg. 2002;50:189–94.

134. Okumura M, Miyoshi S, Fujii Y *et al.* Clinical and functional significance of WHO classification on human thymic epithelial neoplasms: a study of 146 consecutive tumors. *Am J Surg Pathol.* 2001;25:103–10.

135. Sonobe S, Miyamoto H, Izumi H *et al.* Clinical usefulness of the WHO histological classification of thymoma. *Ann Thorac Cardiovasc Surg.* 2005;11:367–73.

136. Moran CA, Suster S. The World Health Organization (WHO) histologic classification of thymomas: a reanalysis. *Curr Treat Options Oncol.* 2008;9:288–99.

137. Suster S, Moran CA. Thymoma, atypical thymoma, and thymic carcinoma. A novel conceptual approach to the classification of thymic epithelial neoplasms. *Am J Clin Pathol.* 1999;111:826–33.

138. Moran CA, Weissferdt A, Kalhor N *et al.* Thymomas I: a clinicopathologic correlation of 250 cases with emphasis on the World Health Organization schema. *Am J Clin Pathol.* 2012;137:444–50.

139. Moran CA, Suster S. Thymic epithelial neoplasms: a comprehensive review of diagnosis and treatment. Preface. *Hematol Oncol Clin North Am.* 2008;22:xi–xii.

140. Marchevsky AM, Wick MR. *Evidence-Based Pathology and Laboratory Medicine.* 2011; New York: Springer.

141. Marchevsky AM, Gupta R, Casadio C *et al.* World Health Organization classification of thymomas provides significant prognostic information for selected stage III patients: evidence from an international thymoma study group. *Hum Pathol.* 2010;41:1413–21.

142. Marchevsky AM, Gupta R, McKenna RJ *et al.* Evidence-based pathology and the pathologic evaluation of thymomas: the World Health Organization classification can be simplified into only 3 categories other than thymic carcinoma. *Cancer.* 2008;112:2780–8.

143. Detterbeck FC, Nicholson AG, Kondo K *et al.* The Masaoka-Koga stage classification for thymic malignancies: clarification and definition of terms. *J Thorac Oncol.* 2011;6:S1710–S1716.

144. Suster S, Moran CA. Spindle cell thymic carcinoma: clinicopathologic and immunohistochemical study of a distinctive variant of primary thymic epithelial neoplasm. *Am J Surg Pathol.* 1999;23:691–700.

145. Weissferdt A, Hernandez JC, Kalhor N *et al.* Spindle cell thymomas: an immunohistochemical study of 30 cases. *Appl Immunohistochem Mol Morphol.* 2011;19:329–35.

146. Eimoto T, Teshima K, Shirakusa T *et al.* Heterogeneity of epithelial cells and reactive components in thymomas: an ultrastructural and immunohistochemical study. *Ultrastruct Pathol.* 1986;10:157–73.

147. Weissferdt A, Moran CA. Pax8 expression in thymic epithelial neoplasms: an immunohistochemical analysis. *Am J Surg Pathol.* 2011;35:1305–10.

148. Cornea R, Cimpean AM, Simu M *et al.* Clinical, morphological and immunohistochemical characterization of a recurrent B1 type thymoma. *Rom J Morphol Embryol.* 2012;53:639–43.

149. Chu PG, Weiss LM. Expression of cytokeratin 5/6 in epithelial neoplasms: an immunohistochemical study of 509 cases. *Mod Pathol.* 2002;15:6–10.

150. Cimpean AM, Raica M, Encica S. Overexpression of cytokeratin 34beta E12 in thymoma: could it be a poor prognosis factor? *Rom J Morphol Embryol.* 1999;45:153–7.

151. Kojika M, Ishii G, Yoshida J *et al.* Immunohistochemical differential diagnosis between thymic carcinoma and type B3 thymoma: diagnostic utility of hypoxic marker, GLUT-1, in thymic epithelial neoplasms. *Mod Pathol.* 2009;22:1341–50.

152. Shiraishi J, Nomori H, Orikasa H *et al.* Atypical thymoma (WHO B3) with neuroendocrine differentiation: report of a case. *Virchows Arch.* 2006;449:234–7.

153. Giaccone G, Rajan A, Ruijter R *et al.* Imatinib mesylate in patients with WHO B3 thymomas and thymic carcinomas. *J Thorac Oncol.* 2009;4:1270–3.

154. Kaira K, Murakami H, Serizawa M *et al.* MUC1 expression in thymic epithelial tumors: MUC1 may be useful marker as differential diagnosis between type B3 thymoma and thymic carcinoma. *Virchows Arch.* 2011;458:615–20.

155. Khoury T, Chandrasekhar R, Wilding G *et al.* Tumour eosinophilia combined with an immunohistochemistry panel is useful in the differentiation of type B3 thymoma from thymic carcinoma. *Int J Exp Pathol.* 2011;92:87–96.

156. Kojika M, Ishii G, Yoshida J *et al.* Immunohistochemical differential diagnosis between thymic carcinoma and type B3 thymoma: diagnostic utility of hypoxic marker, GLUT-1, in thymic epithelial neoplasms. *Mod Pathol.* 2009;22:1341–50.

157. Laeng RH, Eimoto T, Kuo TT *et al.* Corpuscular thymoma: entity or variant of organotypical thymomas WHO B2/B3? *Pathol Res Pract.* 2006;202:697–704.

158. Shiraishi J, Nomori H, Orikasa H *et al.* Atypical thymoma (WHO B3) with neuroendocrine differentiation: report of a case. *Virchows Arch.* 2006;449:234–7.

159. Yoshino N, Kubokura H, Yamauchi S *et al.* Type B3 thymic epithelial tumor in an adolescent detected by immunohistochemical staining for CD5, CD99, and KIT (CD117): a case report. *Ann Thorac Cardiovasc Surg.* 2009;15:324–7.

160. Verghese ET, den Bakker MA, Campbell A *et al.* Interobserver variation in the classification of thymic tumours–a multicentre study using the WHO classification system. *Histopathology.* 2008;53:218–23.

161. Rieker RJ, Muley T, Klein C *et al.* An institutional study on thymomas and thymic carcinomas: experience in 77 patients. *Thorac Cardiovasc Surg.* 2008;56:143–7.

162. Kendall MD. The morphology of perivascular spaces in the thymus. *Thymus.* 1989;13:157–64.

163. Nonaka D, Rosai J. Is there a spectrum of cytologic atypia in type A thymomas analogous to that seen in type B thymomas? A pilot study of 13 cases. *Am J Surg Pathol* 2012;36:889–94.

164. Vladislav IT, Gokmen-Polar Y, Kesler KA, *et al.* The role of histology in predicting recurrence of type A thymomas: a clinicopathologic correlation of 23 cases. *Mod Pathol* 2013 Aug; 26(8):1059–64.

165. Kirchner T, Schalke B, Buchwald J *et al.* Well-differentiated thymic carcinoma. An organotypical low-grade carcinoma with relationship to cortical thymoma. *Am J Surg Pathol.* 1992;16:1153–69.

166. Nobre AR, Albergaria A, Schmitt F. p40: a p63 isoform useful for lung cancer diagnosis – a review of the physiological and pathological role of p63. *Acta Cytol.* 2013;57:1–8.

167. Moran CA, Suster S. On the histologic heterogeneity of thymic epithelial neoplasms. Impact of sampling in subtyping and classification of thymomas. *Am J Clin Pathol.* 2000;114:760–6.

168. Moran CA, Walsh G, Suster S *et al.* Thymomas II: a clinicopathologic correlation of 250 cases with a proposed staging system with emphasis on pathologic assessment. *Am J Clin Pathol.* 2012;137:451–61.

169. Detterbeck FC, Moran C, Huang J *et al.* Which way is up? Policies and procedures for surgeons and pathologists regarding resection specimens of thymic malignancy. *J Thorac Oncol.* 2011;6:S1730–S1738.

170. Marchevsky A, Marx A, Strobel P *et al.* Policies and reporting guidelines for small biopsy specimens of mediastinal masses. *J Thorac Oncol.* 2011;6: S1724–S1729.

171. Cho KJ, Ha CW, Koh JS *et al.* Thymic carcinoid tumor combined with thymoma–neuroendocrine differentiation in thymoma? *J Korean Med Sci.* 1993;8:458–63.

172. Steger C, Steiner HJ, Moser K *et al.* A typical thymic carcinoid tumour within a thymolipoma: report of a case and review of combined tumours of the thymus. *BMJ Case Rep.* 2010. doi:pii: bcr0420102958. 10.1136/bcr.04.2010.2958.

173. Suster S, Moran CA. Primary thymic epithelial neoplasms showing combined features of thymoma and thymic carcinoma. A clinicopathologic study of 22 cases. *Am J Surg Pathol.* 1996;20:1469–80.

174. Suster S, Moran CA, Chan JK. Thymoma with pseudosarcomatous stroma: report of an unusual histologic variant of thymic epithelial neoplasm that may simulate carcinosarcoma. *Am J Surg Pathol.* 1997;21:1316–23.

175. Kang G, Yoon N, Han J *et al.* Metaplastic thymoma: report of 4 cases. *Korean J Pathol.* 2012;46:92–5.

176. Liu B, Rao Q, Zhu Y *et al.* Metaplastic thymoma of the mediastinum. A clinicopathologic, immunohistochemical, and genetic analysis. *Am J Clin Pathol.* 2012;137:261–9.

177. Lu HS, Gan MF, Zhou T *et al.* Sarcomatoid thymic carcinoma arising in metaplastic thymoma: a case report. *Int J Surg Pathol.* 2011;19:677–80.

178. Moritani S, Ichihara S, Mukai K *et al.* Sarcomatoid carcinoma of the thymus arising in metaplastic thymoma. *Histopathology.* 2008;52:409–11.

179. Poorabdollah M, Mehdizadeh E, Mohammadi F *et al.* Metaplastic thymoma: report of an unusual thymic epithelial neoplasm arising in the wall of a thymic cyst. *Int J Surg Pathol.* 2009;17:51–4.

180. Yoneda S, Marx A, Muller-Hermelink HK. Low-grade metaplastic carcinomas of the thymus: biphasic thymic epithelial tumors with mesenchymal metaplasia–an update. *Pathol Res Pract.* 1999;195:555–63.

181. Strobel P, Marino M, Feuchtenberger M *et al.* Micronodular thymoma: an epithelial tumour with abnormal chemokine expression setting the stage for lymphoma development. *J Pathol.* 2005;207:72–82.

182. Suster S, Moran CA. Micronodular thymoma with lymphoid B-cell hyperplasia: clinicopathologic and immunohistochemical study of eighteen cases of a distinctive morphologic variant of thymic epithelial neoplasm. *Am J Surg Pathol.* 1999;23:955–62.

183. El MF, Braham E, Ayadi A *et al.* Micronodular thymoma with lymphoid stroma: report of two cases and particular association with thymic lymphoid hyperplasia in one case. *Pathology.* 2006;38:586–8.

184. Mende S, Moschopulos M, Marx A *et al.* Ectopic micronodular thymoma with lymphoid stroma. *Virchows Arch.* 2004;444:397–9.

185. Moran CA, Koss MN. Rhabdomyomatous thymoma. *Am J Surg Pathol.* 1993;17:633–6.

186. de Queiroga EM, Chikota H, Bacchi CE *et al.* Rhabdomyomatous carcinoma of the thymus. *Am J Surg Pathol.* 2004;28:1245–50.

187. Salih DM, Ceyhan K, Deveci G *et al.* Pericardial rhabdomyomatous spindle cell thymoma with mucinous cystic degeneration. *Histopathology.* 2001;38:479–81.

188. Moran CA, Suster S. "Ancient" (sclerosing) thymomas: a clinicopathologic study of 10 cases. *Am J Clin Pathol.* 2004;121:867–71.

189. Kuo T. Sclerosing thymoma–a possible phenomenon of regression. *Histopathology.* 1994;25:289–91.

190. Weissferdt A, Moran CA. Thymomas with prominent glandular differentiation: a clinicopathologic and immunohistochemical study of 12 cases. *Hum Pathol.* 2013; 44:1612–16.

191. Kalhor N, Suster S, Moran CA. Spindle cell thymomas (WHO Type A) with prominent papillary and pseudopapillary features: a clinicopathologic and immunohistochemical study of 10 cases. *Am J Surg Pathol.* 2011;35:372–7.

192. Onuki T, Iguchi K, Inagaki M *et al.* [Lipofibroadenoma of the thymus]. *Kyobu Geka.* 2009;62:395–8.

193. Moran CA, Suster S, Gil J *et al.* Morphometric analysis of germinal centers in nonthymomatous patients with myasthenia gravis. *Arch Pathol Lab Med.* 1990;114:689–91.

194. Sherer Y, Bardayan Y, Shoenfeld Y. Thymoma, thymic hyperplasia, thymectomy and autoimmune diseases (Review). *Int J Oncol.* 1997;10:939–43.

195. Willcox N, Schluep M, Ritter MA *et al.* Myasthenic and nonmyasthenic thymoma. An expansion of a minor cortical epithelial cell subset? *Am J Pathol.* 1987;127:447–60.

196. Hofmann WJ, Moller P, Otto HF. Thymic hyperplasia. II. Lymphofollicular hyperplasia of the thymus. An immunohistologic study. *Klin Wochenschr.* 1987;65:53–60.

197. Alpert LI, Papatestas A, Kark A *et al.* A histologic reappraisal of the thymus in myasthenia gravis. A correlative study of thymic pathology and response to thymectomy. *Arch Pathol.* 1971;91:55–61.

198. Papatestas AE, Alpert LI, Osserman KE *et al.* Studies in myasthenia gravis: effects of thymectomy. Results on 185 patients with nonthymomatous and thymomatous myasthenia gravis, 1941-1969. *Am J Med.* 1971;50:465–74.

199. Pascoe HR, Miner MS. An ultrastructural study of nine thymomas. *Cancer.* 1976;37:317–26.

200. Pedraza MA. Thymoma immunological and ultrastructural characterization. *Cancer.* 1977;39:1455–61.

201. Bloodworth JM, Jr., Hiratsuka H, Hickey RC et al. Ultrastructure of the human thymus, thymic tumors, and myasthenia gravis. *Pathol Annu.* 1975;10:329–91.

202. Low TL. Biochemical characterization of thymic hormones in thymoma tissues. *Thymus.* 1990;15:93–105.

203. Low TL, Goldstein AL. Thymic hormones: an overview. *Methods Enzymol.* 1985;116:213–19.

204. Chollet P, Plagne R, Fonck Y et al. Thymoma with hypersecretion of thymic hormone. *Thymus.* 1981;3:321–34.

205. Ranelletti FO, Iacobelli S, Carmignani M et al. Glucocorticoid receptors and in vitro corticosensitivity in human thymoma. *Cancer Res.* 1980;40:2020–5.

206. Ranelletti FO, Carmignani M, Marchetti P et al. Estrogen binding by neoplastic human thymus cytosol. *Eur J Cancer.* 1980;16:951–5.

207. Davies SE, Macartney JC, Camplejohn RS et al. DNA flow cytometry of thymomas. *Histopathology.* 1989;15:77–83.

208. Kristoffersson U, Heim S, Mandahl N et al. Multiple clonal chromosome aberrations in two thymomas. *Cancer Genet Cytogenet.* 1989;41:93–8.

209. Abraham KM, Levin SD, Marth JD et al. Thymic tumorigenesis induced by overexpression of p56lck. *Proc Natl Acad Sci U S A.* 1991;88:3977–81.

210. Barthlott T, Keller MP, Krenger W et al. A short primer on early molecular and cellular events in thymus organogenesis and replacement. *Swiss Med Wkly.* 2007;137 Suppl 155:9S–13S.

211. Girard N. Chemotherapy and targeted agents for thymic malignancies. *Expert Rev Anticancer Ther.* 2012;12:685–95.

212. Manley NR. Thymus organogenesis and molecular mechanisms of thymic epithelial cell differentiation. *Semin Immunol.* 2000;12:421–8.

213. Sasaki H, Ide N, Fukai I et al. Gene expression analysis of human thymoma correlates with tumor stage. *Int J Cancer.* 2002;101:342–7.

214. Weissferdt A, Wistuba II, Moran CA. Molecular aspects of thymic carcinoma. *Lung Cancer.* 2012;78:127–32.

215. Girard N. Thymic tumors: relevant molecular data in the clinic. *J Thorac Oncol.* 2010;5:S291–S295.

216. Mentzer SJ, Swanson SJ, DeCamp MM et al. Mediastinoscopy, thoracoscopy, and video-assisted thoracic surgery in the diagnosis and staging of lung cancer. *Chest.* 1997;112:239S–241S.

217. Vilmann P, Puri R. The complete "medical" mediastinoscopy (EUS-FNA + EBUS-TBNA). *Minerva Med.* 2007;98:331–8.

218. Zakkar M, Tan C, Hunt I. Is video mediastinoscopy a safer and more effective procedure than conventional mediastinoscopy? *Interact Cardiovasc Thorac Surg.* 2012;14:81–4.

219. Girard N, Shen R, Guo T et al. Comprehensive genomic analysis reveals clinically relevant molecular distinctions between thymic carcinomas and thymomas. *Clin Cancer Res.* 2009;15:6790–9.

220. Zakowski MF, Huang J, Bramlage MP. The role of fine needle aspiration cytology in the diagnosis and management of thymic neoplasia. *J Thorac Oncol.* 2010;5:S281–S285.

221. Bergh NP, Gatzinsky P, Larsson S et al. Tumors of the thymus and thymic region: I. Clinicopathological studies on thymomas. *Ann Thorac Surg.* 1978;25:91–8.

222. Masaoka A. Staging system of thymoma. *J Thorac Oncol.* 2010;5:S304–S312.

223. Gupta R, Marchevsky AM, McKenna RJ et al. Evidence-based pathology and the pathologic evaluation of thymomas: transcapsular invasion is not a significant prognostic feature. *Arch Pathol Lab Med.* 2008;132:926–30.

224. Blumberg D, Port JL, Weksler B et al. Thymoma: a multivariate analysis of factors predicting survival. *Ann Thorac Surg.* 1995;60:908–13.

225. Koppitz H, Rockstroh JK, Schuller H et al. State-of-the-art classification and multimodality treatment of malignant thymoma. *Cancer Treat Rev.* 2012;38:540–8.

226. Lucchi M, Mussi A. Surgical treatment of recurrent thymomas. *J Thorac Oncol.* 2010;5:S348–S351.

227. Detterbeck FC. Evaluation and treatment of stage I and II thymoma. *J Thorac Oncol.* 2010;5:S318–S322.

228. Eng TY, Thomas CR, Jr. Radiation therapy in the management of thymic tumors. *Semin Thorac Cardiovasc Surg.* 2005;17:32–40.

229. Gomez D, Komaki R. Technical advances of radiation therapy for thymic malignancies. *J Thorac Oncol.* 2010;5:S336–S343.

230. Mangi AA, Wain JC, Donahue DM et al. Adjuvant radiation of stage III thymoma: is it necessary? *Ann Thorac Surg.* 2005;79:1834–9.

231. Vasamiliette J, Hohenberger P, Schoenberg S et al. Treatment monitoring with 18F-FDG PET in metastatic thymoma after 90Y-Dotatoc and selective internal radiation treatment (SIRT). *Hell J Nucl Med.* 2009;12:271–3.

232. Weksler B, Shende M, Nason KS et al. The role of adjuvant radiation therapy for resected stage III thymoma: a population-based study. *Ann Thorac Surg.* 2012;93:1822–8.

233. Chahinian AP. Chemotherapy of thymomas and thymic carcinomas. *Chest Surg Clin N Am.* 2001;11:447–56.

234. Chahinian AP, Holland JF, Bhardwaj S. Chemotherapy for malignant thymoma. *Ann Intern Med.* 1983;99:736.

235. Dosios T, Nikou GC, Toubanakis C et al. Multimodality treatment of neuroendocrine tumors of the thymus. *Thorac Cardiovasc Surg.* 2005;53:305–9.

236. Filosso PL, Actis Dato GM, Ruffini E et al. Multidisciplinary treatment of advanced thymic neuroendocrine carcinoma (carcinoid): report of a successful case and review of the literature. *J Thorac Cardiovasc Surg.* 2004;127:1215–19.

237. Loehrer PJ, Sr., Wang W, Johnson DH et al. Octreotide alone or with prednisone in patients with advanced thymoma and thymic carcinoma: an Eastern Cooperative Oncology Group Phase II Trial. *J Clin Oncol.* 2004;22:293–9.

238. Loehrer PJ, Sr., Wick MR. Thymic malignancies. *Cancer Treat Res.* 2001;105:277–302.

239. Schmitt J, Loehrer PJ, Sr. The role of chemotherapy in advanced thymoma. *J Thorac Oncol.* 2010;5:S357–S360.

240. Nikolic DM, Nikolic AV, Lavrnic DV et al. Childhood-onset myasthenia gravis with thymoma. *Pediatr Neurol.* 2012;46:329–31.

241. Iorio R, Evoli A, Lauriola L et al. A B3 type-thymoma in a 7-year-old child

with myasthenia gravis. *J Thorac Oncol.* 2012;7:937–8.

242. Dehner LP, Martin SA, Sumner HW. Thymus related tumors and tumor-like lesions in childhood with rapid clinical progression and death. *Hum Pathol.* 1977;8:53–66.

243. Welch KJ, Tapper D, Vawter GP. Surgical treatment of thymic cysts and neoplasms in children. *J Pediatr Surg.* 1979;14:691–8.

244. Bowie PR, Teixeira OH, Carpenter B. Malignant thymoma in a nine-year-old boy presenting with pleuropericardial effusion. *J Thorac Cardiovasc Surg.* 1979;77:777–81.

Chapter 7

High-grade malignant epithelial tumors of the thymus: primary thymic carcinomas

Mark R. Wick, MD, Alberto M. Marchevsky, MD, and Saul Suster, MD

Until roughly 35 years ago, concepts pertaining to the existence of malignant thymic neoplasms were muddled. It was often stated at that time that tumors with true thymic epithelial differentiation could only be defined as malignant by their behavior, rather than by their morphological attributes. Furthermore, prior to the advent of immunohistology, the diagnostic distinction between such entities as intrathymic germ-cell tumors or lymphomas and thymic epithelial lesions was also made in an inconsistent fashion.

Currently, it is well accepted that although they are rare, high-grade malignant epithelial tumors of the thymus, primary thymic carcinomas (PTCs) do, in fact, exist, and several distinct variants of such neoplasms have been described (Table 7.1) [1-8]. This review presents a synopsis of current thought regarding PTCs.

Definitions, presentations, and etiologies for primary thymic carcinomas

Grossly, thymic carcinomas (also termed "type II malignant thymomas" in some reports) usually lack encapsulation or internal fibrous septation [2]. They have firm to hard or gritty and white-gray cut surfaces, with frequent foci of necrosis and hemorrhage (Fig. 7.1). Some thymic carcinomas (particularly the basaloid squamous type) may demonstrate a close association with remnants of a multilocular thymic cyst on macroscopic examination (Fig. 7.2). Other types, including mucinous and mucoepidermoid thymic carcinoma, often have a gelatinous cut surface (Fig. 7.3) [3-6,8].

Conceptually and microscopically, PTCs are related to, but, at the same time, distinct from, ordinary thymomas. Both of these groups of tumors have a thymic epithelial lineage, but the former lesions have lost the structured, organotypical pattern of differentiation that typifies the normal thymus gland and is retained in thymomas [7]. As such, thymomas are characteristically more bland cytologically than are PTCs; they also contain a variably dense but consistent intratumoral infiltrate of CD99+, terminal deoxynucleotidyl transferase (TDT) and lymphocytes (Fig. 7.4) that are absent in thymic

carcinomas [9,10]. Regional necrosis, nucleolar prominence, and high nucleocytoplasmic ratios are not observed in ordinary thymomas, whereas they are important diagnostic findings in most forms of PTC.

As implied in the foregoing comments, it must be acknowledged that thymoma and PTC are in the same morphological spectrum, albeit at opposite poles of it. Uncommonly, individual thymic lesions are encountered that represent the central zone of this histological continuum, and which demonstrate a mixture of

Table 7.1. Primary thymic carcinomas

Intermediate-grade thymic malignant epithelial neoplasms

Well-differentiated squamous cell carcinoma

  Keratinizing

  Non-keratinizing

Well-differentiated mucoepidermoid carcinoma

High-grade thymic malignant epithelial neoplasms

Lymphoepithelioma-like thymic carcinoma

Adenosquamous carcinoma

Clear-cell carcinoma

Papillary adenocarcinoma

Basaloid squamous cell carcinoma

Sarcomatoid carcinoma

Anaplastic carcinoma

Rhabdoid carcinoma

Mucinous carcinoma

Micronodular lymphoid-rich carcinoma

Primary thymic carcinomas associated with other lesions (grade depends on carcinoma cell type)

Multilocular thymic cysts

Thymoma

Thymolipoma

Pathology of the Mediastinum, ed. Alberto M. Marchevsky and Mark R. Wick. Published by Cambridge University Press.
© Cambridge University Press 2014.

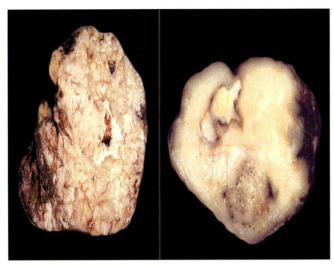

Fig. 7.1 Gross photographs of primary thymic carcinomas, showing fleshy tan-pink masses containing zones of necrosis. No internal fibrous bands are visible.

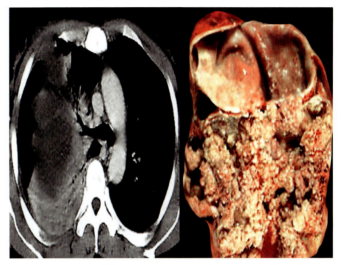

Fig. 7.2 Carcinoma of the thymus arising in a thymic cyst, as shown in a computed tomogram (left) and a gross photograph (right). A remnant of the cyst is visible at the top of the right-sided image.

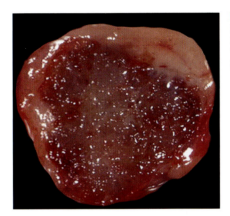

Fig. 7.3 Primary mucinous carcinoma of the thymus has a "gelatinous" cut surface, as shown here.

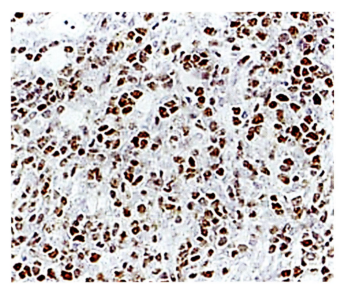

Fig. 7.4 Thymomas are permeated by thymocytes – shown here with an immunostain for terminal deoxynucleotidyl transferase – whereas that type of lymphocyte is lacking in thymic carcinomas.

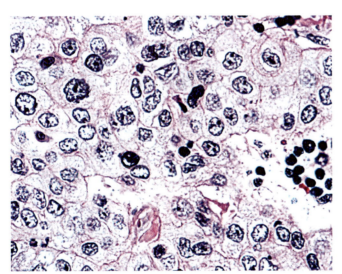

Fig. 7.5 Lymphocyte-depleted with atypia thymomas show nuclear aberrancy in excess of that seen in ordinary thymomas, as depicted here. However, they retain all of the architectural features of the latter tumors, including formation of perivascular serum lakes (right of figure). Thymic carcinomas do not manifest the microarchitectural structure of thymomas.

histological features typifying both thymomas and PTCs. These tumors have been termed "atypical thymomas" by Suster and Moran ("B3" tumors in the World Health Organization scheme); they lack sufficient microscopic criteria (non-organotypical growth, high nucleocytoplasmic ratios, nucleolation, and immuno-nonegativity for CD99 and TDT in intralesional lymphocytes) for an outright diagnosis of carcinoma, but they display more cytological aberrancy than banal thymomas do (Fig. 7.5) [11,12]. Other neoplasms clearly show an admixture of thymoma and PTC in the same mass (see below), implying probable clonal evolution of the latter tumor type from the former [13–15].

Theoretical and nosological problems sometimes arise in distinguishing PTCs from those rare thymomas that

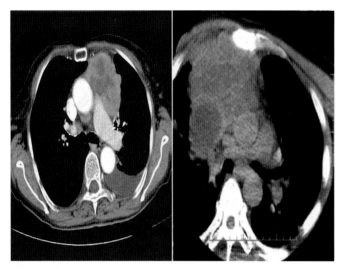

Fig. 7.6 These two computed tomograms demonstrate the obviously-infiltrative nature of most thymic carcinomas.

metastasize outside the thorax. However, because the latter lesions retain their histological identity and are not cytologically anaplastic, the authors prefer the simple and descriptive term of "metastasizing thymoma" to label them.

Another important facet of the pathological definition of PTCs concerns their separation from intrathymic germ cell tumors such as seminoma, embryonal carcinoma, and yolk-sac tumor, all of which show epithelial but not thymic epithelial differentiation. Germ cell lesions usually have characteristic histological appearances that are generally distinct from those of PTCs, and they also manifest immunoreactivity for such cell products as placental-like alkaline phosphatase (PLAP), alpha-fetoprotein (AFP), and beta-human chorionic gonadotropin that are consistently absent in PTCs [16–19]. Both PTCs and germ cell malignancies are reactive for keratin proteins (unlike lymphoma, another important differential diagnostic consideration) but they differ in their synthesis of epithelial membrane antigen (EMA). PTC is generally EMA-positive and germ cell tumors are usually EMA-negative [16,17].

Clinical findings associated with PTCs are relatively nondescript, generally taking the form of chest pain, dyspnea, or the superior vena cava syndrome. Patients with thymic carcinomas are typically middle-aged or elderly adults, with a slight predominance of males. A significant proportion of such tumors are paradoxically discovered incidentally on chest radiographs that are obtained during routine health assessments (Fig. 7.6), but none of these lesions has, to date, been convincingly associated with the paraneoplastic syndromes (e.g., myasthenia gravis, pure red cell aplasia, acquired hypogammaglobulinemia, muco-cutaneous candidiasis) that are seen in conjunction with thymomas [1–8,20].

Tumor size at the time of diagnosis varies considerably, from < 1 cm in serendipitously-discovered masses to > 10 cm. Although the overwhelming majority of PTCs arise in the anterior mediastinum, we have encountered rare "ectopic" examples in other mediastinal compartments, and intrathyroidal or

cervical lesions have been well-described also in the context of the "CASTLE" (carcinoma with thymic-like differentiation) paradigm that was introduced by Chan and Rosai [21].

Etiologic factors for PTCs are almost totally unknown. There is no apparent racial predilection for these lesions, only anecdotal support for possible familial expression, and no consistent association with environmental factors [5,8]. A subgroup of PTCs – namely, some lymphoepithelioma-like carcinomas – may demonstrate integration of Epstein-Barr virus (EBV)-derived nucleic acid into the tumor cell genome, but this has been an inconstant observation and one that is not dispositively related to causation of the lesion [22–25,26].

Specific histologic forms of primary thymic carcinoma

Thymic carcinomas assume a variety of histological images, which will be discussed in the following sections.

Keratinizing squamous cell carcinoma of the thymus

Keratinizing squamous cell carcinoma (KSCC) of the thymus is comparable to histologically-similar tumors of the skin, aerodigestive system, and genitourinary tract [5,8,14,15,27–29]. It is composed of large polygonal cells arranged in groups and cords, and intercellular bridges may occasionally be observed. Nuclei are vesicular or hyperchromatic, typically with easily-seen nucleoli. Cytoplasm is eosinophilic, and keratin "pearls" are, by definition, present at least focally (Fig. 7.7), but it must be emphasized that these can be seen occasionally in ordinary thymomas and do not, in and of themselves, equate with a diagnosis of KSCC [1,30]. Spontaneous "geographic" necrosis and invasion of stromal angiolymphatic spaces are commonly observed as well. The stroma of these tumors is sometimes markedly fibrous (recognized with the name "desmoplastic thymic carcinoma" (Fig. 7.8)), and they commonly extend through the thymic capsule to involve adjacent anatomic structures [8].

Non-keratinizing squamous cell thymic carcinoma

Non-keratinizing SCC (NKSCC), a variant of squamous PTC, differs from KSCC of the thymus because it shows less differentiation [4,5]. The obvious morphological hallmarks of a squamous neoplasm are absent, yielding a tumor that shows angular but cohesive cellular nests with distinct cell membranes, in a fibrous stroma (Fig. 7.9) [5,8,14]. This image differs from that of thymoma because of a greater degree of cytological anaplasia and a lack of distinct intratumoral fibrous septa. Cytoplasm is amphophilic, and associated inflammatory infiltrates, if present at all, are typically sparse.

Lymphoepithelioma-like thymic carcinoma

At this point, few would dispute the fact that "lymphoepitheliomas" of various viscera are, in reality, high-grade and distinctive forms of non-small-cell carcinoma (usually with

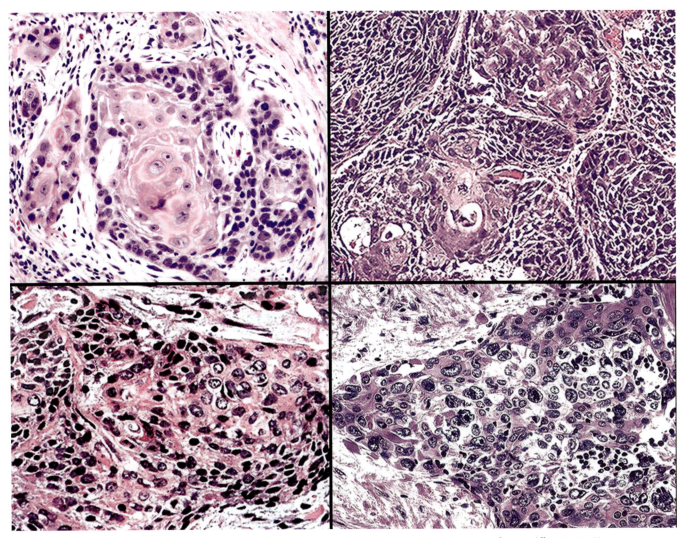

Fig. 7.7 Keratinizing squamous cell carcinoma of the thymus is depicted in these four images, which show a range of tumor differentiation. However, all of these tumors contain obvious keratinization, at least focally.

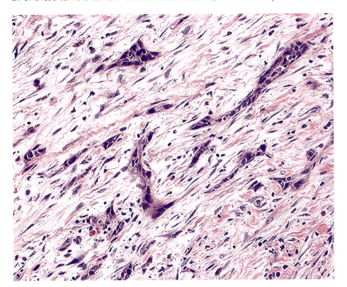

Fig. 7.8 Desmoplastic thymic carcinoma demonstrates a highly-collagenized stroma and narrow cords of tumor cells. It is likely a variant of non-keratinizing squamous carcinoma.

squamous features), and this statement also applies to those lesions that arise in the thymus. Lymphoepithelioma-like thymic carcinoma (LETC) has a histological appearance which, in prototypical form, differs from that of KSCC or NKSCC. It is made up of syncytial sheets of polygonal cells with indistinct membranes, round, uniformly vesicular nuclei, large eosinophilic nucleoli, amphophilic cytoplasm, and a consistent intratumoral population of mature lymphocytes (Fig. 7.10) [5,8,30]. The lesional matrix is usually represented by thin septa of fibrovascular tissue. Areas of regional necrosis are also potentially seen. In some individual cases, the microscopic image of LETC is seen to merge with that of NKSCC.

Adenosquamous and mucoepidermoid thymic carcinomas

Rare PTCs assume histological configurations like those of mucoepidermoid carcinoma of the salivary glands or pulmonary adenosquamous carcinomas [3,30–35]. Both obviously

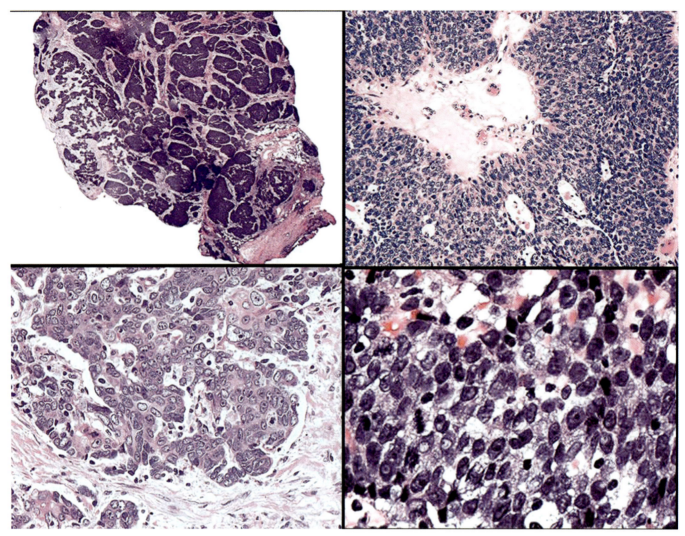

Fig. 7.9 The cells of non-keratinizing squamous cell thymic carcinoma are compact. They show distinct cell borders, the presence of nucleoli, and usually-brisk mitotic activity. No obvious keratinization is present.

exhibit partial squamous differentiation. In mucoepidermoid carcinoma (MEC), areas resembling well-differentiated KSCC are intermingled with others showing goblet cell epithelium disposed around mucinous microcysts (Fig. 7.11). The stroma is generally fibrous, and may be markedly so in some examples. Adenosquamous carcinoma is a high-grade neoplasm that most closely resembles NKSCC microscopically (Fig. 7.12). However, the former of these two tumor types shows definite glandular spaces, often containing mucin, throughout the neoplastic cell population [30].

Clear-cell carcinoma of the thymus

Relatively few cases of clear-cell PTC have been reported [3,36-38]. The lesions show a relatively uniform composition by polyhedral cells with round, vesicular nuclei, discernible nucleoli, and lucent cytoplasm (Fig. 7.13). The latter feature may be ascribed to copious cytoplasmic glycogen, or, in some lesions,

to hydropic cellular degeneration [36,37]. Clear-cell PTC has a vaguely organoid growth pattern and contains delicate fibrovascular stromal septa. Lesional vascularity is inconspicuous, and there are no collections of blood cells in this neoplasm as would be expected in metastatic clear-cell carcinoma of the kidney (Fig. 7.14) [39].

Papillary adenocarcinoma of the thymus

A small number of cases of papillary adenocarcinoma of the thymus have been reported. These tumors showed a mixture of solid and micropapillary growth (Fig. 7.15), with or without focal psammomatous calcification, and were immunoreactive for carcinoembryonic antigen (CEA) but not for thyroid transcription factor-1 (TTF1) [8,30,40,41]. The latter findings are helpful in separating papillary adenocarcinomas of the thymus from ectopic papillary thyroid carcinomas (which are typically CEA-negative and TTF1-positive) diagnostically [40].

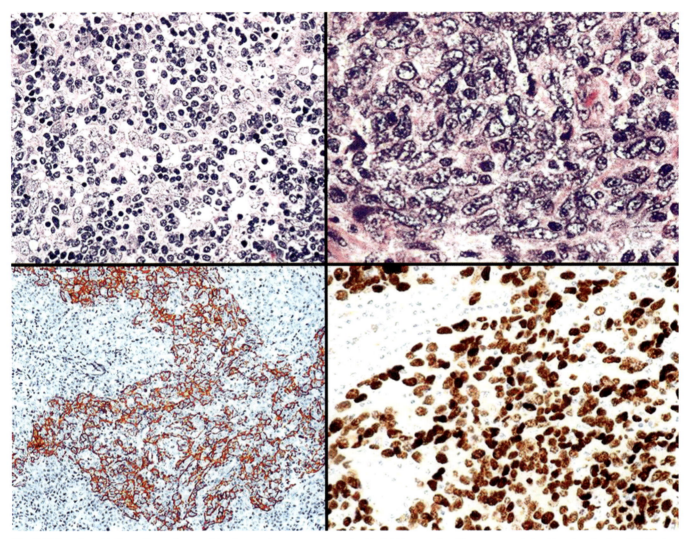

Fig. 7.10 Lymphoepithelioma-like carcinoma of the thymus shows a syncytium of epithelioid tumor cells with numerous admixed lymphocytes (top left). Nuclear chromatin is open, and nucleoli are prominent (top right). A distinctive "interlocking" pattern is seen in keratin immunostains on this tumor type (bottom left); the neoplastic cells are also labeled for p63 protein (bottom right).

Basaloid squamous cell carcinoma of the mediastinum

Basaloid carcinoma (BC) of the thymus is also uncommon. It is composed of groups of compact polygonal cells with high nucleocytoplasmic ratios, little cytoplasm, hyperchromatic round nuclei, and numerous mitotic figures. However, this neoplasm shows no nuclear molding. In addition, it often contains areas with gland-like spaces containing stromal mucin; these produce a vague resemblance to adenoid cystic carcinomas (Fig. 7.16). Moreover, globular eosinophilic deposits of basement membrane or squamous differentiation – rarely, with keratin pearls – are potentially seen in BSCC [3,5,6,8,15,30]. Several cases reported as primary in the thymus have shown a tendency to originate in multilocular thymic cysts [6,30,42–45].

Sarcomatoid thymic carcinoma

A sparse number of sarcomatoid PTCs have been documented. Microscopically, this neoplasm manifests irregularly-arranged fascicles of spindled and pleomorphic tumor cells (Fig. 7.17). Nuclei are usually hyperchromatic, and nucleoli are seen in most cases. Numerous mitoses are seen in sarcomatoid PTCs, and abnormal division figures can be observed as well. Cytoplasm is amphophilic or eosinophilic. Some reported cases have shown small foci in which nondescript epithelioid cell nests were intermingled with the spindle cell elements, and it should be reiterated that obviously squamous, adeno-carcinomatous, or neuroendocrine elements have also been seen in sarcomatoid PTCs [46–48]. Snover *et al.* and Eimoto and colleagues have documented cases of sarcomatoid thymic carcinoma with partial rhabdomyogenic features, including

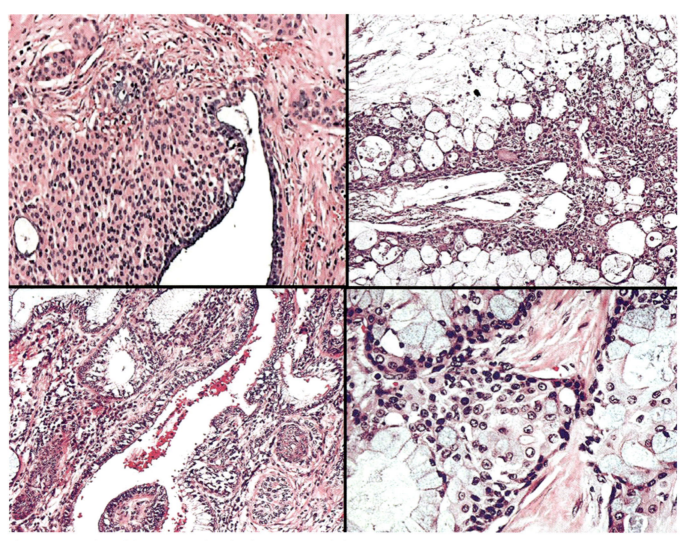

Fig. 7.11 Mucoepidermoid thymic carcinoma has a histologic appearance which is analogous to that of tumors in the salivary glands and lungs. It comprises compact polygonal ("intermediate") cells; obviously-keratinizing foci, and interspersed mucin-producing goblet cells (all four images). Cystic change is common.

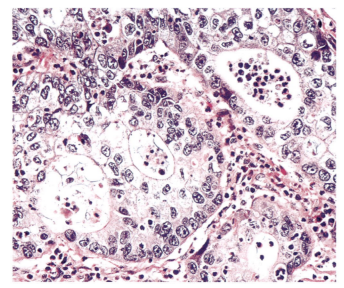

Fig. 7.12 Adenosquamous thymic carcinoma represents a microscopic composite of squamous cell carcinoma and adenocarcinoma, with the formation of glandular lumina.

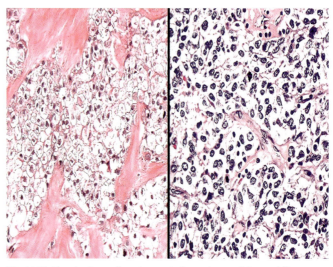

Fig. 7.13 Thymic clear-cell carcinoma is shown here, exhibiting diffuse cytoplasmic lucency and obvious nuclear atypicality. No vascular "lakes" are present in this tumor.

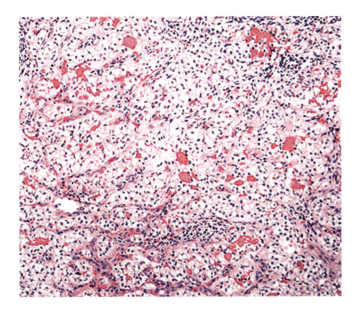

Fig. 7.14 Metastatic clear-cell renal-cell carcinoma (RCC) could be mistaken diagnostically for thymic clear-cell carcinoma. Nevertheless, RCC regularly contains many blood "lakes," as shown here, which are absent in clear-cell carcinoma of the thymus.

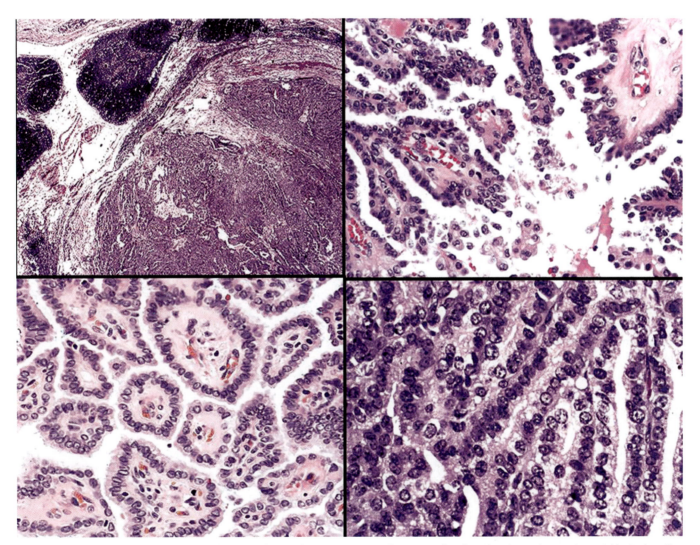

Fig. 7.15 Primary papillary adenocarcinoma of the thymus has a striking microscopic similarity to papillary thyroid carcinoma. It comprises variably-sized papillae which are mantled by compact cuboidal epithelium (top and bottom left panels). Areas of more solid growth are commonly present as well (bottom right).

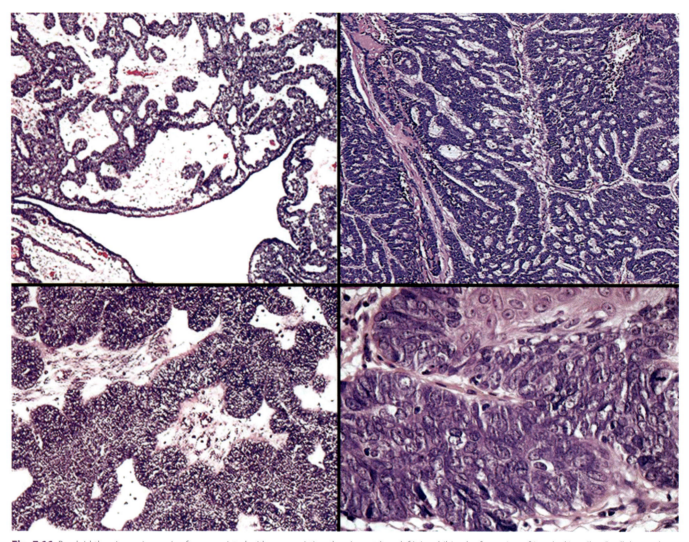

Fig. 7.16 Basaloid thymic carcinoma is often associated with a pre-existing thymic cyst (top, left). It exhibits the formation of interlocking, "lacy" cellular cords which are composed of compact epithelioid cells with high nucleocytoplasmic ratios (top right and bottom panels). Mitotic activity is easily seen in such tumors.

cytoplasmic cross-striations [3,48,49]. Suster and Moran also described examples of this neoplasm in which a transition from pre-existing spindle cell thymoma was found, and others have observed an association with pre-existing "metaplastic" thymoma ("thymoma with pseudosarcomatous stroma") [47,50,51].

Anaplastic carcinoma of the thymus

Weissferdt and Moran documented six examples of anaplastic thymic carcinoma in five women and one man, all of whom were middle-aged to elderly adults [52]. All patients presented with generic symptoms of an anterior mediastinal mass, including shortness of breath, chest pain, and cough. Histologically, the lesions were characterized by infiltrative growth and marked cytologic atypia with bizarre tumor giant cells and atypical mitoses (Fig. 7.18). None of the neoplasms showed patterns of more differentiated forms of thymic carcinoma.

Immunohistochemically, all tumors were labeled for pankeratin, 40% expressed PAX8, and none was reactive for TTF1 or β-human chorionic gonadotropin. Surveillance revealed that three patients had died, at 14, 22, and 63 months respectively after diagnosis, and one was alive at four months. Anecdotal reports of anaplastic PTC have also been made by other authors [52,53].

Rhabdoid thymic carcinoma

Rhabdoid thymic carcinoma is characterized by large cells with eccentric nuclei, prominent nucleoli, and prominent, glassy, eosinophilic, paranuclear cytoplasmic inclusions (Fig. 7.19) [8,54–57]. Immunohistochemical and electron microscopic studies show the presence of filamentous paranuclear cytoplasmic inclusions that label for both pancytokeratin and vimentin. This subtype of PTC is analogous to primary rhabdoid carcinomas of the lung, kidney, and other

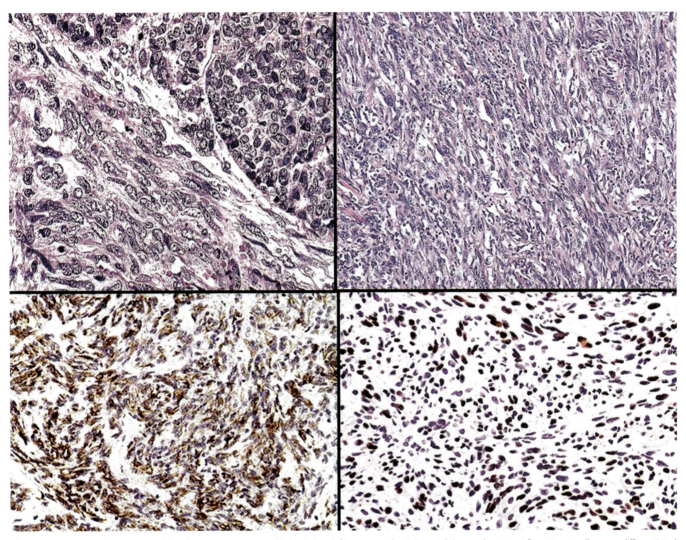

Fig. 7.17 Sarcomatoid carcinoma of the thymus may assume a biphasic (top left) or monophasic (top right) growth pattern. Constituent cells are undifferentiated morphologically, but they exhibit immunoreactivity for pankeratin (bottom left) and often for p63 protein (bottom right) as well.

anatomic sites, and its morphotype equates *de facto* with biological aggressiveness[58,59].

Mucinous carcinoma of the thymus

Mucinous thymic carcinomas resemble mucinous (colloid) adenocarcinomas of other organs, such as the breast and colon (Fig. 7.20) [8,60–63]. They are composed of islands of relatively-bland epithelioid tumor cells suspended in pools of extracellular mucin that label with Best's mucicarmine method, the digested periodic acid-Schiff stain, and the colloidal iron or alcian blue techniques (Fig. 7.21) [62]. As true of papillary PTC, psammoma bodies may sometimes be present in these lesions. Immunohistochemically, the tumor cells are positive for keratin 7 but negative for CD5 [60,61]. An origin in unilocular or multilocular thymic cysts may be seen [42,63]. Mucinous carcinomas of the thymus are immunoreactive for PAX2 and PAX8, but not for mammaglobin, estrogen receptor protein, progesterone receptor protein, or CDX2 (an enteric marker) [60–63].

Micronodular lymphoid-rich thymic carcinoma

Micronodular lymphoid-rich thymic carcinomas (MLRTC) represent the malignant counterparts of micronodular thymoma with lymphoid hyperplasia [64,65,66]. Affected patients are middle-aged to elderly adults, in whom the lesions may be found incidentally on chest radiographs or be associated with chest pain or shortness of breath. These tumors range in size from 3 to 10 cm and are often infiltrative masses that involve adjacent anatomic structures. MLRTCs are composed of epithelial tumor cells arranged in a micronodular growth pattern, set in a stroma exhibiting florid lymphoid hyperplasia (Fig. 7.22). Their epithelial components show overt cytological malignancy and brisk mitotic activity. Immunohistochemical

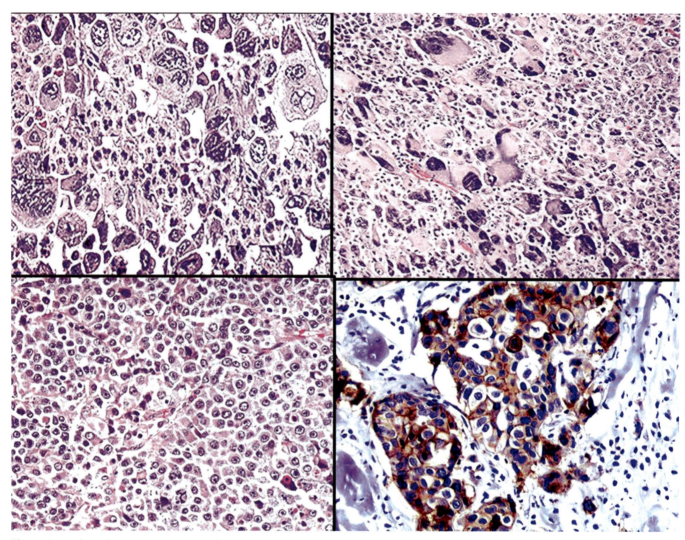

Fig. 7.18 Anaplastic thymic carcinoma contains bizarre, large, pleomorphic tumor cells in most instances (top panels), such that diagnostic consideration may be given to the possibility of a pleomorphic sarcoma. Some of these tumors are composed of only undifferentiated polygonal cells (bottom left). All anaplastic carcinomas are immunoreactive for pankeratin (bottom right), unlike sarcomas.

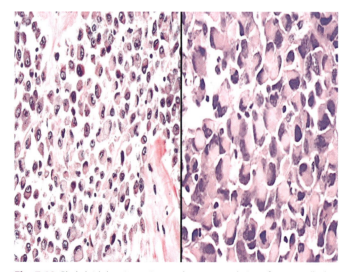

Fig. 7.19 Rhabdoid thymic carcinoma shows a population of tumor cells that contain eccentric nuclei and densely eosinophilic cytoplasm (left), with formation of paranuclear "globules" (right).

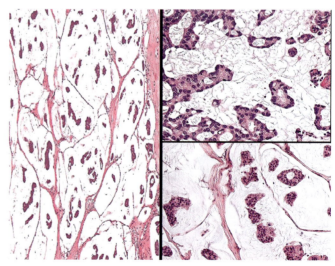

Fig. 7.20 Mucinous carcinoma of the thymus is identical morphologically to "colloid carcinomas" of the breast or gut. They show variably-sized nests of compact polygonal tumor cells that are suspended in pools of epithelial mucin (all panels).

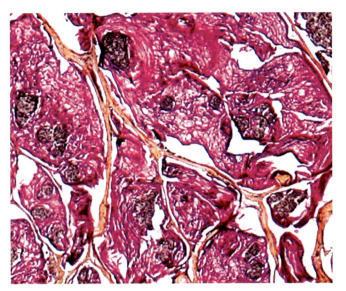

Fig. 7.21 Best's mucicarmine stain can be used to highlight the epithelial mucin in mucinous thymic carcinomas.

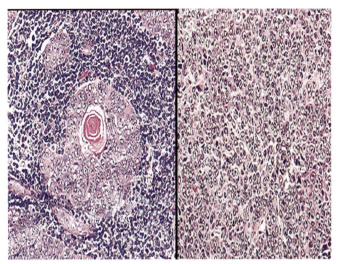

Fig. 7.22 Micronodular thymic carcinoma (MTC) with hyperplastic lymphoid stroma is shown here. It has microarchitectural features which are comparable to those of micronodular "Castlemanoid" thymoma. However, MTC differs from that tumor by manifesting overt cytological anaplasia with high nucleocytoplasmic ratios and prominent nucleoli (both panels).

studies reveal that the lymphoid components are of mixed B- and T-cell lineage [64].

Thymic carcinomas arising from pre-existing lesions

There are three circumstances wherein thymic carcinomas can be a superimposed, complicating component in a pre-existing anterior mediastinal lesion. The first setting concerns thymic cysts – especially multilocular ones – in which several examples of PTC have reportedly arisen [6,42,63,67,68]. Those tumors were of several histological types; however, among them, basaloid squamous carcinoma was over-represented. The other two possibly-antecedent lesions for thymic carcinoma are thymoma and thymolipoma [13,47,50,51,69,70]. Through the process of clonal evolution, histologically-typical thymoma or thymolipoma is juxtaposed to a cytologically-malignant proliferation in the same mass. Immunohistochemical analyses have shown that these are related lesions, but yet definitely distinct from one another. The existence of "secondary" PTC in other thymic neoplasms justifies thorough histopathologic sampling of large tumors because the overtly-malignant components in them may be focal.

Cytopathologic features of thymic carcinomas

The cytopathologic characteristics of thymic carcinomas have not been extensively described in the pertinent literature, in reference to the histologic subtypes outlined above [71–82]. Broadly speaking, the tumor cells in such lesions differ from those of thymoma in showing coarser chromatin, prominent nucleoli, and higher nuclear-to-cytoplasmic ratios (Fig. 7.23). Orangeophilic keratinization may be observed in the cytoplasm in overtly squamous neoplasms. In extrapolation of

surgical pathologic findings, occasional cases of "atypical" thymoma demonstrate relative nucleolar prominence and nuclear enlargement in cytological samples, but their overall images are not fully diagnostic of thymic carcinoma [83].

Adjunctive pathological findings in thymic carcinomas

Ultrastructurally, one encounters several reproducible findings in evaluation of the variants of primary thymic carcinomas considered here. In purely squamous tumors or those with partial squamous differentiation, these include well-formed desmosome-like junctions between the tumor cells and cytoplasmic tonofilaments that often insert into the junctional complexes (Fig. 7.24) [1–4,27,30,72,82,83]. On the other hand, manifestly glandular neoplasms or those with admixed adenocarcinomatous components demonstrate microvillous plasmalemmal differentiation and may contain cytoplasmic mucin droplets as well (Fig. 7.25) [30,40]. Predictably, thymic carcinomas exhibiting a mixture of morphotypes at a light microscopic level will also show admixtures of electron microscopic findings [48]. Interestingly, some publications have described neuroendocrine features, at a subcellular level only, in thymic carcinomas that have few if any endocrine morphological characteristics (e.g., KSCCs, NKSCCs, sarcomatoid carcinomas) [85,86]. This is an example of so-called "occult" neuroendocrine differentiation (Fig. 7.26), and is represented by the presence of neurosecretory granules in the tumors in question.

As in other anatomic sites, sarcomatoid carcinomas of the thymus may show ultrastructural evidence of partial mesenchymal-like differentiation. As cited above, for example, Snover *et al.* documented the presence of

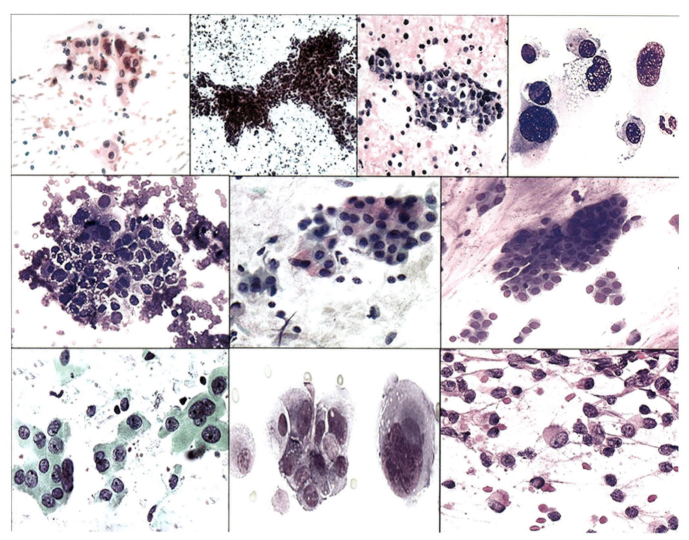

Fig. 7.23 Fine-needle aspiration biopsy images are shown here for several forms of thymic carcinoma. From top to bottom, and left to right, they are represented by keratinizing squamous cell carcinoma; non-keratinizing squamous cell carcinoma; lymphoepithelioma-like carcinoma; sarcomatoid carcinoma; clear-cell carcinoma; mucoepidermoid carcinoma; mucinous carcinoma; papillary adenocarcinoma; anaplastic carcinoma; and rhabdoid carcinoma.

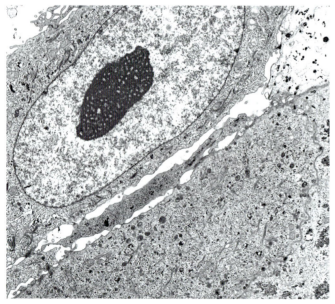

Fig. 7.24 This electron photomicrograph of a thymic squamous cell carcinoma shows the presence of cytoplasmic tonofibrils, inserting into intercellular desmosomes (left lower portion of the image).

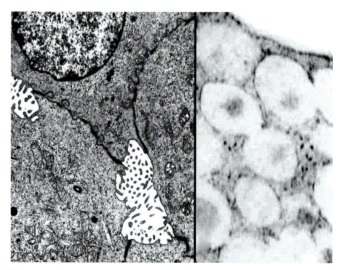

Fig. 7.25 Ultrastructurally, adenocarcinomas and adenosquamous carcinomas of the thymus contain intercellular lumina and microvillous cell projections (left); mucinous carcinomas also manifest numerous mucin droplets in the cytoplasm (right).

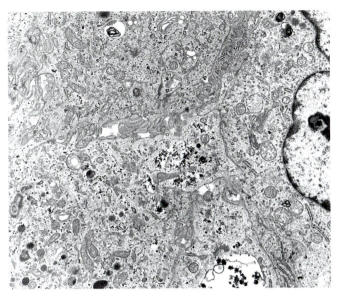

Fig. 7.26 Thymic carcinomas with "occult" neuroendocrine differentiation do not have the histological appearance of a neuroendocrine tumor, but they contain cytoplasmic neurosecretory granules at a subcellular level (lower left portion of the image).

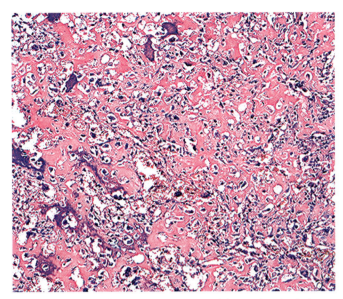

Fig. 7.27 Sarcomatoid thymic carcinoma may exhibit a striking level of divergent differentiation histologically. This particular tumor has the appearance of an osteosarcoma.

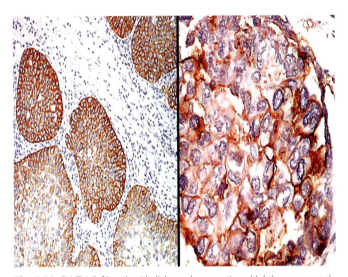

Fig. 7.28 GLUT-1 (left) and epithelial membrane antigen (right) are commonly seen immunohistochemically in thymic carcinoma variants.

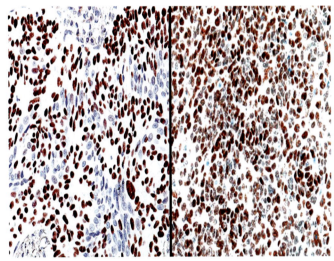

Fig. 7.29 p63 protein (left) and PAX8 (right) represent additional markers that typify thymic carcinomas.

rhabdomyogenous features, complete with cytoplasmic sarcomeres, in one lesion that was studied using electron microscopy [3]. We similarly have encountered occasional sarcomatoid PTCs with divergent striated-muscular, chondro-osseous, smooth muscular, and vascular endothelial differentiation (Fig. 7.27).

Rhabdoid PTC shows prominent, whorled, perinuclear aggregates of intermediate filaments ultrastructurally [56]. This image comports with that of malignant rhabdoid tumors in other anatomic locations [87].

Undifferentiated-anaplastic carcinomas of the thymus manifest only the basic fine structural markers of epithelial differentiation, such as intercellular attachment complexes.

They have no additional morphologic indicators of a particular cellular lineage [88].

Immunohistologic studies of primary thymic carcinomas uniformly show reactivity for keratin proteins, and most of these tumors likewise are labeled by antibodies to EMA, GLUT-1, p63, PAX2, and PAX8 (Figs. 7.28 and 7.29) [71,89–95]. CEA, CD15, MOC31, and the TAG-72 antigen (recognized by antibody B72.3) can be seen as well, especially in lesions with overt or ultrastructural glandular differentiation [17]. Vimentin is variably seen in most subtypes of thymic carcinoma, but is virtually always present in sarcomatoid PTC (SPTC) [92]. SPTC may also manifest reactivity for actin, desmin, S100 protein, and other cell

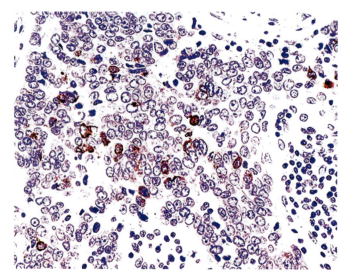

Fig. 7.30 "Occult" neuroendocrine differentiation in a non-keratinizing squamous thymic carcinoma is shown here, reflected by the presence of scattered tumor cells that are immunoreactive for chromogranin-A.

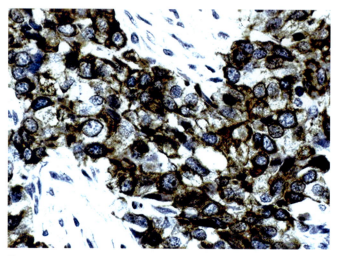

Fig. 7.31 CD5 is often present in thymic carcinomas.

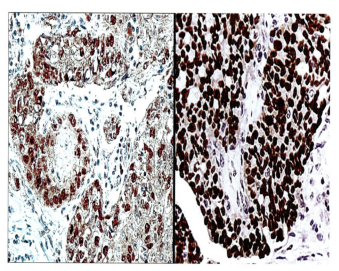

Fig. 7.33 Mutant p53 protein is often present in thymic carcinomas. Keratinizing (left) and non-keratinizing (right) squamous cell carcinomas are shown here, both of which were labeled for that marker.

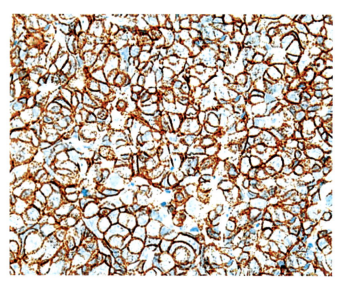

Fig. 7.32 CD117 is another marker that is over-represented in thymic carcinomas; it is not seen in thymomas or in metastatic carcinomas of the thymic region.

products that are usually associated with mesenchymal tissues, because of divergent differentiation in sarcomatoid tumors [96]. Neuroendocrine markers – such as CD56, CD57, synaptophysin, chromogranin-A, and neurofilament protein – are present in those neoplasms that have occult neuroendocrine differentiation (Fig. 7.30) [85,86]. Paradoxically, they are often lacking in small cell neuroendocrine carcinomas because of the primitive nature of those lesions. However, the presence of sharp globular perinuclear immunoreactivity for keratin in such tumors is distinctive and allows for a specific diagnosis even in the absence of other markers [97]. Rhabdoid carcinomas also exhibit prominent localized perinuclear immunolabeling for pankeratin, or vimentin, or both [87].

Several studies have considered the presence of CD5 in the epithelial cells of non-neuroendocrine thymic carcinoma [89,98–102]. In general, those publications reported that CD5 is seen in overtly malignant epithelial tumors of the thymus (Fig. 7.31), but not in thymomas or carcinomas involving the anterior mediastinum by metastasis. However, that paradigm must be qualified somewhat, because atypical epithelial-predominant thymomas (those exhibiting cytological atypia that does not reach the threshold for an interpretation of outright carcinoma) likewise express CD5 in a minority of cases [101]. CD70, CD117, GLUT-1, and mutant p53 protein are also overrepresented in carcinomatous primary thymic tumors (Figs. 7.32 and 7.33), in comparison with thymomas [103–108]. Conjoint immunoreactivity for p63, PAX8, and/or PAX2 is common in PTCs, and helps to exclude the possibility of a metastasis to the mediastinum from somewhere else, as well as ruling out a germ cell tumor or a hematolymphoid lesion.

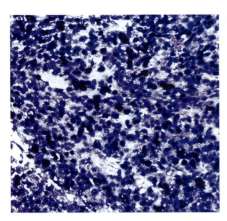

Fig. 7.34 A subset of lymphoepithelioma-like thymic carcinomas show the presence of integrated nucleic acid from the Epstein–Barr virus, as demonstrated in this RNA in-situ hybridization study.

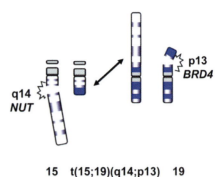

Fig. 7.35 Midline *NUT* carcinomas of the mediastinum feature the presence of a balanced t(15;19) chromosomal translocation, producing a *NUT-BRD* ¾ fusion gene.

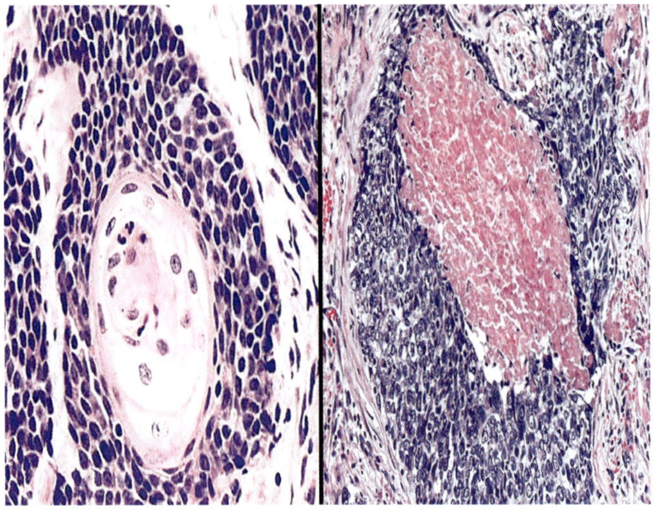

15   t(15;19)(q14;p13)   19

Fig. 7.36 Midline *NUT* carcinomas show variable degrees of squamous differentiation, as shown in these two images.

Chan and colleagues reported that both thymic carcinomas and metastatic carcinomas in the anterior mediastinum are devoid of CD99-reactive, TDT+ lymphocytes [9].

Utilizing in-situ hybridization and probes to Epstein-Barr virus early ribonucleic acid-l (EBER-l) or *BZLFI* transactivator, some workers have demonstrated genomic integration of EBV nucleic acid sequences in a minority of thymic carcinomas of the lymphoepithelioma-like type (Fig. 7.34) [24,109]. Nevertheless, those findings do not have much diagnostic usefulness for three reasons: the frequency of positive results is small; lymphoepithelioma-like carcinomas arising in extrathymic locations (especially the nasopharynx) are also potentially EBV-positive; and other mediastinal tumors besides lymphoepithelioma-like PTCs have been largely unstudied for EBV-related markers. Comparable statements apply to *bcl*-2 protein and the *mcl*-l gene product – both of which affect the regulation of programmed cell death – in PTCs [110].

In the early 1990s, several investigators recognized a peculiar subset of primary carcinomas that arose in midline locations, including the thymic region, often in adolescents or

young adults [111–113]. The lesions were unified by a balanced t(15;19) chromosomal translocation, and they demonstrated a squamoid morphological appearance (Figs. 7.35 and 7.36). Further studies by French and colleagues showed that the operative cytogenetic abnormalities in most cases were fusions of the Bearded (*BRD*) 3 or *BRD4* genes with the Nuclear Protein in Testis (*NUT*) gene, which resides at chromosomal locus 15q14 [114]. Alternatively, *NUT* rearrangements are found in the absence of an association with *BRD* genes in a subset of tumors [115]. The majority of *NUT* midline carcinomas show an aggressive biological behavior with a poor response to conventional treatments [116–119].

Differential diagnosis of thymic carcinomas

The differential diagnosis of primary carcinomas of the thymus is paramount in importance, owing to the rarity of these tumors and the likelihood that most lesions thought possibly to be PTCs are not. A wide array of other neoplasms must be considered interpretatively in this context, as discussed below.

Metastatic mediastinal carcinomas

It cannot be stated too strongly that metastatic lesions comprise nearly all malignant somatic epithelial tumors of the anterior mediastinum. These usually arise in the respiratory or upper alimentary tracts (Fig. 7.37), but other sites of origin (e.g., kidney; breast; ovary; prostate) are seen in some instances [120]. Therefore, some skepticism is encouraged before rushing to a diagnosis of PTC. Attending physicians must be told to undertake thorough imaging studies of other organs to exclude a primary malignant extrathymic lesion.

No macroscopic, microscopic, or ultrastructural findings can be used to identify PTCs with absolute certainty [69]. Immunohistochemical studies have some potential for greater definition, as mentioned above. Especially when selected cell products are detected that are known to be absent in PTCs (e.g., thyroglobulin, TTF1, prostate-specific antigen, S100 protein, placental-like alkaline phosphatase [PLAP], OCT 3/4,

119

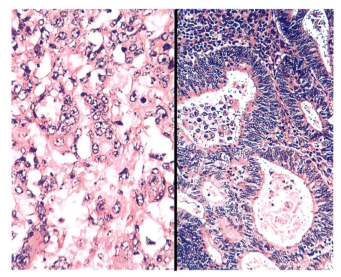

Fig. 7.37 The majority of metastatic carcinomas of the thymic region originate in the lungs (left) or the upper gastrointestinal tract (right).

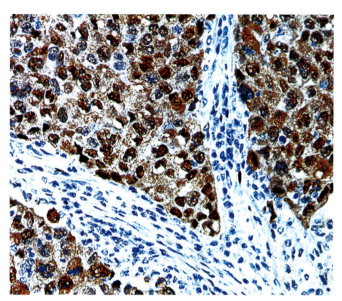

Fig. 7.38 Sometimes, the presence of particular immunohistologic markers will allow for exclusion of thymic carcinoma as a diagnostic possibility. That is true of S100 protein, as seen here in a metastatic ductal breast carcinoma.

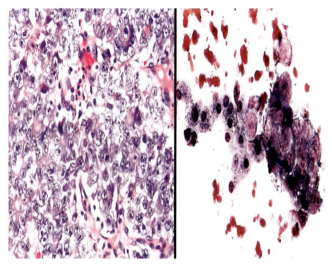

Fig. 7.39 "Solid" embryonal carcinoma of the anterior mediastinum has a histologic (left) and cytologic (right) appearance which is closely similar to that of non-keratinizing squamous carcinoma or undifferentiated-anaplastic carcinoma of the thymus. Those lesions must be separated with adjunctive studies.

Accordingly, the application of ultrastructural studies, immunohistology, fluorescence in situ hybridization (FISH) for isochromosome 12p (which is seen in the majority of germ-cell tumors), or all of these methods, is a necessity in this situation. Non-choriocarcinomatous germ-cell tumors lack tonofilaments as well as fully-developed glandular differentiation, and instead may demonstrate an elaborate nucleolar substructure or cytoplasmic inclusions of AFP by electron microscopy. The great majority of germ-cell malignancies are immunoreactive for PLAP, or OCT ¾, or both, with or without CD30 (Fig. 7.41), and the majority of them lack EMA, whereas PTCs show the converse of that profile [16,17].

Non-Hodgkin lymphomas are devoid of intercellular junctional complexes ultrastructurally, and manifest immunolabeling for CD45 (Fig. 7.42), regardless of whether they are small cell or large cell in nature. Syncytial Hodgkin's lymphoma (Fig. 7.43) has similar electron microscopic attributes, and is keratin-negative but reactive for CD30, in contrast to PTCs [127–129].

CDX2, CA19–9, or CA-125) (Fig. 7.38), one should conclude that a somatic carcinoma is metastatic rather than primary, or, that a germ cell neoplasm is present [18,19,121].

Germ-cell tumors and malignant lymphomas

Germ-cell tumors and malignant lymphomas of the thymic region are both important alternative diagnoses in reference to PTC [18,19,122–126]. In particular, some examples of solid embryonal carcinoma of the thymus and large-cell lymphoma of the anterior mediastinum may be virtually indistinguishable from PTC on conventional microscopy alone (Figs. 7.39 and 7.40).

Malignant melanomas

Very rarely, metastases of nonpigmented malignant melanomas in the mediastinum are the first clinical sign of those neoplasms [130]. Because of this, and the fact that melanoma is a *de facto* inclusion in the differential diagnosis of poorly-differentiated tumors anywhere, it must also be considered in the evaluation of a putative PTC. Electron microscopy may be helpful in that setting because roughly 50% of amelanotic melanocytic malignancies will still demonstrate the presence of cytoplasmic premelanosomes [131]. Immunostains of melanomas are positive for vimentin, S100 protein, and the

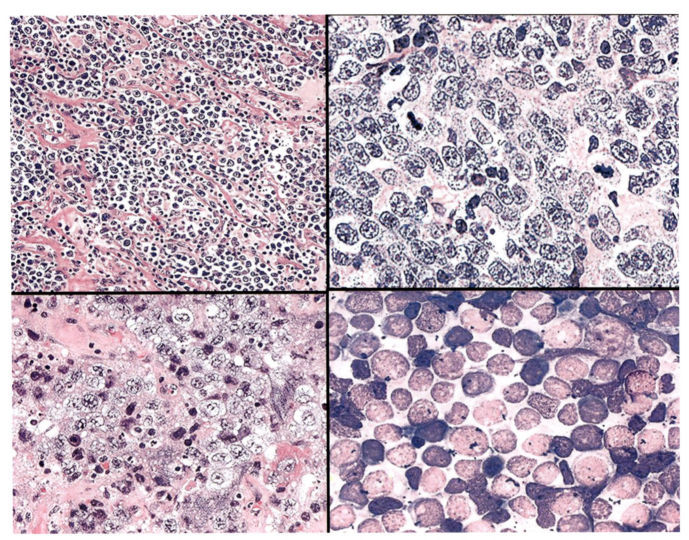

Fig. 7.40 Large-cell non-Hodgkin lymphoma of the anterior mediastinum may be "compartmentalized" by fibrous tissue (upper left), producing a histologic appearance which mimics that of carcinomas. At a cellular level, the tumor cells are undifferentiated histologically (top right and bottom left) and cytologically (bottom right – fine needle aspiration biopsy).

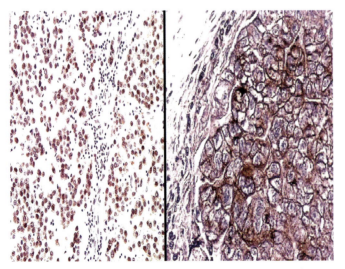

Fig. 7.41 OCT ¾ (left) and CD30 (right) are both immunodeterminants that may be seen in mediastinal germ cell tumors; they are absent in thymic carcinomas.

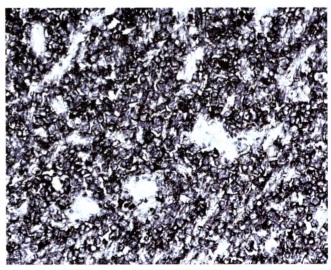

Fig. 7.42 Leukocyte common antigen (CD45) is present in the great majority of non-Hodgkin lymphomas of the mediastinum. It is not seen in thymic carcinomas.

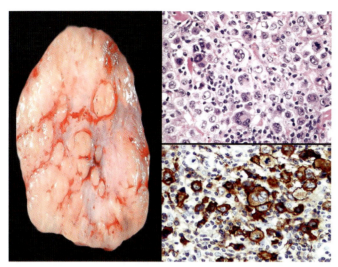

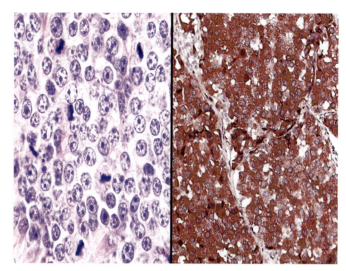

Fig. 7.43 An uncommon variant of nodular sclerosing Hodgkin lymphoma (left) is its "syncytial" subtype. It features sheets of large, atypical tumor cells (top right) which may be confused with those of carcinomas. However, CD30 is consistently present in syncytial Hodgkin lymphoma (bottom right).

Fig. 7.44 Amelanotic melanoma may exceptionally present with metastasis to the anterior mediastinum, simulating the appearance of anaplastic-undifferentiated thymic carcinoma. However, melanoma expresses S100 protein and melan-A (right), both of which are absent in thymic tumors.

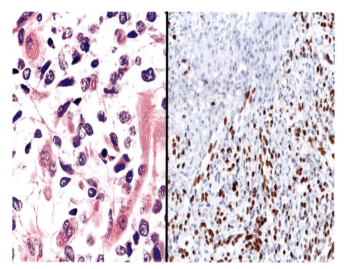

Fig. 7.45 Sarcomatoid carcinomas of the thymus with divergent differentiation may contain tumor cells with striated muscle differentiation (left). These can be labeled for myogenin (right), but other constituents of such lesions are reactive for keratin.

HMB-45, PNL2, or MART-1/Melan-A antigens (Fig. 7.44), whereas keratin and EMA are usually lacking [132].

Sarcomas

Sarcomatoid PTCs may be confused with true sarcomas, even at ultrastructural or immunohistochemical levels of evaluation. That is because of the capacity they have for divergent mesenchymal-like differentiation (Fig. 7.45), as cited above. In general, it should be remembered that a spindle cell or pleomorphic malignancy of the thymic region showing well-formed intercellular junctions by electron microscopy, or keratin immunoreactivity, or both, is overwhelmingly likely to be a carcinoma rather than a sarcoma. A notable exception to this rule is represented by synovial sarcoma, which has indeed been reported in the anterior mediastinum [133–137]. The latter neoplasm shares many of the histological, ultrastructural, and immunohistological features of sarcomatoid PTC (Fig. 7.46). Fortunately, using appropriate probes and the fluorescence in-situ hybridization technique, polymerase chain reaction-based blotting methods, or conventional cytogenetic procedures, the t(X; 18) chromosomal translocation that typifies synovial sarcoma can be identified and used in differential diagnosis; it has not been found in sarcomatoid PTCs [134,135,138]. Both synovial sarcoma and sarcomatoid PTC may label for CD99, but, generally speaking, only PTCs are reactive for p63 [139]. Conversely, nuclear immunolabeling for transducin-like enhancer protein-1 (TLE-1) typifies synovial sarcomas but not PTCs (Fig. 7.47) [140].

Mesotheliomas

Because the pleural surfaces reflect at the boundaries of the mediastinum, various mesothelial lesions may be seen in the thymic region, including mesothelioma (Fig. 7.48) [141,142]. That neoplasm has several potential microscopic appearances, including solid-epithelioid, tubulopapillary-epithelioid, biphasic, sarcomatoid, small-cell, clear-cell, and lymphohistiocytoid variants [143]. Each of those could conceivably imitate the appearance of one PTC subtype or another, as described previously.

Immunohistologic studies are helpful in resolving this particular differential diagnosis, but some important pitfalls are attached to them. Pan et al. reported that one-third of thymic carcinomas are positive for calretinin, or mesothelin, or both, like mesotheliomas [144]. Similarly, thymic carcinomas are frequently positive for CK 5/6 and HBME-1; podoplanin represents another shared determinant in both PTC and

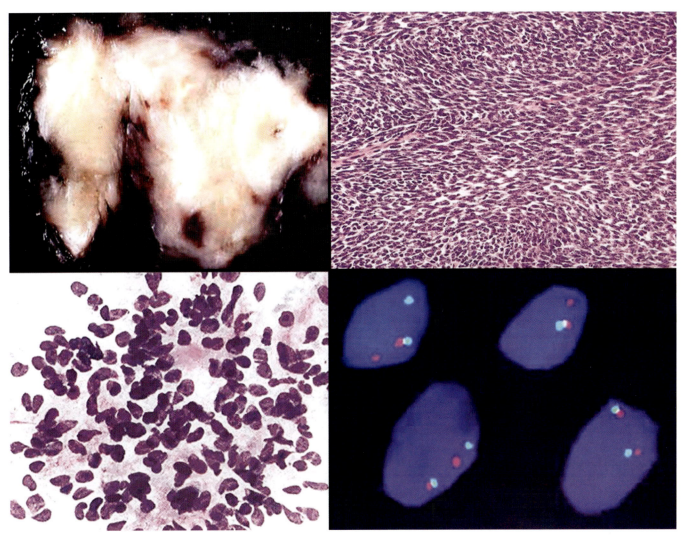

Fig. 7.46 Monophasic synovial sarcoma (MSS) (top panels and bottom left [fine needle aspiration biopsy]) can closely imitate the appearance of sarcomatoid thymic carcinoma. However, MSS shows a t(X;18) chromosomal translocation, represented in an in-situ hybridization study with probes to the *SYT* (green) and *SSX* (red) genes.

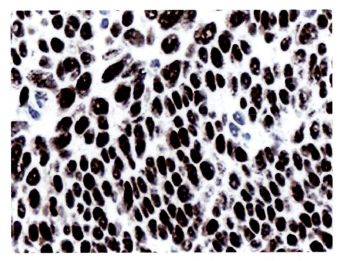

Fig. 7.47 Diffuse nuclear immunoreactivity for *TLE*-1 protein, shown here, is typical of synovial sarcoma but is not seen in sarcomatoid thymic carcinoma.

mesothelioma. In contradistinction to mesotheliomas, PTCs are typically non-reactive for WT1 and thrombomodulin, > 70% of them are positive for Ber-EP4, BG8, and CD15, and virtually all tumors show nuclear reactivity for p63 [144]. The last of those markers is consistently absent in mesotheliomas. Hence labeling for p63, but not for thrombomodulin or WT1, favors the diagnosis of PTC over one of mesothelioma.

Staging of thymic carcinomas

Staging systems for PTCs are still in evolution. In our experience, the Masaoka scheme that is widely used in reference to thymoma does not have similar predictive value for the behavior of cytologically-malignant thymic epithelial tumors [145]. This impression has been validated by the results of Blumberg *et al.* (Fig. 7.49) and Weissferdt and Moran (Fig. 7.50) [146,147,148]. Moreover, the latter authors

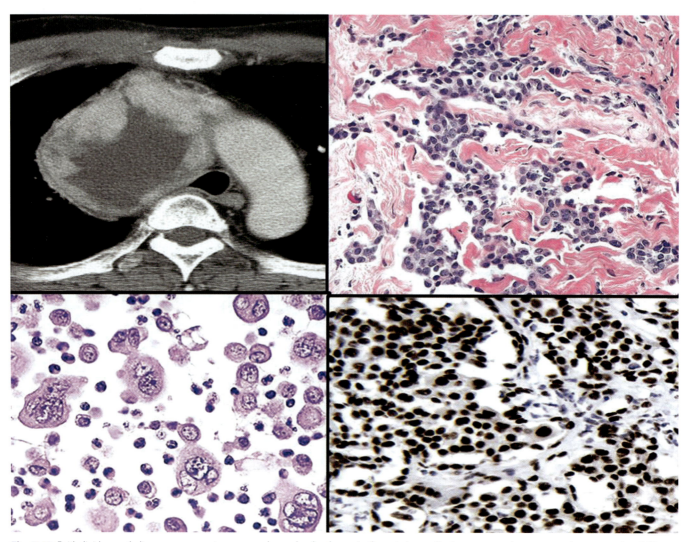

Fig. 7.48 Epithelioid mesothelioma may present uncommonly as a localized mass in the anterior mediastinum, as seen in a computed tomogram (top left). Histologically (top right) and cytologically (bottom left [fine needle aspiration biopsy]), this tumor can simulate thymic carcinoma. Nuclear labeling for WT1 (bottom right) is expected in mesotheliomas but not in carcinomas of the thymus.

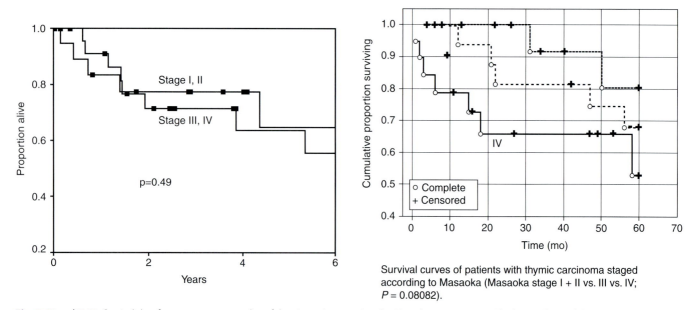

Survival curves of patients with thymic carcinoma staged according to Masaoka (Masaoka stage I + II vs. III vs. IV; $P = 0.08082$).

Fig. 7.49 and 7.50 Survival data from two separate studies of thymic carcinoma, using the Masaoka staging system. The latter scheme did not separate the stages of thymic carcinoma in a statistically significant prognostic manner in either evaluation.

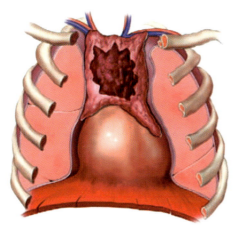

Proposed stage T1, tumor limited to the thymic gland.

Fig. 7.51 Schematic of Weissferdt-Moran Stage pT1 thymic carcinomas.

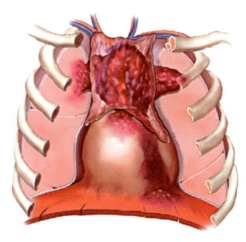

Proposed Stage T2, tumor invading any one or a combination of these structures – visceral pleura, lung, pericardium, great vessels, chest wall, or diaphragm.

Fig. 7.52 Schematic of Weissferdt-Moran Stage pT2 thymic carcinomas.

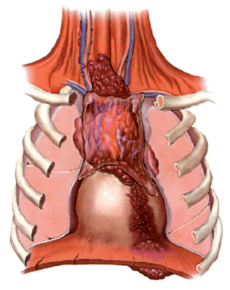

Proposed stage T3, direct (continuous) extrathoracic tumor extension, beyond the thoracic inlet (consisting of the manubrium, first thoracic vertebra, and first ribs and their cartilages) or below the diaphragm

Fig. 7.53 Schematic of Weissferdt-Moran Stage pT3 thymic carcinomas.

found similar deficiencies in a TNM-type staging system that had been proposed by Tsuchiya and co-workers for PTCs [149].

Based on a study of tumors that had been treated at the M.D. Anderson Cancer Center, Weissferdt and Moran recently have devised a novel staging system for PTCs. In that scheme, stage T1 lesions are confined to the thymus; pT2 tumors involve the visceral pleura, lung, pericardium, great vessels, chest wall, or diaphragm; and pT3 PTCs show direct extrathoracic extension beyond the thoracic inlet or diaphragm (Figs. 7.51–7.53). Paired with lymph nodal findings and the status of distant organ sites, those strata were used to construct a 3-tiered TNM system that performed in a statistically meaningful manner prognostically (Figs. 7.54 and 7.55) [148]. A prospective multi-institutional effort is still needed to further test the merits of the Weissferdt-Moran staging system, because of the rarity of thymic carcinomas and the difficulty in accumulating a suitably-powered study group.

Management of thymic carcinomas

Not long ago, it was thought that all non-neuroendocrine PTCs were almost uniformly fatal [150,151]. Nonetheless, one can now predict the clinical course of such lesions with more precision. Some forms of PTC may be cured by surgical excision alone, including well-differentiated KSCC, muco-epidermoid carcinoma, and intracystic basaloid carcinoma. Suster and Rosai observed no deaths in patients with those three tumor types in a retrospective evaluation of 60 PTC cases [152]. Kuo *et al.* and Truong and co-workers obtained similar results [27,28]. Weissferdt and Moran found no meaningful impact of morphotypes on the prognosis of PTC, but they did stipulate that their series was devoid of low-grade carcinomas [147,148]. Another study by Lin and colleagues found that patients with lymphoepithelioma-like (LEL) PTC had the best survival, and those with anaplastic tumors had the worst [153]. They, along with others, supported a primarily-surgical approach to the management of all PTC variants, but they stressed that chemotherapy also was of benefit for LEL-PTC [154,155].

Description

T1	Tumor limited to thymus gland
T2	Tumor invading visceral pleura, lung, pericardium, grea vessels, chest wall, or diaphragm
T3	Direct extrathoracic tumor extension, beyond thoracic inlet (consisting of the manubrium, the first thoracic vertebra, and the first ribs and their cartilages) or diaphragm
N0	No lymph node metastasis
N1	Lymph node metastasis to intrathoracic lymph nodes
M0	No distant metastasis
M1	Distant metastasis (indirect tumor spread, including metastasis to extrathoracic lymph nodes)

Stage groupings

Stage I	T1N0M0
Stage II	T2N0M0
Stage III	T3N0M0
	Any T, N1, M0
	Any T, any N, M1

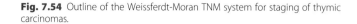

Fig. 7.54 Outline of the Weissferdt-Moran TNM system for staging of thymic carcinomas.

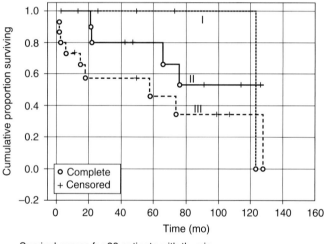

Survival curves for 33 patients with thymic carcinoma according to the Weissferdt-Moran staging system (Kaplan-Meier).

Fig. 7.55 The Weissferdt-Moran staging scheme for thymic carcinoma demonstrated a statistically significant prognostic separation of tumor stages for thymic carcinomas, as shown here.

References

1. Shimosato Y, Kameya T, Nagai K, Suemasu K: Squamous cell carcinoma of the thymus: An analysis of eight cases. *Am J Surg Pathol* 1977;1:109–21.

2. Levine GD, Rosai J: Thymic hyperplasia and neoplasia: A review of current concepts. *Hum Pathol* 1978;9:495–515.

3. Snover DC, Levine GD, Rosai J: Thymic carcinoma: Five distinctive histological variants. *Am J Surg Pathol* 1982;6:451–70.

4. Wick MR, Weiland LH, Scheithauer BW, Bernatz PE: Primary thymic carcinomas. *Am J Surg Pathol* 1982;6:612–30.

5. Suster S, Moran CA: Thymic carcinoma: Spectrum of differentiation and histologic types. *Pathology* 1998;30:111–22.

6. Iezzoni IC, Nass LB: Thymic basaloid carcinoma: A case report and review of the literature. *Mod Pathol* 1996;9:21–5.

7. Marino M, Muller-Hermelink HK: Thymoma and thymic carcinoma: Relation of thymoma epithelial cells to the cortical and medullary differentiation of thymus. *Virchows Arch* 1985;407:119–49.

8. Suster S: Thymic carcinoma: update of current diagnostic criteria and histologic types. *Semin Diagn Pathol* 2005;22:198–212.

9. Chan JKC, Tsang WY, Seneviratne S, Pau MY: The MIC2 antibody 013: Practical application for the study of thymic epithelial tumors. *Am J Surg Pathol* 1995; 19:1115–23.

10. Robertson PB, Neiman RS, Worapongpaiboon S, et al.: 013 (CD99) positivity in hematologic proliferations correlates with TdT positivity. *Mod Pathol* 1997;10:277–82.

11. Suster S, Moran CA: Thymoma, atypical thymoma, and thymic carcinoma: A novel conceptual approach to the classification of neoplasms of thymic epithelium. *Am J Clin Pathol* 1999;111:826–33.

12. Travis WD, Brambilla E, Muller-Hermelink HK, et al. (Eds): *Pathology & Genetics of Tumors of the Lung, Pleura, Thymus, & Heart.* In: World Health Organization Classification of Tumors, Lyon, IARC Press, 2004.

13. Suster S, Moran CA: Primary thymic epithelial neoplasms with combined features of thymoma and thymic carcinoma: A clinicopathologic study of 22 cases. *Am J Surg Pathol* 1996;20:1469–80.

14. Suster S, Moran CA: Primary thymic epithelial neoplasms: spectrum of differentiation & histologic features. *Semin Diagn Pathol* 1999;16:2–17.

15. Suster S, Moran CA: Thymic carcinoma: spectrum of differentiation and histologic types. *Pathology* 1998;30:111–22.

16. Niehans GA, Manivel IC, Copland GT, et al.: Immunohistochemistry of germ cell and trophoblastic neoplasms. *Cancer* 1988;62:1113–23.

17. Wick MR, Simpson RW, Niehans GA, Scheithauer BW: Anterior mediastinal tumors: A clinicopathologic study of 100 cases, with emphasis on immunohistochemical analysis. *Prog Surg Pathol* 1990;11:79–119.

18. Moran CA, Suster S: Germ-cell tumors of the mediastinum. *Adv Anat Pathol* 1998;5:1–15.

19. Suster S, Moran CA, Dominguez-Malagon H, Quevedo-Blanco P: Germ cell tumors of the mediastinum and testis: a comparative immunohistochemical study of 120 cases. *Hum Pathol* 1998;29;737–42.

20. Tormoehlen LM, Pascuzzi RM: Thymoma, myasthenia gravis, and other paraneoplastic syndromes. *Hematol Oncol Clin North Am* 2008;22;509–26.

21. Chan JKC, Rosai I: Tumors of the neck showing thymic or related branchial pouch differentiation: A unifying concept. *Hum Pathol* 1991;22:349–67.

22. Leyvraz S, Henle W, Cahinian AP, et al.: Association of Epstein-Barr virus with thymic carcinoma. *N Engl J Med* 1985;312:1296–9.

23. Dimery IW, Lee JS, Blick M, et al.: Association of the Epstein-Barr virus with lymphoepithelioma of the thymus. *Cancer* 1988;61:2475–80.

24. Wu TC, Kuo TT: Study of Epstein-Barr virus early RNA-1 (EBER1) expression by in-situ hybridization in thymic epithelial tumors of Chinese patients in Taiwan. *Hum Pathol* 1993;24:235–8.

25. Chan PC, Pan CC, Yang AH, et al.: Detection of Epstein-Barr virus genome within thymic epithelial tumors in Taiwanese patients with nested PCR, PCR in-situ hybridization, and RNA in-situ hybridization. *J Pathol* 2002;197:684–8.

26. Engel PJH: Absence of latent Epstein-Barr virus in thymic epithelial tumors as demonstrated by Epstein-Barr-encoded RNA (EBER) in-situ hybridization. *APMIS* 2000;108:393–7.

27. Truong LD, Mody DR, Cagle PT, et al.: Thymic carcinoma: a clinicopathologic study of 13 cases. *Am J Surg Pathol* 1990;14:151–66.

28. Kuo TT, Chang JP, Lin FJ, et al.: Thymic carcinomas: histopathologic varieties and immunohistochemical study. *Am J Surg Pathol* 1990;14:24–34.

29. Chlabreysse L, Etienne-Mastroianni B, Adeleine P, et al.: Thymic carcinoma: a clinicopathological and immunohistochemical study of 19 cases. *Histopathology* 2004;44:367–74.

30. Shimosato Y, Mukai K: *Tumors of the Mediastinum*, In: Rosai J (ed), Atlas of Tumor Pathology, Series 3, Fascicle 21, Washington, DC, Armed Forces Institute of Pathology, 1997;pp 33–273.

31. Weiss LM, Gaffey MI, Shibata D: Lymphoepithelioma-like carcinoma and its relationship to Epstein-Barr virus. *Am J Clin Pathol* 1991;96:156–8.

32. Tanaka M, Shimokawa R, Matsubara O, et al.: Mucoepidermoid carcinoid of the thymic region. *Acta Pathol Jpn* 1982;32:703–12.

33. Moran CA, Suster S: Mucoepidermoid carcinoma of the thymus: A clinicopathologic study of six cases. *Am J Surg Pathol* 1995;19:826–34.

34. Brightman I, Morgan JA, Kunze WP, et al.: Primary mucoepidermoid carcinoma of the thymus: a rare cause of mediastinal tumor. *Thorac Cardiovasc Surg* 1991;40:90–1.

35. Nonaka D, Klimstra D, Rosai J: Thymic mucoepidermoid carcinomas: a clinicopathologic study of 10 cases and review of the literature. *Am J Surg Pathol* 2004;28:1526–31.

36. Wolfe JT Jr, Wick MR, Scheithauer BW, Banks PM: Clear cell carcinoma of the thymus. *Mayo Clin Proc* 1983;58:365–70.

37. Hasserjian RP, Klimstra DS, Rosai J: Carcinoma of the thymus with clear cell features: report of eight cases and review of the literature. *Am J Surg Pathol* 1995;19:835–41.

38. Stephens M, Khalin J, Gibbs AR: Primary clear cell carcinoma of the thymus gland. *Histopathology* 1987;11:763–5.

39. Mattana J, Jurtz B, Miah A, Singhal PC: Renal cell carcinoma presenting as a solitary anterior superior mediastinal mass. *J Med* 1996;27:205–10.

40. Matsuno Y, Morozumi N, Hirohashi S, et al.: Papillary carcinoma of the thymus: Report of four cases of a new microscopic type of thymic carcinoma. *Am J Surg Pathol* 1998;22:873–80.

41. Makino Y, Asada M, Suzuki T, et al.: A case of adenocarcinoma of the thymus. *Jpn J Thorac Cardiovasc Surg* 1998;46:1168–71.

42. Weissferdt A, Moran CA: Thymic carcinoma associated with multilocular thymic cyst: a clinicopathologic study of 7 cases. *Am J Surg Pathol* 2011;35:1074–9.

43. Kawashima O, Kamiyoishihara M, Skata S, et al.: Basaloid carcinoma of the thymus. *Ann Thorac Surg* 1999;68:1863–5.

44. Natsuo T, Hayashida R, Kobayashi K, et al.: Thymic basaloid carcinoma with hepatic metastases. *Ann Thorac Surg* 2002;74:579–82.

45. Tanimura S, Tomoyasu H, Kohno T, et al.: Basaloid carcinoma originating from the wall of a thymic cyst presenting as pericardial and thoracic effusion; report of a case. *Kyobu Geka [Jpn J Thorac Surg]* 2002;55:571–5.

46. Nishimura M, Kodama T, Nishiyama H, et al.: A case of sarcomatoid carcinoma of the thymus. *Pathol Int* 1997;47:260–3.

47. Suster S, Moran CA: Spindle-cell carcinoma: clinicopathologic and immunohistochemical study of a distinctive variant of primary thymic epithelial neoplasm. *Am J Surg Pathol* 1999;23:691–700.

48. Paties C, Zangrandi A, Vassallo G, *et al.*: Multidirectional carcinoma of the thymus with neuroendocrine and sarcomatoid components and carcinoid syndrome. *Pathol Res Pract* 1991;187:170–7.

49. Eimoto T, Kitaoka M, Ogawa H, *et al.*: Thymic sarcomatoid carcinoma with skeletal muscle differentiation: report of two cases, one with cytogenetic analysis. *Histopathology* 2002;40:46–57.

50. Moritani S, Ichihara S, Mukai K, *et al.*: Sarcomatoid carcinoma of the thymus arising in metaplastic thymoma. *Histopathology* 2008;52:409–11.

51. Lu HS, Gan MF, Zhou T, Wang SZ: Sarcomatoid thymic carcinoma arising in metaplastic thymoma: a case report. *Int J Surg Pathol* 2011;19:677–80.

52. Weissferdt A, Moran CA: Anaplastic thymic carcinoma: a clinicopathologic and immunohistochemical study of 6 cases. *Hum Pathol* 2012;43:874–7.

53. Hsu CP, Chen CY, Chen CL, *et al.*: Thymic carcinoma: ten years' experience in twenty patients. *J Thorac Cardiovasc Surg* 1994;107:615–20.

54. Thomas-de-Montpréville V, Ghigna MR, *et al.*: Thymic carcinomas: clinicopathologic study of 37 cases from a single institution. *Virchows Arch* 2013;462:307–13.

55. Falconieri G, Moran CA, Pizzolito S, *et al.*: Intrathoracic rhabdoid carcinoma: a clinicopathologic, immunohistochemical, and ultrastructural study of 6 cases. *Ann Diagn Pathol* 2005;9:279–83.

56. Moreira-deq-Ueiroga E, Chikota H, Bacchi CE, *et al.*: Rhabdomyomatous carcinoma of the thymus. *Am J Surg Pathol* 2004;28:1245–50.

57. Toprani TH, Tamboli P, Amim MB, *et al.*: Thymic carcinoma with rhabdoid features. *Ann Diagn Pathol* 2003;7:106–11.

58. Cavazza A, Colby TV, Tsokos M, Rush W, Travis WD: Lung tumors with a rhabdoid phenotype. *Am J Clin Pathol* 1996;105:182–8.

59. Gokden N, Nappi O, Swanson PE, *et al.*: Renal cell carcinoma with rhabdoid features. *Am J Surg Pathol* 2000;34:1329–38.

60. Choi WWL, Lui YH, Lau WH, *et al.*: Adenocarcinoma of the thymus: report of two cases, including a previously-undescribed mucinous subtype. *Am J Surg Pathol* 2003;27:124–130.

61. Takahashi F, Tsuta K, Matsuno Y, *et al.*: Adenocarcinoma of the thymus: mucinous subtype. *Hum Pathol* 2005;36:219–23.

62. Matsuno Y, Mukai K, Noguchi M, *et al.*: Histochemical and immunohistochemical evidence of glandular differentiation in thymic carcinoma. *Acta Pathol Jpn* 1989;39:433–38.

63. Babu MK, Nirmala V: Thymic carcinoma with glandular differentiation arising in a congenital thymic cyst. *J Surg Oncol* 1994;57:277–9.

64. Weissferdt A, Moran CA: Micronodular thymic carcinoma with lymphoid hyperplasia: a clinicopathological and immunohistochemical study of five cases. *Mod Pathol* 2012;25:993–9.

65. Nonaka D, Rodriguez J, Rollo JL, *et al.*: Undifferentiated large cell carcinoma of the thymus associated with Castleman-like reaction: a distinctive type of thymic neoplasm characterized by an indolent behavior. *Am J Surg Pathol* 2005;29:490–5.

66. Suster S, Moran CA: Micronodular thymoma with lymphoid B-cell hyperplasia: clinicopathologic and immunohistochemical study of 18 cases of a distinctive variant of thymic epithelial neoplasm. *Am J Surg Pathol* 1999;23:955–62.

67. Leong ASY, Brown JH: Malignant transformation in a thymic cyst. *Am J Surg Pathol* 1984;8:471–5.

68. Fukayama M, Nihei Z, Takizawa T, *et al.*: A case of squamous cell carcinoma of the thymus, probably originating from thymic cyst. *Lung Cancer* 1984;24:415–20.

69. Moran CA, Suster S: Thymic carcinoma: current concepts and histologic features. *Hematol Oncol Clin North Am* 2008;22:393–407.

70. Haddad H, Joudeh A, El-Taani H, *et al.*: Thymoma and thymic carcinoma arising in a thymolipoma: report of a unique case. *Int J Surg Pathol* 2009;17:55–9.

71. Kuo TT, Chan JKC: Thymic carcinoma arising in thymoma is associated with alterations in immunohistochemical profile. *Am J Surg Pathol* 1998;22:1474–81.

72. Finley JL, Silverman JF, Strausbauch PH, *et al.*: Malignant thymic neoplasms: diagnosis by fine-needle aspiration biopsy with histologic, immunocytochemical, and ultrastructural confirmation. *Diagn Cytopathol* 1986;2:118–25.

73. Kaw YT, Esparza AR: Fine needle aspiration cytology of primary squamous cell carcinoma of the thymus: a case report. *Acta Cytol* 1993;37:735–9.

74. Geisinger KR. Differential diagnostic considerations and potential pitfalls in fine-needle aspiration biopsies of the mediastinum. *Diagn Cytopathol* 1995;13:436–42.

75. Lucchi M, Mussi A, Ambrogi M, *et al.*: Thymic carcinoma: a report of 13 cases. *Eur J Surg Oncol* 2001;27:636–40.

76. Wakely PE Jr: Cytopathology-histopathology of the mediastinum: epithelial, lymphoproliferative, and germ cell neoplasms. *Ann Diagn Pathol* 2002;6:30–43.

77. Wakely PE Jr: Cytopathology of thymic epithelial neoplasms. *Semin Diagn Pathol* 2005;22:213–22.

78. Assaad MW, Pantanowitz L, Otis CN. Diagnostic accuracy of image-guided percutaneous fine needle aspiration biopsy of the mediastinum. *Diagn Cytopathol* 2007;35:705–9.

79. Wakely PE Jr. Fine needle aspiration in the diagnosis of thymic epithelial neoplasms. *Hematol Oncol Clin North Am* 2008;22:433–42.

80. Zakowski MF, Huang J, Bramlage MP. The role of fine needle aspiration cytology in the diagnosis and management of thymic neoplasia. *J Thorac Oncol* 2010;5 (10 Suppl 4): S281–S285.

81. Singhal M, Lal A, Srinivasan R, Duggal R, Khandelwal N. Thymic carcinoma developing in a multilocular thymic cyst. *J Thorac Dis* 2012;4:512–15.

82. Posliqua L, Ylagan L: Fine-needle aspiration cytology of thymic basaloid carcinoma: case studies and review of

the literature. *Diagn Cytopathol* 2006;34:358–66.

83. Riazmontazer N, Bedayat C, Izadi B: Epithelial cytologic atypia in a fine needle aspirate of an invasive thymoma: a case report. *Acta Cytol* 1992;36:387–90.

84. Walker AN, Mills SE, Fechner RE: Thymomas and thymic carcinomas. *Semin Diagn Pathol* 1990;7:250–65.

85. Lauriola L, Erlandson RA, Rosai J: Neuroendocrine differentiation is a common feature of thymic carcinoma. *Am J Surg Pathol* 1998;22:1059–66.

86. Hishima T, Fukayama M, Hayashi Y, *et al.*: Neuroendocrine differentiation in thymic epithelial tumors with special reference to thymic carcinoma and atypical thymoma. *Hum Pathol* 1998;29:330–8.

87. Wick MR, Ritter JH, Dehner LP: Malignant rhabdoid tumors: a clinicopathologic review and conceptual discussion. *Semin Diagn Pathol* 1995;12:233–48.

88. Kuzume T, Kubonishi I, Takeuchi S, *et al.*: Establishment and characterization of a thymic carcinoma cell line (Ty-82) carrying t(15;19) (q15;p13) chromosome abnormality. *Int J Cancer* 1992;50:259–64.

89. Kojika M, Ishii G, Yoshida J, *et al.*: Immunohistochemical differential diagnosis between thymic carcinoma and type B3 thymoma: diagnostic utility of hypoxic marker, GLUT-1, in thymic epithelial neoplasms. *Mod Pathol* 2009;22:1341–50.

90. Saad RS, Landreneau RJ, Liu Y, *et al.*: Utility of immunohistochemistry in separating thymic neoplasms from germ cell tumors and metastatic lung cancer involving the anterior mediastinum. *Appl Immunohistochem Mol Morphol* 2003;11:107–12.

91. Brown JG, Bamiliari U, Papotti M, *et al.*: Thymic basaloid carcinoma: a clinicopathologic study of 12 cases, with a general discussion of basaloid carcinoma and its relationship with adenoid cystic carcinoma. *Am J Surg Pathol* 2009;33:1113–24.

92. Rosai J. The pathology of thymic neoplasia. *Monogr Pathol* 1987;29:161–83.

93. Pomplun S, Wotherspoon AC, Shah G, *et al.*: Immunohistochemical markers in the differentiation of thymic and pulmonary neoplasms. *Histopathology* 2002;40:152–8.

94. Weissferdt A, Moran CA: PAX8 expression in thymic epithelial neoplasms: an immunohistochemical analysis. *Am J Surg Pathol* 2011;35:1305–10.

95. Laury AR, Perets R, Piao H, *et al.*: A comprehensive analysis of PAX8 expression in human epithelial tumors. *Am J Surg Pathol* 2011;35:816–26.

96. Wick MR, Swanson PE: "Carcinosarcomas:" current perspectives and an historical review of nosological concepts. *Semin Diagn Pathol* 1993;10:118–27.

97. Wick MR: Immunohistology of neuroendocrine and neuroectodermal tumors. *Semin Diagn Pathol* 2000;17:194–203.

98. Dorfman DM, Shahsafaei A, Chan JKC: Thymic carcinomas, but not thymomas and carcinomas of other sites, show CD5 immunoreactivity. *Am J Surg Pathol* 1997;21:936–40.

99. Kornstein MJ, Rosai J: CD5 labeling of thymic carcinomas and other nonlymphoid neoplasms. *Am J Clin Pathol* 1998;109:722–6.

100. Hishima T, Fukayama M, Fujisawa M, *et al.*: CD5 expression in thymic carcinoma. *Am J Pathol* 1994;145:268–75.

101. Tateyama H, Eimoto T, Tada T, *et al.*: Immunoreactivity of a new CD5 antibody with normal epithelium and malignant tumors, including thymic carcinomas. *Am J Clin Pathol* 1999;111:235–40.

102. Berezowski K, Grimes MM, Gal A, *et al.*: CD5 immunoreactivity of epithelial cells in thymic carcinoma and CASTLE using paraffin-embedded tissue. *Am J Clin Pathol* 1996;106:483–6.

103. Hishima T, Fukayama M, Hayashi Y, *et al.*: CD70 expression in thymic carcinoma. *Am J Surg Pathol* 2000;24:742–6.

104. Pan CC, Chen PC, Chieng H: *Kit* (CD117) is frequently overexpressed in thymic carcinomas but is absent in thymomas. *J Pathol* 2004;202:375–81.

105. Schirosi L, Nannini N, Nicoli D, *et al.*: Activating c-*kit* mutations in a subset of thymic carcinoma and response to different c-*kit* inhibitors. *Ann Oncol* 2012;23:2409–14.

106. Miettinen M, Lasota J: *Kit* (CD117): a review on expression in normal and neoplastic tissues, and mutations and their clinicopathologic correlation. *Appl Immunohistochem Mol Morphol* 2005;13:205–20.

107. Tateyama H, Eimoto T, Tada T, *et al.*: p53 protein expression and p53 gene mutation in thymic epithelial tumors: an immunohistochemical and DNA sequencing study. *Am J Clin Pathol* 1995;104:375–81.

108. Nino H, Kondo K, Miyoshi T, *et al.*: High frequency of p53 protein expression in thymic carcinoma and atypical thymoma. *Hum Pathol* 1998;29:330–8.

109. Patton DF, Ribeiro RC, Jenkins Jf, Sixbey JW: Thymic carcinoma with a defective Epstein-Barr virus encoding the BZLFI trans-activator. *J Infect Dis* 1994;170:7–12.

110. Dorfman DM, Shahsafaei A, Miyauchi A: Immunohistochemical staining for *bcl*-2 and *mcl*-1 in intrathyroidal epithelial thymoma (ITET)/carcinoma showing thymus-like differentiation (CASTLE) and cervical thymic carcinoma. *Mod Pathol* 1998;11:989–94.

111. Vargas SO, French CA, Faul PN, *et al.*: Upper respiratory tract carcinoma with chromosomal translocation 15;19. Evidence for a distinct disease entity of young patients with a rapidly fatal outcome. *Cancer* 2001;92:1195–1203.

112. Kees UR, Mulcahy MT, Willoughby MLN: Intrathoracic carcinoma in an 11 year old girl showing a translocation t (15;19). *Am J Ped Hematol Oncol* 1991;13:459 64.

113. Lee ACW, Kwong YI, Fu KH, *et al.*: Disseminated mediastinal carcinoma with chromosomal translocation (15;19). A distinctive clinicopathologic syndrome. *Cancer* 1993;72:2273–6.

114. French CA, Miyoshi I, Aster JC, *et al.*: *BRD* 4 bromodomain gene rearrangement in aggressive carcinoma with translocation t(15;19). *Am J Pathol* 2001;159:1987–92.

115. French CA. Pathogenesis of *NUT* midline carcinoma. *Annu Rev Pathol* 2012;7:247–65.

116. French CA. *NUT* midline carcinoma. *Cancer Genet Cytogenet* 2010;203:16–20.

117. Petrini P, French CA, Rajan A, *et al.*: *NUT* rearrangement is uncommon in human thymic epithelial tumors. *J Thorac Oncol* 2012;7:744–50.

118. Evans AG, French CA, Cameron MJ, *et al.*: Pathologic characteristics of *NUT* midline carcinoma arising in the mediastinum. *Am J Surg Pathol* 2012;36:1222–7.

119. Bauer DE, Mitchell CM, Strait KM, *et al.*: Clinicopathologic features and long-term outcomes of *NUT* midline carcinoma. *Clin Cancer Res* 2012;18:5773–9.

120. Hayashi S, Hamanaka Y, Sueda T, *et al.*: Thymic metastasis from prostatic carcinoma: Report of a case. *Surg Today* 1993;23:632–4.

121. DeYoung BR, Wick MR: Immunohistologic evaluation of metastatic carcinomas of unknown origin: an algorithmic approach. *Semin Diagn Pathol* 2000;17:184–93.

122. Knapp RH, Hurt RD, Payne WS, *et al.*: Malignant germ cell tumors of the mediastinum. *J Thorac Cardiovasc Surg* 1985;89:82–9.

123. Dehner LP: Germ cell tumors of the mediastinum. *Semin Diagn Pathol* 1990;7:266–84.

124. Montresor E, Nifosii F, Lupi A, *et al.*: Primary germinal tumors of the mediastinum. *Chir Ital* 1994; 46:46–52.

125. Strickler JG, Kurtin PJ: Mediastinal lymphoma. *Semin Diagn Pathol* 1991;8:2–13.

126. Suster S: Primary large-cell lymphomas of the mediastinum. *Semin Diagn Pathol* 1999;16:51–64.

127. Stanley MW, Powers CN: Syncytial variant of nodular sclerosing Hodgkin's disease: fine-needle aspiration findings in two cases. *Diagn Cytopathol* 1997;17:477–9.

128. Pai NB, Kim S, Pathak R, *et al.*: Syncytial variant of nodular sclerosing Hodgkin lymphoma. *Lymphology* 1999;32:75–9.

129. Park IS, Kim L, Han JY, *et al.*: Syncytial variant of nodular sclerosis Hodgkin's lymphoma assessed by fine needle aspiration cytology. *Cytopathology* 2008;19:394–397.

130. Feldman L, Kricun ME: Malignant melanoma presenting as a mediastinal mass. *JAMA* 1979;241:396–7.

131. Mackay B, Lichteiger B, Tessmer CF, Chang JP: The pathologic diagnosis of metastatic malignant melanoma. *Cancer Bull* 1971;23:30–45.

132. Prieto VG, Shea CR: Immunohistochemistry of melanocytic proliferations. *Arch Pathol Lab Med* 201;135:853–9.

133. Witkin GB, Miettinen M, Rosai J: A biphasic tumor of the mediastinum with features of synovial sarcoma: a report of four cases. *Am J Surg Pathol* 1989;13:490–9.

134. Trupiano JK, Rice TW, Herzog K, *et al.*: Mediastinal synovial sarcoma: report of two cases with molecular genetic analysis. *Ann Thorac Surg* 2002;73:628–30.

135. Yano M, Toyooka S, Tsukuda K, *et al.*: *SYT-SSX* fusion genes in synovial sarcoma of the thorax. *Lung Cancer* 2004;44:391–7.

136. Suster S, Moran CA. Primary synovial sarcomas of the mediastinum: a clinicopathologic, immunohistochemical, and ultrastructural study of 15 cases. *Am J Surg Pathol* 2005;29:569–78.

137. Katakura H, Fukuse T, Shiraishi I, *et al.*: Mediastinal synovial sarcoma. *Thorac Cardiovasc Surg* 2009;57:183–5.

138. DeLeeuw B, Suijkerbuijk RF, Olde-Weghuis D, *et al.*: Distinct Xpl1.2 breakpoint regions in synovial sarcoma revealed by metaphase and interphase FISH: Relationship to histologic subtypes. *Cancer Genet Cytogenet* 1994;73:89–94.

139. Jo VY, Fletcher CDM: p63 immunohistochemical staining is limited in soft tissue tumors. *Am J Clin Pathol* 2011;136:762–6.

140. Foo WC, Cruise MW, Wick MR, Hornick JL: Immunohistochemical staining for *TLE*1 distinguishes synovial sarcoma from histologic mimics. *Am J Clin Pathol* 2011;135:839–44.

141. Shrivastava CP, Devgarha S, Ahlawat V: Mediastinal tumors: a clinicopathological analysis. *Asian Cardiovasc Thorac Ann* 2006;14:102–4.

142. Ng CS, Munden RF, Libshitz HI: Malignant pleural mesothelioma: the spectrum of manifestations on CT in 70 cases. *Clin Radiol* 1999;54:415–21.

143. Wick MR, Mills SE: Mesothelial proliferations: an increasing morphologic spectrum. *Am J Clin Pathol* 2000;113:619–22.

144. Pan CC, Chen PC, Chou TY, Chiang H. Expression of calretinin and other mesothelioma-related markers in thymic carcinoma and thymoma. *Hum Pathol* 2003;34:1155–62.

145. Masaoka A, Monden Y, Nakahara K, *et al.*: Follow-up study of thymomas with special reference to their clinical stages. *Cancer* 1981;48:2485–92.

146. Blumberg D, Burt ME, Bains MS, *et al.*: Thymic carcinoma: current staging does not predict prognosis. *J Thorac Cardiovasc Surg* 1998;115:303–8.

147. Weissferdt A, Moran CA. Thymic carcinoma, part 1: a clinicopathologic and immunohistochemical study of 65 cases. *Am J Clin Pathol* 2012;138:103–14.

148. Weissferdt A, Moran CA. Thymic carcinoma, part 2: a clinicopathologic correlation of 33 cases with a proposed staging system. *Am J Clin Pathol* 2012;138:115–21.

149. Tsuchiya R, Koga K, Matsuno Y, *et al.*: Thymic carcinoma: Proposal for pathological TNM and staging. *Pathol Int* 1994;44:505–12.

150. Weide LG, Ulbright TM, Loehrer PJ Sr, Williams SD. Thymic carcinoma. A distinct clinical entity responsive to chemotherapy. *Cancer* 1993;71:1219–23.

151. Chung DA. Thymic carcinoma: analysis of nineteen clinicopathological studies. *Thorac Cardiovasc Surg* 2000;48:114–19.

152. Suster S, Rosai J: Thymic carcinoma: a clinicopathologic study of 60 cases. *Cancer* 1991;67:1025–32.

153. Lin JT, Wei-Shu W, Yen CC, *et al.*: Stage IV thymic carcinoma: a study of 20 patients. *Am J Med Sci* 2005;330:172–5.

154. Bott MJ, Wang H, Travis W, *et al.*: Management and outcomes of relapse after treatment for thymoma and thymic carcinoma. *Ann Thorac Surg* 2011;92:1984–91.

155. Okuma Y, Hosomi Y, Takagi Y, *et al.*: Clinical outcomes with chemotherapy for advanced thymic carcinoma. *Lung Cancer* 2013;80:75–80.

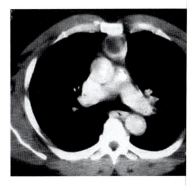

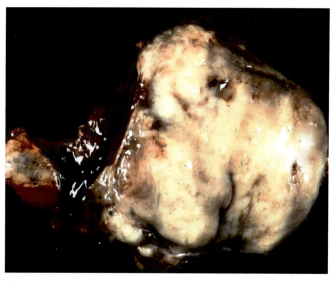

Fig. 8.5 Neuroendocrine carcinoma grade I of the thymus (typical carcinoid tumor). The tumor appears as a large, partially encapsulated yellow-tan mass. No necrosis is seen.

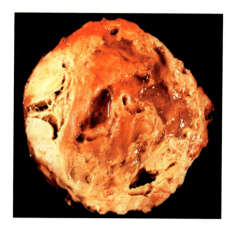

Fig. 8.6 Neuroendocrine carcinoma grade II of the thymus (atypical carcinoid tumor) with cystic change.

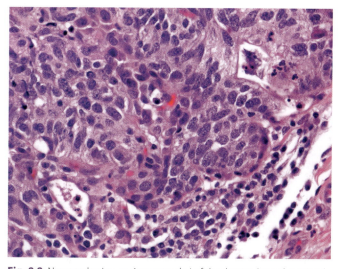

Fig. 8.8 Neuroendocrine carcinoma grade I of the thymus (typical carcinoid tumor) showing nesting pattern. The tumor cells have round nuclei with stippled chromatin pattern and inconspicuous nucleoli. The cytoplasm is amphophilic. No significant anisocytosis, necrosis, or mitotic activity is seen (H&E 200x).

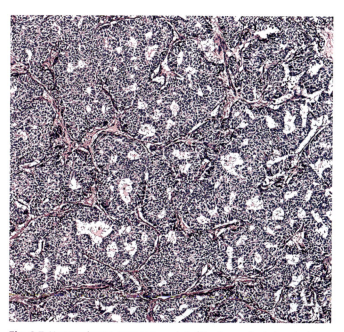

Fig. 8.7 Neuroendocrine carcinoma grade I of the thymus (typical carcinoid tumor). The tumor shows a low-power microscopy anastomosing cords, ribbons and cellular nests surrounded by a thin, highly vascularized septa (H&E 20x).

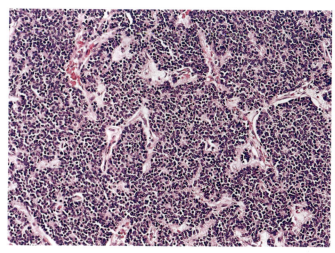

Fig. 8.9 Neuroendocrine carcinoma grade I of the thymus (typical carcinoid tumor) showing characteristic organoid appearance at low-power microscopy (H&E 20x).

diagnosed on asymptomatic patien (Fig. 8.1) in about one third of p 20–50% of patients present with Cushing's syndrome and Multiple being the most frequent [16,21-23]. Tl sent with non-specific symptoms fever, rarely polyarthropathy or dig pathy, and peripheral myopathy. caused by displacement of media plasm and include chest or inter cough, and/or manifestations of drome [24]. Rarely, mediastinal NEC ical carcinoid tumors) rupture w hemothorax and mediastinal enlar

Endocrine abnormalities are fr grade I and II (typical, atypical ca of patients present with endoc Cushing's syndrome, inappropri parathyroidism, acromegaly of growth hormone-releasing syndrome [5,6,8,12,15,16,18,22,23,25,26]

Cushing's syndrome, caused by the neoplasm, is the most frequ studies have confirmed the preser extracts and in tumor cells. Occ patients with thymic NEC grad carcinoid tumors) and Cushing's ence of several other polypeptide β-endorphin, Met-enkephalin, an with radioimmunoassay [16].

About 19% of patients with (carcinoid, atypical carcinoid tur ations of MEN type I (Wermer's is inherited as an autosomal d penetrance and is characterized b thyroidism resulting from parath single) or hyperplasia, islet cell tu ary adenoma, and, less frequen lung, intestine, and/or thymus. adrenal neoplasms (adenomas o omas, and multiple neuromas. In *et al.* of patients with MEN syndr

can raise the diagnostic possibility of a neuroendocrine neoplasm that can be readily identified with the use of appropriate immunostains. NEC grade I and II (typical, atypical carcinoid tumors) with sclerotic stroma need to be distinguished from extra thyroidal medullary carcinoma, as the tumor can rarely occur in the mediastinum. Congo red stain to demonstrate that the sclerotic material is indeed amyloid and immunostain for calcitonin are needed to establish the correct diagnosis [34].

NEC grade I (typical carcinoid) are distinguished from NEC grade II (atypical carcinoid) based on the same criteria developed for pulmonary neuroendocrine lesions, although

Neuroendocrine carcinomas of the thymus

Alberto M. Marchevsky, MD, Saul Suster, MD, and Mark R. Wick, MD

(a)

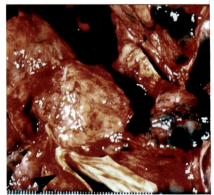

(c)

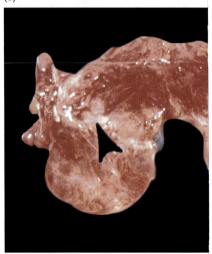

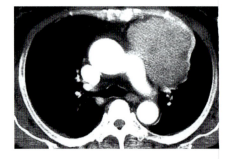

cribriform pattern (Fig. 8.13), and solid c
thymic NEC grade I and II (typic
tumors) [33,34]. The cribriform pattern is f
small acinar spaces or rosette-like form;
rather uniform cells with round or oval n
lymphoid infiltrates and other features s

The thymus gland can be the organ of origin of neuroendo-crine carcinomas (NEC) that generally have a more aggressive clinical behavior than their pulmonary counterparts and have been classified by the World Health Organization (WHO) and the Armed Forces Institute of Pathology (AFIP) as carcinoid tumors and neuroendocrine carcinomas [1,2].

Thymomas are derived from endodermal thymic epithelial cells, whereas NEC are presumed to originate from thymic neu-roendocrine cells of neural crest origin [1]. This view is supported by morphologic and ultrastructural similarities between NEC grade I (carcinoid tumors) and neuroendocrine cells and by the frequent presence of multiple endocrine neoplasms (MEN) in patients with these neoplasms. The presence of normal neuroen-docrine cells has been demonstrated in the thymus of chickens, reptiles, and other animals and the presence of calcitonin produ-cing cells has been shown in the human thymus [1,3,4].

However, this theory does not entirely explain the patho-genesis of NEC grade III, neoplasms that are currently con-sidered as probably having a different histogenesis in the lung than carcinoid tumors, and does not fully account for the development of combined thymic neoplasms that exhibit com-bined features of thymoma and neuroendocrine carcinoma.

Classification of thymic neuroendocrine carcinomas

Kay and Willson described in 1970 a patient with Cushing's syndrome and a "thymoma" [5]. Two years later, in 1972, Rosai el al. recognized that this type of neoplasm had neuroendocrine histopathologic features, different than those of a thymoma, and reported eight carcinoid tumors of the thymus [6]. The same year they also described a patient with mediastinal endocrine neoplasm associated with MEN [6]. A small number of patients with small cell carcinoma and large cell neuroendocrine carcin-oma of the thymus where subsequently described [7–13].

NEC of the thymus comprise less than 5% of all anterior mediastinal neoplasms and are currently classified by WHO and AFIP using similar terminology and diagnostic criteria to pulmonary neuroendocrine neoplasms, as carcinoid, atypical

Table 8.1. Neuroendocrine carcinomas of the thymus

Neuroendocrine carcinoma grade I
Typical carcinoid tumor
  Spindle cell carcinoid
  Pigmented carcinoid
  Carcinoid with mucinous trauma
  Oncocytic carcinoid
  Angiomatoid carcinoid

Neuroendocrine carcinoma grade II
Atypical carcinoid tumor

Neuroendocrine carcinoma grade III
Small cell carcinoma
Large cell carcinoma

Neuroendocrine carcinoma with grades I–III growth features

Neuroendocrine carcinoma combined with other neoplastic components

  Carcinoid tumor with sarcomatous changes
  Carcinoid tumor with thymoma
  Goblet cell carcinoid with mature teratoma
  Carcinoid with thymolipoma
  High-grade neuroendocrine carcinoma with other thymic carcinoma components

carcinoid, small cell carcinoma and large cell neuroendocrine carcinoma. In other organs, such as the gastrointestinal tract, the term NEC is currently used and will be used in this chapter to emphasize that all neuroendocrine neoplasms of the thymus are malignant (Table 8.1) [1,2].

Thymic neuroendocrine carcinomas grades I and II
Typical and atypical carcinoid tumors

NEC grades I and II (thymic carcinoids and atypical carcinoids) are more frequent in male patients in their fifth decade of life (median age of diagnosis, 43 years; age range: 9 to 100 years old) [14]. They are more common in males (3:1). They are

Neuroendocrine carcinomas of the thymus

Alberto M. Marchevsky, MD, Saul Suster, MD, and Mark R. Wick, MD

The thymus gland can be the organ of origin of neuroendocrine carcinomas (NEC) that generally have a more aggressive clinical behavior than their pulmonary counterparts and have been classified by the World Health Organization (WHO) and the Armed Forces Institute of Pathology (AFIP) as carcinoid tumors and neuroendocrine carcinomas [1,2].

Thymomas are derived from endodermal thymic epithelial cells, whereas NEC are presumed to originate from thymic neuroendocrine cells of neural crest origin [1]. This view is supported by morphologic and ultrastructural similarities between NEC grade I (carcinoid tumors) and neuroendocrine cells and by the frequent presence of multiple endocrine neoplasms (MEN) in patients with these neoplasms. The presence of normal neuroendocrine cells has been demonstrated in the thymus of chickens, reptiles, and other animals and the presence of calcitonin producing cells has been shown in the human thymus [1,3,4].

However, this theory does not entirely explain the pathogenesis of NEC grade III, neoplasms that are currently considered as probably having a different histogenesis in the lung than carcinoid tumors, and does not fully account for the development of combined thymic neoplasms that exhibit combined features of thymoma and neuroendocrine carcinoma.

Classification of thymic neuroendocrine carcinomas

Kay and Willson described in 1970 a patient with Cushing's syndrome and a "thymoma" [5]. Two years later, in 1972, Rosai el al. recognized that this type of neoplasm had neuroendocrine histopathologic features, different than those of a thymoma, and reported eight carcinoid tumors of the thymus [6]. The same year they also described a patient with mediastinal endocrine neoplasm associated with MEN [6]. A small number of patients with small cell carcinoma and large cell neuroendocrine carcinoma of the thymus where subsequently described [7–13].

NEC of the thymus comprise less than 5% of all anterior mediastinal neoplasms and are currently classified by WHO and AFIP using similar terminology and diagnostic criteria to pulmonary neuroendocrine neoplasms, as carcinoid, atypical

Table 8.1. Neuroendocrine carcinomas of the thymus

Neuroendocrine carcinoma grade I
    Typical carcinoid tumor
        Spindle cell carcinoid
        Pigmented carcinoid
        Carcinoid with mucinous trauma
        Oncocytic carcinoid
        Angiomatoid carcinoid

Neuroendocrine carcinoma grade II
    Atypical carcinoid tumor

Neuroendocrine carcinoma grade III
    Small cell carcinoma
    Large cell carcinoma

Neuroendocrine carcinoma with grades I–III growth features

Neuroendocrine carcinoma combined with other neoplastic components

    Carcinoid tumor with sarcomatous changes
    Carcinoid tumor with thymoma
    Goblet cell carcinoid with mature teratoma
    Carcinoid with thymolipoma
    High-grade neuroendocrine carcinoma with other thymic carcinoma components

carcinoid, small cell carcinoma and large cell neuroendocrine carcinoma. In other organs, such as the gastrointestinal tract, the term NEC is currently used and will be used in this chapter to emphasize that all neuroendocrine neoplasms of the thymus are malignant (Table 8.1) [1,2].

Thymic neuroendocrine carcinomas grades I and II

Typical and atypical carcinoid tumors

NEC grades I and II (thymic carcinoids and atypical carcinoids) are more frequent in male patients in their fifth decade of life (median age of diagnosis, 43 years; age range: 9 to 100 years old) [14]. They are more common in males (3:1). They are

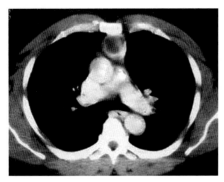

Fig. 8.1 Thymic neuroendocrine carcinomas grade I and II (carcinoid, atypical carcinoid) are often found as an incidental mass on routine chest X-rays. This patient had an abnormality that on chest CT scan appears as a well circumscribed mass in the anterior mediastinum, with focal cystic change.

diagnosed on asymptomatic patients on routine imaging studies (Fig. 8.1) in about one third of patients [15–20]. Approximately 20–50% of patients present with endocrine syndromes, with Cushing's syndrome and Multiple Endocrine Neoplasia (MEN) being the most frequent [16,21–23]. The remainder of patients present with non-specific symptoms, including fatigue, malaise, fever, rarely polyarthropathy or digital clubbing, proximal myopathy, and peripheral myopathy. Local thoracic symptoms are caused by displacement of mediastinal structures by the neoplasm and include chest or interscapular back pain, dyspnea, cough, and/or manifestations of the superior vena cava syndrome [24]. Rarely, mediastinal NEC grade I and II (typical, atypical carcinoid tumors) rupture with hemorrhage resulting in hemothorax and mediastinal enlargement.

Endocrine abnormalities are frequent in patients with NEC grade I and II (typical, atypical carcinoid tumors). About 50% of patients present with endocrine disturbances including Cushing's syndrome, inappropriate ADH secretion, hyperparathyroidism, acromegaly due to ectopic secretion of growth hormone-releasing hormone, and/or a MEN syndrome [5,6,8,12,15,16,18,22,23,25,26].

Cushing's syndrome, caused by hypersecretion of ACTH by the neoplasm, is the most frequent abnormality, and several studies have confirmed the presence of the hormone in tumor extracts and in tumor cells. Occasionally, tumor extracts of patients with thymic NEC grade I and II (typical, atypical carcinoid tumors) and Cushing's syndrome exhibit the presence of several other polypeptide hormones including α-MSH, β-endorphin, Met-enkephalin, and somatostatin when studied with radioimmunoassay [16].

About 19% of patients with thymic NEC grade I and II (carcinoid, atypical carcinoid tumors) present with manifestations of MEN type I (Wermer's syndrome) [18]. This condition is inherited as an autosomal dominant trait with variable penetrance and is characterized by the presence of hyperparathyroidism resulting from parathyroid adenomas (multiple or single) or hyperplasia, islet cell tumors of the pancreas, pituitary adenoma, and, less frequently, carcinoid tumors of the lung, intestine, and/or thymus. These patients can also have adrenal neoplasms (adenomas or carcinomas), thyroid adenomas, and multiple neuromas. In a prospective study by Gibril et al. of patients with MEN syndrome, approximately 8% were

found to have a thymic NEC grade I and II (carcinoid, atypical carcinoid tumors) [27].

A patient reported by Marchevsky et al. had a thymic NEC grade I (typical carcinoid tumor) (Fig. 8.2a–b) associated with an incomplete Sipple's syndrome including medullary carcinoma of the thyroid (Fig. 8.2c), parathyroid hyperplasia, carcinoid tumors in multiple organs (including the intestine, stomach, and gallbladder), and an adrenal neuroma [28].

Warren described a rare patient with an aggressive carcinoid tumor of the mediastinum arising after initially successful treatment of a germ cell tumor [29].

No association with myasthenia gravis, aplastic anemia, hypogammaglobulinemia, or other systemic syndromes encountered in patients with thymomas has been described.

Yen et al. have recently reported that patients with thymic NEC grade I and II (carcinoid, atypical carcinoid tumors) have an increased risk of extra thymic malignancies, including hepatocellular carcinoma, colorectal cancer, breast cancer, and cervical cancer [30].

Imaging findings

Thymic NEC grade I and II (carcinoid, atypical carcinoid tumors) are usually large, solid, lobulated anterior mediastinal masses that occasionally exhibit focal stippled calcification [31]. Computed tomographic (CT) scans may show the infiltrative character of the lesion (Fig. 8.3). Positron emission tomography (PET) usually exhibits activity in thymic neuroendocrine carcinomas (Fig. 8.4), particularly in high-grade lesions, and is very helpful to detect metastases. Bone scans and roentgenograms are useful in detecting metastases, which are usually multifocal and osteoblastic.

Pathology

Grossly, thymic NEC grade I and II (carcinoid, atypical carcinoid tumors) are solid, usually large, and exhibit an incompletely lobulated tan-gray or yellow-tan surface with focal areas of calcification that can give a "sandy", gritty appearance (Fig. 8.5) [1,2,20,32]. They vary in size from small lesions that are smaller than 3 cm in diameter to large 20 cm in greatest dimension tumors. Focal areas of necrosis can be seen in NEC grade II (atypical carcinoids). The neoplasms are frequently locally invasive and do not have the typical encapsulation and compartmentalization characteristic of thymomas. They rarely undergo cystic degeneration (Fig. 8.6), a frequent finding in thymomas.

Histologically, thymic NEC grade I and II (typical, atypical carcinoid tumors) are composed of cords, anastomosing ribbons and festoons (Fig. 8.7), islands ("balls") (Fig. 8.8), irregular nests with an organoid appearance (Fig. 8.9), and/or rosette-like formations (Fig. 8.10) composed of oval to round cells with amphophilic or eosinophilic cytoplasm and uniform nuclei, inconspicuous nucleolus, and stippled chromatin pattern (Fig. 8.11). Some neoplasms do not readily exhibit an organoid insular or trabecular growth feature. For example, Wick et al. described the presence of a sclerotic stroma (Fig. 8.12), "indian-file" growth pattern,

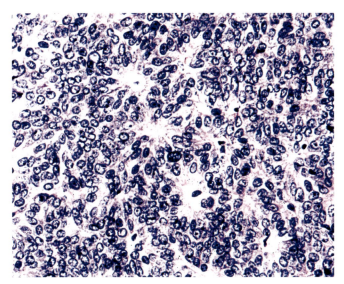

Fig. 8.10 Neuroendocrine carcinoma grade I of the thymus (typical carcinoid tumor) showing multiple rosette-like formations (H&E 40x).

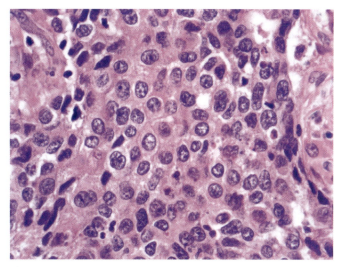

Fig. 8.11 Neuroendocrine carcinoma grade I of the thymus (typical carcinoid tumor). The tumor cells have round nuclei with stippled chromatin pattern, inconspicuous nucleoli, and abundant amphophilic cytoplasm. No significant anisocytosis, necrosis, or mitoses are seen (H&E 400x).

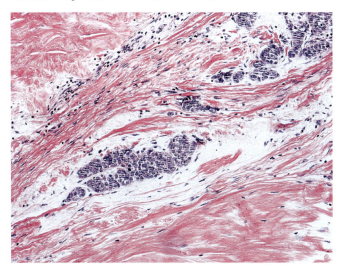

Fig. 8.12 Neuroendocrine carcinoma grade I of the thymus (typical carcinoid tumor) with a sclerotic stroma (H&E 40x).

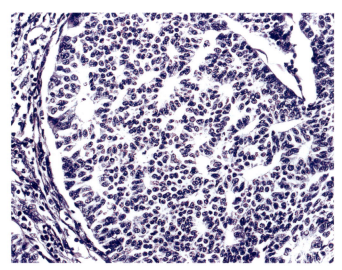

Fig. 8.13 Neuroendocrine carcinoma grade I of the thymus (typical carcinoid tumor) with a cribriform pattern (H&E 40x).

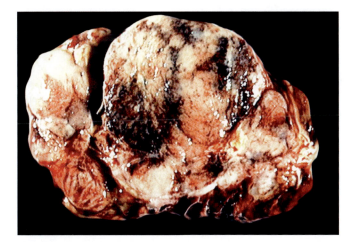

Fig. 8.14 Neuroendocrine carcinoma grade II of the thymus (atypical carcinoid tumor) presenting as a large, poorly encapsulated, yellow-gray mass with areas of hemorrhage and focal necrosis.

there are no systematic studies correlating mitoses, necrosis (Figs. 8.14 and 8.15), cytologic atypia and other pathologic features with prognosis [2]. Mitoses are infrequent in NEC grade I (typical carcinoid tumors); less than 3 mitoses in 10 high-power fields (HPF). These neoplasms also lack necrosis. The tumors with 3–10 mitoses in 10 HPF and/or areas of punctate necrosis are classified as NEC grade II (atypical carcinoid). Thymic NEC grade I and II (typical, atypical carcinoid tumors) lack a significant lymphocytic component, perivascular spaces, compartmentalization, and other features encountered in thymomas [14].

Histochemical and immunohistochemical features

The tumor cells of thymic NEC grade I and II (typical, atypical carcinoid tumors) have argyrophilic intracytoplasmic granules that can be detected with the Grimelius,

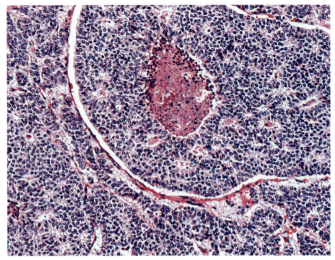

Fig. 8.15 Neuroendocrine carcinoma grade II of the thymus (atypical carcinoid tumor) showing characteristic focal, punctate necrosis (H&E 40x).

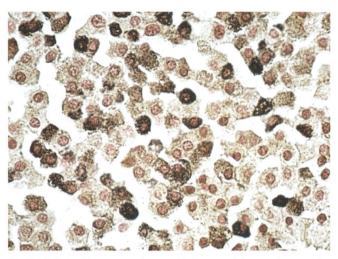

Fig. 8.16 Sevier-Munger stain showing black, argyrophilic granules in a neuroendocrine carcinoma grade I of the thymus (typical carcinoid tumor) (200x).

(a)

(b)

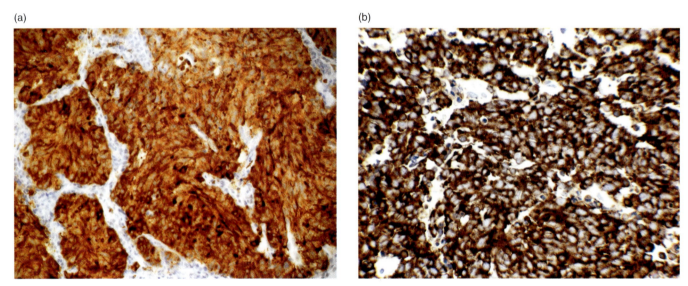

Fig. 8.17 (a) Neuroendocrine carcinoma grade II of the thymus (atypical carcinoid tumor) showing intense chromogranin cytoplasmic immunoreactivity (PAP 100x). **(b)** Neuroendocrine carcinoma grade II of the thymus (atypical carcinoid tumor) showing synaptophysin immunoreactivity (PAP 100x).

Sevier-Munger (Fig. 8.16), and other silver stains but usually lack argentaffin cells [1].

The tumor cells of NEC grade I and II (typical, atypical carcinoid tumors) exhibit characteristic dot-like paranuclear immunoreactivity for keratin AE1/AE3, and more diffuse cytoplasmic immunoreactivity for keratin CAM 5.2, and neuroendocrine markers such as chromogranin (Fig. 8.17a), synaptophysin (Fig. 8.17b), and CD56 [1,2]. Most lesions, particularly NEC grade III, also exhibit nuclear immunoreactivity for TTF-1 (Fig. 8.18), so this feature is not helpful to distinguish thymic NEC from their pulmonary counterparts. Immuno stains for Ki-67 can provide information about the proliferative activity of the tumor cells, although there is

limited evidence regarding how to use this information for the evaluation of thymic NEC. NEC grade I (typical tumor) exhibit low Ki-67 nuclear immunoreactivity (Fig. 8.19) while NEC grade III (small cell carcinoma, large cell neuroendocrine carcinoma) usually exhibit over 25% nuclear immunoreactivity. Cardillo et al. recently reported that Ki-67 index >10% had negative prognostic impact [35].

The tumor cells of thymic NEC grade I and II (typical, atypical carcinoid tumors) can also exhibit immunoreactivity for a variety of hormonal products. For example, Wick and associates reported 13 thymic NEC grade I and II (typical, atypical carcinoid tumors) stained with anti-sera to serotonin, gastrin, ACTH, and calcitonin [33]. Four tumors in their study

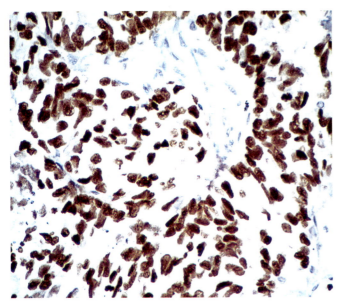

Fig. 8.18 Neuroendocrine carcinoma grade III of the thymus, large cell neuroendocrine carcinoma variant showing nuclear TTF-1 immunoreactivity (PAP 200x).

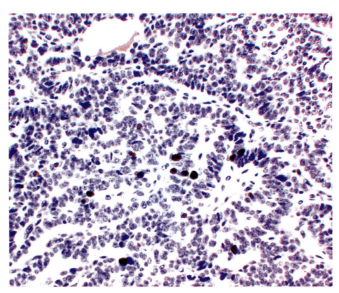

Fig. 8.19 Neuroendocrine carcinoma grade I of the thymus (typical carcinoid tumor) showing scanty cells with nuclear immunoreactivity for Ki-67, consistent with low proliferative activity (PAP 100x).

exhibited ACTH-like immunoreactivity, and three of these patients had Cushing's syndrome. Two tumors exhibited focal serotonin-like immunoreactivity; no gastrin or calcitonin was found in any of the thymic carcinoids. Herbst and associates reported cholecystokinin, neurotensin, ACTH, calcitonin, chromogranin A, and neuron-specific enolase immunoreactivity in NEC grade I and II (typical, atypical carcinoid tumors) of the thymus [36]. The study also demonstrated that each tumor reacted slightly differently with the various markers, emphasizing the need for the use of a panel of reagents for diagnostic purposes. In addition, the presence of peptide immunoreactivity in the tumor cells did not correlate well with endocrine symptoms in several patients.

Immunostain for S100 protein, present in sustentacular cells, schwann cells, and other cellular structures is usually but not always negative in thymic NEC grade I and II (carcinoid, atypical carcinoid tumors) [1]. This feature, when absent, can be helpful to distinguish NEC from paragangliomas, another neoplasm that exhibits a nesting growth pattern that can closely resemble an insular growth pattern and is composed of cells that exhibit neuroendocrine marker immunoreactivity.

Recent studies have shown the expression of PAX-8 in a thymic NEC grade I and II (typical, atypical carcinoid tumors) [37]. PAX (paired box) genes encode a family of transcription factors important for organogenesis and have been recognized in neuroendocrine tumors of the pancreas and other sites.

Ultrastructural features

Ultrastructural studies have been helpful in the past to establish the diagnosis of thymic NEC grade I and II (typical, atypical carcinoid tumors) [5]. Indeed, in a study at the Mayo Clinic, 4 of 11 tumors that were initially classified as thymic

carcinoids on the basis of light microscopic features had to be reclassified as thymomas after ultrastructural studies demonstrated the lack of neurosecretory granules in the cytoplasm of the tumor cells, which exhibited, instead, numerous desmosomes, tonofilaments, and cytoplasmic processes [38]. Thymic NEC grade I and II (typical, atypical carcinoid tumors) have ultrastructurally a population of polyhedral and/or spindle cells with clear cytoplasm admixed with smaller electron-dense ("dark") cells [1]. The latter are probably undergoing degeneration. The tumor cells have a round to oval nucleus with a central small nucleolus and fine chromatin pattern. The cytoplasm has a well-developed Golgi apparatus, granular endoplasmic reticulum, polyribosomes, microtubules, characteristic membrane-bound dense-core neurosecretory granules ranging in size from 100 to 300 nm, easily discernible smooth endoplasmic reticulum, rare exocytoses of neurosecretory granules, and rare rudimentary cilia (Fig. 8.20).

Larger pleomorphic granules measuring up to 450 nm in diameter can also be seen [1]. The cytoplasm can also have intracellular type I and II microfilaments measuring 5 to 7 nm that are arranged in whorls and are usually closely associated with dense-core granules. In unusual instances, they can become so prominent in thymic NEC grade I and II (typical, atypical carcinoid tumors) as to be visible by light microscopy as 1- to 4-μm eosinophilic argyrophilic intracytoplasmic inclusions.

Fetissof and associates classified a lesion with those features as microfilamentous carcinoid of the thymus [39]. This tumor had numerous intermediate-type 10-nm filaments arranged in whorls and bundles associated with neurosecretory granules. Similar filaments have been designated as type II microfilaments and have been described in normal endocrine cells of the gastroenteropancreatic system (D cells secreting somatostatin)

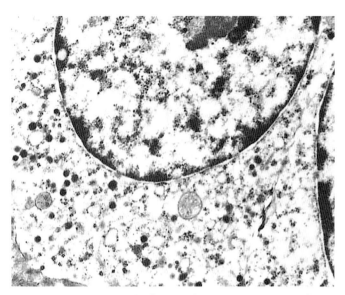

Fig. 8.20 Electron micrograph of neuroendocrine carcinoma grade I of the thymus (typical carcinoid tumor) showing dense core granules.

and in carcinoid tumors of the lung, stomach, rectum, and duodenum that are now believed to have an endodermal origin. The presence of intracytoplasmic whorls of microfilaments in thymic carcinoids has been suggested to be evidence that these tumors may also have an endodermal origin.

Differential diagnosis

Thymic NEC grade I and II (typical, atypical carcinoid tumors) should be distinguished from thymomas, thymic carcinomas, germ cell tumors, and malignant lymphomas. The neuroendocrine lesions are usually not encapsulated as thymomas and lack their lobular configuration. Histologically, they exhibit the organoid features described previously and lack the presence of a prominent lymphoid component. The cells of NEC grade I and II (typical, atypical carcinoid tumors) are smaller and less pleomorphic than those of germ cell tumors and thymic carcinomas. Immunocytochemical studies with a battery of markers, particularly chromogranin, neuron-specific enolase, and neuropeptides can be very helpful to confirm the epithelial and neuroendocrine nature of thymic carcinoids. Ultrastructurally, thymic NEC grade I and II (typical, atypical carcinoid tumors) exhibit prominent dense-core granules, smooth endoplasmic reticulum, and type I and II microfilaments. Although it is rare, thymic carcinomas can have ultrastructural features similar to those of carcinoid tumors; however, these tumors are more pleomorphic under light microscopy and probably represent more primitive carcinomas with neuroendocrine differentiation.

Treatment and prognosis

Thymic NEC grade I and II (typical, atypical carcinoid tumors) invade contiguous mediastinal structures and metastasize in a higher proportion than similar tumors arising in the lung and other sites [25,40,41]. Recent European Society of Medical Oncology (ESMO) guidelines for neuroendocrine bronchial and thymic tumors recommend that these patients be staged with contrast enhanced chest CT or MRI [42]. Biochemical evaluation for plasma chromogranin A, plasma neuron specific enolase, and in selected cases plasma ACTH and other hormones is also recommended.

Patients with thymic NEC grade I and II (typical, atypical carcinoid tumors) are treated primarily with wide local excision [15–17,20]. Postoperative radiotherapy can be of value in instances of persistent or recurrent disease.

Thymic NEC grade I and II (typical, atypical carcinoid tumors) are more aggressive than their pulmonary counterparts, with a higher incidence of associated endocrine syndromes, more frequent local recurrence and distant metastases and high mortality [43]. For example, Wick and associates reported Cushing's syndrome or MEN syndrome in 35% of patients with neuroendocrine neoplasms of the thymus and distant metastases in 30–40% of them. Metastatic sites included mediastinal and cervical lymph nodes, liver, bone, skin, and lungs [44]. Bone metastases were usually osteoblastic. The overall cure rate in patients followed for at least five years was 13%. The mean survival rate of patients with metastasis was 3 years after the diagnosis of extrathymic disease. Adjuvant chemotherapy did not influence the prognosis. In a more recent study of 21 thymic neuroendocrine tumors, including 18 atypical carcinoids, Ahn *et al.* reported that all patients died with systemic metastases [45]. Unresectability and advanced clinical stage are generally associated with decreased survival [46]. Cardillo *et al.* reported the multicenter experience in Italian hospitals with 35 patients with primary neuroendocrine carcinomas of the thymus stage stratified by Masaoka stage and reported 10 year survival rates of 100%, 66.7%, 61.9%, 25%, and 0% in stages I, II, III, IVa and IVb respectively. The histologic type, presence of paraneoplastic syndrome, Masaoka staging, presence of metastatic disease at diagnosis, and postoperative radiation therapy had a significant impact on prognosis.

Recent studies have shown promising results with novel agents such as somatostatin inhibitors, sunitinib, a thyrosine kinase inhibitor and everolimus, an mTOR inhibitor, combined with capecitabine and temozolomide chemotherapy in patients with neuroendocrine tumors [21,31,47,48].

Patients with thymic NEC grade I and II (typical, atypical carcinoid tumors) have a very prolonged clinical course and need to be followed for many years before they are considered cured. Patients with thymic NEC grade I and II (typical, atypical carcinoid tumors) and associated endocrine syndromes such as Cushing's or MEN type I have a worse prognosis [12,15,16,25,27,49,50]. Most individuals reported in the literature with these associations died with tumor and/or metabolic abnormalities secondary to the secretory activities of the endocrine neoplasms.

Unusual variants of NEC grades I and II (typical and atypical carcinoid tumors)

Spindle cell carcinoid

Thymic NEC grade I (typical carcinoid) (Fig. 8.21) and NEC grade II (atypical carcinoid) (Fig. 8.22a and b) can be composed of spindle cells, akin to pulmonary spindle cell carcinoids [51,52]. The patient reported by Kuo had a spindle cell pigmented carcinoid tumor of the thymus [53]. Spindle cell NEC grade I and II (typical, atypical carcinoid tumors) can be

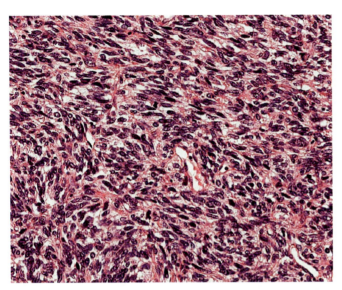

Fig. 8.21 Low-grade spindle cell carcinoid tumor of the thymus (NEC grade I). The tumor is composed of cells with spindle-shaped nuclei, indistinct amphophilic cytoplasm arranged in solid sheets with vague nodular growth features. Immunostains for chromogranin, synaptophysin or other neuroendocrine markers are necessary to distinguish this lesion from a spindle cell thymoma (WHO A thymoma) (H&E 100x).

difficult to distinguish on routine histopathology from spindle cell thymomas (WHO A) as they tend not to exhibit the typical growth features described above for NEC composed of round or polygonal cells [2]. Immunostains for synaptophysin, chromogranin, and other neuroendocrine markers are probably indicated for the diagnosis of thymic spindle cell neoplasm, as the prognosis and treatment of NEC grade I and II (typical, atypical carcinoid tumors) and thymomas is quite different.

Pigmented carcinoid

A few studies have reported another unusual feature in thymic NEC: the presence of prominent pigmentation in the lesion [1,53,54]. Some neoplasms have melanin containing dendritic melanocytes and macrophages admixed with a nest of neuroendocrine neoplastic cells [1,55]. The pigmented cells are stained with Fontana-Masson stain and exhibit immunoreactivity for S100 protein. Iron stain and HMB45 immunostains are negative. In other pigmented NEC (carcinoids), the tumor cells exhibited intracytoplasmic melanin and/or lipofuscin pigment. Ho and Ho reported a pigmented carcinoid in which melanin was demonstrated histochemically and ultrastructurally in the cytoplasm of non-neoplastic cells that probably represented hyperplastic thymic melanoblasts stimulated by the neoplasm [54]. The patient with pigmented carcinoid tumor of the thymus reported by Kuo had associated Cushing's syndrome [53].

Carcinoid with mucinous stroma

Suster described four patients with a distinctive variant of thymic NEC (carcinoid) characterized by the presence of abundant extracellular connective tissue mucin that was not

(a)

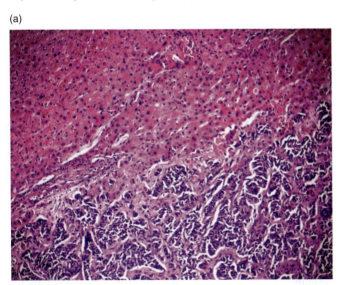

(b)

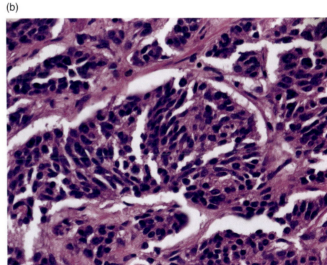

Fig. 8.22 **(a)** Neuroendocrine carcinoma grade II of the thymus (atypical carcinoid) metastatic to liver (H&E 40x). **(b)** The tumor is composed of spindle-shaped cells forming cellular nests surrounded by vascularized thin septa. Mild nuclear anisocytosis, focal necrosis, and moderate mitotic activity (4 mitoses/10 HPF) were present (H&E 200x).

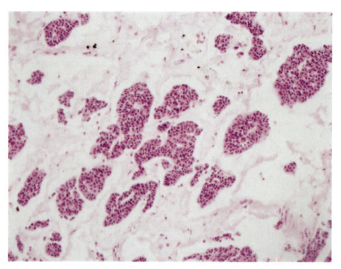

Fig. 8.23 NEC grade I (carcinoid tumor) with mucinous stroma (H&E 40x).

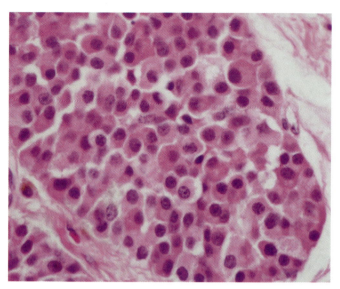

Fig. 8.24 Oncocytic NEC grade I (carcinoid tumor). The cells have abundant, granular, eosinophilic cytoplasm (H&E 400x).

(a)

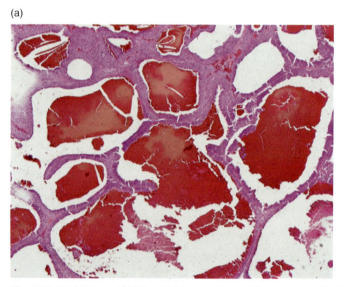

(b)

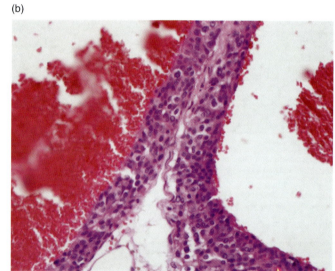

Fig. 8.25 (a) Angiomatoid NEC grade I (carcinoid tumor) showing blood-filled lakes (H&E 20x). **(b)** The blood lakes are lined by tumor cells rather than by endothelial cells (H&E 400x).

produced by the tumor cells [56]. The tumor cells are negative with mucicarmine stains and no goblet cells are seen, as in goblet cell carcinoid tumor (Fig. 8.23).

Oncocytic carcinoid

Moran and Suster have described 22 cases of thymic oncocytic carcinoid tumors composed of medium to large size neoplastic cells with eosinophilic, granular cytoplasm (Fig. 8.24) [57]. Ultrastructural studies demonstrated the presence of numerous mitochondria in the cytoplasm of the tumor cells [57]. A few of these cases were associated with MEN I syndrome and Cushing's syndrome.

Angiomatoid carcinoid

Moran and Suster described three neuroendocrine carcinomas of the thymus showing features of carcinoid tumor and prominent blood-filled cystic spaces lined by tumor cells rather than by endothelial cells (Fig. 8.25a and b) [58].

Neuroendocrine carcinoma grade III
Small cell carcinoma variant

Primary carcinomas of the thymus exhibiting pathologic features similar to those of small cell carcinoma of the lung and other organs have been described by Wick and Scheithauer in 1982 and others thereafter [7,8,20,33]. This is a difficult diagnosis

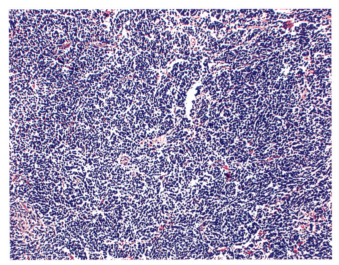

Fig. 8.26 Neuroendocrine carcinoma, grade III, small cell variant of the thymus. The tumor exhibits a vague nesting pattern at low-power microscopy (H&E 20x).

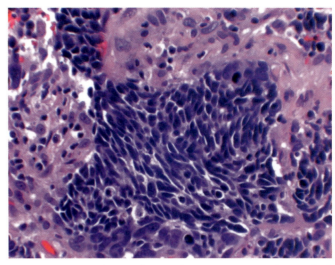

Fig. 8.27 Needle core biopsy of neuroendocrine carcinoma, grade III, small cell variant of the thymus. The tumor cells show round- to oval-shaped nuclei with nuclear molding. Mitoses are present (H&E 400x).

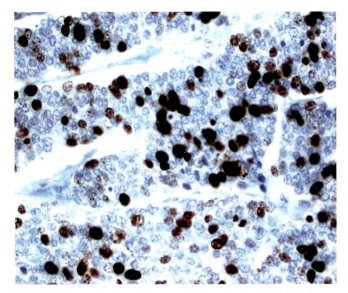

Fig. 8.28 Neuroendocrine carcinoma, grade III, small cell variant of the thymus showing high Ki-67 proliferative index. Please contrast this finding with the proliferative index of neuroendocrine carcinoma grade I (typical carcinoid) of the thymus shown in Fig. 8.19 (PAP 100x).

that can be rendered only after careful exclusion of the possibility of a primary small cell carcinoma of the lung, a neoplasm that can be small and particularly difficult to visualize on imaging studies.

Thymic NEC grade III, small cell carcinoma variant is composed of small to intermediate sized cells exhibiting round or ovoid hyperchromatic nuclei with a "salt-and-pepper" chromatin pattern and scanty cytoplasm (Fig. 8.26) [20]. The tumor cells are arranged in solid sheets with focal nesting and trabecular growth features. Focal rosettes can be present. Prominent nuclear molding (Fig. 8.27), necrosis, and necrotic activity

higher than ten mitoses/ten HPF are characteristic of small cell carcinomas.

The tumor cells of thymic NEC grade III, small cell carcinoma variant exhibit faint cytoplasmic immunoreactivity with antibodies to keratin AE1/AE3 and CAM 5.2 and cytoplasmic immunoreactivity for synaptophysin, chromogranin and CD 56 [1]. The tumor cells can exhibit TTF-1 immunoreactivity and this feature is not helpful to distinguish primary thymic NEC grade III, small cell carcinoma variant from metastatic carcinoma of pulmonary origin. In contrast with NEC grade I and II (typical and atypical carcinoids), thymic NEC grade III, small cell carcinoma variant exhibit a high Ki-67 proliferative index (Fig. 8.28). Ultrastructural studies, currently seldom performed in clinical practice, show the presence of intracytoplasmic 100 to 200 nm dense core granules, characteristic of neuroendocrine differentiation [1].

Large cell neuroendocrine carcinoma

A few patients with thymic NEC grade III, large cell neuroendocrine carcinoma variant have been described [9,10,12,13,20]. This is a diagnosis by exclusion of a pulmonary neuroendocrine carcinoma.

NEC grade III, large cell neuroendocrine carcinoma variant appear as large, solid, well-circumscribed but usually not encapsulated tumors with a yellow-gray, somewhat lobulated, granular surface (Fig. 8.29) [20]. They can be adherent to the lung, raising the question as to the tumor origin. In lesions when the bulk of the tumor is extrapulmonary with only focal lung involvement, the possibility of a mediastinal origin is generally favored.

NEC grade III, large cell neuroendocrine carcinoma variant are composed of large-sized cells exhibiting round or ovoid hyperchromatic nuclei with prominent nucleoli

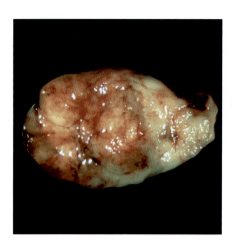

Fig. 8.29 Neuroendocrine carcinoma, grade III, large cell variant of the thymus. The tumor is encapsulated with a tan-gray surface showing areas of necrosis and focal cystic degeneration.

and amphophilic or clear cytoplasm (Fig. 8.30a and b) [2]. The tumor cells are arranged in a growth pattern reminiscent of an NEC grade II (atypical carcinoid tumor) with solid sheets with focal nesting and trabecular growth features (Fig. 8.30a). Focal rosettes can be present (Fig. 8.30a). Nuclear atypia with anisocytosis and presence of prominent nucleoli in the tumor cells, necrosis, and mitotic activity higher than 10 mitoses/10 HPF allow for the distinction between NEC grade III, large cell neuroendocrine carcinoma variant and NEC grade II (atypical carcinoid). The tumors exhibit similar immunophenotype to other neuroendocrine carcinomas of the thymus (Fig. 8.30c) and can exhibit TTF-1 nuclear immunoreactivity [1]. NEC grade III in general can exhibit less prominent immunoreactivity for keratin and neuroendocrine markers than NEC grade I and II.

(a)

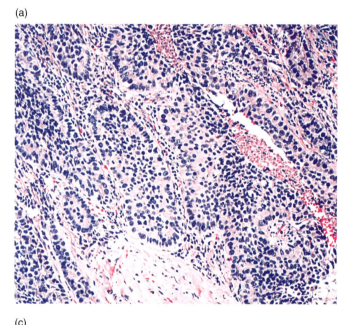

(b)

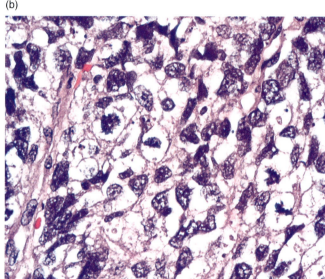

(c)

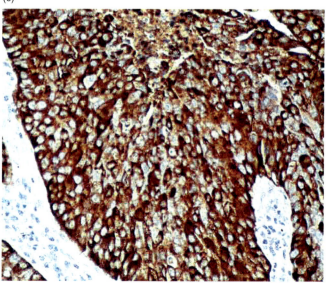

Fig. 8.30 (a) Neuroendocrine carcinoma, grade III, large cell variant of the thymus showing nesting pattern, characteristic of neuroendocrine differentiation and focal areas of necrosis. The lesion had high mitotic activity (20 mitoses/10 HPF) (H&E 40x). **(b)** Neuroendocrine carcinoma, grade III, large cell variant of the thymus composed of large, somewhat pleomorphic cells with hyperchromatic nuclei, focal nucleoli, and clear cytoplasm. Several mitoses are present (H&E 400x). **(c)** Neuroendocrine carcinoma, grade III, large cell variant of the thymus showing chromogranin cytoplasmic immunoreactivity (PAP 100x).

Treatment and prognosis of thymic neuroendocrine carcinoma grade III, large cell neuroendocrine carcinoma variant

NEC grade III, large cell neuroendocrine carcinoma variant are very aggressive neoplasms that frequently recur, metastasize widely, and are fatal in most patients [17,21,47,59–61]. Patients are treated with surgery, radiation therapy, and chemotherapy protocols similar to those used in patients with pulmonary high-grade neuroendocrine carcinoma, with poor results [62].

Neuroendocrine carcinoma with heterologous grades I-III features

Most textbooks describe the pathologic features of thymic typical carcinoids, atypical carcinoids, small cell carcinoma and large cell neuroendocrine carcinoma as distinct neoplasms, but not infrequently these tumors exhibit focal areas with morphological features reminiscent of a typical or an atypical carcinoid tumor that blend imperceptibly with the areas of high-grade neoplasm [1,2]. In addition, the distinction between small cell neuroendocrine carcinoma and large cell neuroendocrine carcinoma is often difficult, due to overlap of the nuclear size and cytologic features (Fig. 8.28) between the two neoplastic components. This diagnostic difficulty results in interobserver diagnostic variability, a problem that has been well-documented for pulmonary high-grade neuroendocrine carcinomas, and favors the classification of these lesions as thymic NEC grade III, with description of the prevalent variant [63].

Neuroendocrine carcinoma combined with other tumors

Carcinoid with sarcomatoid changes

This rare variant of thymic neuroendocrine carcinoma shows areas of carcinoid tumor admixed with a sarcomatoid component that shows fibrosarcoma, osteogenic sarcoma or chondrosarcoma differentiation [64,65].

Thymic neuroendocrine carcinoma combined with thymoma

A few examples of thymic neoplasms showing areas of NEC grade I–III combined with a thymoma have been described [1,66]. Mizuno et al. described a unique patient with a carcinoid tumor in one lobe of the thymus and a thymoma in the other [67].

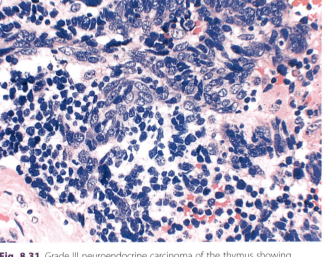

Fig. 8.31 Grade III neuroendocrine carcinoma of the thymus showing tumor cells of variable size and cytologic features. Please note the presence of small cells with hyperchromatic nuclei and scanty cytoplasm, consistent with small cell carcinoma features admixed with considerably larger cells with round hyperchromatic nuclei and more abundant amphophilic cytoplasm, consistent with large cell carcinoma features. The variability in morphology often results in interobserver differences in the manner grade III neuroendocrine carcinoma are classified by different pathologists (H&E 400x).

Nagata reported the association of a large cell neuroendocrine thymic carcinoma with a large WHO type AB thymoma [11].

Goblet cell carcinoid combined with a mature teratoma

Lancaster et al. reported a unique case of goblet cell carcinoid of the thymus associated with a mature teratoma [68].

Carcinoid combined with a thymolipoma

Steger et al. reported a unique patient with a typical thymic carcinoid arising within a thymolipoma [69].

Neuroendocrine carcinoma grade III of the thymus with other thymic carcinoma components

Thymic neoplasms can also exhibit combined areas of NEC grade III with squamous cell carcinoma, and less often other variants of thymic carcinoma [1,2,70,71]. These neoplasms are classified by WHO as either small cell carcinoma, combined type, or large cell carcinoma, combined type [2]. The different neoplastic components can be closely admixed with each other or be present in different areas of the neoplasm [1].

References

1. Shimosato Y, Mukai K, Matsuno Y. *Tumors of the Mediastinum.* 2010; Washington: American Registry of Pathology.

2. Travis WD, Brambilla E, Muller-Hermelink HK, *et al. Tumours of the Lung, Pleura, Thymus and Heart.* 2004; Lyon: IARC Press.

3. Botham CA, Jones GV, Kendall MD. Immuno-characterisation of neuroendocrine cells of the rat thymus gland in vitro and in vivo. *Cell Tissue Res.* 2001;303:381–9.

4. Moll UM, Lane BL, Robert F, *et al.* The neuroendocrine thymus. Abundant occurrence of oxytocin-, vasopressin-, and neurophysin-like peptides in epithelial cells. *Histochemistry.* 1988;89:385–90.

5. Kay S, Willson MA. Ultrastructural studies of an ACTH-secreting

thymic tumor. *Cancer.* 1970;26:445–2.

6. Rosai J, Higa E, Davie J. Mediastinal endocrine neoplasm in patients with multiple endocrine adenomatosis. A previously unrecognized association. *Cancer.* 1972;29:1075–83.

7. Gal AA, Kornstein MJ, Cohen C, *et al.* Neuroendocrine tumors of the thymus: a clinicopathological and prognostic study. *Ann Thorac Surg.* 2001;72:1179–82.

8. Hekimgil M, Hamulu F, Cagirici U, *et al.* Small cell neuroendocrine carcinoma of the thymus complicated by Cushing's syndrome. Report of a 58-year-old woman with a 3-year history of hypertension. *Pathol Res Pract.* 2001;197:129–33.

9. Chetty R, Batitang S, Govender D. Large cell neuroendocrine carcinoma of the thymus. *Histopathology.* 1997;31:274–6.

10. Mega S, Oguri M, Kawasaki R, *et al.* Large-cell neuroendocrine carcinoma in the thymus. *Gen Thorac Cardiovasc Surg.* 2008;56:566–9.

11. Nagata Y, Ohno K, Utsumi T, *et al.* Large cell neuroendocrine thymic carcinoma coexisting within large WHO type AB thymoma. *Jpn J Thorac Cardiovasc Surg.* 2006;54:256–9.

12. Saito T, Kimoto M, Nakai S, *et al.* Ectopic ACTH syndrome associated with large cell neuroendocrine carcinoma of the thymus. *Intern Med.* 2011;50:1471–5.

13. Yoon YH, Kim JH, Kim KH, *et al.* Large cell neuroendocrine carcinoma of the thymus: a two-case report. *Korean J Thorac Cardiovasc Surg.* 2012;45:60–4.

14. Moran CA, Suster S. Neuroendocrine carcinomas (carcinoid tumor) of the thymus. A clinicopathologic analysis of 80 cases. *Am J Clin Pathol.* 2000;114:100–10.

15. Arora R, Gupta R, Sharma A, *et al.* Primary neuroendocrine carcinoma of thymus: a rare cause of Cushing's syndrome. *Indian J Pathol Microbiol.* 2010;53:148–51.

16. de Perrott M, Spiliopoulos A, Fischer S, *et al.* Neuroendocrine carcinoma (carcinoid) of the thymus associated with Cushing's syndrome. *Ann Thorac Surg.* 2002;73:675–81.

17. Dosios T, Nikou GC, Toubanakis C, *et al.* Multimodality treatment of neuroendocrine tumors of the thymus. *Thorac Cardiovasc Surg.* 2005;53:305–9.

18. Ferolla P, Falchetti A, Filosso P, *et al.* Thymic neuroendocrine carcinoma (carcinoid) in multiple endocrine neoplasia type 1 syndrome: the Italian series. *J Clin Endocrinol Metab.* 2005;90:2603–9.

19. Klemm KM, Moran CA. Primary neuroendocrine carcinomas of the thymus. *Semin Diagn Pathol.* 1999;16:32–41.

20. Moran CA, Suster S. Neuroendocrine carcinomas (carcinoid tumor) of the thymus. A clinicopathologic analysis of 80 cases. *Am J Clin Pathol.* 2000;114:100–10.

21. Filosso PL, Actis Dato GM, Ruffini E, *et al.* Multidisciplinary treatment of advanced thymic neuroendocrine carcinoma (carcinoid): report of a successful case and review of the literature. *J Thorac Cardiovasc Surg.* 2004;127:1215–19.

22. Ruffini E, Oliaro A, Novero D, *et al.* Neuroendocrine tumors of the thymus. *Thorac Surg Clin.* 2011;21:13–23.

23. Goudet P, Murat A, Cardot-Bauters C, *et al.* Thymic neuroendocrine tumors in multiple endocrine neoplasia type 1: a comparative study on 21 cases among a series of 761 MEN1 from the GTE (Groupe des Tumeurs Endocrines). *World J Surg.* 2009;33:1197–1207.

24. Komoda S, Komoda T, Knosalla C, *et al.* A giant neuroendocrine tumor of the thymus gland causing superior vena cava syndrome. *Gen Thorac Cardiovasc Surg.* 2012;60:863–7.

25. Neary NM, Lopez-Chavez A, Abel BS, *et al.* Neuroendocrine ACTH-producing tumor of the thymus–experience with 12 patients over 25 years. *J Clin Endocrinol Metab.* 2012;97:2223–30.

26. Rosai J, Higa E. Mediastinal endocrine neoplasm, of probable thymic origin, related to carcinoid tumor. Clinicopathologic study of 8 cases. *Cancer.* 1972;29:1061–74.

27. Gibril F, Schumann M, Pace A, *et al.* Multiple endocrine neoplasia type 1 and Zollinger-Ellison syndrome: a prospective study of 107 cases and comparison with 1009 cases from the literature. *Medicine (Baltimore).* 2004;83:43–83.

28. Marchevsky AM, Dikman SH. Mediastinal carcinoid with an incomplete Sipple's syndrome. *Cancer.* 1979;43:2497–2501.

29. Warren JS, Yum MN. Carcinoid tumor arising in a treated primary germ cell tumor of the mediastinum. *South Med J.* 1987;80:259–61.

30. Yen YT, Lai WW, Wu MH, *et al.* Thymic neuroendocrine carcinoma and thymoma are both associated with increased risk of extrathymic malignancy: a 20-year review of a single institution. *Ann Thorac Surg.* 2011;91:219–25.

31. Li H, Wang DL, Liu XW, *et al.* Computed tomography characterization of neuroendocrine tumors of the thymus can aid identification and treatment. *Acta Radiol.* 2013;54:175–80.

32. Marchevsky AM, Kaneko M. *Surgical Pathology of the Mediastinum.* 1991; New York: Raven Press.

33. Wick MR, Carney JA, Bernatz PE, *et al.* Primary mediastinal carcinoid tumors. *Am J Surg Pathol.* 1982;6:195–205.

34. Wick MR, Rosai J. Neuroendocrine neoplasms of the mediastinum. *Sem Diagn Pathol.* 1991;8:31–51.

35. Cardillo G, Rea F, Lucchi M, *et al.* Primary neuroendocrine tumors of the thymus: a multicenter experience of 35 patients. *Ann Thorac Surg.* 2012;94:241–5.

36. Herbst WM, Kummer W, Hofmann W, *et al.* Carcinoid tumors of the thymus. An immunohistochemical study. *Cancer.* 1987;60:2465–70.

37. Haynes CM, Sangoi AR, Pai RK. PAX8 is expressed in pancreatic well-differentiated neuroendocrine tumors and in extrapancreatic poorly differentiated neuroendocrine carcinomas in fine-needle aspiration biopsy specimens. *Cancer Cytopathol.* 2011;119:193–201.

38. Wick MR, Scott RE, Li CY, *et al.* Carcinoid tumor of the thymus: a clinicopathologic report of seven cases with a review of the literature. *Mayo Clin Proc.* 1980;55:246–54.

39. Fetissof F, Boivin F, Jobard P, *et al.* Microfilamentous carcinoid of the thymus: correlation of ultrastructural study with Grimelius stain. *Ultrastruct Pathol.* 1982;3:9–15.

40. Tiffet O, Nicholson AG, Ladas G, *et al.* A clinicopathologic study of 12 neuroendocrine tumors arising in the thymus. *Chest.* 2003;124:141–6.

41. Chaer R, Massad MG, Evans A, *et al.* Primary neuroendocrine tumors of the thymus. *Ann Thorac Surg.* 2002;74:1733–40.

42. Oberg K, Hellman P, Ferolla P, *et al.* Neuroendocrine bronchial and thymic tumors: ESMO Clinical Practice Guidelines for diagnosis, treatment and follow-up. *Ann Oncol.* 2012;23 Suppl 7: vii120–vii123.

43. Gaur P, Leary C, Yao JC. Thymic neuroendocrine tumors: a SEER database analysis of 160 patients. *Ann Surg.* 2010;251:1117–21.

44. Wick MR, Rosai J. Neuroendocrine neoplasms of the thymus. *Pathol Res Pract.* 1988;183:188–99.

45. Ahn S, Lee JJ, Ha SY, *et al.* Clinicopathological analysis of 21 thymic neuroendocrine tumors. *Korean J Pathol.* 2012;46:221–5.

46. Gal AA, Kornstein MJ, Cohen C, *et al.* Neuroendocrine tumors of the thymus: a clinicopathological and prognostic study. *Ann Thorac Surg.* 2001;72:1179–82.

47. Saranga-Perry V, Morse B, Centeno B, *et al.* Treatment of metastatic neuroendocrine tumors of the thymus with capecitabine and temozolomide: a case series. *Neuroendocrinology.* 2013;97:318–21.

48. Savino W, Dardenne M. Neuroendocrine interactions in the thymus: from physiology to therapy. *Neuroimmunomodulation.* 2011;18:263.

49. Cardillo G, Rea F, Lucchi M, *et al.* Primary neuroendocrine tumors of the thymus: a multicenter experience of 35 patients. *Ann Thorac Surg.* 2012;94:241–5.

50. Gal AA, Kornstein MJ, Cohen C *et al.* Neuroendocrine tumors of the thymus: a clinicopathological and prognostic study. *Ann Thorac Surg.* 2001;72:1179–82.

51. Levine GD, Rosai J. A spindle cell varient of thymic carcinoid tumor. A clinical, histologic, and fine structural study with emphasis on its distinction

from spindle cell thymoma. *Arch Pathol Lab Med.* 1976;100:293–300.

52. Moran CA, Suster S. Spindle-cell neuroendocrine carcinomas of the thymus (spindle-cell thymic carcinoid): a clinicopathologic and immunohistochemical study of seven cases. *Mod Pathol.* 1999;12:587–91.

53. Kuo TT. Pigmented spindle cell carcinoid tumour of the thymus with ectopic adrenocorticotropic hormone secretion: report of a rare variant and differential diagnosis of mediastinal spindle cell neoplasms. *Histopathology.* 2002;40:159–65.

54. Ho FC, Ho JC. Pigmented carcinoid tumour of the thymus. *Histopathology.* 1977;1:363–9.

55. Lagrange W, Dahm HH, Karstens J, *et al.* Melanocytic neuroendocrine carcinoma of the thymus. *Cancer.* 1987;59:484–8.

56. Suster S, Moran CA. Thymic carcinoid with prominent mucinous stroma. Report of a distinctive morphologic variant of thymic neuroendocrine neoplasm. *Am J Surg Pathol.* 1995;19:1277–85.

57. Moran CA, Suster S. Primary neuroendocrine carcinoma (thymic carcinoid) of the thymus with prominent oncocytic features: a clinicopathologic study of 22 cases. *Mod Pathol.* 2000;13:489–94.

58. Moran CA, Suster S. Angiomatoid neuroendocrine carcinoma of the thymus: report of a distinctive morphological variant of neuroendocrine tumor of the thymus resembling a vascular neoplasm. *Hum Pathol.* 1999;30:635–9.

59. Cardillo G, Treggiari S, Paul MA, *et al.* Primary neuroendocrine tumours of the thymus: a clinicopathologic and prognostic study in 19 patients. *Eur J Cardiothorac Surg.* 2010;37:814–18.

60. Habbe N, Waldmann J, Bartsch DK, *et al.* Multimodal treatment of sporadic and inherited neuroendocrine tumors of the thymus. *Surgery.* 2008;144:780–5.

61. Oberg K, Hellman P, Ferolla P, *et al.* Neuroendocrine bronchial and thymic tumors: ESMO Clinical Practice Guidelines for diagnosis, treatment and

follow-up. *Ann Oncol.* 2012;23 Suppl 7: vii120–vii123.

62. Levine GD. Primary thymic seminoma–a neoplasm ultrastructurally similar to testicular seminoma and distinct from epithelial thymoma. *Cancer.* 1973;31:729–41.

63. Travis WD, Gal AA, Colby TV, *et al.* Reproducibility of neuroendocrine lung tumor classification. *Hum Pathol.* 1998;29:272–9.

64. Kuo TT. Carcinoid tumor of the thymus with divergent sarcomatoid differentiation: report of a case with histogenetic consideration. *Hum Pathol.* 1994;25:319–23.

65. Paties C, Zangrandi A, Vassallo G, *et al.* Multidirectional carcinoma of the thymus with neuroendocrine and sarcomatoid components and carcinoid syndrome. *Pathol Res Pract.* 1991;187:170–7.

66. Miller BS, Rusinko RY, Fowler L. Synchronous thymoma and thymic carcinoid in a woman with multiple endocrine neoplasia type 1: case report and review. *Endocr Pract.* 2008;14:713–16.

67. Mizuno T, Masaoka A, Hashimoto T, *et al.* Coexisting thymic carcinoid tumor and thymoma. *Ann Thorac Surg.* 1990;50:650–2.

68. Lancaster KJ, Liang CY, Myers JC, *et al.* Goblet cell carcinoid arising in a mature teratoma of the mediastinum. *Am J Surg Pathol.* 1997;21:109–13.

69. Steger C, Steiner HJ, Moser K. *et al.* A typical thymic carcinoid tumour within a thymolipoma: report of a case and review of combined tumours of the thymus. *BMJ Case Rep.* 2010. bcr0420102958. doi: 10.1136/bcr.04.2010.2958

70. Kuo TT. Frequent presence of neuroendocrine small cells in thymic carcinoma: a light microscopic and immunohistochemical study. *Histopathology.* 2000;37: 19–26.

71. Kuo TT, Chang JP, Lin FJ, *et al.* Thymic carcinomas: histopathological varieties and immunohistochemical study. *Am J Surg Pathol.* 1990;14:24–34.

Germ cell tumors of the mediastinum

Sean R. Williamson, MD, and Thomas M. Ulbright, MD

Introduction and general features

Most germ cell tumors occur in the gonads; however, their development in extragonadal sites is an intriguing and recognized phenomenon [1], estimated to account for about 1–6% of all cases [1–5]. Of the extragonadal sites, the mediastinum is the most common [1,6–8], encompassing 50–70% of adult extragonadal germ cell tumors [9]. Conversely, germ cell tumors comprise approximately 10–20% of primary anterior mediastinal tumors (the compartment where they almost exclusively occur) in adults, with the additional primary considerations for this population in this location being thymic lesions, lymphomas, and endocrine tumors (Fig. 9.1) [9–14]. The predominance of mediastinal cases in adults with extragonadal germ cell tumors contrasts with the situation in children where the mediastinum gives rise to only 4–7% of the extragonadal germ cell tumors [9,15,16], and the sacrococcygeal region and central nervous system are more common sites of origin [15,17,18]. However, germ cell tumors are still estimated to make up as much as 24% of primary anterior mediastinal tumors and 8–18% of primary mediastinal tumors as a whole in children since primary epithelial tumors of the thymus are uncommon in the pediatric population (Fig. 9.2) [9,19–21]. Therefore, mediastinal germ cell tumors occur over a wide age range, from neonates to the eighth decade of life [8,10,22]. Median and mean ages vary from 23–40 years, reflecting their predominant occurrence in young adults, particularly men [8,10,22]. Histologic features of mediastinal germ cell tumors are largely similar to those that occur in the testis and ovary, although they exhibit a number of unique clinicopathologic features and occasional characteristic findings that distinguish them from those of the gonads. In this chapter, we will discuss the incidence, distribution, and pathologic features of the individual histologic types of mediastinal germ cell tumors, with particular emphasis on the most important differential diagnostic considerations related to the mediastinum and points of contrast between these tumors and those of the gonads.

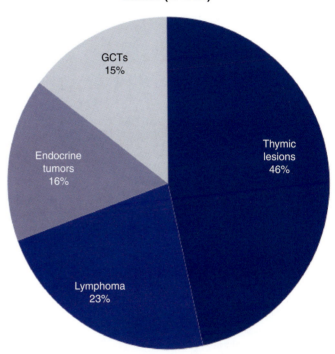

Fig. 9.1 Distribution of primary anterior mediastinal tumors in adults based on data from reference 14. (GCTs – germ cell tumors)

Location

Most mediastinal germ cell tumors occur in the anterior or anterosuperior mediastinum [23–25], within the thymus or adjacent to it. Less commonly, germ cell tumors arise in the posterior mediastinum [23–25]. Intrapericardial cases have also been described, including: yolk sac tumor [26] and teratoma (Fig. 9.3) [27–29]. Rarely, examples of myocardial germ cell tumors, including yolk sac tumor [15], have also been reported. At surgery, other structures are often also found to be involved, including the pericardium, lung, or great vessels [25].

Pathology of the Mediastinum, ed. Alberto M. Marchevsky and Mark R. Wick. Published by Cambridge University Press.
© Cambridge University Press 2014.

Primary anterior mediastinal tumors in children (N=179)

Mesenchymal tumors 14%

Thymic lesions 17%

Lymphoma 45%

GCTs 24%

(a)

Primary mediastinal tumors in children (N=127)

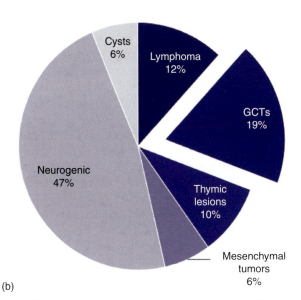

Cysts 6%

Lymphoma 12%

GCTs 19%

Neurogenic 47%

Thymic lesions 10%

Mesenchymal tumors 6%

(b)

Fig. 9.2 Distribution of primary anterior mediastinal tumors **(a)** and mediastinal tumors in general **(b)** in children based on data from references 14 and 12, respectively. (GCTs – germ cell tumors)

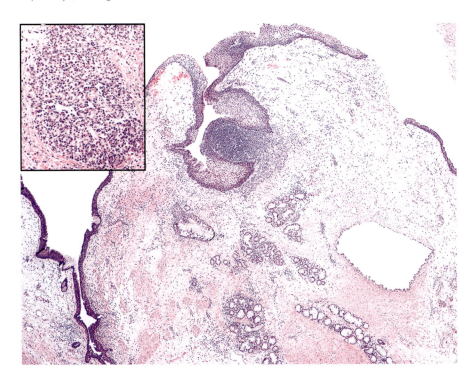

Fig. 9.3 Intrapericardial teratoma with lobular clusters of glands around a central cystic cavity lined by squamous and respiratory epithelium. Pancreatic tissue (inset) was also present.

In contrast to primary mediastinal germ cell tumors, metastases to the mediastinum from a tumor of testicular origin most commonly involve the middle or "visceral" mediastinum, which is attributable to drainage through the thoracic duct. Only a small fraction (7%) involves the anterior mediastinum or paravertebral sulcus (16%), and involvement of the anterior mediastinum as the only site of metastasis is highly unusual [30].

Clinical features and diagnostic techniques

Presenting symptoms of mediastinal germ cell tumors are often related to their location within the chest, including: chest pain, shortness of breath, cough, and superior vena cava obstruction. However, systemic symptoms also occur, and some patients are asymptomatic [8,31,32], with the tumors typically discovered on chest radiographs performed for other reasons. Children have a higher likelihood of being symptomatic [23]. Since the mediastinum is not easily surgically accessed, the frequently limited biopsy material that is available for the diagnosis of mediastinal germ cell tumors represents a departure from what is typically available for the evaluation of gonadal germ cell tumors. Therefore, biopsy specimens may be limited in size and also artifactually distorted, making careful attention to light microscopic morphology critically important and increasing the dependence on immunohistochemistry in supporting the diagnosis. A significant help in the diagnosis of these neoplasms is the availability of serum tumor markers to the extent that many clinicians do not feel biopsy is necessary in certain circumstances. If a young man presents with an anterior mediastinal mass and significantly elevated serum levels of either α-fetoprotein (AFP) or human chorionic gonadotropin (hCG), that patient has an established diagnosis of a non-seminomatous germ cell tumor and platinum-based chemotherapy can be initiated. On the other hand, if serum tumor markers are normal or only minimally elevated (a situation that may be seen in a variety of tumors apart from germ cell tumors) then a tissue diagnosis is required. The first approach is usually with percutaneous needle biopsy. Unfortunately, those samples are susceptible to interpretive problems due to extensive tumor necrosis, crush artifact, limited specimen size and sampling of non-lesional tissue. These problems can be lessened by on-site cytologic evaluation of the specimen to ensure the presence of non-necrotic neoplastic tissue. Still some efforts at needle biopsy fail, and in that circumstance it may be necessary to perform either mini-mediastinotomy or video-assisted thoracoscopic sampling to acquire diagnostic tissue.

Theories regarding pathogenesis

The pathogenesis of mediastinal germ cell tumors is interesting and not entirely understood. Early after their recognition [33], they were considered metastases from an occult primary tumor in the testis [9]. Later, the teratomas were accepted as a primary phenomenon because their benign appearance and behavior made it untenable for them to be considered metastases. Subsequently, non-teratomatous germ cell tumors were recognized as primary neoplasms [6], supported by studies finding no identifiable tumor in the testis or even evidence of a scar to support regression of a putative primary lesion [9,34]. Various hypotheses are offered for their mediastinal origin, none definitively proven [1,6,7,11,35,36]. The most prevalent one posits origin from misplaced germ cells within the thymus, abnormally localized during embryonic migration [1,35,37]. In normal development, primordial germ cells are formed in the epiblast during the second week and are localized within the wall of the yolk sac close to the allantois. They migrate along the dorsal mesentery of the hindgut to arrive at the primitive gonads [38]. As such, the possibility that

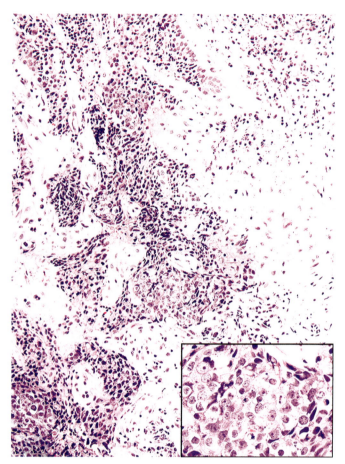

Fig. 9.4 Thymic epithelium containing aggregates of seminoma-like cells. Inset shows higher magnification of seminoma-like cells admixed with thymic epithelial cells.

extragonadal germ cell tumors arise from primordial germ cells that failed to migrate properly has been raised. However, this fails to explain development within the thymus or anterior mediastinum, which is not generally considered to be along this migration path. It also fails to explain why these structures are preferentially involved by extragonadal germ cell tumors compared to other midline structures. Another theory suggests that a number of tissues are normally hosts to germ cells that are distributed during embryogenesis, where they serve incompletely understood regulatory or other functions [9]. Since normal germ cells are not identified within the thymus, their transformation into a somatic cell, such as a myoid cell, has been suggested, particularly since thymic myoid cells, in contrast to the epithelial cells and lymphoid cells, have an incompletely understood origin and function [35]. Still other authors again raise the possibility of gonadal origin [36]. Thymic stem cells, on the other hand, may represent an attractive potential source for these tumors, supported by the finding in some cases of non-invasive seminoma-like cells within nests of thymic epithelium (Fig. 9.4). Regardless of whether or not such a pathogenesis would qualify a neoplasm of "germ cell" origin, historical precedence and treatment considerations mandate continued classification as such.

Epidemiology

Factors leading to the development of mediastinal germ cell tumors are not entirely understood. One interesting association with their development is Klinefelter syndrome, the constellation of hypergonadotropic hypogonadism, infertility, gynecomastia, abnormal body habitus, and mild developmental abnormalities, usually attributable to the constitutional chromosomal abnormality 47, XXY [39–42]. At least 8% of men with primary mediastinal germ cell tumors have Klinefelter syndrome based upon review of cases in the literature [43], and as many as 21–23% when patients are prospectively screened with karyotyping [39,44]. A significant number of children with primary mediastinal germ cell tumors are also subsequently found to have extra copies of the X chromosome [45]. In contrast, men with primary testicular germ cell tumors lack numerical abnormalities of the X chromosome [44]. Klinefelter syndrome has also been associated with malignancies of several organ systems, including leukemia, lymphoma, and carcinoma of the breast and lung [42,46], although a definitive pathogenetic link and the precise risk for development of germ cell tumors and other malignancies is not well established [45]. Since Klinefelter syndrome has a range of clinical features, it may be unrecognized in some men. It has therefore been suggested that patients with mediastinal germ cell tumors be reflexively evaluated for extra copies of the X chromosome [39]. Likewise, suspicious symptoms involving the chest in patients with known Klinefelter syndrome have been suggested to trigger evaluation for a possible mediastinal germ cell tumor [39]. One explanation for the association of Klinefelter syndrome with mediastinal germ cell tumors is an abnormal hormonal milieu during embryonic development, resulting in either increased frequency of aberrant migration of primordial germ cells [39,44] or an increased malignant potential of hormonally induced dysgenetic germ cells [39]. The possibility that the hypergonadotropism of Klinefelter syndrome produces a stimulatory effect has also been raised [40,45]; however, there does not appear to be an increased risk for gonadal germ cell tumors in Klinefelter syndrome [45], which might otherwise be expected.

Other environmental or other factors contributing to the development of mediastinal germ cell tumors are not well characterized. In an analysis of additional, non-germinal malignancies in patients with extragonadal germ cell tumors, mediastinal germ cell tumors were not found to be associated with a significantly increased risk of developing other malignancies, with the exception of hematopoietic neoplasms (discussed later in conjunction with yolk sac tumor) [47].

Genetics

Similar to testicular germ cell tumors, gain of chromosome 12p, often in the form of isochromosome 12p, appears to be a key event in the pathogenesis of malignant mediastinal germ cell tumors in postpubertal patients [45]. Benign mediastinal teratomas in both prepubertal and postpubertal patients usually show no genetic gains or losses, at least in young patients

in whom these genetic alterations have been most thoroughly studied [45,48,49]. Genetic alterations in malignant mediastinal germ cell tumors of prepubertal patients (predominantly yolk sac tumor) are largely similar to those of testicular or sacrococcygeal tumors in this age group [36,50,51], with frequent gains of chromosomes 1q, 3, or 20q and loss of chromosomes 1p, 4q, or 6q, but lacking 12p amplification [45]. The chromosomal region Xq27 has recently been noted as a possible susceptibility locus for testicular germ cell neoplasms [52] suggesting that gain of an extra copy of the X chromosome may play a role in development of these tumors in patients with Klinefelter syndrome. However, subsequent investigation of genetic links has not supported a strong association with this chromosomal region in most cases, suggesting that if genes at this site are involved in the pathogenesis of germ cell tumors they are only involved in a small proportion of cases [53].

Distribution of histologic subtypes of mediastinal germ cell tumors

It is important to separate the mediastinal germ cell tumors by gender and pubertal status since, as will become apparent and has already been alluded to in the preceding section concerning genetics, the pathogenesis and likely behavior differ significantly according to these parameters.

Mediastinal germ cell tumors in postpubertal male patients

Similar to germ cell tumors of the testis, mediastinal germ cell tumors may be composed of variable admixtures of seminoma, yolk sac tumor, embryonal carcinoma, choriocarcinoma, and teratoma [1,9]. Since most occur in male patients, especially malignant germ cell tumors, of which greater than 90% occur in men [9,10,23–25,54], it might be expected that the distribution of histologic subtypes would closely mirror that of the testis. However, several striking differences contrast mediastinal germ cell tumors with those of the testis, supporting the idea that differing pathogenetic mechanisms are at play [36]. As one such example, teratoma is a common subtype of mediastinal germ cell tumor, even in male patients, while pure teratoma is infrequent in the testis (approximately 4% of germ cell tumors) [55].

Along these lines, teratoma and seminoma comprise the largest fractions of mediastinal germ cell tumors in postpubertal male patients, with the more predominant of the two varying somewhat between large series [10,23–25,54]. Among the 322 tumors reported by Moran and Suster (Fig. 9.5), the great majority of which were from postpubertal male patients, there were 138 that had a teratoma component; those included 87 pure mature teratomas, 6 immature teratomas, and 45 cases of teratoma with additional malignant components, including 19 with one or more additional germ cell tumor components (what we would consider a mixed germ cell tumor); 13 with one or more additional germ cell tumor components and sarcoma; 7 with sarcoma; 4 with carcinoma; and 2 with

Mediastinal germ cell tumors - AFIP Series (N=322)

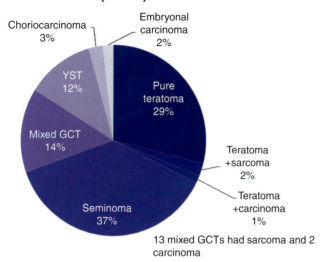

Fig. 9.5 Distribution of primary mediastinal germ cell tumor subtypes, based on data from the Armed Forces Institute of Pathology series of 322 patients (reference 10; GCT – germ cell tumor; YST – yolk sac tumor)

Mediastinal germ cell tumors in postpubertal female patients (N=128)

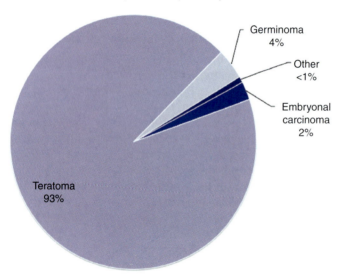

Fig. 9.7 Distribution of subtypes of primary mediastinal germ cell tumors in postpubertal female patients, estimated based on data from references 10, 23, 24, 25, 54, and 56.

one or more germ cell tumor components with carcinoma. The remaining tumors included 120 seminomas, 38 yolk sac tumors, 12 mixed germ cell tumors, 8 choriocarcinomas, and 6 embryonal carcinomas [10]. Therefore, teratoma either pure or as a component of a mixed germ cell tumor is likely the most common element, while either seminoma or teratoma is likely the most common pure tumor.

In the series of Japanese patients reported by Takeda and colleagues, teratoma was the most common mediastinal germ cell tumor in male patients (36 cases), more significantly

Mediastinal germ cell tumors in postpubertal male patients (N=519)

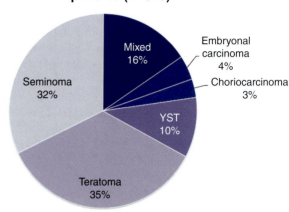

Fig. 9.6 Distribution of subtypes of primary mediastinal germ cell tumors in postpubertal male patients, estimated based on data from references 10, 23, 24, 25, 54, and 56. (YST – yolk sac tumor)

outnumbering seminomas (13 cases), although pre- and postpubertal cases were not discriminated. Almost all of the malignant mediastinal germ cell tumors in that series occurred in postpubertal male patients [12,23]. In the French experience of Dulmet et al., teratomas also outnumbered seminomas and other non-seminomatous germ cell tumors [24]. Other studies, in contrast, have found a greater proportion of seminomas than teratomas [8]. Pure yolk sac tumors, embryonal carcinomas, and choriocarcinomas comprise smaller fractions of mediastinal germ cell tumors in postpubertal male patients. Interestingly, pure yolk sac tumor comprises approximately 10% of mediastinal germ cell tumors in this population [7,10,23,24,54], a substantially greater frequency than pure yolk sac tumor of the testis (approximately 1%) [7,55]. Mixed germ cell tumors in the testis encompass a significant fraction of cases (approximately one third), whereas primary mediastinal mixed germ cell tumors make up a smaller number (approximately 15% based on our estimation from several large series of mediastinal germ cell tumors) [10,23–25,54,56]. The proportions of other subtypes, in contrast, appear to be relatively similar in the testis and mediastinum (Fig. 9.6) [55,56]. Notably, testicular germ cell tumors are over-represented in Caucasian men compared to other ethnic groups; however, extragonadal germ cell tumors do not appear to share this characteristic, with a more uniform distribution across races [5].

Mediastinal germ cell tumors in postpubertal female patients

Mediastinal germ cell tumors in women are uncommon and those that do occur are usually teratomas (Fig. 9.7), with an approximately equal number of teratomas in male and female patients [23–25] or even a female predominance [24]. In the series of Moran and Suster [10], only 2 of 322 primary mediastinal germ cell tumors occurred in women, both of which were teratomas associated with other malignant components, although selection bias for malignant cases and military-derived cases likely played a role for this finding in

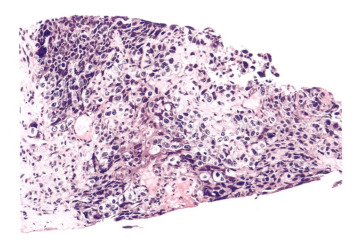

Fig. 9.8 Primary mediastinal choriocarcinoma in a young woman in a needle biopsy showing admixture of mononucleated trophoblast cells with less conspicuous syncytiotrophoblasts having denser cytoplasm and smudged nuclear chromatin. The latter were highlighted by an hCG immunostain and the post-chemotherapy resection had a yolk sac tumor component.

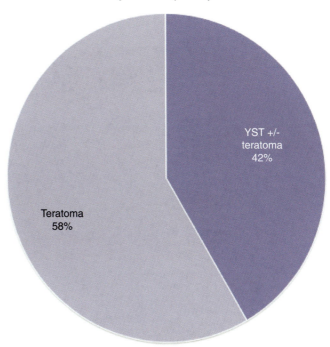

Mediastinal germ cell tumors in prepubertal patients (N=48)

YST +/- teratoma 42%

Teratoma 58%

Fig. 9.9 Distribution of subtypes of primary mediastinal germ cell tumors in prepubertal patients, estimated based on data from references 15 and 64. (YST – yolk sac tumor)

that study. The marked predilection for malignant mediastinal germ cell tumors to occur in young men has also been observed in other large series [9,10,23–25,54]; but, a small number of non-teratomatous germ cell tumors have been reported in women, including: yolk sac tumor [57], dysgerminoma [23,24,54,58,59], embryonal carcinoma [23,54,60], and choriocarcinoma (Fig. 9.8) [61].

Mediastinal germ cell tumors in prepubertal patients

In prepubertal children, mediastinal germ cell tumors generally consist of teratoma and yolk sac tumor (Fig. 9.9) [7,15,62] and unlike in postpubertal patients, they occur in the prepubertal group with at least equal frequency in female as male patients [15,63]. Schneider *et al.* reported equal numbers of teratoma and "secreting" germ cell tumors (either yolk sac tumor or predominantly yolk sac tumor) among 34 patients 0–9 years of age with mediastinal germ cell tumors [15]. Similarly, in a study of 21 children with mediastinal germ cell tumors, Lack *et al.* [64] reported 11 pure teratomas (6 girls and 5 boys) and 3 yolk sac tumors (2 boys and 1 girl), one of which also included a teratomatous component. (The single non-teratomatous tumor in a girl was referred to as "embryonal carcinoma," [64] although based on the description it likely would be considered a yolk sac tumor in a more current classification scheme.) In both of these studies, all tumors in infants under 1 year of age were teratoma [15,64].

Essentially all malignant tumors in girls are yolk sac tumor, and this is also true for younger boys, with the great majority of cases occurring in those 4 years of age or less [62,63]. In older children, boys, but not girls, may develop other malignant germ cell tumor types, but seminoma is rarely if ever seen in those less than 10 years of age [15,21,23,32,49], contrasting with adults.

Staging of mediastinal germ cell tumors

Based on the outcomes from their large series of primary mediastinal germ cell tumors, Moran and Suster proposed a staging system specific for mediastinal germ cell tumors, distinct from that used for primary thymic epithelial neoplasms [10]. Their recommendation divides tumors into four groups: Stage I encompasses well-circumscribed tumors that may have pleural or pericardial adhesions but do not demonstrate invasion of adjacent structures. Stage II, in contrast, includes tumors that are confined to the mediastinum but which do exhibit invasion (microscopic or macroscopic) of adjacent structures, such as the pleura, pericardium, or great vessels. Stage III is divided into two groups: IIIa for tumors with intrathoracic metastasis (such as lymph node or lung), and IIIb for tumors with extrathoracic metastases [10,65].

Individual tumor types

Seminoma

Primary mediastinal seminoma is one of the two most common subtypes of mediastinal germ cell tumor, usually ranked just below or just above teratoma in frequency in most studies [8,12,23,32]. As with malignant mediastinal germ cell tumors in general, pure seminomas almost always occur in men and there is a tendency for development in slightly older patients than testicular seminoma [22,23,32], with a mean age up to 47 years [32]. Like its gonadal counterparts, primary

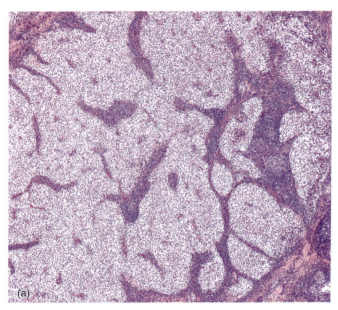
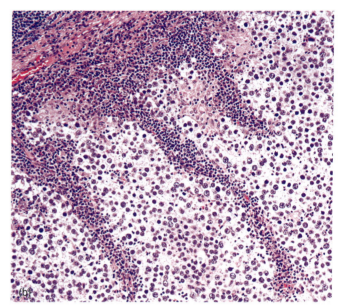

Fig. 9.10 Primary mediastinal seminoma showing characteristic fibrous septa with lymphocytes separating islands of tumor cells **(a)** and having associated epithelioid granulomas **(b)**.

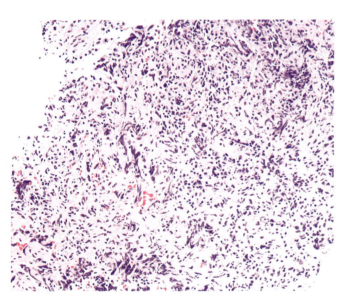
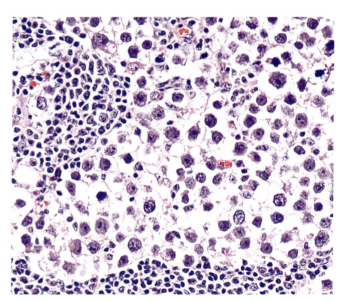

Fig. 9.11 Mediastinal seminoma in a core biopsy specimen with prominent "crush" or "squeezing" artifact that obscures the cytologic features of the tumor cells, a common finding that causes diagnostic difficulty.

Fig. 9.12 Characteristic cytologic features of seminoma, including rounded or squared nuclear contours, abundant clear cytoplasm, prominent cell borders, and conspicuous central nucleoli.

mediastinal seminoma grossly forms a large, soft, tan mass, often with a lobulated contour and sometimes with gross necrosis or hemorrhage [32]. Microscopically, the growth pattern is often nested or lobulated, with tumor nests separated by fibrovascular septa often containing infiltrates of lymphocytes. (Fig. 9.10a) Epithelioid granulomas are scattered throughout in many cases, (Fig. 9.10b) sometimes with giant cells of Langhans type. Tumors may also include foci of necrosis, which may limit the amount of viable tumor tissue in needle biopsy specimens, and seminoma is especially susceptible to "squeezing" artifact in core biopsy, yielding elongated thread-like distortion of tumor cells (Fig. 9.11). Similar to their

testicular counterparts, primary mediastinal seminomas also include scattered syncytiotrophoblastic cells in some cases, which may be a helpful diagnostic feature [32]. Approximately a quarter of cases also include remnants of thymic tissue, within the mass or at its periphery [66]. Cytologically, the cells of seminoma characteristically have clear cytoplasm and prominent cell borders, (Fig. 9.12) although eosinophilic or scant cytoplasm can also be seen (Fig. 9.13), potentially causing concern for a non-seminomatous germ cell tumor such as yolk sac tumor or embryonal carcinoma or a primary thymic carcinoma. Characteristic features include enlarged nuclei with rounded or squared-off contours, clumped nuclear chromatin, and prominent, often single nucleoli (Fig. 9.12).

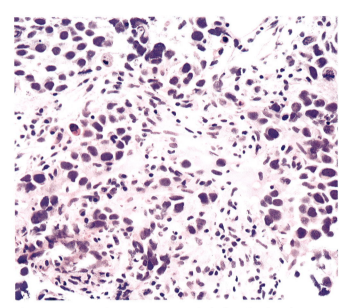

Fig. 9.13 Mediastinal seminoma composed of cells with enlarged, hyperchromatic nuclei and scant to moderate eosinophilic cytoplasm.

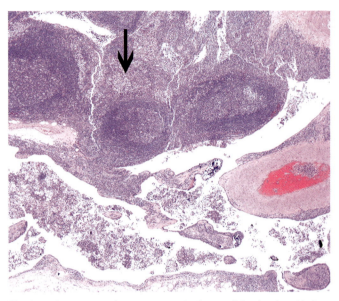

Fig. 9.14 Seminoma with prominent cystic change of the thymic epithelium, resembling a thymic cyst. Seminoma cells (arrow) may be inconspicuously dispersed within the prominent lymphocytic infiltrate.

An interesting feature of primary mediastinal seminoma is prominent cystic change of the thymic epithelium, reported to occur in approximately 10% of tumors (Fig. 9.14) [66]. This phenomenon can be so striking that it leads to a misdiagnosis of a benign thymic cyst, both clinically and pathologically. Moran and Suster reported ten such seminomas [66]. Grossly, they formed multilocular cystic masses with relatively small foci of gray-white induration on the cut surfaces of the cyst walls. Microscopically, some of these cyst walls have areas of nodularity accompanied by a brisk inflammatory infiltrate and granulomas, providing clues to the presence of the seminoma cells, evident at higher magnification [66]. Hence, these findings stress the importance of careful gross examination, thorough sampling, and attentive microscopic examination of mediastinal tumors with a multilocular cystic growth pattern. Hodgkin lymphoma is also prone to such change, as well as thymoma [67].

Differential diagnosis

The morphologic characteristics of seminomas raise a number of differential diagnostic considerations in the mediastinum that differ from those of the testis. Hodgkin lymphoma, particularly the nodular sclerosing subtype (which involves the mediastinum in approximately 80% of cases) [68] may be a prime consideration in the differential diagnosis since both neoplasms are composed of a population of large cells with abundant cytoplasm and prominent nucleoli and often intermingled with mature lymphoid cells and epithelioid histiocytes. Aggregates of lacunar cells in Hodgkin lymphoma can also morphologically resemble granulomatous inflammation [68]. The presence of binucleate cells with genuine Reed-Sternberg cell morphology is a tremendous aid and can guide the prudent use of immunohistochemical studies. Large B-cell lymphoma may also enter the differential diagnosis, in which case the more ovoid nuclear shape and frequently irregular nuclear contours may be helpful distinguishing features, triggering application of lymphoid immunohistochemical markers.

Metastatic melanoma is another neoplasm often composed of non-cohesive cells demonstrating prominent nucleoli and having varied cytoplasmic characteristics. A known clinical history of melanoma [32] and characteristic morphologic features that may include intracellular pigment, mixed spindle-shaped and epithelioid cells and eccentrically-located nuclei with prominent eosinophilic nucleoli, are helpful and should prompt immunohistochemical confirmation. Like seminoma and Hodgkin lymphoma, thymic epithelial neoplasms also frequently include a lymphocytic component. Features of thymomas that may point to the correct diagnosis include thick bands of fibrous connective tissue, a calcified capsule, and prominently lobulated architecture, evident even at the gross level. Perivascular spaces containing proteinaceous material, blood, or inflammatory cells are also a characteristic microscopic feature [32]. In contrast, although seminomas may have a vaguely lobulated appearance grossly, they usually have more delicate fibrous septa that are not visible grossly. The epithelial cell nuclei in thymoma sometimes possess nucleoli, although generally their chromatin is fine compared to the coarse chromatin with prominent nucleoli of seminoma [69]. Expression of cytokeratin in thymoma and the absence of more specific markers of seminoma (see below) are major diagnostic aids. Thymic carcinoma generally shows morphologic features similar to carcinomas of other sites, including more cohesive arrangements and greater pleomorphism than most seminomas. In particular, the clear cell variant of thymic carcinoma, however, may more closely mimic seminoma, although its lack of the ancillary features associated with seminoma (intimate lymphocytic infiltrates, granulomatous inflammation, or syncytiotrophoblastic cells [32]) may be helpful in resolving this differential diagnosis.

Other subtypes of mediastinal germ cell tumors may also be considered in the differential diagnosis of seminoma.

Table 9.1. Most common patterns of immunoreactivity for neoplasms in the differential diagnosis of mediastinal germ cell tumors*

Diagnosis	Cytokeratin AE1/AE3	EMA	CK7	OCT4	PLAP	c-KIT (CD117)	Podoplanin	SOX2	SOX17	SALL4	HCG	CD30	Glypican-3	AFP	Other markers
Seminoma	+/−	−	+/−	+	+	+	+	−	+	+	−	−	−	−	
Yolk sac tumor	+	−	−	−	+	+/−	−	−	+/−	+	−	−	+	+/−	
Embryonal carcinoma	+	−	+/−	+	+	−	−	+	−	+	−	+	+/−	−	
Chorio-carcinoma	+	+/−	+	−	+	−	+/−	−	−	+/−	+	−	+	−	p63, inhibin
Thymoma	+	+	+/−	−	−	−	+/−	−	ND	−	ND	ND	ND	ND	PAX8
Thymic carcinoma	+	+/−	+/−	−	−	+	ND	−	ND	−	ND	ND	ND	ND	CD5, PAX8
Large cell lymphoma	−	−	−	−	−	+/−	−	−	ND	−	ND	+/−	ND	ND	Lymphoid markers
Metastatic carcinoma	+	+/−	+/−	−	+/−	+/−	+/−	ND	ND	+/−	+/−	−	+/−	+/−	Origin dependent

* Although the table provides a synopsis of the usual immunoreactivity patterns of various neoplasms for several antigens, it is important to be aware that occasional exceptions to these patterns do occur. Abbreviations: EMA – epithelial membrane antigen, CK7 – cytokeratin 7, PLAP – placental alkaline phosphatase, HCG – human chorionic gonadotropin, AFP – alpha fetoprotein, ND – no data or limited data available.

Since primary mediastinal seminomas sometimes contain scattered syncytiotrophoblastic cells [32], care must be taken to avoid misdiagnosis of choriocarcinoma, which includes associated populations of mononucleated trophoblasts and syncytiotrophoblasts. Choriocarcinoma, in contrast to seminoma, lacks a stromal component (fibrous septa), lymphocytes, and granulomatous response and has a more diffusely hemorrhagic background than the punctate hemorrhagic foci that typifies seminoma with trophoblast cells. Additionally, the mononucleated trophoblast cells of choriocarcinoma are usually significantly more pleomorphic than seminoma cells. Contrasting immunohistochemical features (see below) are also present. Some seminomas may have an increased degree of nuclear pleomorphism; however, in contrast to embryonal carcinomas, the nuclei usually show little overlap and lack epithelial structures (glands, papillae). Problematic cases may be resolved with immunohistochemistry. When a slightly lesser degree of cytologic atypia is present, solid-pattern yolk sac tumor may also be considered in the differential diagnosis with seminoma (Fig. 9.15a). Admixture of other characteristic patterns of yolk sac tumor, most commonly microcystic/reticular, and the presence of intercellular basement membrane material or intracellular hyaline globules may be helpful clues to the correct diagnosis in such cases [70]. Serum AFP levels and immunohistochemistry should resolve this differential.

Immunohistochemistry

Although antibody to placental alkaline phosphatase (PLAP) used to be the most frequently recommended immunohistochemical marker for the diagnosis of seminoma, its specificity is limited, with frequent reactivity in a number of

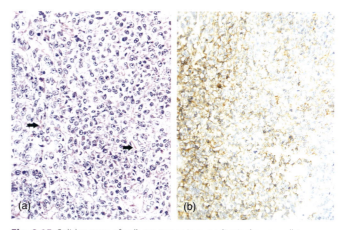

Fig. 9.15 Solid pattern of yolk sac tumor in a mediastinal germ cell tumor resembling seminoma but with deposition of intercellular basement membrane material (arrows) **(a)**. Membrane staining for CD117, a potential diagnostic pitfall **(b)**.

other tumors, including lung and intestinal carcinomas (Table 9.1) [71]. Interestingly, however, primary mediastinal seminoma has been reported to have an increased likelihood of showing a positive reaction for PLAP (93%) compared to testicular seminoma (50%) [72,73]. More recently, stem cell-directed immunohistochemical markers such as OCT4 and SALL4 have begun to assume a more substantial role in confirming the germ cell origin of primary and metastatic tumors. As in the testis, these two markers have a high sensitivity for primary mediastinal seminomas and embryonal carcinomas [73,74], with OCT4 being specific, with only rare non-small-cell carcinomas of the lung and renal cell carcinomas showing positivity [75]. Yolk sac tumor, in contrast, is positive for

SALL4 but negative for OCT4. Antibody to CD117 (c-KIT) frequently labels seminoma cells and usually is negative in embryonal carcinoma; however, positive staining is not restricted to seminomas, also showing positive reactivity in yolk sac tumors (Fig. 9.15b) [70,76], as well as other neoplasms [77]. Limited or negative staining for cytokeratin (AE1/AE3) and CD30 and positivity for podoplanin also support a diagnosis of seminoma over embryonal carcinoma. It should be kept in mind, however, that mediastinal seminomas, although generally considered to have limited cytokeratin reactivity, may show frequent (80%) paranuclear, dot-like positivity with antibody to cytokeratin CAM 5.2 that contrasts with 20% reactivity in testicular cases [72]. Otherwise, cytokeratin expression is generally limited to a minority of the tumor cells [73]. More recently, antibody to SOX2 has also been utilized as a positive marker of embryonal carcinoma, distinguishing it from seminoma. As in the testis, it appears useful in labeling primary mediastinal embryonal carcinomas, although positive expression is also sometimes seen in carcinomas originating in other organs [74].

Teratoma

Teratoma, either in pure form or as a component of a mixed germ cell tumor, usually ranks as the most common type of mediastinal germ cell tumor. As in other sites, mediastinal teratomas are frequently composed of a mixture of mature and/or immature histologic tissue types that recapitulate the differentiation of multiple germinal layers (ectoderm, mesoderm, or endoderm) [7]. They occur over a wide age range, with one large series spanning patients from 1 month to 73 years old (mean, 28 years) [25]. During the first year of life, teratoma is the predominant type of mediastinal tumor [7].

An area of contrast between pure teratomas of the mediastinum and postpubertal testis is the important distinction between mature and immature phenotypes in the mediastinum [1]. In the postpubertal testis almost all teratomas are malignant, even those that are composed of mature tissues, due to their development from intratubular germ cell neoplasia, unclassified-type through various forms of non-teratomatous germ cell tumor [55]. This pathogenesis negates the impact of immaturity, with the common occurrence of metastases in patients with pure "mature" testicular teratomas. However, mature teratomas of the mediastinum, including those of adult men, behave in a benign manner [1]. Immaturity, which requires the presence of embryonic type tissue in the teratoma, needs therefore to be recognized in mediastinal teratomas because of its possible negative impact on clinical behavior, although in children it has been thought that immaturity, *per se*, is not the direct cause of such behavior but rather its tendency to correlate with aggressively acting yolk sac tumor elements [78].

Mature teratoma

Pure (mature, benign) mediastinal teratomas tend to exhibit pathologic characteristics that contrast with those of malignant mixed germ cell tumors with a teratoma component. Grossly and by imaging studies, benign teratomas often form a large, single, cystic cavity or multiple cystic spaces. Calcification, either of the wall of the mass or in the form of bone or tooth structures, can be a helpful radiographic feature leading to their recognition [25]. Grossly, bone or hair is more commonly a feature of mature teratoma than teratoma as a component of a mixed germ cell tumor [10]. Microscopically, the cystic cavities are often lined by squamous epithelium and frequently associated with cutaneous adnexal elements in an organoid architecture around the cyst (Fig. 9.16); other epithelial components, such as enteric and respiratory-type glands [10], are common and may form organoid arrangements with mesenchymal tissues that often include smooth muscle, adipose tissue, cartilage and bone (Fig. 9.17) [25]. Mature glial tissue is also frequent. Interestingly, pancreatic tissue is common, (Fig. 9.18) contrasting with

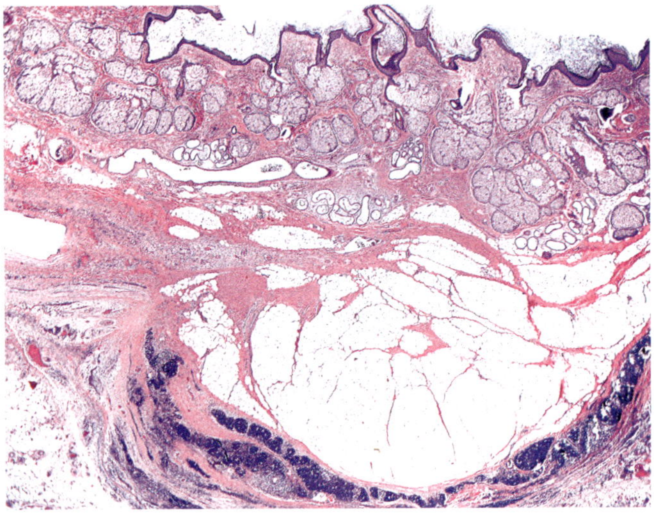

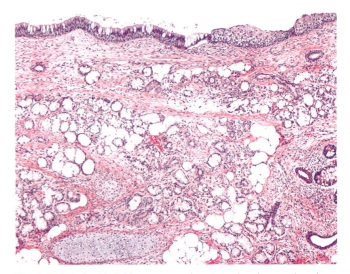

Fig. 9.16 Organoid arrangement of sebaceous glands and cutaneous adnexal elements around a squamous-lined central cystic cavity in a mature mediastinal teratoma. Adipose and residual thymic tissue are also present (bottom).

Fig. 9.17 Mixed epithelial (squamous and respiratory) and mesenchymal elements (cartilage, adipose tissue, and smooth muscle) in a mediastinal teratoma.

its less frequent presence in gonadal teratomas [37,79–81]. In keeping with the high degree of differentiation of these tissue types, it often contains not only acinar structures but also pancreatic islets [25], including a mixture of the normal islet cell types (alpha, beta, delta cells) [82,83] and ductal structures. In some cases, pancreatic differentiation is such a prominent component of the teratoma that proteolytic enzymes can be detected by aspiration of the contents of the cyst cavity, proposed to have diagnostic utility in some circumstances [84]. This enzyme production has also been hypothesized to be at least partly responsible for the tendency of mediastinal teratomas to be inflamed [85] and in some cases to rupture. A graph showing the relative frequencies of various tissue types in mature mediastinal teratoma is provided in Fig. 9.19.

Immature teratoma

Immature teratoma in contrast is composed, at least in part, of embryonic-type tissues that may show differentiation along several pathways, but most commonly manifest as immature neuroectodermal elements. These often form primitive neural tubules (Fig. 9.20) but other arrangements, including rosettes, pseudorosettes, and diffuse growth, may also occur. A diagnostic pitfall with regard to an immature component is the discrimination of mature ependymal structures from true immature neuroectodermal elements [1]. Mature ependymal tubules are lined by cuboidal or columnar ciliated cells arranged around a true lumen, typically associated with other mature glial tissues, in contrast to immature neuroepithelial

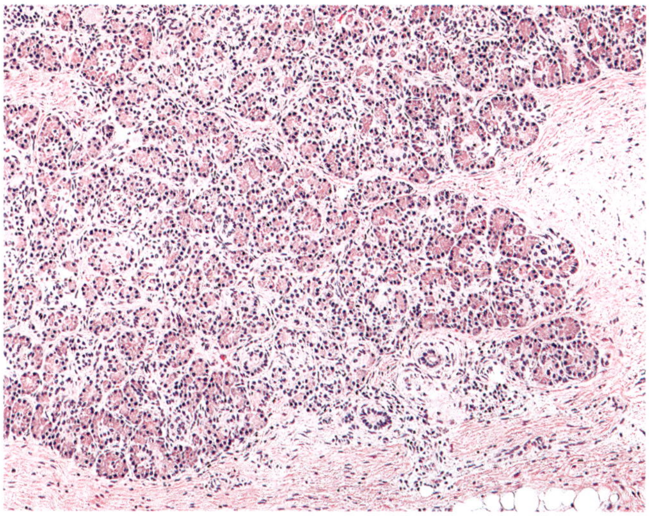

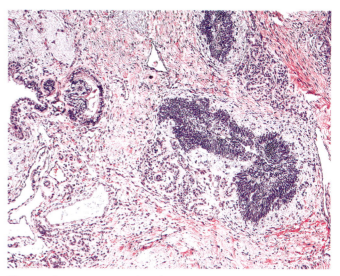

Fig. 9.20 Primitive neuroectodermal tissue in an immature mediastinal teratoma.

Fig. 9.18 Pancreatic tissue in a mediastinal teratoma, including acini and ducts.

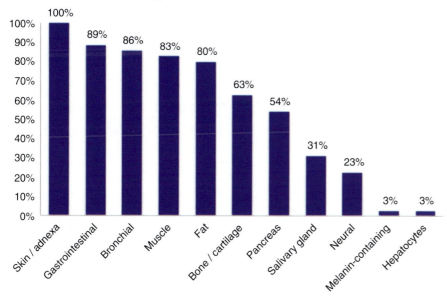

Tissue types in mature mediastinal teratomas

Skin / adnexa 100%
Gastrointestinal 89%
Bronchial 86%
Muscle 83%
Fat 80%
Bone / cartilage 63%
Pancreas 54%
Salivary gland 31%
Neural 23%
Melanin-containing 3%
Hepatocytes 3%

Fig. 9.19 Most common tissue types in mature teratomas of the mediastinum, based on data from references 80 and 81.

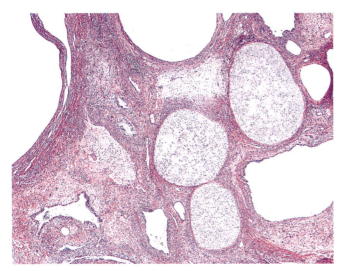

Fig. 9.21 Haphazard arrangement of mesenchymal, epithelial, and glial elements in the teratomatous component of a mixed mediastinal germ cell tumor.

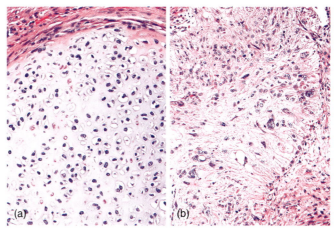

Fig. 9.22 Increased cellularity and cytologic atypia in the cartilaginous (**a**) and glial (**b**) teratomatous components of a mixed mediastinal germ cell tumor.

rosettes, which often have readily identifiable mitotic figures embedded in a background of cellular mesenchymal stroma [1]. Other immature elements in teratoma may include blastemal-like stromal cells, and primitive tubules resembling structures seen in nephroblastoma.

Grading of immature teratomas, as performed for ovarian tumors [86], has not been found to have established prognostic value in the mediastinum; however, reporting an estimated percentage of immature elements is generally recommended for mediastinal cases [1,87]. In prepubertal children, immaturity appears to correlate with a higher likelihood of a yolk sac tumor component [1,78] and in postpubertal patients an immature component is associated with an increased likelihood that the teratoma is a component of a malignant mixed germ cell tumor and has chromosome 12p amplification, including isochromosome 12p [87].

Teratomatous components in mixed germ cell tumors

When a teratomatous component is present in association with other germ cell tumor types (seminoma, yolk sac tumor, embryonal carcinoma, choriocarcinoma), it is classified as a mixed germ cell tumor with a teratomatous component [87]. Although these teratomatous components also demonstrate multiple tissue types recapitulating those of the germinal layers, the well-differentiated, organoid architecture that typifies the mature, histologically benign form of teratoma is lacking. The tissue elements themselves often possess a more disorganized, haphazard arrangement (Fig. 9.21) and are associated with areas of hemorrhage or necrosis [10] and frequently show an increased degree of cytologic atypia (Fig. 9.22a and b).

Somatic-type malignancy of germ cell tumor origin

Somatic-type malignancies arising from mediastinal germ cell tumors are well-established and include sarcomas, carcinomas, malignant glial tumors, and hematopoietic-like

malignancies [10,88-90]. The terminology "teratoma with malignant transformation" has often been used for this phenomenon [91], although this nomenclature is not ideal since this event is likely to develop in association with a mixed germ cell tumor and the teratomatous component of a mixed germ cell tumor should not be considered "benign". Additionally, although such neoplasms have been hypothesized to derive from teratoma, perhaps through acquisition of additional genetic alterations, origin from other germ cell tumor components or a malignant common progenitor cell are also distinct possibilities. Not surprisingly, the development of somatic-type malignancies in mediastinal germ cell tumors is almost exclusively confined to postpubertal patients with malignant germ cell tumors, with both their conventional tumor and somatic-type malignancy sharing chromosome 12p abnormalities [90,92]. Most of these somatic-type malignancies are sarcomas, which are discussed in greater detail below in conjunction with yolk sac tumor. The distinction of somatic-type malignancies from atypical teratomatous elements (which are a usual finding in the postpubertal germ cell tumors of males) can be problematic. What we require, for sarcomas, is overgrowth of a pure lesion exceeding a 4× microscopic field. The diagnosis of carcinomas depends upon identifying destructive, infiltrative growth by cytologically malignant epithelial cells, often accompanied by a desmoplastic reaction, as in carcinomas of other sites (Fig. 9.23).

Differential diagnosis

Multilocular thymic cyst, because of its multiple cystic spaces lined by cuboidal, ciliated, or squamous epithelium (Fig. 9.24), may mimic teratoma. In contrast to teratoma, heterologous elements such as pancreatic tissue, neuroglia, cartilage, or other tissues foreign to the thymus are not found in multilocular thymic cysts. Sebaceous glands and parathyroid tissue are occasionally seen within the thymus and thought to be related to anomalous thymic development rather than indicative of teratoma [93]. The fibrous septa between the spaces of

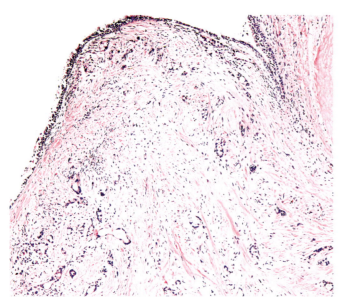

Fig. 9.23 Adenocarcinoma, composed of infiltrative glands in a desmoplastic stroma, developing as a secondary somatic-type malignancy in a mediastinal teratoma.

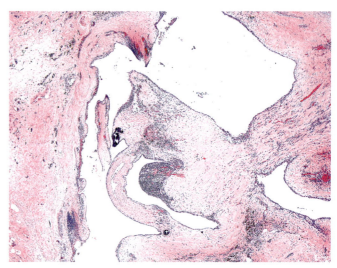

Fig. 9.24 Multilocular thymic cyst composed of multiple cystic spaces within a fibrous stroma containing inflammatory cells and siderophages and resembling teratoma but lacking heterologous tissue types.

multilocular thymic cyst are typically thick and inflamed. Although residual thymic tissue can be observed adjacent to a teratoma, it is usually not as prominent as in multilocular thymic cyst, lacks the frequently inflammatory background of the latter, and may show intervening mesenchymal stromal elements. Likewise, enteric [94,95] and bronchogenic cysts enter the differential diagnosis of a mediastinal teratoma. The former, however, always occur in the posterior mediastinum and are composed of a two-layered smooth muscle wall surrounding an enteric-type glandular lumen [95]. Some features of bronchogenic cysts overlap with those of teratoma, particularly in the composition by respiratory epithelium, smooth muscle, and cartilage. However, the absence of non-bronchial components and their bronchus-like appearance are helpful distinguishing features [1,95]. Additionally, malignant neoplasms having spindled and epithelioid components, such as synovial sarcoma [96] or biphasic mesothelioma, may also be considered in the differential diagnosis [1], but they lack the heterogeneity of teratoma and have overtly malignant features.

Yolk sac tumor

Yolk sac tumor is the predominant malignant germ cell tumor in prepubertal patients [7,15,62,64], found in some studies to have a female predominance [45]. In adults, primarily men, pure yolk sac tumor comprises 3 to 18% of mediastinal germ cell tumors (Figs. 9.5 and 9.6) [7,10,23,24,54], overall a greater proportion than pure yolk sac tumor of the testis. It is also frequently a component of mediastinal mixed germ cell tumors, where it admixes with teratoma in prepubertal patients [45] or other germ cell tumor types in postpubertal patients [56]. Grossly, yolk sac tumors usually form large, partially encapsulated anterior

mediastinal masses with a rounded to nodular contour. The cut surface may be solid and tan colored, myxoid, or cystic, often containing areas of hemorrhage, congestion, or necrosis. If present in a mixed germ cell tumor, teratomatous components may also be recognizable grossly [97]. As is the case with other neoplasms involving the thymus, including lymphoma, seminoma, or thymoma, yolk sac tumor may occasionally cause multilocular cystic change of the thymic epithelium imparting resemblance to multilocular thymic cyst [98].

Microscopically, similar to yolk sac tumor of the testis, the reticular or microcystic pattern is the most common one, comprising a net-like or web-like arrangement of cells with intracellular vacuoles and thin, interconnecting strands of cytoplasm (Figs. 9.25 and 9.26) [56]. A myxomatous or myxoid pattern is often intimately intermingled with microcystic elements (Figs. 9.25 and 9.26) [56]. The endodermal sinus pattern is also seen in mediastinal tumors, so-named for the formation of endodermal sinus-like structures or Schiller–Duval bodies, composed of a central vessel surrounded by a layer of fibrous tissue and a rim of tumor cells that is recessed in a cystic space, lined by flattened epithelium at its periphery (Fig. 9.27) [97]. Other yolk sac tumor patterns, including papillary (Fig. 9.28) and glandular (Fig. 9.29), can also be seen in mediastinal cases [97]. The solid pattern (Figs. 9.15a and 9.30), composed of sheet-like arrangements of frequently clear or pale cells, may be a particular source of differential diagnostic difficulty, especially in the mediastinum [70]. In gonadal tumors, ample histologic sampling of the tumor usually reveals other yolk sac tumor patterns admixed with the solid growth. In the mediastinum, however, small biopsies are often performed, and differentiation from other tumors may be more challenging. Other key features facilitating recognition of solid yolk sac tumor include the formation of hyaline globules (Fig. 9.31) and deposition of basement membrane material (Fig. 9.30), a feature shared by many patterns of yolk sac tumor, including solid ones [70,97].

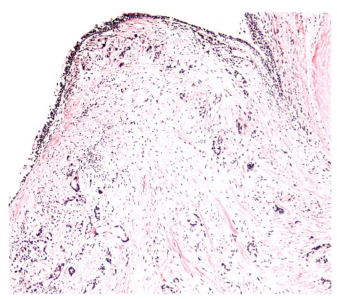

Fig. 9.23 Adenocarcinoma, composed of infiltrative glands in a desmoplastic stroma, developing as a secondary somatic-type malignancy in a mediastinal teratoma.

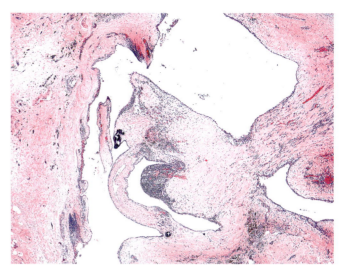

Fig. 9.24 Multilocular thymic cyst composed of multiple cystic spaces within a fibrous stroma containing inflammatory cells and siderophages and resembling teratoma but lacking heterologous tissue types.

multilocular thymic cyst are typically thick and inflamed. Although residual thymic tissue can be observed adjacent to a teratoma, it is usually not as prominent as in multilocular thymic cyst, lacks the frequently inflammatory background of the latter, and may show intervening mesenchymal stromal elements. Likewise, enteric [94,95] and bronchogenic cysts enter the differential diagnosis of a mediastinal teratoma. The former, however, always occur in the posterior mediastinum and are composed of a two-layered smooth muscle wall surrounding an enteric-type glandular lumen [95]. Some features of bronchogenic cysts overlap with those of teratoma, particularly in the composition by respiratory epithelium, smooth muscle, and cartilage. However, the absence of non-bronchial components and their bronchus-like appearance are helpful distinguishing features [1,95]. Additionally, malignant neoplasms having spindled and epithelioid components, such as synovial sarcoma [96] or biphasic mesothelioma, may also be considered in the differential diagnosis [1], but they lack the heterogeneity of teratoma and have overtly malignant features.

Yolk sac tumor

Yolk sac tumor is the predominant malignant germ cell tumor in prepubertal patients [7,15,62,64], found in some studies to have a female predominance [45]. In adults, primarily men, pure yolk sac tumor comprises 3 to 18% of mediastinal germ cell tumors (Figs. 9.5 and 9.6) [7,10,23,24,54], overall a greater proportion than pure yolk sac tumor of the testis. It is also frequently a component of mediastinal mixed germ cell tumors, where it admixes with teratoma in prepubertal patients [45] or other germ cell tumor types in postpubertal patients [56]. Grossly, yolk sac tumors usually form large, partially encapsulated anterior

mediastinal masses with a rounded to nodular contour. The cut surface may be solid and tan colored, myxoid, or cystic, often containing areas of hemorrhage, congestion, or necrosis. If present in a mixed germ cell tumor, teratomatous components may also be recognizable grossly [97]. As is the case with other neoplasms involving the thymus, including lymphoma, seminoma, or thymoma, yolk sac tumor may occasionally cause multilocular cystic change of the thymic epithelium imparting resemblance to multilocular thymic cyst [98].

Microscopically, similar to yolk sac tumor of the testis, the reticular or microcystic pattern is the most common one, comprising a net-like or web-like arrangement of cells with intracellular vacuoles and thin, interconnecting strands of cytoplasm (Figs. 9.25 and 9.26) [56]. A myxomatous or myxoid pattern is often intimately intermingled with microcystic elements (Figs. 9.25 and 9.26) [56]. The endodermal sinus pattern is also seen in mediastinal tumors, so-named for the formation of endodermal sinus-like structures or Schiller–Duval bodies, composed of a central vessel surrounded by a layer of fibrous tissue and a rim of tumor cells that is recessed in a cystic space, lined by flattened epithelium at its periphery (Fig. 9.27) [97]. Other yolk sac tumor patterns, including papillary (Fig. 9.28) and glandular (Fig. 9.29), can also be seen in mediastinal cases [97]. The solid pattern (Figs. 9.15a and 9.30), composed of sheet-like arrangements of frequently clear or pale cells, may be a particular source of differential diagnostic difficulty, especially in the mediastinum [70]. In gonadal tumors, ample histologic sampling of the tumor usually reveals other yolk sac tumor patterns admixed with the solid growth. In the mediastinum, however, small biopsies are often performed, and differentiation from other tumors may be more challenging. Other key features facilitating recognition of solid yolk sac tumor include the formation of hyaline globules (Fig. 9.31) and deposition of basement membrane material (Fig. 9.30), a feature shared by many patterns of yolk sac tumor, including solid ones [70,97].

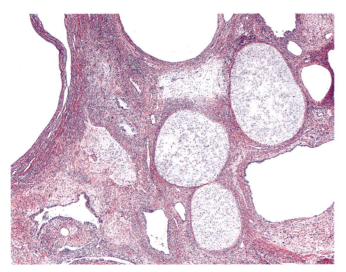

Fig. 9.21 Haphazard arrangement of mesenchymal, epithelial, and glial elements in the teratomatous component of a mixed mediastinal germ cell tumor.

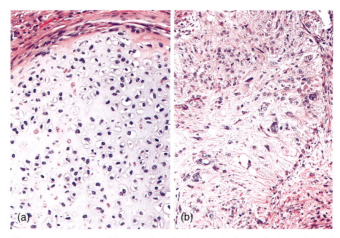

Fig. 9.22 Increased cellularity and cytologic atypia in the cartilaginous **(a)** and glial **(b)** teratomatous components of a mixed mediastinal germ cell tumor.

rosettes, which often have readily identifiable mitotic figures embedded in a background of cellular mesenchymal stroma [1]. Other immature elements in teratoma may include blastemal-like stromal cells, and primitive tubules resembling structures seen in nephroblastoma.

Grading of immature teratomas, as performed for ovarian tumors [86], has not been found to have established prognostic value in the mediastinum; however, reporting an estimated percentage of immature elements is generally recommended for mediastinal cases [1,87]. In prepubertal children, immaturity appears to correlate with a higher likelihood of a yolk sac tumor component [1,78] and in postpubertal patients an immature component is associated with an increased likelihood that the teratoma is a component of a malignant mixed germ cell tumor and has chromosome 12p amplification, including isochromosome 12p [87].

Teratomatous components in mixed germ cell tumors

When a teratomatous component is present in association with other germ cell tumor types (seminoma, yolk sac tumor, embryonal carcinoma, choriocarcinoma), it is classified as a mixed germ cell tumor with a teratomatous component [87]. Although these teratomatous components also demonstrate multiple tissue types recapitulating those of the germinal layers, the well-differentiated, organoid architecture that typifies the mature, histologically benign form of teratoma is lacking. The tissue elements themselves often possess a more disorganized, haphazard arrangement (Fig. 9.21) and are associated with areas of hemorrhage or necrosis [10] and frequently show an increased degree of cytologic atypia (Fig. 9.22a and b).

Somatic-type malignancy of germ cell tumor origin

Somatic-type malignancies arising from mediastinal germ cell tumors are well-established and include sarcomas, carcinomas, malignant glial tumors, and hematopoietic-like malignancies [10,88–90]. The terminology "teratoma with malignant transformation" has often been used for this phenomenon [91], although this nomenclature is not ideal since this event is likely to develop in association with a mixed germ cell tumor and the teratomatous component of a mixed germ cell tumor should not be considered "benign". Additionally, although such neoplasms have been hypothesized to derive from teratoma, perhaps through acquisition of additional genetic alterations, origin from other germ cell tumor components or a malignant common progenitor cell are also distinct possibilities. Not surprisingly, the development of somatic-type malignancies in mediastinal germ cell tumors is almost exclusively confined to postpubertal patients with malignant germ cell tumors, with both their conventional tumor and somatic-type malignancy sharing chromosome 12p abnormalities [90,92]. Most of these somatic-type malignancies are sarcomas, which are discussed in greater detail below in conjunction with yolk sac tumor. The distinction of somatic-type malignancies from atypical teratomatous elements (which are a usual finding in the postpubertal germ cell tumors of males) can be problematic. What we require, for sarcomas, is overgrowth of a pure lesion exceeding a 4× microscopic field. The diagnosis of carcinomas depends upon identifying destructive, infiltrative growth by cytologically malignant epithelial cells, often accompanied by a desmoplastic reaction, as in carcinomas of other sites (Fig. 9.23).

Differential diagnosis

Multilocular thymic cyst, because of its multiple cystic spaces lined by cuboidal, ciliated, or squamous epithelium (Fig. 9.24), may mimic teratoma. In contrast to teratoma, heterologous elements such as pancreatic tissue, neuroglia, cartilage, or other tissues foreign to the thymus are not found in multilocular thymic cysts. Sebaceous glands and parathyroid tissue are occasionally seen within the thymus and thought to be related to anomalous thymic development rather than indicative of teratoma [93]. The fibrous septa between the spaces of

Hematopoietic neoplasms associated with mediastinal germ cell tumors

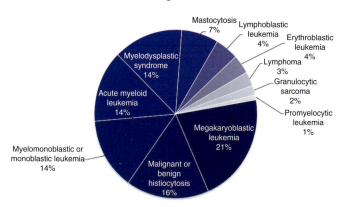

Fig. 9.37 Distribution of hematopoietic neoplasms associated with mediastinal germ cell tumors, based on reference 89.

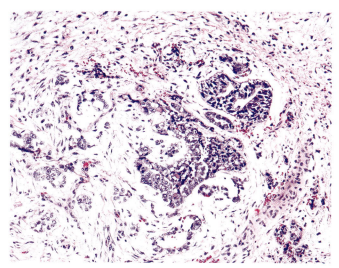

Fig. 9.39 Embryonal carcinoma in a mixed mediastinal germ cell tumor, associated with teratomatous and yolk sac tumor components.

histiocytosis, myelomonoblastic leukemia, monoblastic leukemia, other acute myeloid leukemias, myelodysplastic syndrome, mastocytosis, acute lymphoblastic leukemia, erythroblastic leukemia, lymphoma, myeloid (granulocytic) sarcoma, and promyelocytic leukemia (Fig. 9.37) [89]. The prognosis for these acute leukemias is poor, with a survival spanning from a few months to 2 years [89,113,119]. The hematopoietic neoplasms may involve the mediastinal tumor itself [121,122], or hematopoietic sites such as bone marrow, spleen and so on, without evident involvement of the mediastinal mass [121].

Differential diagnosis and immunohistochemistry

Due to the number of patterns that yolk sac tumors may assume, a variety of other neoplasms may be considered in the differential diagnosis. We have already mentioned the differential posed between solid pattern yolk sac tumor and seminoma, with guidelines for its resolution. The most useful immunostaining panel is OCT4 and glypican-3 [74], which are negative and positive in yolk sac tumor (including the solid

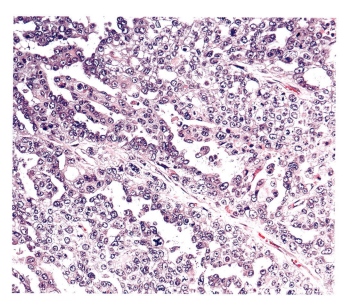

Fig. 9.38 Yolk sac tumor showing increased nuclear pleomorphism and prominent nucleoli, resembling embryonal carcinoma. Immunohistochemical staining for OCT4 was entirely negative in this neoplasm, supporting classification as yolk sac tumor.

pattern), respectively, and have opposite reactivities in seminoma. Staining for AFP has been a long-used marker of yolk sac tumor; however, caution must be exercised in interpretation of positive staining, since some malignancies of non-germ cell type may also show positive reactivity and, furthermore, AFP is a relatively insensitive marker, especially in the solid pattern [70,74]. In some cases, a high degree of nuclear pleomorphism in yolk sac tumor may lead to confusion with embryonal carcinoma (Fig. 9.38), although, as in seminoma, OCT4 positivity or positivity for other novel stem-cell-directed markers such as SOX2 can distinguish embryonal carcinoma from yolk sac tumor [74].

Given the location within the chest, metastatic carcinomas also enter the differential diagnosis with yolk sac tumor. SALL4, a novel stem-cell-directed marker is of particular value in this situation because of its high sensitivity for yolk sac tumor and infrequent positivity in carcinomas [74]; it should be supplemented by more specific yolk sac tumor markers (glypican-3, AFP) because of occasional SALL4 reactivity in high-grade carcinomas. Absence of immunoreactivity for epithelial membrane antigen (EMA) and CK7 are also helpful in supporting yolk sac tumor over metastatic carcinoma [100]. When the hepatoid pattern is present, the absence of the canalicular pattern with polyclonal antibody to carcinoembryonic antigen (CEA) also contrasts with metastatic hepatocellular carcinoma [100], which is also SALL4 negative [101,102], unlike yolk sac tumor.

Embryonal carcinoma

Pure embryonal carcinoma is an uncommon subtype of primary mediastinal germ cell tumor [10,23,24,54], and in our experience, many tumors originally considered to be mediastinal embryonal carcinomas actually represent yolk sac tumors with

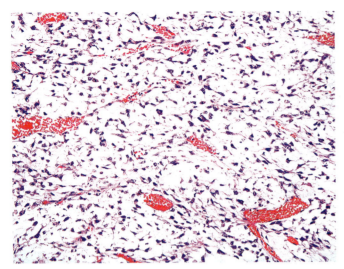

Fig. 9.33 Sarcomatoid yolk sac tumor has spindle-shaped cells in a myxoid stroma. Despite the sarcomatoid appearance, expression of cytokeratin, glypican-3, and SALL4 are often present, similar to other patterns of yolk sac tumor. Note prominent vascularity.

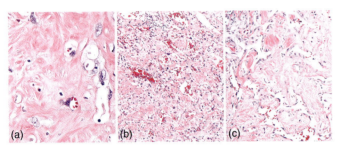

Fig. 9.35 Neoplastic stromal cells show vasoformative capacity as they develop lumina (lower center) and merge to form primitive vessels **(a)**. Highly atypical stromal cells are distributed around thin-walled vessels having mild to moderately atypical endothelium **(b)**. Irregular vessels are lined by atypical cells, with similar cells in adjacent fibrous stroma **(c)**.

Distribution of sarcoma types in mediastinal germ cell tumors

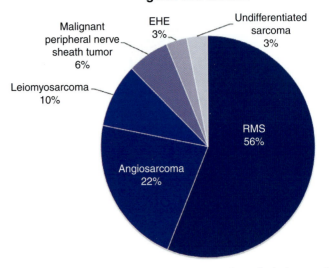

Fig. 9.34 Most common sarcomatous components in mediastinal germ cell tumors, based on data from references 88 and 107. (EHE – epithelioid hemangioendothelioma; RMS – rhabdomyosarcoma.)

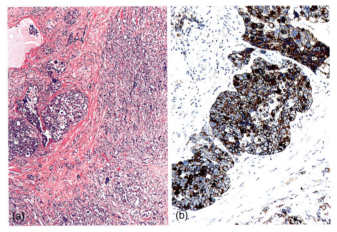

Fig. 9.36 Megakaryoblastic leukemia **(a)** with intravascular and stromal invasive components in a mediastinal germ cell tumor. There is diffuse positivity for CD42b in the megakaryoblasts **(b)**.

unclear reasons. In our opinion, the myxoid/mesenchymal foci of yolk sac tumor (termed by Teilum the "magma reticulare") give rise to such neoplasms. It has vasoformative capacity and its dysplastic spindled and epithelioid cells appear to excavate the stroma and condense into vessels (Fig. 9.35a). Thus, undifferentiated spindle-shaped and epithelioid cells are seen in a myxomatous to fibrous stroma adjacent to abortive to well formed vessels having variable degrees of cytological atypia (Figs 9.35b and c). This entire tissue component represents an angiodysplastic mesenchyme within which a spectrum of endothelial cell atypia may be identified [104,107].

Hematopoietic neoplasms

An intriguing aspect of mediastinal germ cell tumors is their unique association with malignant hematopoietic neoplasms, almost exclusively restricted to those with a yolk sac tumor component. This is not a feature of germ cell tumors of non-mediastinal origin [89,108–119] and is not treatment-related. Although this association is not completely understood, an interesting correlate is that in embryogenesis the first blood

cells arise in the wall of the yolk sac, although adult or definitive hematopoiesis is thought to later derive from the mesoderm of the aorta-gonad-mesonephros region [38,120]. Additionally, in some affected patients, hematopoietic blasts can also be identified by immunohistochemistry within the yolk sac tumor, particularly the vascular-rich, myxoid zones. Derivation of these malignancies from the germ cell tumor receives strong support from the identification of isochromosome 12p in the leukemic cells [113]. The genetic abnormalities typical of the particular subtype of hematopoietic neoplasia also are often present [121], likely determining its phenotype. Megakaryoblastic leukemia (Figs 9.36a and b) is particularly prone to arise in this context, although a spectrum of neoplasms has been reported, including malignant and benign

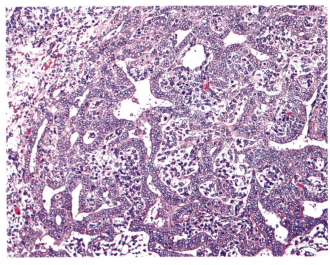

Fig. 9.29 Glandular pattern in a mediastinal yolk sac tumor with intervening solid nests.

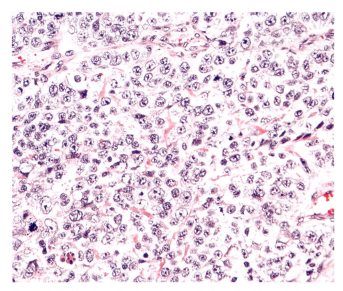

Fig. 9.30 Solid pattern of yolk sac tumor with deposits of intercellular eosinophilic basement membrane, a finding that assists with the differentiation from seminoma.

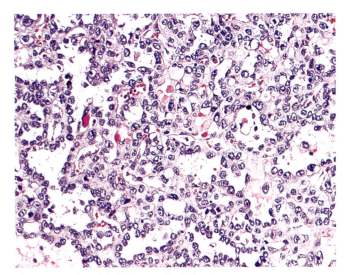

Fig. 9.31 Hyaline globules in a mediastinal yolk sac tumor.

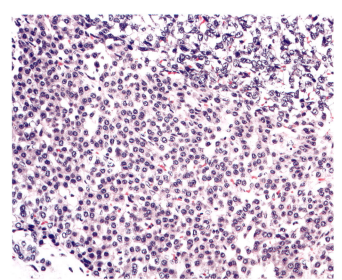

Fig. 9.32 Hepatoid yolk sac tumor composed of cells with eosinophilic cytoplasm and central, round nuclei, arranged in sheets and trabecular structures resembling liver. There is transition to a microcystic pattern (bottom).

embedded in a myxoid to collagenous stroma (Fig. 9.33), there is positivity for cytokeratin [103,104] and often for SALL4 and glypican-3 (personal observations) but usually not AFP. More typical patterns of yolk sac tumor sometimes intermingle with these areas [103], and even when a more readily recognizable yolk sac tumor pattern is not identified, most patients have a history of yolk sac tumor, supporting derivation of sarcomatoid tumor from yolk sac tumor [104]. Transition of relatively low-grade sarcomatoid foci to high-grade areas and the acquisition of specific forms of differentiation, most commonly rhabdomyosarcomatous but occasionally angiosarcomatous or osteosarcomatous or others, support both the high malignant potential of such elements as well as their pluripotential capacity [103–105].

In a study of germ cell tumors with sarcomatous components [88], embryonal rhabdomyosarcoma was the most common sarcoma, followed by angiosarcoma, leiomyosarcoma, and

individual cases of malignant peripheral nerve sheath tumor, epithelioid hemangioendothelioma, and undifferentiated sarcoma (Fig. 9.34) [88]. Liposarcoma and osteosarcoma have also been reported [10]. Although 10% of germ cell tumors originate in the mediastinum, 30% of cases with sarcomatous elements originate there, perhaps because the mediastinal tumors are larger and therefore more likely of longer duration than at other sites [106], or because of inherent properties of the mediastinal cases. We require overgrowth of a 4× microscopic field to distinguish atypical mesenchymal elements of teratoma from sarcoma.

The development of angiosarcoma or other vascular neoplasms is largely restricted to mediastinal germ cell tumors, for

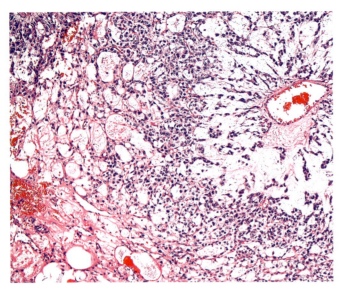

Fig. 9.25 Microcystic and reticular (top) pattern in a mediastinal yolk sac tumor.

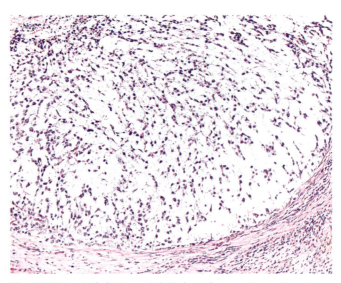

Fig. 9.26 Intermingled microcystic/reticular and myxomatous patterns in a mediastinal yolk sac tumor.

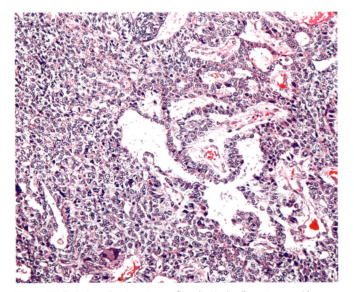

Fig. 9.27 Endodermal sinus pattern of mediastinal yolk sac tumor with Schiller–Duval bodies (upper half), characterized by a central blood vessel, surrounded by a rim of fibrous, edematous tissue and a layer of tumor cells recessed in a cystic space. Areas of solid growth are also present (bottom).

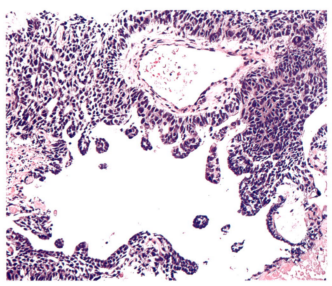

Fig. 9.28 Papillary pattern in a mediastinal yolk sac tumor.

The hepatoid pattern of yolk sac tumor is uncommon and represented by solid to trabecular or pseudoglandular growth of cells with abundant eosinophilic cytoplasm, and prominent round or oval nucleoli (Fig. 9.32), resulting in an appearance similar to liver parenchyma (fetal or adult) or hepatocellular carcinoma. Similar to the cases originally described in the ovary [99], hepatoid yolk sac tumor also occurs in mediastinal tumors, sometimes leading to confusion with metastatic carcinoma. In a series of four such cases, the tumors were notable for their predominant composition by this pattern, leading some to be misdiagnosed as metastatic carcinoma from an unknown primary site [100]. They, like other yolk sac tumor patterns, are positive for the stem cell marker SALL4 (see below), which distinguishes them from metastatic hepatocellular carcinomas, but such reactivity is also seen in hepatoid carcinomas of visceral origin [101,102].

Sarcomatoid yolk sac tumor and sarcoma of germ cell tumor origin

Yolk sac tumors with spindle-shaped cells (sarcomatoid) are recognized both in patients with testicular and mediastinal germ cell tumors [103,104]. Despite the sarcomatoid appearance, typically represented by cells with elongated nuclei and variable degrees of cellularity and nuclear pleomorphism

increased nuclear atypia, as evidenced by their lack of immunoreactivity for OCT4 (Fig. 9.38). When present, embryonal carcinoma is often a component of a mixed germ cell tumor (Fig. 9.39). Gross features include frequent necrosis and hemorrhage [81]. As in the testis, primary mediastinal embryonal carcinomas can show several architectural growth patterns including solid sheets, tubular or glandular structures [56], and papillary formation. Cytologically, the tumor cells show a higher degree of nuclear pleomorphism than yolk sac tumor or seminoma, with nuclei that have single or multiple prominent nucleoli and that are frequently crowded, appearing to abut or overlap. Embryonal carcinomas lack the hyaline globules and basement membrane deposits of yolk sac tumor and usually the granulomatous inflammation of seminoma.

Differential diagnosis and immunohistochemistry

The differential diagnosis of mediastinal embryonal carcinoma encompasses poorly differentiated malignancies, including thymic carcinoma, metastatic carcinoma from another organ, and direct extension of poorly differentiated carcinoma from the lung. Compounding this difficulty, it is not unusual for mediastinal embryonal carcinomas to invade adjacent structures, including the lung [56]. A relatively young patient age and absence of a known malignancy of another organ may be helpful in pointing to embryonal carcinoma [56]. Embryonal carcinomas express cytokeratin and CD30 [74], although this combination is not entirely specific. The lack of immunohistochemical staining for EMA is also helpful and contrasts with many carcinomas of other organs. Of most value is positive staining for OCT4 and SALL4 [74], a pattern shared only by seminoma. Positive staining for CD5 in combination with epithelial markers supports thymic carcinoma [1].

Expression of CD30 by embryonal carcinoma overlaps with anaplastic large cell lymphoma [123], which may uncommonly manifest as a pleomorphic malignant neoplasm involving the mediastinum. Additional immunohistochemical markers resolve this differential diagnosis. Both in the testis and mediastinum, distinguishing embryonal carcinoma from choriocarcinoma may occasionally be challenging. Degenerated, hyperchromatic embryonal carcinoma cells at the periphery of tumor cell nests may mimic the syncytiotrophoblasts of choriocarcinoma, and some areas of embryonal carcinoma show a syncytial-like growth pattern [56]. Unlike choriocarcinoma, embryonal carcinoma usually lacks the background of diffuse hemorrhage typical of the former and its cells are negative when stained with antibody to hCG. Additionally, choriocarcinoma is negative for OCT4, unlike embryonal carcinoma. As noted above, yolk sac tumors composed of glandular elements or with solid growth may show increased nuclear atypia and prominent nucleoli that cause confusion with embryonal carcinoma. Positive reactivity for SALL4 but not OCT4 in such yolk sac tumors can be a helpful combination in supporting this interpretation (Fig. 9.38).

Choriocarcinoma

Choriocarcinoma is likely the rarest form of primary mediastinal germ cell tumor; it is associated with highly aggressive behavior and very short survival after diagnosis, usually only a few months in the absence of effective treatment [56,124]. Mediastinal choriocarcinoma almost always occurs in men, although rare cases in women (Fig. 9.8) have been thought to represent a primary mediastinal neoplasm [61] rather than the more common occurrence of metastatic gestational choriocarcinoma. Grossly, mediastinal choriocarcinomas form large, soft, extensively hemorrhagic and necrotic masses. Like choriocarcinomas of other sites, they are microscopically composed

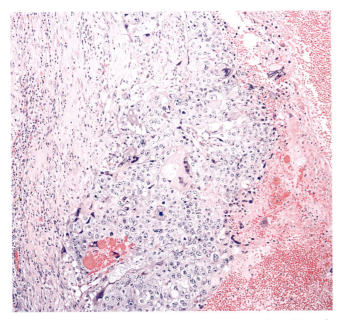

Fig. 9.40 Mediastinal choriocarcinoma composed of a mixed population of syncytiotrophoblasts and mononucleated trophoblasts. Note prominent hemorrhage.

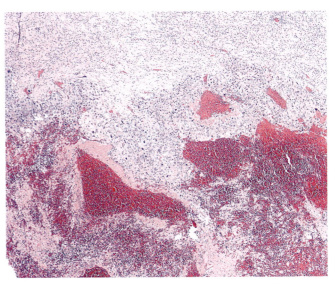

Fig. 9.41 Arrangement of viable choriocarcinoma cells in a rim-like layer surrounding an area of hemorrhage and necrosis.

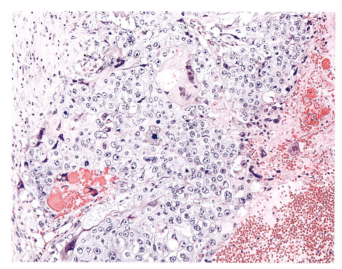

Fig. 9.42 Mono-nucleated trophoblasts with lightly eosinophilic cytoplasm, irregular nuclear contours and prominent nucleoli admixed with syncytiotrophoblasts with denser, eosinophilic cytoplasm and smudged nuclei.

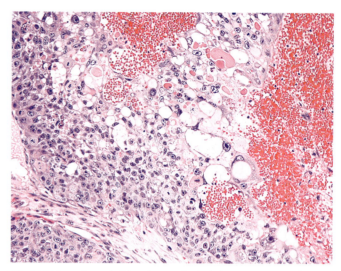

Fig. 9.43 Syncytio-trophoblasts in a mediastinal choriocarcinoma with cytoplasmic cystic spaces or lacunae containing eosinophilic material and blood.

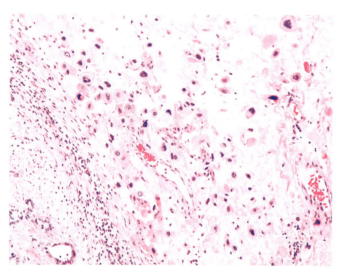

Fig. 9.44 A placental site trophoblastic tumor-like component in a mediastinal germ cell tumor composed of intermediate trophoblasts in a fibrous stroma.

Differential diagnosis and immunohistochemistry

Seminoma with scattered syncytiotrophoblastic cells [32], a more common lesion, may be mistaken for choriocarcinoma. The less uniform nature of the mononucleated cell population, prominent hemorrhage, absence of ancillary seminoma features (lymphocytes, granulomas, fibrous septa) and negative reactivity for OCT4 [74] in choriocarcinoma serve to distinguish these two neoplasms.

The mononuclear trophoblastic component of choriocarcinoma can sometimes appear squamoid. Given the location in the chest, carcinoma originating from the lung or another organ is a stronger consideration in the mediastinum than in gonadal tumors. Along these lines, choriocarcinomas frequently are positive with broad-spectrum cytokeratin antibodies, CAM5.2 and p63, which may also suggest a squamous tumor [72,125], although co-expression of other markers, such as CD10 and inhibin are supportive of choriocarcinoma [125]. Unfortunately, squamoid mononucleated trophoblasts are usually hCG negative, so this stain may not serve to distinguish these entities.

Other tumors

Less commonly, other forms of germ cell tumor also occur primarily in the mediastinum. For example, a case of placental site trophoblastic tumor has been reported in a 14 year-old boy two years after resection of a mature mediastinal teratoma [126], and we have seen a similar case (Fig. 9.44). In contrast to choriocarcinoma, placental site trophoblastic tumor lacks the biphasic population of trophoblast cells, but has a more homogeneous population of intermediate trophoblasts with an infiltrative growth pattern and fibrinoid deposits involving blood vessel walls [126]. By immunohistochemistry, antibody to HLA-G is a helpful positive marker of intermediate trophoblasts that is negative in the syncytiotrophoblasts and the mononucleated trophoblasts with cytotrophoblastic

of a dual population of mononucleated trophoblasts and syncytiotrophoblastic cells (Fig. 9.40) [56,124], often arranged at the periphery of large foci of hemorrhage and necrosis (Fig. 9.41). The mononuclear cells usually possess clear or lightly eosinophilic cytoplasm, while the multinucleated (syncytiotrophoblastic) cells have more voluminous, dense, eosinophilic cytoplasm and several nuclei that vary from well-defined to hyperchromatic with smudged chromatin (Fig. 9.42). The syncytiotrophoblastic cells sometimes contain cystic cavities or lacunae within their cytoplasm, either empty-appearing or containing eosinophilic material (Fig. 9.43). Sometimes the mononucleated trophoblast cells have a distinctly squamoid appearance. These two cellular populations admix either randomly or sometimes with the syncytiotrophoblast cells "capping" the mononucleated trophoblast cells in a pattern similar to that seen on placental villi.

differentiation of choriocarcinoma [126,127]. Additionally, placental site trophoblastic tumor lacks the diffuse hemorrhage typically seen in choriocarcinoma. Likewise, the polyembryoma pattern, resulting in the formation of embryoid bodies composed of embryonal carcinoma and yolk sac tumor, has been rarely reported to also occur in primary mediastinal germ cell tumors [128]. Notably, spermatocytic seminoma has not been reported to occur outside of the testis [129].

Metastatic germ cell tumor to the mediastinum

Generally the most critical information for determining whether a germ cell tumor is a primary mediastinal tumor or a metastasis from the testis is correlation with other clinical parameters. Metastasis to the mediastinum as an isolated lesion, particularly the anterior mediastinum alone without clinical evidence of involvement of other sites such as retroperitoneal lymph nodes, is highly unusual [124]. As such, the areas of involvement are a helpful clue in resolving this differential diagnosis. Since testicular germ cell tumors may undergo spontaneous regression, a clinically evident testicular primary may not be evident. Still, careful palpation and testicular ultrasound may reveal subtle testicular abnormalities, including small, scarred foci. When metastatic germ cell tumors do involve the anterior mediastinum, these metastases are usually present in conjunction with additional involvement of the middle or visceral mediastinum [30].

Acknowledgments

The authors would like to thank Tracey Bender for excellent clerical assistance.

References

1. McKenney JK, Heerema-McKenney A, Rouse RV. Extragonadal germ cell tumors: a review with emphasis on pathologic features, clinical prognostic variables, and differential diagnostic considerations. *Adv Anat Pathol.* 2007;14:69–92.

2. Hainsworth JD, Greco FA. Extragonadal germ cell tumors and unrecognized germ cell tumors. *Semin Oncol.* 1992;19:119–27.

3. Nichols CR, Saxman S, Williams SD, *et al.* Primary mediastinal nonseminomatous germ cell tumors. A modern single institution experience. *Cancer.* 1990;65:1641–6.

4. Collins DH, Pugh RC. Classification and frequency of testicular tumours. *Br J Urol.* 1964;36:Suppl:1–11.

5. Stang A, Trabert B, Wentzensen N, *et al.* Gonadal and extragonadal germ cell tumours in the United States, 1973–2007. *Int J Androl.* 2012;35:616–25.

6. Moran CA, Suster S. Germ-cell tumors of the mediastinum. *Adv Anat Pathol.* 1998;5:1–15.

7. Wick M, Perlman E, Orazi A, *et al.* Germ cell tumors of the mediastinum. In: Travis WD, Brambilla E, Müller-Hermelink H, Harris C, editors. *Pathology and genetics of tumours of the lung, pleura, thymus and heart.* Lyon: IARC Press; 2004. 198–201.

8. Goss PE, Schwertfeger L, Blackstein ME, *et al.* Extragonadal germ cell tumors. A 14-year Toronto experience. *Cancer.* 1994;73:1971–9.

9. Nichols CR. Mediastinal germ cell tumors. Clinical features and biologic correlates. *Chest.* 1991;99:472–9.

10. Moran CA, Suster S. Primary germ cell tumors of the mediastinum: I. Analysis of 322 cases with special emphasis on teratomatous lesions and a proposal for histopathologic classification and clinical staging. *Cancer.* 1997;80:681–90.

11. Weidner N. Germ-cell tumors of the mediastinum. *Semin Diagn Pathol.* 1999;16:42–50.

12. Takeda S, Miyoshi S, Akashi A, *et al.* Clinical spectrum of primary mediastinal tumors: a comparison of adult and pediatric populations at a single Japanese institution. *J Surg Oncol.* 2003;83:24–30.

13. Dubashi B, Cyriac S, Tenali SG. Clinicopathological analysis and outcome of primary mediastinal malignancies – A report of 91 cases from a single institute. *Ann Thorac Med.* 2009;4:140–2.

14. Mullen B, Richardson JD. Primary anterior mediastinal tumors in children and adults. *Ann Thorac Surg.* 1986;42:338–45.

15. Schneider DT, Calaminus G, Reinhard H, *et al.* Primary mediastinal germ cell tumors in children and adolescents: results of the German cooperative protocols MAKEI 83/86, 89, and 96. *J Clin Oncol.* 2000;18:832–9.

16. Harms D, Janig U. Germ cell tumours of childhood. Report of 170 cases including 59 pure and partial yolk-sac tumours. *Virchows Arch A Pathol Anat Histopathol.* 1986;409:223–39.

17. De Backer A, Madern GC, Pieters R, *et al.* Influence of tumor site and histology on long-term survival in 193 children with extracranial germ cell tumors. *Eur J Pediatr Surg.* 2008;18:1–6.

18. Harms D, Zahn S, Gobel U, *et al.* Pathology and molecular biology of teratomas in childhood and adolescence. *Klin Padiatr.* 2006;218:296–302.

19. Gun F, Erginel B, Unuvar A, *et al.* Mediastinal masses in children: experience with 120 cases. *Pediatr Hematol Oncol.* 2012;29:141–7.

20. Tansel T, Onursal E, Dayloglu E, *et al.* Childhood mediastinal masses in infants and children. *Turk J Pediatr.* 2006;48:8–12.

21. Temes R, Allen N, Chavez T, *et al.* Primary mediastinal malignancies in children: report of 22 patients and comparison to 197 adults. *Oncologist.* 2000;5:179–84.

22. Bokemeyer C, Nichols CR, Droz JP, *et al.* Extragonadal germ cell tumors of the mediastinum and retroperitoneum: results from an international analysis. *J Clin Oncol.* 2002;20:1864–73.

23. Takeda S, Miyoshi S, Ohta M, *et al.* Primary germ cell tumors in the mediastinum: a 50-year experience at a single Japanese institution. *Cancer.* 2003;97:367–76.

24. Dulmet EM, Macchiarini P, Suc B, *et al.* Germ cell tumors of the mediastinum. A 30-year experience. *Cancer.* 1993;72:1894–901.

25. Lewis BD, Hurt RD, Payne WS, *et al.* Benign teratomas of the mediastinum. *J Thorac Cardiovasc Surg.* 1983;86:727–31.

26. Bath LE, Walayat M, Mankad P, *et al.* Stage IV malignant intrapericardial germ cell tumor: a case report. *Pediatr Hematol Oncol.* 1997;14:451–5.

27. Meissner A, Kirch W, Regensburger D, *et al.* Intrapericardial teratoma in an adult. *Am J Med.* 1988;84:1089–90.

28. Laquay N, Ghazouani S, Vaccaroni L, *et al.* Intrapericardial teratoma in newborn babies. *Eur J Cardiothorac Surg.* 2003;23:642–4.

29. Bitar FF, el-Zein C, Tawil A, *et al.* Intrapericardial teratoma in an adult: a rare presentation. *Med Pediatr Oncol.* 1998;30:249–51.

30. Kesler KA, Brooks JA, Rieger KM, *et al.* Mediastinal metastases from testicular nonseminomatous germ cell tumors: patterns of dissemination and predictors of long-term survival with surgery. *J Thorac Cardiovasc Surg.* 2003;125:913–23.

31. De Backer A, Madern GC, Hakvoort-Cammel FG, *et al.* Mediastinal germ cell tumors: clinical aspects and outcomes in 7 children. *Eur J Pediatr Surg.* 2006;16:318–22.

32. Moran CA, Suster S, Przygodzki RM, *et al.* Primary germ cell tumors of the mediastinum: II. Mediastinal seminomas–a clinicopathologic and immunohistochemical study of 120 cases. *Cancer.* 1997;80:691–8.

33. Gordon JA. Case of tumor in the anterior mediastinum, containing bone and teeth. *Med Chir Trans.* 1827;13:12–6.

34. Lynch MJ, Blewitt GL. Choriocarcinoma arising in the male mediastinum. *Thorax.* 1953;8:157–61.

35. Rosai J, Parkash V, Reuter VE. The origin of mediastinal germ cell tumors in men. *Int J Surg Pathol.* 1994;2:73–8.

36. Chaganti RS, Rodriguez E, Mathew S. Origin of adult male mediastinal germ-cell tumours. *Lancet.* 1994;343:1130–2.

37. Schlumberger HG. Teratoma of the anterior mediastinum in the group of military age: a study of 16 cases, and a review of theories of genesis. *Arch Pathol (Chic).* 1946;41:398–444.

38. Sadler TW, Langman J. *Langman's medical embryology.* Philadelphia: Wolters Kluwer Health/Lippincott Williams & Wilkins; 2012

39. Nichols CR, Heerema NA, Palmer C, *et al.* Klinefelter's syndrome associated with mediastinal germ cell neoplasms. *J Clin Oncol.* 1987;5:1290–4.

40. Volkl TM, Langer T, Aigner T, *et al.* Klinefelter syndrome and mediastinal germ cell tumors. *Am J Med Genet A.* 2006;140:471–81.

41. Hasle H, Jacobsen BB. Origin of male mediastinal germ-cell tumours. *Lancet.* 1995;345:1046.

42. Hasle H, Mellemgaard A, Nielsen J, *et al.* Cancer incidence in men with Klinefelter syndrome. *Br J Cancer.* 1995;71:416–20.

43. Hasle H, Jacobsen BB, Asschenfeldt P, *et al.* Mediastinal germ cell tumour associated with Klinefelter syndrome. A report of case and review of the literature. *Eur J Pediatr.* 1992;151:735–9.

44. Dexeus FH, Logothetis CJ, Chong C, *et al.* Genetic abnormalities in men with germ cell tumors. *J Urol.* 1988;140:80–4.

45. Schneider DT, Schuster AE, Fritsch MK, *et al.* Genetic analysis of mediastinal nonseminomatous germ cell tumors in children and adolescents. *Genes Chromosomes Cancer.* 2002;34:115–25.

46. Zon R, Orazi A, Neiman RS, *et al.* Benign hematologic neoplasm associated with mediastinal mature teratoma in a patient with Klinefelter's syndrome: a case report. *Med Pediatr Oncol.* 1994;23:376–9.

47. Hartmann JT, Nichols CR, Droz JP, *et al.* The relative risk of second nongerminal malignancies in patients with extragonadal germ cell tumors. *Cancer.* 2000;88:2629–35.

48. Hoffner L, Deka R, Chakravarti A, *et al.* Cytogenetics and origins of pediatric germ cell tumors. *Cancer Genet Cytogenet.* 1994;74:54–8.

49. Bussey KJ, Lawce HJ, Olson SB, *et al.* Chromosome abnormalities of eighty-one pediatric germ cell tumors: sex-, age-, site-, and histopathology-related differences–a Children's Cancer Group study. *Genes Chromosomes Cancer.* 1999;25:134–46.

50. Perlman EJ, Hu J, Ho D, *et al.* Genetic analysis of childhood endodermal sinus tumors by comparative genomic hybridization. *J Pediatr Hematol Oncol.* 2000;22:100–5.

51. Perlman EJ, Cushing B, Hawkins E, *et al.* Cytogenetic analysis of childhood endodermal sinus tumors: a Pediatric Oncology Group study. *Pediatr Pathol.* 1994;14:695–708.

52. Rapley EA, Crockford GP, Teare D, *et al.* Localization to Xq27 of a susceptibility gene for testicular germ-cell tumours. *Nat Genet.* 2000;24:197–200.

53. Crockford GP, Linger R, Hockley S, *et al.* Genome-wide linkage screen for testicular germ cell tumour susceptibility loci. *Hum Mol Genet.* 2006;15:443–51.

54. Knapp RH, Hurt RD, Payne WS, *et al.* Malignant germ cell tumors of the mediastinum. *J Thorac Cardiovasc Surg.* 1985;89:82–9.

55. Ulbright TM. Germ cell tumors of the gonads: a selective review emphasizing problems in differential diagnosis, newly appreciated, and controversial issues. *Mod Pathol.* 2005;18 Suppl 2: S61–79.

56. Moran CA, Suster S, Koss MN. Primary germ cell tumors of the mediastinum: III. Yolk sac tumor, embryonal carcinoma, choriocarcinoma, and combined nonteratomatous germ cell tumors of the mediastinum–a clinicopathologic and immunohistochemical study of 64 cases. *Cancer.* 1997;80:699–707.

57. Coskun U, Gunel N, Yildirim Y, *et al.* Primary mediastinal yolk sac tumor in a 66-year-old woman. *Med Princ Pract.* 2002;11:218–20.

58. Shimizu J, Yazaki U, Kinoshita T, *et al.* Primary mediastinal germ cell tumor in a middle-aged woman: case report and literature review. *Tumori.* 2001;87:269–71.

59. Brown K, Collins JD, Batra P, *et al.* Mediastinal germ cell tumor in a young woman. *Med Pediatr Oncol.* 1989;17:164–7.

60. Morishima Y, Satoh H, Ohtsuka M, *et al.* Primary mediastinal nonseminomatous germ cell tumour in an adult female. *Respir Med.* 1998;92:882–4.

61. Rivera C, Poingt M, Vandenbossche F, *et al.* A mediastinal germ cell tumor mimicking an ectopic pregnancy. *J Gynecol Oncol.* 2011;22:288–91.

62. Billmire D, Vinocur C, Rescorla F, *et al.* Malignant mediastinal germ cell tumors: an intergroup study. *J Pediatr Surg.* 2001;36:18–24.

63. Schneider DT, Calaminus G, Koch S, *et al.* Epidemiologic analysis of 1,442 children and adolescents registered in the German germ cell tumor protocols. *Pediatr Blood Cancer.* 2004;42:169–75.

64. Lack EE, Weinstein HJ, Welch KJ. Mediastinal germ cell tumors in childhood. A clinical and pathological study of 21 cases. *J Thorac Cardiovasc Surg.* 1985;89:826–35.

65. Weissferdt A, Moran CA. Staging of primary mediastinal tumors. *Adv Anat Pathol.* 2013;20:1–9.

66. Moran CA, Suster S. Mediastinal seminomas with prominent cystic changes. A clinicopathologic study of 10 cases. *Am J Surg Pathol.* 1995;19:1047–53.

67. Suster S, Rosai J. Cystic thymomas. A clinicopathologic study of ten cases. *Cancer.* 1992;69:92–7.

68. Stein H, von Wasielewski R, Poppema S, *et al.* Nodular sclerosis classical Hodgkin lymphoma. In: Swerdlow SH, Campo E, Harris NL, Jaffe ES, Pileri S, Stein H, *et al.*, editors. *WHO classification of tumours of haematopoietic and lymphoid tissues.* Lyon, France: International Agency for Research on Cancer; 2008. 330.

69. Levine GD, Rosai J. Thymic hyperplasia and neoplasia: a review of current concepts. *Hum Pathol.* 1978;9:495–515.

70. Kao CS, Idrees MT, Young RH, *et al.* Solid pattern yolk sac tumor: a morphologic and immunohistochemical study of 52 cases. *Am J Surg Pathol.* 2012;36:360–7.

71. Wick MR, Swanson PE, Manivel JC. Placental-like alkaline phosphatase reactivity in human tumors: an immunohistochemical study of 520 cases. *Hum Pathol.* 1987;18:946–54.

72. Suster S, Moran CA, Dominguez-Malagon H, *et al.* Germ cell tumors of the mediastinum and testis: a comparative immunohistochemical study of 120 cases. *Hum Pathol.* 1998;29:737–42.

73. Sung MT, Maclennan GT, Lopez-Beltran A, *et al.* Primary mediastinal seminoma: a comprehensive assessment integrated with histology, immunohistochemistry, and fluorescence in situ hybridization for chromosome 12p abnormalities in 23 cases. *Am J Surg Pathol.* 2008;32:146–55.

74. Liu A, Cheng L, Du J, *et al.* Diagnostic utility of novel stem cell markers SALL4, OCT4, NANOG, SOX2, UTF1, and TCL1 in primary mediastinal germ cell tumors. *Am J Surg Pathol.* 2010;34:697–706.

75. Looijenga LH, Stoop H, de Leeuw HP, *et al.* POU5F1 (OCT3/4) identifies cells with pluripotent potential in human germ cell tumors. *Cancer Res.* 2003;63:2244–50.

76. Trinh DT, Shibata K, Hirosawa T, *et al.* Diagnostic utility of CD117, CD133, SALL4, OCT4, TCL1 and glypican-3 in malignant germ cell tumors of the ovary. *J Obstet Gynaecol Res.* 2012;38:841–8.

77. Arber DA, Tamayo R, Weiss LM. Paraffin section detection of the c-kit gene product (CD117) in human tissues: value in the diagnosis of mast cell disorders. *Hum Pathol.* 1998;29:498–504.

78. Heifetz SA, Cushing B, Giller R, *et al.* Immature teratomas in children: pathologic considerations: a report from the combined Pediatric Oncology Group/Children's Cancer Group. *Am J Surg Pathol.* 1998;22:1115–24.

79. Suda K, Mizuguchi K, Hebisawa A, *et al.* Pancreatic tissue in teratoma. *Arch Pathol Lab Med.* 1984;108:835–7.

80. Shimosato Y, Mukai K. *Tumors of the mediastinum.* Washington, D.C.: Armed Forces Institute of Pathology; 1997

81. Shimosato Y, Mukai K, Matsuno Y. *Tumors of the mediastinum.* Washington, D.C.: American Registry of Pathology in collaboration with the Armed Forces Institute of Pathology; 2010

82. Dunn PJ. Pancreatic endocrine tissue in benign mediastinal teratoma. *J Clin Pathol.* 1984;37:1105–9.

83. Bordi C, De Vita O, Pollice L. Full pancreatic endocrine differentiation in a mediastinal teratoma. *Hum Pathol.* 1985;16:961–4.

84. Kallis P, Treasure T, Holmes SJ, *et al.* Exocrine pancreatic function in mediastinal teratomata: an aid to preoperative diagnosis? *Ann Thorac Surg.* 1992;54:741–3.

85. Sommerlad BC, Cleland WP, Yong NK. Physiological activity in mediastinal teratomata. *Thorax.* 1975;30:510–15.

86. Gonzalez-Crussi F. *Extragonadal teratomas.* Washington, D.C.: Armed Forces Institute of Pathology under the auspices of Universities Associated for Research and Education in Pathology; 1982

87. Wick M, Perlman E, Göbel U, *et al.* Teratoma. In: Travis WD, Brambilla E,

Müller-Hermelink H, Harris C, editors. *Pathology and genetics of tumours of the lung, pleura, thymus and heart.* Lyon: IARC Press; 2004. 210–12.

88. Malagon HD, Valdez AM, Moran CA, *et al.* Germ cell tumors with sarcomatous components: a clinicopathologic and immunohistochemical study of 46 cases. *Am J Surg Pathol.* 2007;31:1356–62.

89. Zhao GQ, Dowell JE. Hematologic malignancies associated with germ cell tumors. *Expert Rev Hematol.* 2012;5:427–37.

90. Motzer RJ, Amsterdam A, Prieto V, *et al.* Teratoma with malignant transformation: diverse malignant histologies arising in men with germ cell tumors. *J Urol.* 1998;159:133–8.

91. Wick M, Perlman E, Ströbel P, *et al.* Germ cell tumors with somatic-type malignancy. In: Travis WD, Brambilla E, Müller-Hermelink H, Harris C, editors. *Pathology and genetics of tumours of the lung, pleura, thymus and heart.* Lyon: IARC Press; 2004. 216–18.

92. Kum JB, Ulbright TM, Williamson SR, *et al.* Molecular genetic evidence supporting the origin of somatic-type malignancy and teratoma from the same progenitor cell. *Am J Surg Pathol.* 2012;36:1849–56.

93. Wolff M, Rosai J, Wright DH. Sebaceous glands within the thymus: report of three cases. *Hum Pathol.* 1984;15:341–3.

94. Chitale AR. Gastric cyst of the mediastinum. A distinct clinicopathological entity. *J Pediatr.* 1969;75:104–10.

95. Salyer DC, Salyer WR, Eggleston JC. Benign developmental cysts of the mediastinum. *Arch Pathol Lab Med.* 1977;101:136–9.

96. Suster S, Moran CA. Primary synovial sarcomas of the mediastinum: a clinicopathologic, immunohistochemical, and ultrastructural study of 15 cases. *Am J Surg Pathol.* 2005;29:569–78.

97. Truong LD, Harris L, Mattioli C, *et al.* Endodermal sinus tumor of the mediastinum. A report of seven cases and review of the literature. *Cancer.* 1986;58:730–9.

98. Moran CA, Suster S. Mediastinal yolk sac tumors associated with prominent multilocular cystic changes of thymic

epithelium: a clinicopathologic and immunohistochemical study of five cases. *Mod Pathol*. 1997;10:800–3.

99. Prat J, Bhan AK, Dickersin GR, *et al*. Hepatoid yolk sac tumor of the ovary (endodermal sinus tumor with hepatoid differentiation): a light microscopic, ultrastructural and immunohistochemical study of seven cases. *Cancer*. 1982;50:2355–68.

100. Moran CA, Suster S. Hepatoid yolk sac tumors of the mediastinum: a clinicopathologic and immunohistochemical study of four cases. *Am J Surg Pathol*. 1997;21:1210–14.

101. Ikeda H, Sato Y, Yoneda N, *et al*. alpha-Fetoprotein-producing gastric carcinoma and combined hepatocellular and cholangiocarcinoma show similar morphology but different histogenesis with respect to SALL4 expression. *Hum Pathol*. 2012;43:1955–63.

102. Ushiku T, Shinozaki A, Shibahara J, *et al*. SALL4 represents fetal gut differentiation of gastric cancer, and is diagnostically useful in distinguishing hepatoid gastric carcinoma from hepatocellular carcinoma. *Am J Surg Pathol*. 2010;34:533–40.

103. Moran CA, Suster S. Yolk sac tumors of the mediastinum with prominent spindle cell features: a clinicopathologic study of three cases. *Am J Surg Pathol*. 1997;21:1173–7.

104. Ulbright TM, Michael H, Loehrer PJ, *et al*. Spindle cell tumors resected from male patients with germ cell tumors. A clinicopathologic study of 14 cases. *Cancer*. 1990;65:148–56.

105. Michael H, Ulbright TM, Brodhecker CA. The pluripotential nature of the mesenchyme-like component of yolk sac tumor. *Arch Pathol Lab Med*. 1989;113:1115–19.

106. Ulbright TM, Loehrer PJ, Roth LM, *et al*. The development of non-germ cell malignancies within germ cell tumors. A clinicopathologic study of 11 cases. *Cancer*. 1984;54:1824–33.

107. Manivel C, Wick MR, Abenoza P, *et al*. The occurrence of sarcomatous components in primary mediastinal germ cell tumors. *Am J Surg Pathol*. 1986;10:711–17.

108. Sales LM, Vontz FK. Teratoma and Di Guglielmo syndrome. *South Med J*. 1970;63:448–50.

109. Wang SE, Fligiel S, Naeim F. Acute megakaryocytic leukemia following chemotherapy for a malignant teratoma. *Arch Pathol Lab Med*. 1984;108:202–5.

110. Irie J, Kawai K, Ueno Y, *et al*. Malignant germ cell tumor of the anterior mediastinum with leukemia-like infiltration. *Acta Pathol Jpn*. 1985;35:1561–70.

111. Mihal V, Dusek J, Jarosova M, *et al*. Mediastinal teratoma and acute megakaryoblastic leukemia. *Neoplasma*. 1989;36:739–47.

112. Orazi A, Wick M, Hartmann JT, *et al*. Germ cell tumors with associated haematologic malignancies. In: Travis WD, Brambilla E, Müller-Hermelink H, Harris C, editors. *Pathology and genetics of tumours of the lung, pleura, thymus and heart*. Lyon: IARC Press; 2004. 219–20.

113. Ladanyi M, Samaniego F, Reuter VE, *et al*. Cytogenetic and immunohistochemical evidence for the germ cell origin of a subset of acute leukemias associated with mediastinal germ cell tumors. *J Natl Cancer Inst*. 1990;82:221–7.

114. Chariot P, Monnet I, Gaulard P, *et al*. Systemic mastocytosis following mediastinal germ cell tumor: an association confirmed. *Hum Pathol*. 1993;24:111–12.

115. Nichols CR, Hoffman R, Einhorn LH, *et al*. Hematologic malignancies associated with primary mediastinal germ-cell tumors. *Ann Intern Med*. 1985;102:603–9.

116. DeMent SH, Eggleston JC, Spivak JL. Association between mediastinal germ cell tumors and hematologic malignancies. Report of two cases and review of the literature. *Am J Surg Pathol*. 1985;9:23–30.

117. Nichols CR, Roth BJ, Heerema N, *et al*. Hematologic neoplasia associated with primary mediastinal germ-cell tumors. *N Engl J Med*. 1990;322:1425–9.

118. de Ment SH. Association between mediastinal germ cell tumors and hematologic malignancies: an update. *Hum Pathol*. 1990;21:699–703.

119. Hartmann JT, Nichols CR, Droz JP, *et al*. Hematologic disorders associated with primary mediastinal nonseminomatous germ cell tumors. *J Natl Cancer Inst*. 2000;92:54–61.

120. Medvinsky A, Rybtsov S, Taoudi S. Embryonic origin of the adult hematopoietic system: advances and questions. *Development*. 2011;138:1017–31.

121. Orazi A, Neiman RS, Ulbright TM, *et al*. Hematopoietic precursor cells within the yolk sac tumor component are the source of secondary hematopoietic malignancies in patients with mediastinal germ cell tumors. *Cancer*. 1993;71:3873–81.

122. Saito A, Watanabe K, Kusakabe T, *et al*. Mediastinal mature teratoma with coexistence of angiosarcoma, granulocytic sarcoma and a hematopoietic region in the tumor: a rare case of association between hematological malignancy and mediastinal germ cell tumor. *Pathol Int*. 1998;48:749–53.

123. Delsol G, Falini B, Müller-Hermelink HK, *et al*. Anaplastic large cell lymphoma (ALCL), ALK-positive. In: Swerdlow SH, Campo E, Harris NL, Jaffe ES, Pileri S, Stein H, *et al*., editors. *WHO classification of tumours of haematopoietic and lymphoid tissues*. Lyon, France: International Agency for Research on Cancer; 2008. 312–16.

124. Moran CA, Suster S. Primary mediastinal choriocarcinomas: a clinicopathologic and immunohistochemical study of eight cases. *Am J Surg Pathol*. 1997;21:1007–12.

125. Kalhor N, Ramirez PT, Deavers MT, *et al*. Immunohistochemical studies of trophoblastic tumors. *Am J Surg Pathol*. 2009;33:633–8.

126. Went PT, Dirnhofer S, Stallmach T, *et al*. Placental site trophoblastic tumor of the mediastinum. *Hum Pathol*. 2005;36:581–4.

127. Singer G, Kurman RJ, McMaster MT, *et al*. HLA-G immunoreactivity is specific for intermediate trophoblast in gestational trophoblastic disease and can serve as a useful marker in differential diagnosis. *Am J Surg Pathol*. 2002;26:914–20.

128. Beresford L, Fernandez CV, Cummings E, *et al*. Mediastinal polyembryoma associated with Klinefelter syndrome. *J Pediatr Hematol Oncol*. 2003;25:321–3.

129. Eble JN. Spermatocytic seminoma. *Hum Pathol*. 1994;25:1035–42.

Parathyroid lesions, paragangliomas, thyroid tumors, and pleomorphic adenomas of the mediastinum

Chapter 10

Mark R. Wick, MD, and Alberto M. Marchevsky, MD

Because of the developmental association that the thymus has with other foregut-derived structures, a diversity of pathologic epithelial lesions other than thymic or germ cell tumors may arise in the anterior mediastinum. In addition, the thorax is the second most common site (after the retroperitoneum) in which paragangliomas arise, and most of them are seen in either the anterior or posterior mediastinum. This chapter considers the attributes of those lesions.

Parathyroid tumors of the mediastinum

In light of the intimate embryological relationship between the thymus and the parathyroid glands, it should not be surprising that parathyroid neoplasms may be encountered in the mediastinum. Readers will recall that the third branchial pouch gives rise to the thymus and the inferior pair of parathyroid glands, whereas the superior parathyroids are derived from the fourth branchial pouch. During the fifth week of gestation, these structures begin their ventral-inferior descent from the upper cervical region into the lower neck or anterior mediastinum. If abnormalities occur in this migratory process, portions of the thymus may be left in the supraclavicular cervical region; conversely, the parathyroids may descend into the parathymic tissues or the posterior mediastinal compartment [1]. Also, up to 6.5% of otherwise normal individuals have supernumerary, ectopic parathyroids (in addition to four retrothyroidal glands) within the thoracic confines [2].

Historical considerations

Surprisingly, the developmental considerations just cited were not well recognized until the early part of the twentieth century. The migration of branchial pouch derivatives was delineated in the 1920s, and the first example of a surgically-managed mediastinal parathyroid tumor was reported in the United States in 1932. The remarkable patient in this case was a retired sea captain, Charles Martell (Fig. 10.1). After several unsuccessful neck explorations at the Massachusetts General Hospital, he immersed himself in the medical literature then extant on hyperparathyroidism and insisted to his

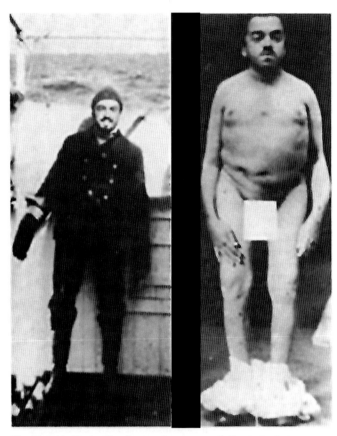

Fig. 10.1 Mr. Charles Martell, a merchant seaman (left), was the first person to undergo successful excision of an intramediastinal parathyroid adenoma after it had caused significant bony and renal disease (right).

attending physicians that they had likely missed an intrathoracic parathyroid tumor in his previous evaluations! This conclusion proved to be true. After removal of the latter lesion (a 3 cm anterior mediastinal adenoma), Martell improved markedly, but he unfortunately later died of postoperative complications [3].

Since that time, numerous reports have been made on mediastinal parathyroid proliferations [4–10]. These lesions recapitulate all of the hyperplasias and neoplastic conditions

Pathology of the Mediastinum, ed. Alberto M. Marchevsky and Mark R. Wick. Published by Cambridge University Press.
© Cambridge University Press 2014.

(a)

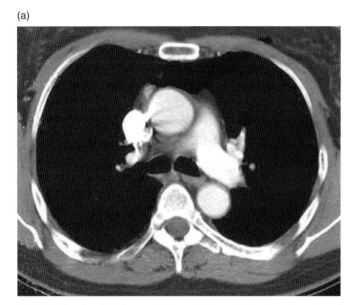

(b)

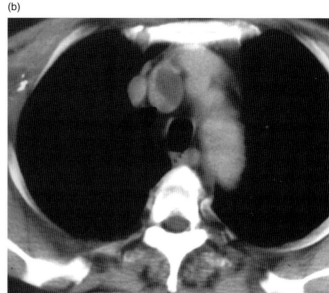

Fig. 10.2 Parathyroid adenomas in the anterior mediastinal are shown here in computed tomograms. The lesion in **(a)** is just to the right of the aortic arch; in **(b)** it is intrathymic.

of the cervical parathyroids and are now familiar to endocrinologic surgeons. Some observers may take issue with our opinion that mediastinal parathyroid lesions are "neuroendocrine" proliferations, because they do differ in many respects from carcinoids, paragangliomas, and other tumors of that type. Nevertheless, several reviews on generic neuroendocrine markers have demonstrated such determinants in parathyroid lesions, and the evolving convention is to classify them accordingly.

Clinical features

Hyperplasia or neoplasia of mediastinal parathyroid glands is observed over a wide age range – extending from childhood into late adult life – and is not an uncommon occurrence; in one large series on parathyroid lesions, 22% were intramediastinal [6]. The most characteristic mode of presentation is with hypercalcemia, inasmuch as the great majority of these lesions manufacture parathyroid hormone (PTH). Calcium levels associated with mediastinal parathyroid tumors are variable, but generally exceed 3 mmol/L; accordingly, PTH values in serum are elevated to a range that is clearly diagnostic of hyperparathyroidism (> 100 pg/ml) in most instances [2,5,6,10].

Other signs and symptoms may reflect secondary effects of the latter condition, including mental obtundation or lethargy, pathologic fractures of the vertebra or long bones, radiographically detected osteopenia, peptic ulcer disease, hypertension, constipation, and the formation of calculi in the urinary tract [2]. Because mediastinal parathyroid tumors tend to be relatively small, it is unusual for clinical complaints to reflect a mass-displacement of intrathoracic structures. In circumstances where the latter symptoms are present (particularly with marked hypercalcemia), the diagnosis of mediastinal parathyroid carcinoma must be considered seriously. Huang *et al.* [11] reported an unusual case in which spontaneous rupture of a

parathyroid adenoma produced significant intrathoracic hemorrhage with airway compromise.

Parathyroid proliferations of the mediastinum may be encountered in patients with multiple endocrine neoplasia syndrome (MEN) types 1 or 2 [12–15]. Persons with MEN 1 are born with one mutated copy of the *MEN*1 gene in each cell. During their lifetimes, the other gene copy is also mutated in a proportion of cells, giving rise to endocrine neoplasms [14]. MEN 2 generally results from a gain-of-function variant of the *RET* gene, producing a similar tumor diathesis [12].

Radiographic findings

Conventional chest radiographs are usually unproductive in the detection of intrathoracic parathyroid tumors, with the exception of rare cases involving uncommonly large adenomas or carcinomas. For this reason, high-resolution computed tomography (CT) and magnetic resonance imaging (MRI) of the thorax are the modalities preferred by radiologists for the localization of ectopic parathyroid lesions [16]. Hyperplastic or adenomatous glands are well circumscribed; 15% are present in the most superior "cuts" of CT or MRI scans, and are usually found in an intrathymic or parathymic location (Fig. 10.2). Less commonly, paraesophageal posterior mediastinal lesions are seen. Rare cases of cystic parathyroid adenoma or lipoadenoma are best delineated with MRI procedures; the invasive nature of parathyroid carcinomas can be elucidated with either CT or MRI (Fig. 10.3) [17].

Macroscopic features

Hyperplasias and adenomas of intramediastinal parathyroid glands manifest themselves as well-circumscribed masses that are often contained within the thymic capsule. Their sizes and weights vary in direct proportion to the serum calcium level, and

(b)

(a)

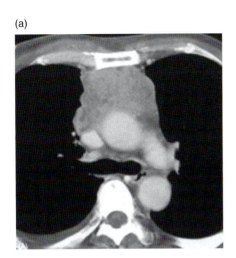

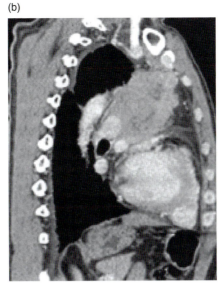

Fig. 10.3 The invasive nature of mediastinal parathyroid carcinoma is seen here in a computed tomogram **(a)** and a magnetic resonance imaging scan **(b)**.

(a)

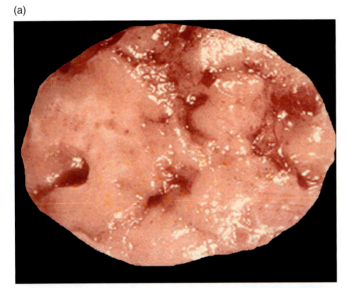

(b)

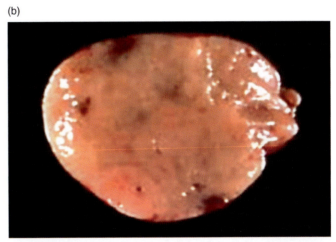

Fig. 10.4 Parathyroid adenomas of the anterior mediastinum are ovoid, variably-solid masses, with a tan pink cut surface **(a and b)**. They may weigh up to 5 gms.

range from less than 1 to 8 cm, or 0.4 to greater than 100 g, respectively. The cut surfaces of these lesions are uniform in appearance and firm, with a tan-brown color (Fig. 10.4). Necrosis and hemorrhage are exceedingly rare, but focal cystic change is not [2]. Indeed, some parathyroid lesions may undergo extensive degeneration and grossly resemble thymic cysts [4].

In contrast, parathyroid carcinomas of the mediastinum are difficult to distinguish from thymic carcinomas or malignant germ cell tumors on macroscopic grounds. They are invasive into contiguous lung tissue or blood vessels, and exhibit white-gray, firm to hard cut surfaces (Fig. 10.5). Necrosis is not unusual [18–24]. These neoplasms may attain large dimensions and weights, such that occasional examples literally fill the anterior mediastinum [25].

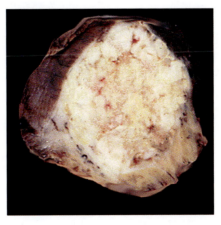

Fig. 10.5 Mediastinal parathyroid carcinomas are large (up to 10 cm in maximal dimension) and white-tan with a gritty cut surface.

(a)

(b)

(c)

(d)

(e)

(f)

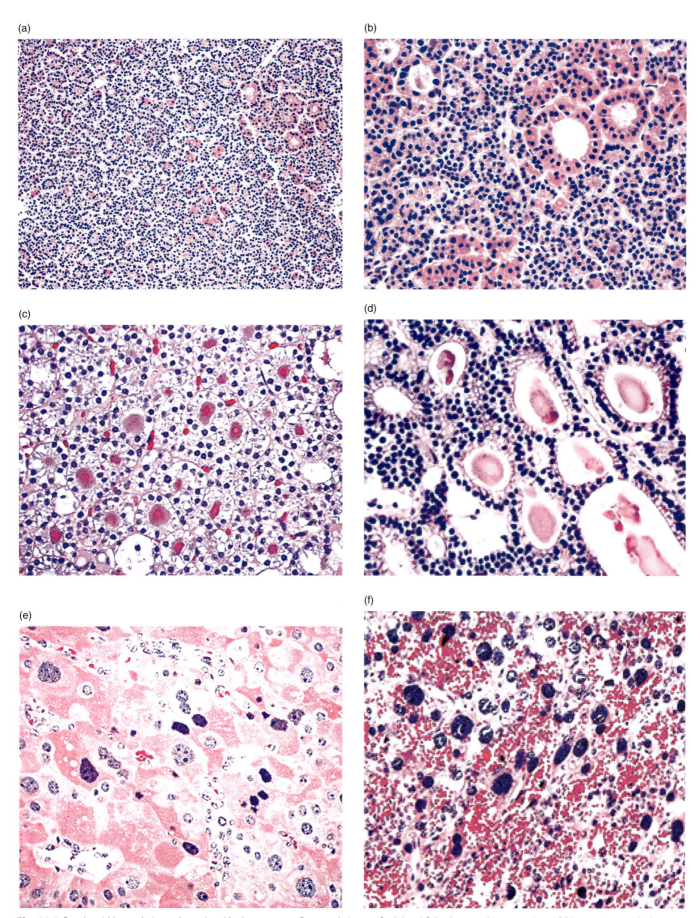

Fig. 10.6 Parathyroid hyperplasias and parathyroid adenomas manifest an admixture of solid and follicular growth patterns **(a and b)**, sometimes with the intraluminal presence of colloid-like secretions **(c and d)**. In rare instances, these lesions can demonstrate striking nuclear pleomorphism and atypicality **(e and f)**.

(a)

(b)

(c)

(d)

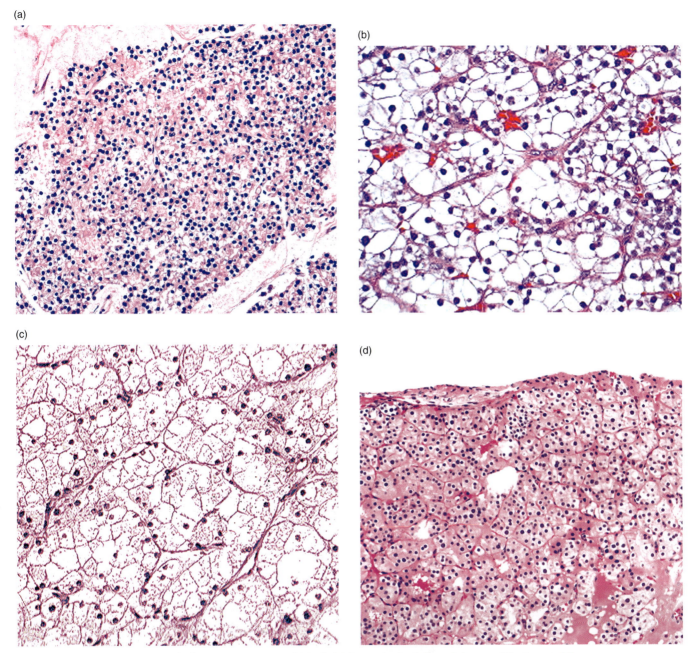

Fig. 10.7 Parathyroid hyperplasias and adenomas may comprise chief cells **(a)**; "water-clear" cells **(b and c)**, or oxyphilic elements **(d)**.

Histologic and cytological characteristics

Parathyroid hyperplasia and parathyroid adenoma share several significant microscopic features, and may be indistinguishable from one another after examination of an isolated gland. Both conditions are bounded by a fibrous capsule, and feature the presence of expansive sheets, nodules, acinae, or trabeculae composed of polyhedral epithelial cells (Fig. 10.6e–f) [2,4,6,7]. Increased cellular density is sometimes seen around supporting stromal blood vessels, which may be numerous. These proliferations most commonly contain bland, round nuclei with evenly dispersed chromatin, but rare cases may

manifest appreciable nuclear pleomorphism and discernible nucleoli [2]. Mitotic activity is usually scanty; however, careful examination will reveal the presence of some division figures in over 50% of cases [26]. The cytoplasmic appearance of the proliferating cells has been used to designate cytomorphologic subtypes of parathyroid lesions, including chief cell, clear cell, and oxyphil cell variants (Fig. 10.7) [2,4]. Nonetheless, these do not seem to correlate with definable differences in behavior, and are of interest only in differential diagnosis.

Past emphasis has been given to the premise that parathyroid lesions bordered by a compressed rim of microscopically normal gland are probably adenomatous, rather than hyperplastic (Fig. 10.8) [2,27]. However, in our experience this finding is evident in only 50% of adenomas and may be seen in nodular hyperplasia as well; hence, it is not a consistently-effective means of separating the two processes. The only indisputable way of doing so is to examine biopsy specimens from the remaining parathyroid glands; if these are unavailable, a diagnosis of "parathyroid proliferative disease" may be the most appropriate.

Lipoadenomas are peculiar growths that differ from adenomas in having a higher content of intratumoral adipose cells (Fig. 10.9) [2,28]. Small biopsies from such lesions may be misinterpreted as normal, but the total epithelial cell volume is definitely appreciated as increased in excision specimens.

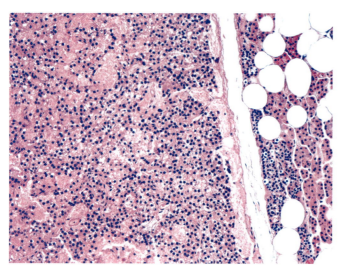

Fig. 10.8 A rim of morphologically normal parathyroid tissue (right of figure) may be seen adjacent to either nodular hyperplasia or adenoma of the parathyroid. Hence, that finding is not helpful in distinguishing between the two entities.

Other peculiar variants of mediastinal parathyroid adenoma were documented by Fallone and co-workers [29], and Elgoweini and Chetty [30], in which many intralesional lymphocytes and hyalinizing stromal fibrosis were present, respectively. The causes of those alterations were unknown.

Mediastinal parathyroid carcinomas contrast with the description just given in manifesting more markedly organoid growth, often with internal fibrous septa. They are unencapsulated and invasive, and regularly contain mitotic figures (Fig. 10.10) [2,24]. Although such lesions commonly exhibit cellular pleomorphism, vascular infiltration, and nuclear atypia, those features are not always present. Differential diagnosis of mediastinal parathyroid proliferations includes thymic neuroendocrine carcinoma (NEC) [31–33] when the lesion has a chief cell appearance; clear cell thymic carcinoma [34], paraganglioma, or seminoma in cases showing a clear cell composition [35]; and paraganglioma or an ectopic thyroid tumor when oxyphil cells predominate [36]. Attention to the biochemical presence of hypercalcemia is the most helpful way of resolving these uncertainties, although unfortunately some tumors are clinically non-functional [37]. In addition, parathyroid lesions typically contain abundant PAS-positive glycogen (Fig. 10.11), whereas some (but not all) of the other diagnostic alternatives do not. Moreover, significant argyrophilia is unusual in parathyroid proliferations but common in NECs and paragangliomas (Fig. 10.12) [33].

Fine needle aspiration biopsies of parathyroid lesions reveal a variably-cohesive population of relatively monomorphic cells with compact ovoid nuclei (Fig. 10.13) [38–42]. Parathyroid carcinomas may manifest slight increases in the nucleocytoplasmic ratio, with some nuclear pleomorphism (Fig. 10.14); however, those changes are not uniform. The stippled chromatin pattern seen in NECs is generally lacking in parathyroid proliferations.

(a)

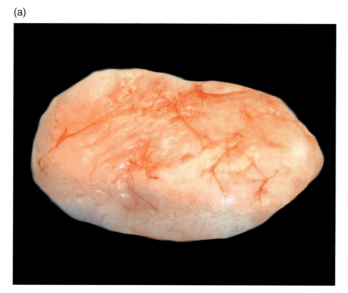

(b)

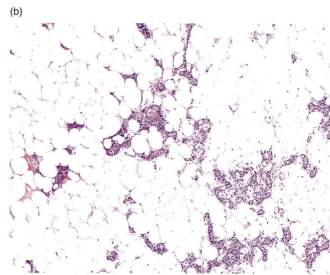

Fig. 10.9 Lipoadenomas are unusual proliferations with a yellowish, soft cut surface **(a)**. They are constituted by parathyroid chief or oxyphil cells in admixture with mature fat, simulating the appearance of a normal parathyroid gland **(b)**.

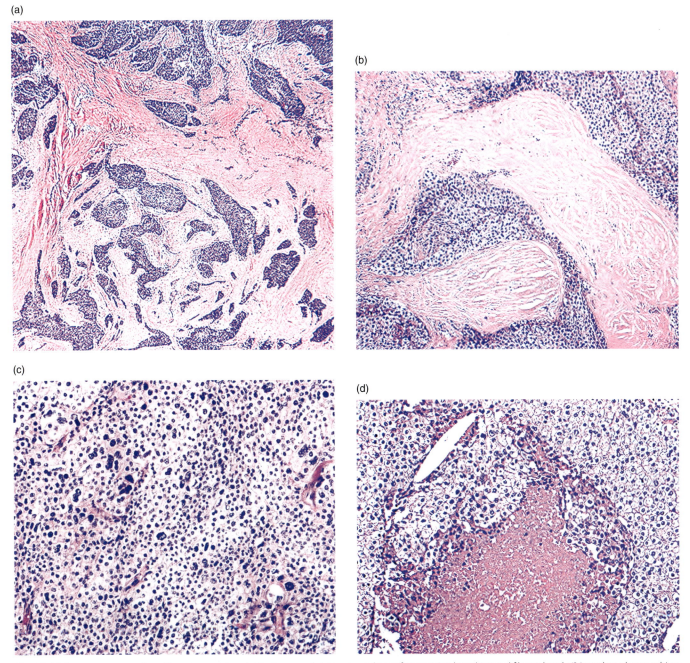

Fig. 10.10 In most cases, parathyroid carcinomas show infiltrative growth into surrounding soft tissues **(a)**; broad internal fibrous bands **(b)**; nuclear pleomorphism and mitotic activity **(c)**; or necrosis **(d)**.

Cytogenetic findings in parathyroid lesions

A spectrum of cytogenetic abnormalities has been documented in parathyroid lesions. Among all of them, the one with greatest potential diagnostic utility is mutation of the *HRPT2* gene [43]. DeLellis has reported differential labeling for the protein product of that gene – called parafibromin (PF) – in parathyroid adenomas and parathyroid carcinomas [44]. The nuclei of adenomatous cells were consistently PF-immunoreactive, whereas that protein was partially or completely lost in carcinomas.

Mediastinal paragangliomas

Paragangliomas (PGs) can be divided into two broad morphological categories, as suggested by Glenner and Grimley [45]. Branchiomeric PGs are associated with tissues related to the ontogenetic gill arches, and include the majority of such tumors that arise in the head and neck or in apposition to large intrathoracic blood vessels. Aorticosympathetic PGs, on the other hand, are anatomically and functionally linked with sympathetic autonomic nervous tissues. Both of these classes of PG occur within the

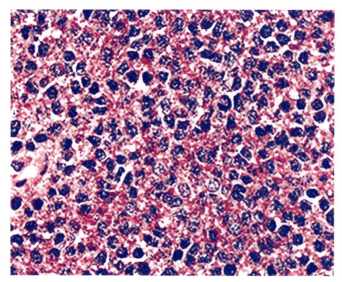

Fig. 10.11 Parathyroid proliferations of all types are often labeled with the periodic acid-Schiff stain, as shown here, because of their content of cytoplasmic glycogen.

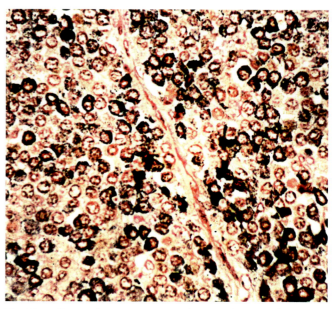

Fig. 10.12 Neuroendocrine carcinomas and paragangliomas are both argyrophilic with such histochemical methods as the Churukian-Schenk stain, shown here. However, parathyroid lesions do not have this property.

(a)

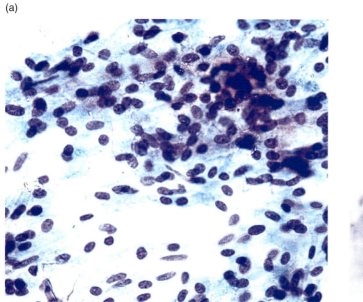

(b)

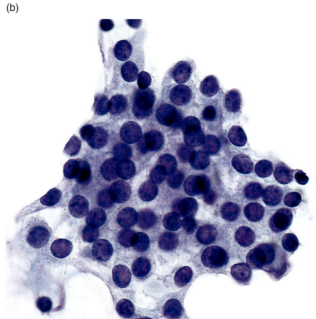

Fig. 10.13 Fine needle aspiration biopsies of parathyroid lesions yield variably-cohesive populations of round to ovoid cells, with relatively monomorphic nuclei **(a and b)**.

mediastinum, in its anterior and posterior compartments, respectively [46–54]. For the sake of clarity, these will be referred to henceforth as aorticopulmonary and paravertebral mediastinal PGs.

Historical considerations

As physiological studies progressed in the 1920s and 1930s, the functions of the paraganglion system became better delineated. With these advances, interest in possible neoplasms of this tissue grew. The first documented case of a human paravertebral paraganglioma (PVPG) was reported by Miller in 1924 [55], and concerned a 39-year-old woman whose posterior mediastinal tumor was an incidental finding at autopsy. The first functional PVPG was described by Philips in 1940 [56], and occurred in a 31-year-old man who had had classical symptoms and signs of catecholamine excess for six years. Postmortem examination showed a posterior mediastinal mass with the histologic features of PG, as well as findings related to chronically uncontrolled hypertension.

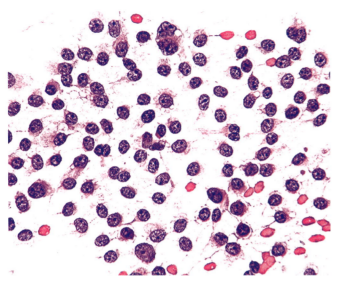

Fig. 10.14 Parathyroid carcinoma may show notable nuclear pleomorphism in fine needle aspiration biopsies.

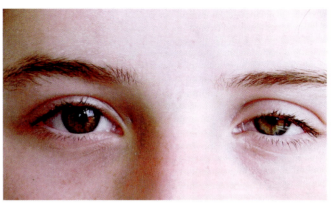

Fig. 10.15 Horner syndrome, typified by ptosis and miosis of the left eye, caused by a thoracic-level paravertebral paraganglioma in an adolescent boy.

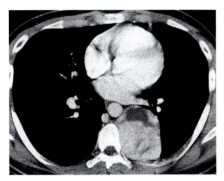

Fig. 10.16 The tumor referenced in Fig. 10.15 is shown here in a computed tomogram; it shows vascular enhancement, helping to characterize it as a paraganglioma.

Aorticopulmonary paragangliomas (APPGs) of the mediastinum were first recognized in animals, as reflected by a report on a pair of dogs with such tumors in 1943 [57]. Seven years thereafter, Lattes described two similar lesions in humans; one tumor was an incidental postmortem finding, whereas the other was an unresectable anterior mediastinal mass [58]. Both occurred in middle-aged adults. Since these seminal communications, over 1,000 mediastinal paragangliomas have been documented [46–54].

Clinical characteristics

Mediastinal PGs are uncommon lesions; the sizable number of reports on such tumors reflects physicians' interest in them, rather than their overall frequency. Anterior mediastinal PGs are seen at an average age of 49 years, with a slight female predilection (1.5:1) [59]. Those located in the paravertebral posterior mediastinal tissues present at a lesser mean age (29 years), and 60% affect males [50,51,53].

Functional and symptomatic aspects of APPG and PVPG also differ. The former neoplasms only infrequently synthesize exportable catecholamines (3%), while PVPGs do so in nearly one-half of all cases [46]. Accordingly, anterior-superior

mediastinal PG typically present with non-specific symptoms and signs of an intrathoracic mass [59–61], whereas PVPG may produce complaints like those associated with adrenal pheochromocytomas [50,51]. Non-secretory PG of the paravertebral mediastinum may present with spinal cord compression, interscapular chest pain, or Horner's syndrome (Fig. 10.15) [50]. A minority of tumors are detected incidentally on chest radiographs. Odze *et al.* [62] suggested that biologically malignant PG in any intrathoracic location are those that are less likely to synthesize catecholamines. Mediastinal PG again may be part of the MEN type 2 syndrome [12,13], and it is also likely that kindreds with these neoplasms exist apart from the latter disorder. For example, a literature review on mediastinal PVPGs by Gallivan *et al.* indicated that over 20% of patients had more than one of these tumors [63]. In addition, Carney [64] has described a peculiar syndromic complex featuring gastric stromal tumors, pulmonary chondromas, and functioning extraadrenal paragangliomas, which chiefly affects young women.

Radiographic findings

Intrathoracic paragangliomas characteristically appear on chest x-rays as opaque, rounded, or irregularly shaped masses in the anterior or posterior mediastinum. In this regard, they are indistinguishable from many other neoplasms on conventional imaging studies [16]. However, high-resolution CT (Fig. 10.16) is capable of narrowing the radiological differential diagnosis considerably, if such imaging procedures are done with and without infusion of contrast materials. Spizarny *et al.* [65] found that PGs were the most common CT-enhancing mediastinal tumors; in that respect, they were similar to NECs and parathyroid adenomas. The common denominator behind this observation is the histological vascularity of those neoplasms.

Macroscopic features

Mediastinal PGs are typically firm, reddish-pink or brown masses (Fig. 10.17), and they are vascular tumors that commonly undergo focal necrosis. The average size of APPG is 7.5 cm, whereas that of PVPG is 6 cm [45]. Partial encapsulation may be observed in either group, but it is more frequently evident in

177

(b)

(a)

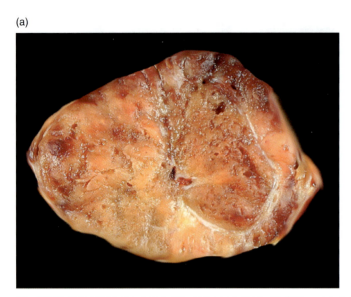

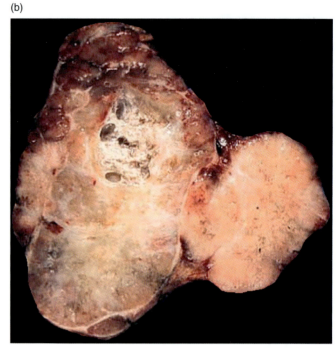

Fig. 10.17 Paragangliomas are tan, pink, or brown tumors with fleshy cut surfaces **(a)**; they may also demonstrate gross invasion into adjacent tissues **(b)**.

paravertebral lesions. APPGs more commonly invade adjacent intrathoracic organs [49,59], and surgical resection specimens in such cases reflect that fact. Extensive cystic change in mediastinal PGs has been reported by Ortega *et al.* [66].

Histological characteristics

The microscopic appearances of PVPG and APPG are similar, but some minor differences between them may indeed be discerned [45–54,67]. Both types of mediastinal paraganglioma are composed of large polygonal cells that are arranged in a characteristic fashion into tightly grouped nests ("Zellballen") of roughly equal size. The supporting stroma is highly vascular, and may contain ectatic blood vessels with an angiomatoid appearance. Nuclei are round or slightly irregular, usually with dispersed chromatin (Fig. 10.18). However, vesicular chromatin may be observed focally, as may prominent nucleoli and sometimes striking nuclear pleomorphism (Fig. 10.19). Mitoses are typically sparse or absent, but rare PGs do contain numerous division figures. Also, areas of spindle cell growth may be evident. Zellballen in APPGs are somewhat subtle, in that less matrical collagen tends to be present between them than that seen in PVPGs; moreover, the former lesions are less likely to manifest cellular pleomorphism.

Plaza and colleagues [68] have described an atypical variant of mediastinal PG which features prominent intralesional sclerosis. Broad internal bands of fibrous tissue transect such tumors, compartmentalizing the neoplastic cells into irregular nests, cords, and islands with angular profiles. That finding, together with the fact that "sclerosing" PG often shows nuclear atypicality, may lead to a mistaken morphological diagnosis of invasive carcinoma.

Another PG subtype that rarely may be encountered in the mediastinum is the gangliocytic form (Fig. 10.20) [69]. In that lesion, one sees areas with histological identity to the appearance of ganglioneuromas, admixed with conventional PG.

A pigmented PVPG was reported by Hofmann *et al.* [70]. That lesion contained melanin, histochemically demonstrable with the Fontana-Masson method.

In fine needle aspiration biopsies of PG, one may see dyshesive cells, or aggregates in clusters or acinar formations. The tumor cells may be round, ovoid, plasmacytoid, or fusiform, with moderately-pleomorphic nuclear contours (Fig. 10.21) [71]. A common finding is the presence of pink cytoplasmic granules in the tumor cells [72].

Some mediastinal PG do have the potential for metastasis, but it is impossible to identify these lesions individually by prospective use of microscopic criteria. Attention to such features as necrosis, mitotic activity, spindle cell change, nuclear pleomorphism, hemorrhage, and vascular invasion (Fig. 10.22) is not consistently effective in this regard [54]. Nevertheless, APPG of the mediastinum commonly cause significant morbidity and mortality through local invasion of contiguous organs; hence, this finding should be noted in diagnostic reports on such lesions if it is apparent microscopically.

Histochemical techniques show argyrophilia in most mediastinal PG, and they are argentaffinic as well if stained with the del Rio Hortega method (Fig. 10.23). PAS stains fail to demonstrate appreciable glycogen in these neoplasms; however, some PG contain ceroid-like material or lipofuscin that is labeled with Schiff-base methods [45]. Mast cells are also common in PGs, and may be enumerated with the toluidine blue procedure or Leder's stain. The reticulin method is particularly useful in highlighting

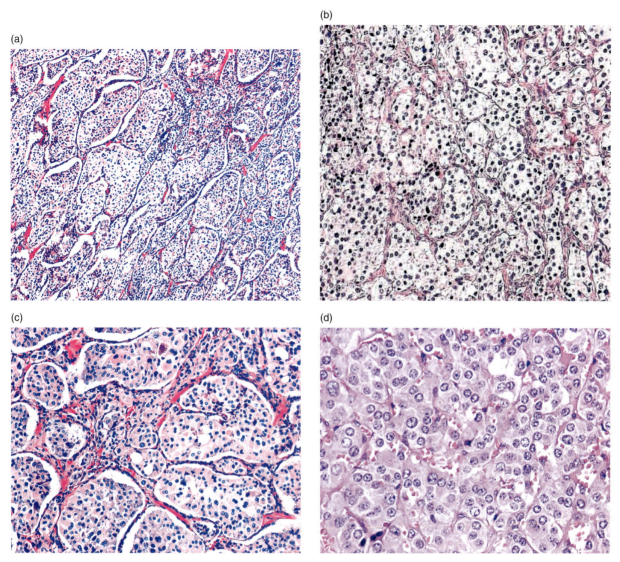

Fig. 10.18 Paragangliomas exhibit an organoid architecture, represented by distinct groups of polygonal cells that are enclosed by fibrovascular stroma – so-called "Zellballen" **(a–c)**. Variable nuclear and cytological pleomorphism is usually apparent in such tumors **(d)**.

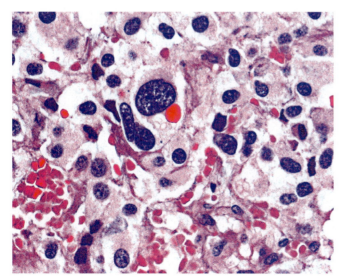

Fig. 10.19 Occasional examples of paraganglioma show marked anisonucleosis, as shown here. This feature is not necessarily a marker of malignancy.

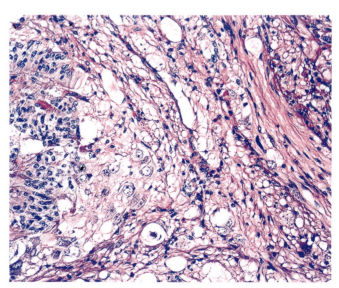

Fig. 10.20 The "gangliocytic" variant of paraganglioma contains elements like those seen in ganglioneuroma (bottom left of figure), admixed with conventional paragangioma.

the intratumoral stroma, and in emphasizing the structure of constituent Zellballen (Fig. 10.24).

Composite paraganglioma–neuroblastoma

A most unusual form of PG is usually encountered in the adrenal gland, in which ordinary paraganglioma is juxtaposed to a second tumor component with the appearance of neuroblastoma [73–76]. These "composite" tumors (PG-NBs) have also been reported rarely in other anatomic sites, including the anterior and posterior mediastinum (Fig. 10.25) [74]. One might expect that children might be exclusively affected by PG-NBs, because of the presence of neuroblastic tissue in such lesions. However, that is not true; several cases have been described in adults as well [77].

Microscopically, one typically sees an abrupt transition between the two histologic components of PG-NBs, with little admixture (Fig. 10.26). The neuroblastic element comprises monotonous, small, round cells, sometimes showing formation of neural rosettes [78].

Comstock *et al.* compared the clinicopathologic and cytogenetic characteristics of PG-NBs with those of "pure" PGs and neuroblastomas [77]. The age range of the patients with composite tumors was 15 to 40 years, and half of them had syndromic lesions. None of the composite PG-NBs showed any amplification of the N-*myc* gene, and none recurred or proved fatal. Among the classic PGs, no case demonstrated any N-*myc* amplification; two tumors recurred, but none caused death. Fifty percent of the pure neuroblastomas manifested amplification of N-*myc* amplification, and half of them also were lethal. Those findings suggest that composite PG-NB is probably a biological variant of PG. Hence, aggressive chemotherapy for neuroblastoma is likely not necessary in such cases.

Genetic findings associated with paragangliomas

Multiple PGs may be seen in several hereditary conditions, including neurofibromatosis, von Hippel-Lindau syndrome, MEN 2, and familial paragangliomatosis [50]. Germline

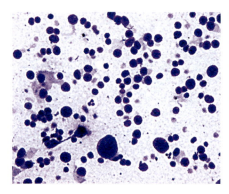

Fig. 10.21 Fine needle aspiration biopsies of paraganglioma commonly show dyshesive tumor cells with obvious nuclear pleomorphism and a moderate amount of amphophilic cytoplasm.

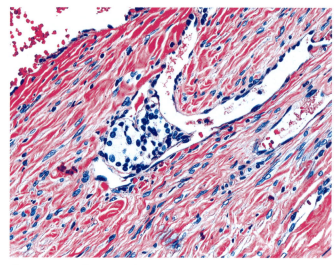

Fig. 10.22 Vascular invasion by paraganglioma is suggestive of biological malignancy, but does not constitute definitive evidence of the same.

(a)

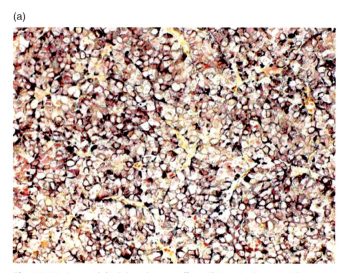

(b)

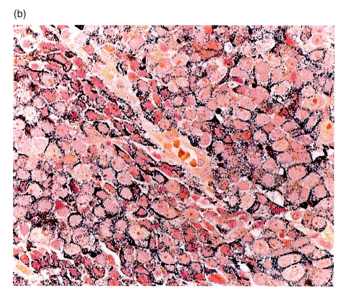

Fig. 10.23 Argyrophilia **(a)** and argentaffinity **(b)** are both potentially seen in mediastinal paragangliomas.

mutations in the succinic dehydrogenase *SDHB* gene can cause the last of those syndromes, or, less frequently, early-onset renal cell carcinoma [79]. Paragangliomas related to *SDHB* mutations have a high rate of biological malignancy (in at least 35% of cases) [80], and commonly arise in an extra-adrenal location. Mutations in the *SDHB* gene that cause disease are observed in exons 1 through 7. Paraganglionic tumor formation comports with the "two hit" hypothesis. The first copy of the gene is mutated in all cells, but the second copy functions normally. When the latter also mutates in certain cells because of random subcellular events, a loss of heterozygosity obtains and functional *SDHB* protein is no longer produced, because the responsible gene is a tumor-suppressor. Neoplasia is then possible. Although succinic dehydrogenase is present throughout most tissues, it is not currently known why paraganglionic cells are principally affected by *SDHB* mutations. Adrenal neuroblastoma and composite extra-adrenal PG-NBs have also been reported in a few patients with this genetic aberration [80]. Some clinical overlap also exists between familial paragangliomatosis and the Cowden syndrome [81].

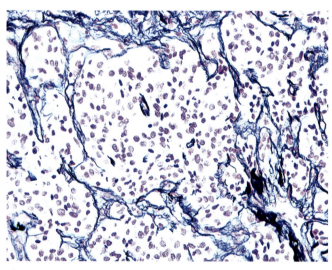

Fig. 10.24 Reticulin stains clearly delineate the boundaries of the cellular nests in paragangliomas.

(a)

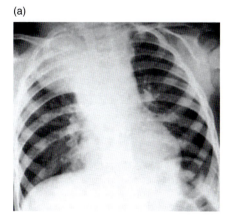

(b)

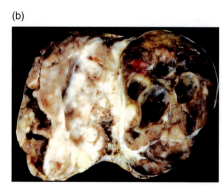

Ultrastructure of parathyroid and paraganglionic tumors

Because of the shared cellular attributes of neuroendocrine neoplasms, neuroendocrine carcinomas, parathyroid lesions, and paragangliomas of the mediastinum have basically similar electron microscopic features [33,45,82]. Tumor cells in such neoplasms are polygonal with limited numbers of blunt cytoplasmic extensions, and they are surrounded by a generally scanty intercellular collagenous matrix. Pericellular basal lamina is variable in its presence, and adjacent cells are connected by desmosomal or macula adherens-type attachment complexes. Nuclei are round to oval with evenly distributed heterochromatin and small nucleoli.

Aside from the usual metabolic organelles and neurosecretory granules, which are present in all mediastinal neuroendocrine tumors, other cytoplasmic constituents merit some consideration in separating them diagnostically. Thymic neuroendocrine carcinomas (NECs) often contain unusually abundant rough endoplasmic reticulum, which may be arranged in a concentric fashion ("Nebenkerns"). In addition, tumors associated with ACTH production may exhibit arrays of smooth endoplasmic reticulum as well. Apoptosis in CTT produces pseudolumina in the midst of cellular nests – a feature that is not common to the other tumors under discussion. Moreover, whorled intermediate filament aggregates are frequently present in a perinuclear location in NECs (Fig. 10.27) [33]; that finding is not observed in parathyroid or paraganglion cell tumors.

Parathyroid tumors may display the presence of true intercellular lumina, lined by blunt microvilli. In addition, they contain glycogen particles in much greater quantity than that seen in carcinoids or PGs [82]. Paragangliomas contain two distinct cell types, making them unique among the mediastinal lesions being considered here. The most prominent are the chief cells, containing numerous neurosecretory granules. They are grouped into the aforementioned Zellballen, and are surrounded by members of the second paragangliomatous constituent – the sustentacular cell population. The latter elements are fusiform and contain few organelles; in particular, neurosecretory granules are uniformly lacking in sustentacular cells [45].

Fig. 10.25 "Composite" paragangliomas, as shown here in the anterosuperior mediastinum in a chest film **(a)**, are more heterogeneous macroscopically than conventional paragangliomas **(b)**. They contain paragangliomatous tissue that is juxtaposed to primitive neuroblastic elements.

(a)

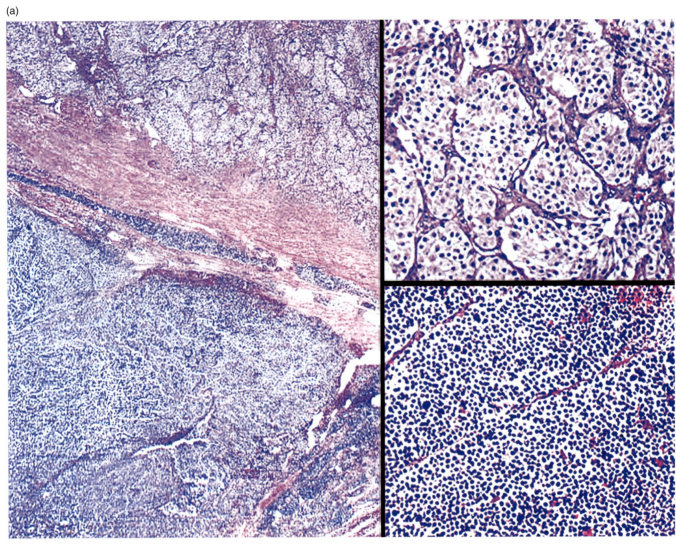

(b)

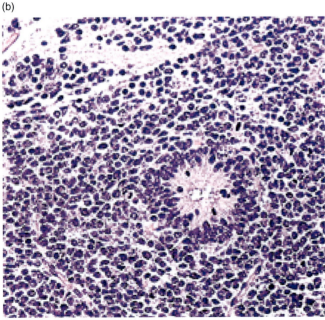

Fig. 10.26 "Composite" paragangliomas **(a)** exhibit an abrupt interface between conventional paraganglioma (top left and top right), and a neuroblastic component (bottom left). The neuroblastic elements may demonstrate formation of neural rosettes **(b)**.

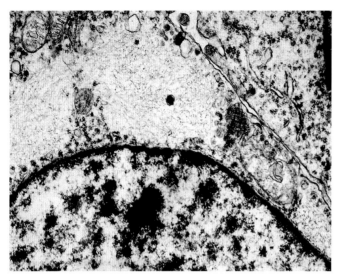

Fig. 10.27 Neuroendocrine carcinomas often contain paranuclear whorls of intermediate filaments ultrastructurally, as shown here. That feature is not shared by paragangliomas or parathyroid lesions.

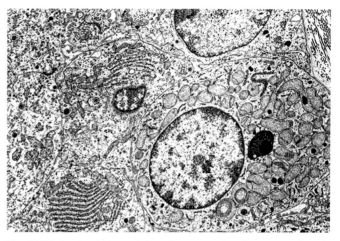

Fig. 10.28 Parathyroid hyperplasias, adenomas, and carcinomas contain only a sparse number of neurosecretory granules by electron microscopy. This particular example – a parathyroid adenoma – shows prominent profiles of rough endoplasmic reticulum.

The quantity and appearance of neurosecretory granules also differs in mediastinal neuroendocrine proliferations. NECs typically contain at least a moderate number of these organelles, which are relatively uniform in shape and density; they range from 100 to 400 nm in size. Neurosecretory granules are quite sparse in parathyroid adenomas (Fig. 10.28), presumably because the latter lesions exhibit extremely active exocytosis. Lastly, the granules in PG are more variable in size and shape, sometimes assuming "dumb-bell" configurations. In addition, those seen in functional paraganglion cell tumors have a pronounced peripheral "halo" with eccentric dense cores (Fig. 10.29)[45].

Immunohistology of parathyroid and paraganglionic tumors

The use of immunohistochemical techniques has contributed greatly to an understanding of the similarities and differences among neuroendocrine tumors of the mediastinum. Thymic NECs and intrathoracic PG share the potential synthesis of several "generic" endocrine proteins, including neuron-specific enolase, CD56, CD57, chromogranin-A, protein gene product 9.5, and synaptophysin (Fig. 10.30)[83–87]. However, these may sometimes not be present in any given lesion, necessitating the concomitant use of antibody panels which are directed at several additional markers for differential diagnosis.

Intermediate filament typing is useful as a means of separating parathyroid proliferations or neuroendocrine carcinomas from paragangliomas. The first two of those lesions are reactive for cytokeratin, whereas PG express neurofilament protein alone or in combination with vimentin[88]. In addition, the sustentacular cells of many paragangliomas can be labeled with antibodies to S100 protein (Fig. 10.31)[89], which is lacking in other mediastinal neuroendocrine neoplasms. Parathyroid

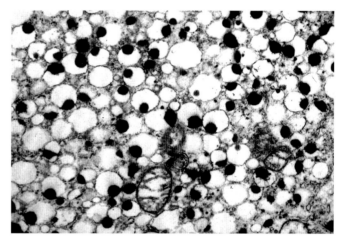

Fig. 10.29 Functional paragangliomas often exhibit the presence of distinctive neurosecretory granules with accentuated internal "haloes" and eccentric dense cores.

tumors are unique among this group in their synthesis of PTH, which can be demonstrated immunohistochemically (Fig. 10.32)[90].

A variety of other neuropeptide hormones and amines has been documented in mediastinal neuroendocrine tumors. Thymic NECs may contain ACTH, enkephalins, endorphins, serotonin, calcitonin, gastrin, cholecystokinin, somatostatin, and neurotensin[91,92]. However, among those products, PG most reproducibly synthesize the enkephalins (Fig. 10.33)[93]. Parathyroid adenomas and parathyroid carcinomas typically lack all neuropeptides except for PTH. Fortunately, that peptide is seen immunohistochemically even in some clinically-non-functional lesions[37,90]. These markers have more than academic significance, because they may account for clinical paraneoplastic syndromes and provide a means of monitoring the response to treatment serologically.

Additional determinants are necessary in differential diagnosis with lesions that may be confused occasionally with

(a)

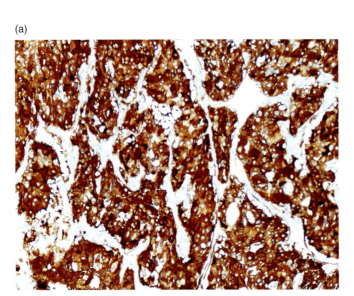

(b)

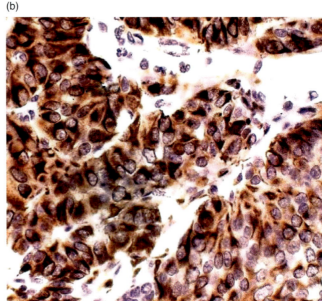

Fig. 10.30 Diffuse immunoreactivity is expected in paragangliomas for chromogranin-A **(a)** and neurofilament protein **(b)**.

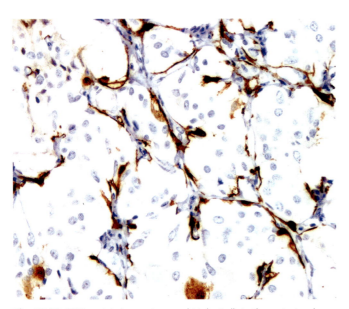

Fig. 10.31 S100 protein is seen immunohistologically in the sustentacular cells of many paragangliomas.

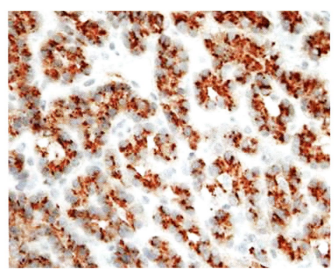

Fig. 10.32 Parathyroid hormone can be demonstrated immunohistochemically in almost all parathyroid lesions, regardless of whether or not they are clinically functional.

neuroendocrine tumors. The most valuable of those are leukocyte common antigen, CD30, OCT ¾, and placental alkaline phosphatase, which are present in lymphomas and/or germ cell tumors but not in neuroendocrine neoplasms [94].

Prognosis and therapy of mediastinal parathyroid and paraganglionic tumors

With the exception of parathyroid hyperplasias and adenomas, all neuroendocrine neoplasms of the mediastinum have the potential for aggressive behavior and should be considered malignant. Relatively few cases of primary mediastinal parathyroid carcinoma have been reported, and the behavioral attributes of that tumor type are therefore vaguely defined. However, many of them are lethal. The clinical course of mediastinal paragangliomas is principally predicated on their sites of origin. Paravertebral tumors rarely invade extensively or metastasize, whereas APPGs do so in a sizable number of cases [46–54]. A review by Olson and Salyer [59] showed that 53% of the latter neoplasms proved fatal, usually because of infiltrative growth and unresectability. Their juxtaposition to the thoracic great vessels largely accounted for surgical difficulties, and was associated with an operative mortality of 10%.

As a general rule, surgery is the mainstay of treatment for malignant mediastinal parathyroid and paraganglionic tumors.

(a)

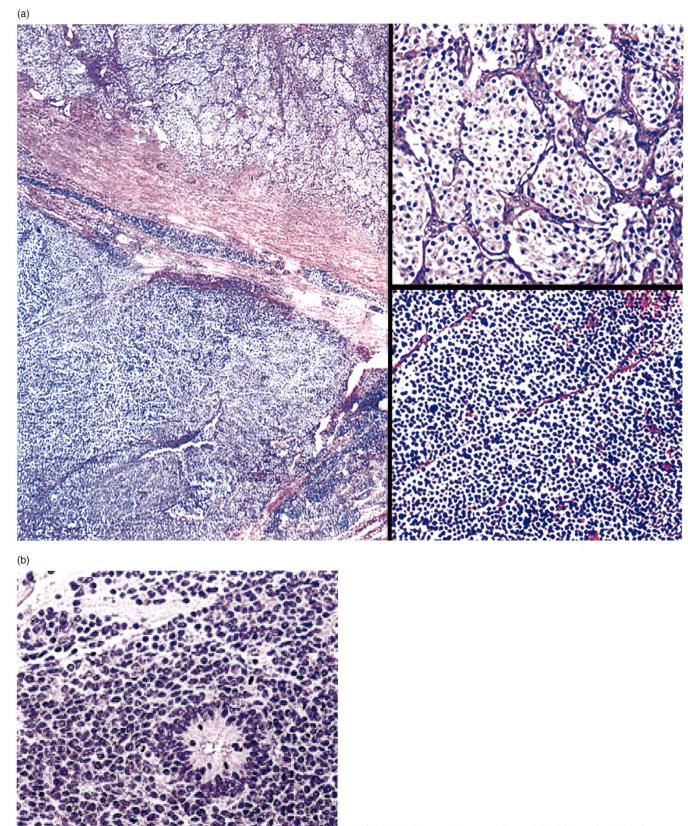

(b)

Fig. 10.26 "Composite" paragangliomas **(a)** exhibit an abrupt interface between conventional paraganglioma (top left and top right), and a neuroblastic component (bottom left). The neuroblastic elements may demonstrate formation of neural rosettes **(b)**.

mutations in the succinic dehydrogenase *SDHB* gene can cause the last of those syndromes, or, less frequently, early-onset renal cell carcinoma [79]. Paragangliomas related to *SDHB* mutations have a high rate of biological malignancy (in at least 35% of cases) [80], and commonly arise in an extra-adrenal location. Mutations in the *SDHB* gene that cause disease are observed in exons 1 through 7. Paraganglionic tumor formation comports with the "two hit" hypothesis. The first copy of the gene is mutated in all cells, but the second copy functions normally. When the latter also mutates in certain cells because of random subcellular events, a loss of heterozygosity obtains and functional *SDHB* protein is no longer produced, because the responsible gene is a tumor-suppressor. Neoplasia is then possible. Although succinic dehydrogenase is present throughout most tissues, it is not currently known why paraganglionic cells are principally affected by *SDHB* mutations. Adrenal neuroblastoma and composite extra-adrenal PG-NBs have also been reported in a few patients with this genetic aberration [80]. Some clinical overlap also exists between familial paragangliomatosis and the Cowden syndrome [81].

Ultrastructure of parathyroid and paraganglionic tumors

Because of the shared cellular attributes of neuroendocrine neoplasms, neuroendocrine carcinomas, parathyroid lesions, and paragangliomas of the mediastinum have basically similar electron microscopic features [33,45,82]. Tumor cells in such neoplasms are polygonal with limited numbers of blunt cytoplasmic extensions, and they are surrounded by a generally scanty intercellular collagenous matrix. Pericellular basal lamina is variable in its presence, and adjacent cells are connected by desmosomal or macula adherens-type attachment complexes. Nuclei are round to oval with evenly distributed heterochromatin and small nucleoli.

Aside from the usual metabolic organelles and neurosecretory granules, which are present in all mediastinal neuroendocrine tumors, other cytoplasmic constituents merit some consideration in separating them diagnostically. Thymic neuroendocrine carcinomas (NECs) often contain unusually abundant rough endoplasmic reticulum, which may be arranged in a concentric fashion ("Nebenkerns"). In addition, tumors associated with ACTH production may exhibit arrays of smooth endoplasmic reticulum as well. Apoptosis in CTT produces pseudolumina in the midst of cellular nests – a feature that is not common to the other tumors under discussion. Moreover, whorled intermediate filament aggregates are frequently present in a perinuclear location in NECs (Fig. 10.27) [33]; that finding is not observed in parathyroid or paraganglion cell tumors.

Parathyroid tumors may display the presence of true intercellular lumina, lined by blunt microvilli. In addition, they contain glycogen particles in much greater quantity than that seen in carcinoids or PGs [82]. Paragangliomas contain two distinct cell types, making them unique among the mediastinal lesions being considered here. The most prominent are the chief cells, containing numerous neurosecretory granules. They are grouped into the aforementioned Zellballen, and are surrounded by members of the second paragangliomatous constituent – the sustentacular cell population. The latter elements are fusiform and contain few organelles; in particular, neurosecretory granules are uniformly lacking in sustentacular cells [45].

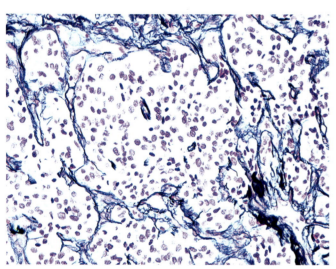

Fig. 10.24 Reticulin stains clearly delineate the boundaries of the cellular nests in paragangliomas.

(a)

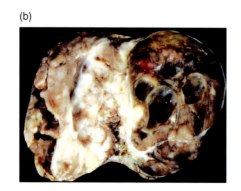

(b)

Fig. 10.25 "Composite" paragangliomas, as shown here in the anterosuperior mediastinum in a chest film (**a**), are more heterogeneous macroscopically than conventional paragangliomas (**b**). They contain paragangliomatous tissue that is juxtaposed to primitive neuroblastic elements.

(a)

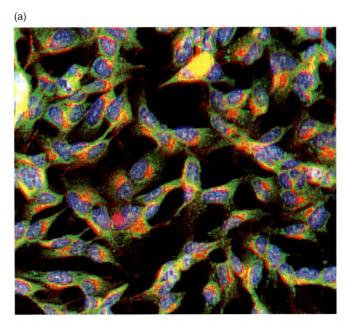

(b)

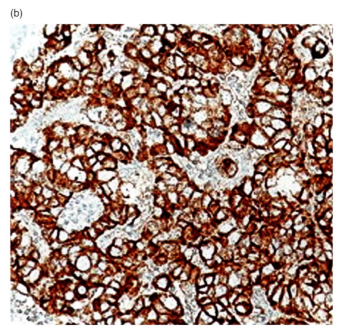

Fig. 10.33 Met- and leu- enkephalins **(a and b)** are often detectable immunohistologically in paragangliomas.

The effects on those lesions of radiotherapy and chemotherapy have been uncertain or unrewarding [95].

Intramediastinal thyroid neoplasms

Intramediastinal goiters are not uncommon, but they usually represent direct extensions of large eutopic glands. More rarely, hyperplasias and neoplasias of the thyroid may be observed in the thorax in patients without cervical disease [96-99]. For the sake of simplicity, we shall confine our comments on these disorders to neoplastic conditions. Primary thyroid carcinomas of the mediastinum are rare, with comparatively few cases having been documented [100-104]. Indeed, one should assume that such tumors are metastatic from a cervical source until proven otherwise.

Mediastinal thyroid adenomas or carcinomas are nearly always located in the anterior compartment, and they typically affect adult patients. Effects of compression of adjacent organs – such as dyspnea, wheezing, chest pain, or cough – are characteristic of intrathoracic thyroid carcinomas. In contrast, many benign neoplasms are discovered incidentally in thoracic radiographs [100].

Chest films show the presence of a dense, variably circumscribed, lobulated mass (Fig. 10.34) that may be partially cystic. CT scans done with contrast material often reveal enhancement of the lesion, as also may be seen with angiograms [65]. Thyroid adenomas of the mediastinum are usually well demarcated from surrounding tissues, whereas carcinomas often invade the lungs, pericardium, or great vessels (Fig. 10.35).

Gross examination of thyroid adenomas and carcinomas in the thorax shows features that are identical to those of corresponding lesions in cervical thyroid glands. Papillary, follicular, and medullary lesions are possible in both sites. However, no

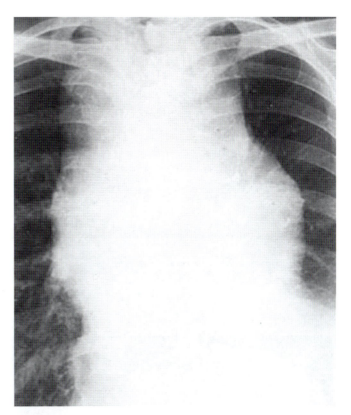

Fig. 10.34 Anterior mediastinal goiters produce widening of that compartment with projection into the lung fields, as shown in this chest film.

well-documented example of primary anaplastic thyroid carcinoma has yet been documented in the mediastinum. Papillary and follicular carcinomas both produce nondescript white-gray masses in the thyroid parenchyma, which efface variable proportions of the gland (Fig. 10.36). On the other

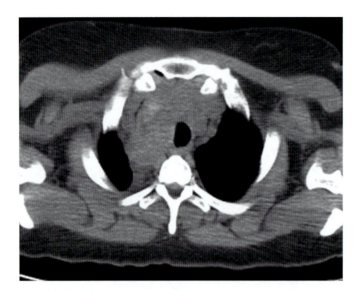

Fig. 10.35 Ectopic thyroid carcinomas in the mediastinum commonly demonstrate invasion of the great vessels and other regional structures, as shown in this computed tomogram.

(a)

(b)

(c)

(d)

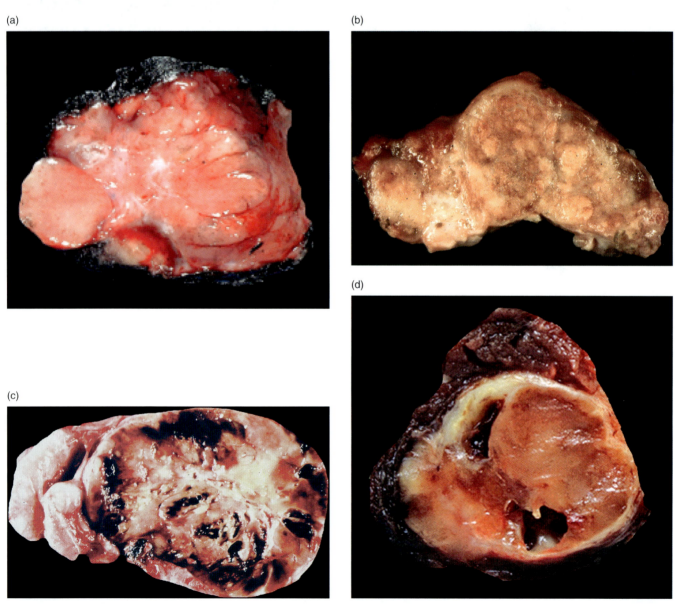

Fig. 10.36 Papillary carcinomas **(a and b)** and follicular carcinomas **(c and d)** produce variable effacement of mediastinal thyroid glands on gross examination.

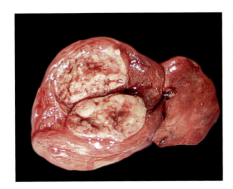

Fig. 10.37 Ectopic medullary thyroid carcinoma in the mediastinum has a yellowish, fleshy cut surface.

hand, medullary carcinoma tends to have a yellowish cut surface (Fig. 10.37), and may be multifocal in syndromic cases.

Microscopically, mediastinal thyroid adenomas are circumscribed tumors that lack evidence of vascular or capsular invasion, just as in eutopic glands. Hence, thorough examination of the lesional boundaries and supporting stroma is essential. These neoplasms may have a macrofollicular, microfollicular, or "fetal" histologic configuration. Multinodular thyroid hyperplasia is similar microscopically, but comprises several intrathyroidal nodules instead of only one (Fig. 10.38) [102].

Papillary carcinomas (PCs) in mediastinal thyroid glands may show classical-papillary, follicular-variant, or tall-cell/columnar configurations histologically (Figs. 10.39 and 10.40) [102,103,104–106].

(a)

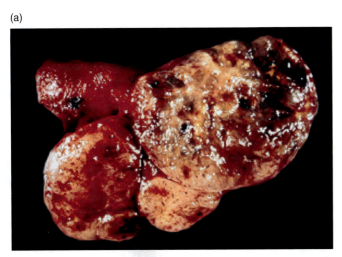

(b)

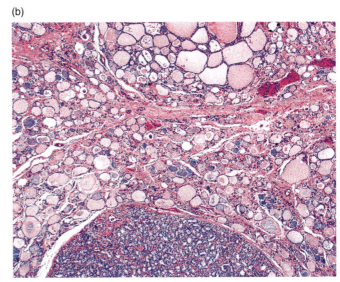

Fig. 10.38 Nodular thyroid hyperplasia in mediastinal thyroid glands is manifest by multinodular distortion of the gland **(a)**. Microscopically, one can see portions of several hyperplastic nodules juxtaposed to one another at scanning power **(b)**.

(a)

(b)

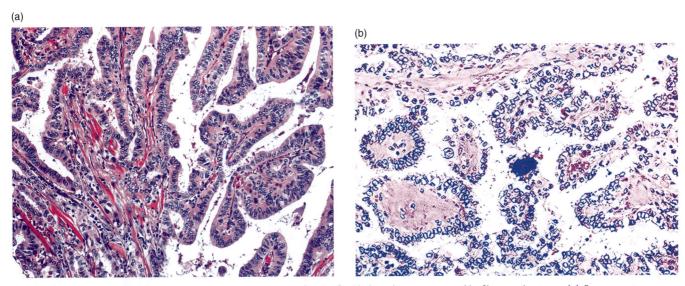

Fig. 10.39 Classical papillary thyroid carcinoma comprises numerous fronds of epithelium that are supported by fibrovascular stroma **(a)**. Psammomatous microcalcification is common **(b)**.

(a)

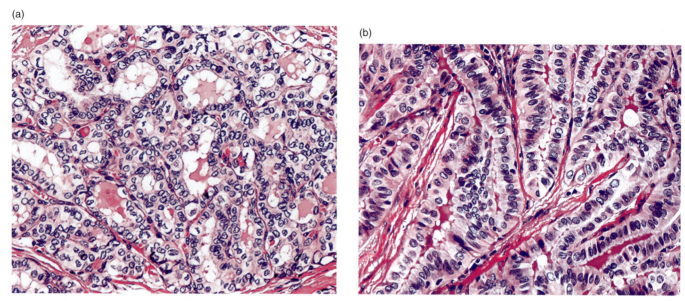

Fig. 10.40 In the follicular variant of papillary thyroid carcinoma, irregularly-shaped cellular microacinae (a) or elongated, tubular epithelial profiles (b) are present.

(b)

(a)

(c)

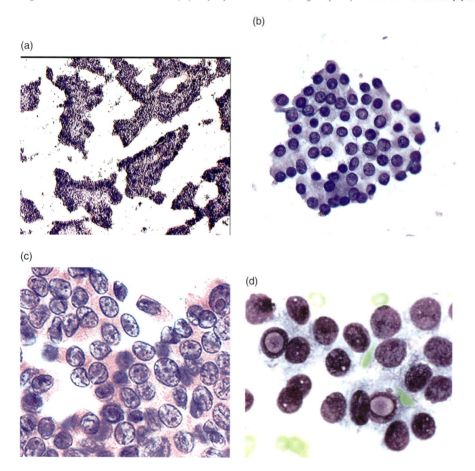

Fig. 10.41 Fine needle aspiration biopsy specimens from papillary carcinoma may show obvious papillae (a) and groups of uniform polygonal cells with nuclear folds, grooves, or cytoplasmic pseudoinclusions (b–d).

(d)

In both tissue sections and fine needle aspirates, the first two of those subtypes are typified by folds and grooves in the nuclear membranes, or intranuclear pseudoinclusions of cytoplasm (Fig. 10.41). Tall-cell/columnar tumors have higher nucleocytoplasmic ratios and a larger cell size, yielding a vaguely-enteric microscopic image (Fig. 10.42). The latter lesions have more aggressive biological potential than other forms of PC do [106].

As mentioned above, follicular carcinomas (FCs) are distinguished from adenomas by showing capsular invasion, vascular permeation, or both (Figs. 10.43 and 10.44) [102,104,107]. They lack the

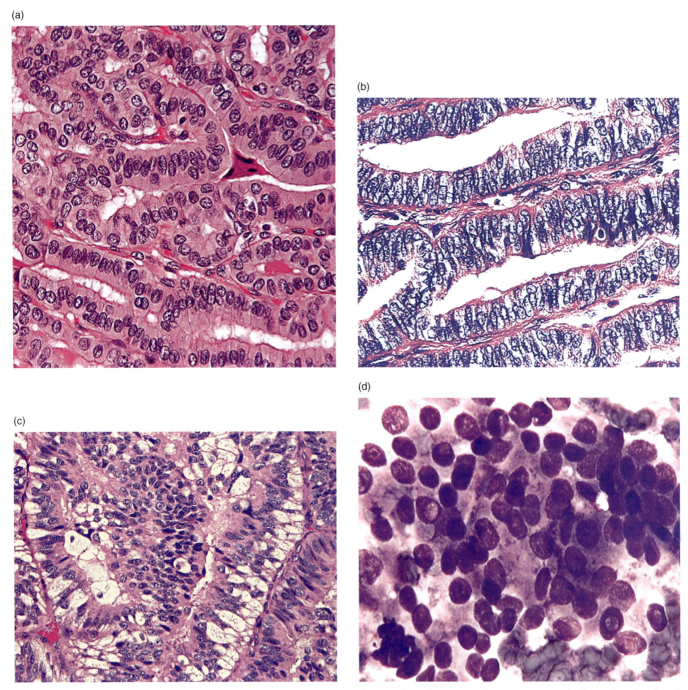

Fig. 10.42 The tall-cell variant of papillary thyroid carcinoma (PTC) comprises cells that are at least three times as long as they are wide. The resulting histological appearance is vaguely enteric **(a and b)**. Columnar-cell papillary carcinoma is similar, except that cytoplasmic vacuolization is common **(c)**. In fine needle aspiration biopsies, both of these histologic variants of PTC exhibit larger cells than those seen in conventional papillary carcinomas **(d)**.

nuclear features of PC. Accordingly, the morphologic findings in fine needle aspirates of FCs cannot be reliably distinguished from those of nodular hyperplasia or follicular adenoma [108]. A rare, poorly-differentiated variant of FC that has been described in cervical thyroids – "insular" carcinoma [109] – has not been reported in the mediastinum to date, but oncocytic ("Hurthle-cell") FC is potentially seen in the thorax (Fig. 10.45) [110]. It is typified by large cells with prominent nucleoli and brightly-eosinophilic cytoplasm in cytological or histologic preparations [108].

Medullary carcinomas (MCs) manifest an organoid growth pattern, like other neuroendocrine tumors. Constituent cells may have an oncocytoid, plasmacytoid, or fusiform configuration; their nuclear chromatin is evenly-dispersed and nuclear pleomorphism is modest (Fig. 10.46) [104,111]. Tumors in MEN 2 patients are usually multiple, and they are also associated with multifocal C-cell hyperplasia in the remainder of the thyroid gland [111]. Deposits of amyloid – which can be labeled with the crystal-violet or Congo-red methods (Fig. 10.47) – are seen in

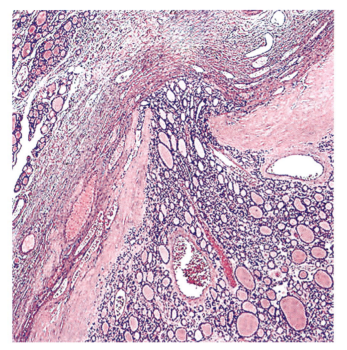

Fig. 10.43 Follicular carcinomas of the thyroid commonly show invasion of their fibrous capsules, with a "mushroom" configuration.

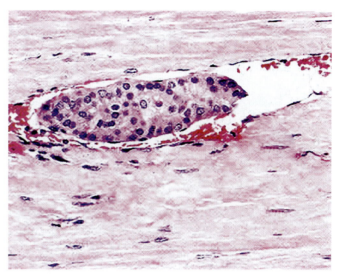

Fig. 10.44 Vascular invasion is also possible in follicular thyroid carcinoma.

(a)

(b)

(c)

(d)

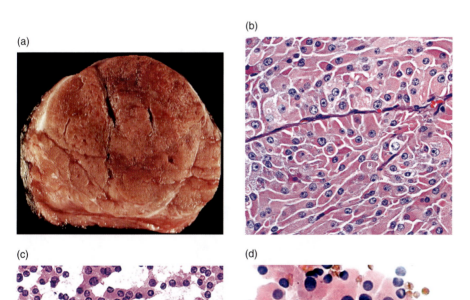

Fig. 10.45 Hurthle-cell (oncocytic) follicular thyroid carcinoma has a brownish cut surface macroscopically **(a)**. Histologically **(b)** and cytologically **(c and d)**, this tumor is constituted by large polygonal cells with prominent nucleoli and relatively-abundant, granular, eosinophilic cytoplasm.

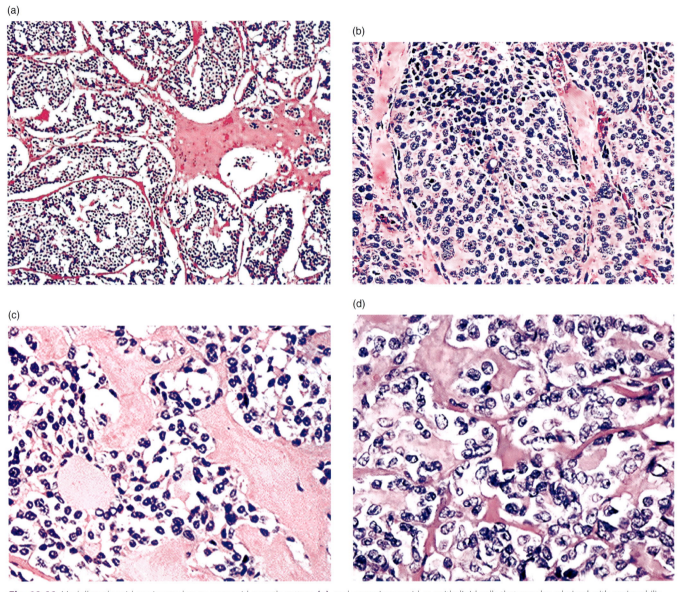

Fig. 10.46 Medullary thyroid carcinoma has an organoid growth pattern **(a)**, and comprises ovoid or epithelioid cells that may be admixed with eosinophilic deposits of amyloid **(b–d)**.

over 50% of MCs. These tumors are also argyrophilic. In fine needle aspirates, only loose cohesion of MC tumor cells is often seen (Fig. 10.48).

Electron microscopic examination of MCs is useful in demonstrating the presence of cytoplasmic neurosecretory granules [109]. Those organelles are not seen in PC or FC. Immunohistologically, MC is reactive for pankeratin, and potentially also for CD56, CD57, chromogranin-A, and synaptophysin [112,113]. Carcinoembryonic antigen (CEA) is consistently present in such lesions as well (Fig. 10.49); that is a useful finding in differential diagnosis with other forms of thyroid carcinoma, because both PC and FC lack CEA. Although the majority of MCs can be labeled for calcitonin (Fig. 10.50), a small number of cases lack that neuropeptide immunohistochemically. Chernyavsky et al. [114] have suggested

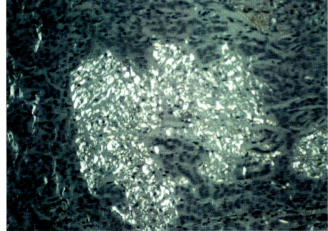

Fig. 10.47 Polarized Congo-red stains of the amyloid in medullary thyroid carcinoma show an "apple-green" birefringent image, as shown here.

(a)

(b)

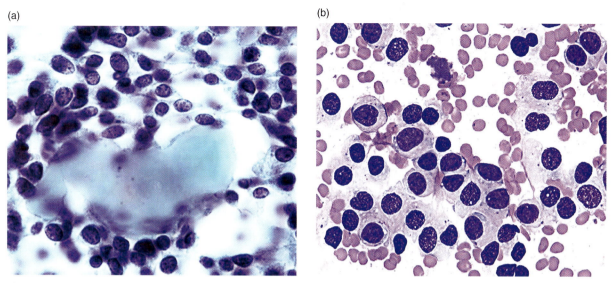

Fig. 10.48 Ovoid or plasmacytoid tumor cells in medullary thyroid carcinoma may be admixed with amyloid **(a)** or seen in loosely-cohesive groups **(b)**.

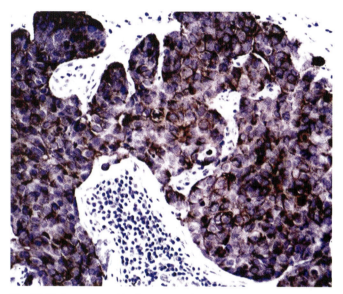

Fig. 10.49 Immunoreactivity for carcinoembryonic antigen is present in virtually all medullary thyroid carcinomas.

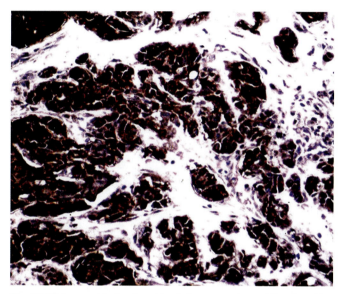

Fig. 10.50 Immunolabeling for calcitonin is common in medullary thyroid carcinoma, but not ubiquitous.

(a)

(b)

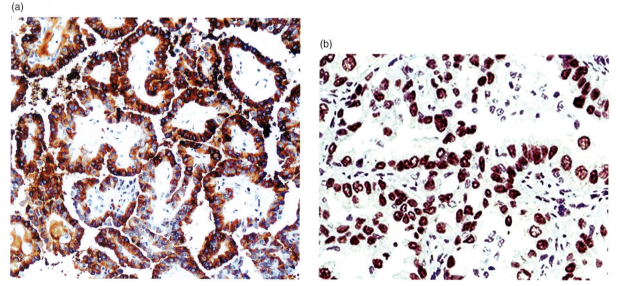

Fig. 10.51 Immunoreactivity for thyroglobulin **(a)** and thyroid transcription factor-1 **(b)** is common to both papillary and follicular thyroid carcinoma variants. In combination, these markers can be valuable in differential diagnosis.

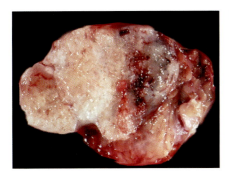

Fig. 10.52 Gross specimens of mediastinal pleomorphic adenoma contain fleshy tan or white-blue firm tissues, as shown in admixture here.

that those lesions should be distinguished diagnostically from MC, but we see little reason to do so.

Immunohistochemical studies are likewise helpful in distinguishing thyroid tumors from large parathyroid adenomas, and in separating primary papillary or follicular thyroid malignancies from metastatic carcinomas of non-thyroidal origins. Among those diagnostic possibilities, only thyroid proliferations are capable of expressing thyroglobulin and thyroid transcription factor-1 (Fig. 10.51), making those markers particularly valuable in this setting [112,113].

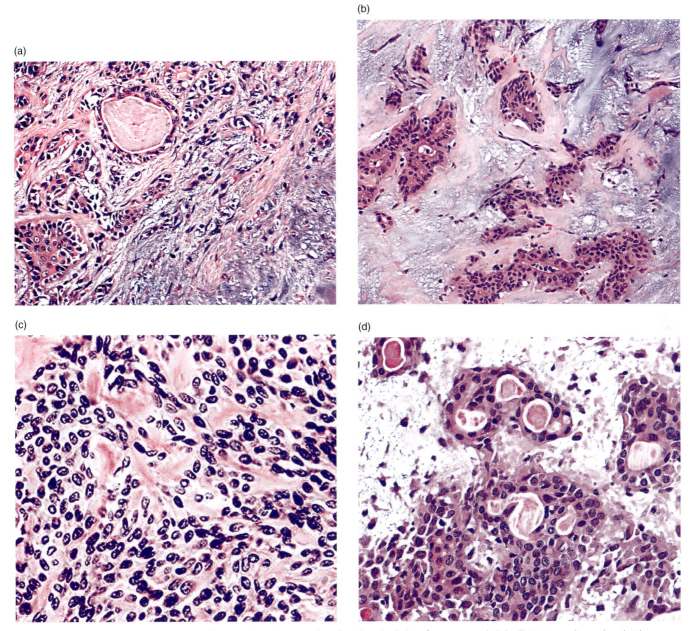

Fig. 10.53 A common microscopic image in pleomorphic adenoma is that of cords and tubules of compact epithelial cells, juxtaposed to a chondroid stroma **(a and b)**. Epithelial-predominant tumors may instead show solid clusters **(c)** or tubular epithelial formations **(d)**, with comparatively little mesenchymal-like stroma.

(a)

(b)

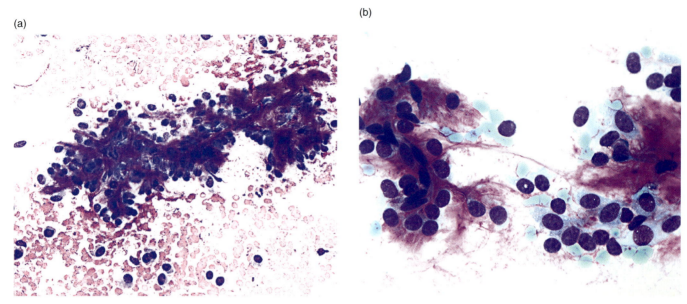

Fig. 10.54 Fine needle aspiration biopsies of pleomorphic adenoma often demonstrate groups of compact, relatively bland epithelial cells, adhering to bright pink stromal material **(a and b)**.

(a)

(b)

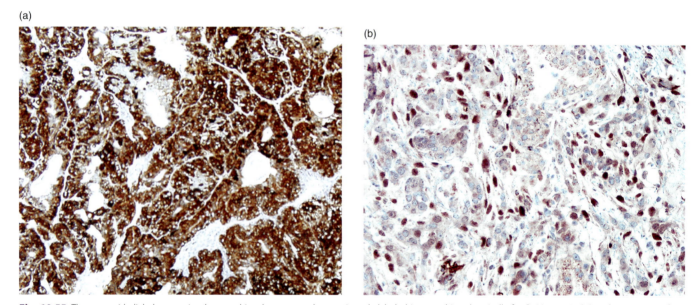

Fig. 10.55 The myoepithelial elements in pleomorphic adenoma can be consistently labeled immunohistochemically for S100 protein **(a)** and p63 protein **(b)**.

Surgical removal of benign mediastinal thyroid lesions is curative. However, no meaningful published data are available on the results of systematic operative approaches to primary intrathoracic thyroid carcinomas. In light of the overall rarity of such tumors, relative survival statistics on them are undocumented at this time.

Pleomorphic adenoma of the mediastinum

Rare examples have been reported of primary intramediastinal pleomorphic adenoma (PA [also known as "mixed tumor"]) in adults [115]. Just as uncommonly, metastasis to the thorax from ordinary PA of the salivary glands also has been described [116,117]. With respect to primary mediastinal tumors

of this type, the precise organ-site of origin is unclear. PA could conceivably arise in the thymus – which can harbor another salivary gland-type tumor (mucoepidermoid carcinoma) – or it could derive from ectopic salivary glandular tissue in other parts of the thorax [115].

Radiographically, there are few if any findings that would allow for a specific diagnosis of mediastinal PA. It is generically expected to present as a lobulated mass of variable density, which may project into either hemithorax.

Grossly, PAs may be fleshy and tan-pink, soft and yellow, or firm and blue-white (Fig. 10.52), depending on the proportions of such constituent tissues as epithelium, fat, fibrous stroma, and cartilaginous matrix. Internal lobulation may be apparent as well.

The microscopic appearances of PA are many, lending support to the use of the term "mixed tumor" in describing them. Generally speaking, these tumors show an admixture of obvious epithelial islands – often containing luminal spaces – with mesenchymal-like tissues resembling muscle, fat, cartilage, or even bone (Fig. 10.53) [118–120]. The neoplastic cells in all of those potential elements are cytologically-bland, and transitions between them can be seen microscopically. In fine needle aspiration biopsies of PAs, one often sees bright pink stromal tissue that is associated with groups of compact epithelial cells with bland nuclei (Fig. 10.54) [121–123].

Immunohistochemical studies show reactivity for pankeratin, potentially in all of the components of PAs. Most tumors are also labeled for S100 protein and p63 protein (Fig. 10.55), as well as vimentin. Alpha-isoform ("smooth-muscle") actin and glial fibrillary acidic protein are present as well in over 50% of cases [124,125]. These determinants are principally used in identifying epithelial-predominant PAs, which conceivably could be confused with other neoplasms histologically.

The behavior of primary mediastinal PA is uncertain, because of the rarity of reported cases.

References

1. Langman J: *Medical Embryology*. Baltimore, MD, Williams & Wilkins, 1969, pp. 245–6.

2. van der Walt J: Pathology of the parathyroid glands. *Diagn Histopathol* 2012; 18: 221–33.

3. Schulte K-M, Roher H-D: History of thyroid and parathyroid surgery, *In*: Oertli D, Udelsman R (eds): *Surgery of the Thyroid & Parathyroid Glands*. Springer, Berlin, 2012; pp. 1–14.

4. Williams ED: Pathology of the parathyroid glands. *Clin Endocrinol Metab* 1974; 3: 285–303.

5. Nathaniels EK, Nathaniels AM, Wang CA: Mediastinal parathyroid tumors: A clinical and pathological study of 84 cases. *Ann Surg* 1970; 171: 165–70.

6. Van Heerden JA, Beahrs OH, Woolner LB: The pathology and surgical management of primary hyperparathyroidism. *Surg Clin North Am* 1977; 57: 557–63.

7. Wang CA, Gaz RD, Moncure AC: Mediastinal parathyroid exploration: A clinical and pathologic study of 47 cases. *World J Surg* 1986; 10: 687–95.

8. Russell CF, Edis AI, Scholz DA: Mediastinal parathyroid tumors: Experience with 38 tumors requiring median sternotomy for removal. *Ann Surg* 1981; 193: 805–9.

9. Massac E, Righini M, Seremetis M: Mediastinal hyperfunctioning parathyroid adenoma. *J Natl Med Assoc* 1982; 74: 385–7.

10. Kay S: Primary hyperparathyroidism as observed over a 22 year period. *Arch Pathol* 1973; 95: 256–9.

11. Huang J, Soskos A, Murad SM, Krawisz BR, Yale SH, Urquhart AC: Spontaneous hemorrhage of a parathyroid adenoma into the mediastinum. *Endocr Pract* 2012; 18: e57–e60.

12. Romei C, Pardi E, Cetani F, Elisei R: Genetic and clinical features of multiple endocrine neoplasia types 1 and 2. *J Oncol* 2012; 2012: 705036 (e-publication).

13. Gulati AP, Krantz B, Moss RA, *et al.*: Treatment of multiple endocrine neoplasia 1/2 tumors: case report and review of the literature. *Oncology* 2013; 84: 127–34.

14. Carroll RW: Multiple endocrine neoplasia type 1 (MEN1): *Asia Pac J Clin Oncol* 2012; December 26 (e-publication).

15. Gaztambide S, Vazquez F, Castano L: Diagnosis and treatment of multiple endocrine neoplasia type 1 (MEN1). *Minerva Endocrinol* 2013; 38: 17–28.

16. Schnyder P, Garnsu G: Computed tomography and magnetic resonance imaging, *In*: Givel J-C (ed): *Surgery of the Thymus*. Berlin, Germany, Springer-Verlag, 1990, pp. 217–25.

17. Phillips CD, Shatzkes DR: Imaging of the parathyroid glands. *Semin Ultrasound CT MR* 2012; 33: 123–9.

18. Peshev ZV, Borisov BB, Genova SN, Danev VH: Parathyroid carcinoma of the mediastinum. *Folia Med* 2012; 54: 80–3.

19. Gawrychowski J, Gabriel A, Kluczewska E, Bula G, Lackowska B: Mediastinial parathyroid carcinoma: a case report. *Endokrynol Pol* 2012; 63: 143–6.

20. Meng Z, Li D, Zhang Y, Zhang P, Tan J: Ectopic parathyroid carcinoma presenting with hypercalcemic crisis, ectopic uptake in bone scan, and obstruction of superior vena cava. *Clin Nucl Med* 2011; 36: 487–90.

21. Nakamura Y, Kataoka H, Sakoda T, Horie Y, Kitano H: Nonfunctional parathyroid carcinoma. *Int J Clin Oncol* 2010; 15: 500–3.

22. Talat N, Schulte KM: Clinical presentation, staging, and long-term evolution of parathyroid cancer. *Ann Surg Oncol* 2010; 17: 2156–74.

23. Vazquez FJ, Aparicio LS, Gallo CG, Diehl M: Parathyroid carcinoma presenting as a giant mediastinal retrotracheal functioning cyst. *Singapore Med J* 2007; 48: e304–e307.

24. Moran CA, Suster S: Primary parathyroid tumors of the mediastinum: a clinicopathologic and immunohistochemical study of 17 cases. *Am J Clin Pathol* 2005; 124: 749–54.

25. Avramides A, Papamargaritis K, Antoniadis A, Gakis D, Leontsini M: Large parathyroid functioning carcinoma (1200 g) presenting as a substernal goiter. *J Endocrinol Invest* 1992; 15: 39–42.

26. Snover DC, Foucar K: Mitotic activity in benign parathyroid disease. *Am J Clin Pathol* 1981; 75: 345–7.

27. Lawrence DAS: A histological comparison of adenoma to hyperplastic parathyroid glands. *J Clin Pathol* 1978; 31: 626–32.

28. Wolff M, Goodman EN: Functioning lipoadenoma of a supernumerary parathyroid gland in the mediastinum. *Head Neck Surg* 1980; 2: 302–7.

29. Fallone E, Bourne PA, Watson TJ, Ghossein RA, Travis WD, Xu H: Ectopic (mediastinal) parathyroid adenoma with prominent lymphocytic infiltration. *Appl Immunohistochem Mol Morphol* 2009; 17: 82–4.

30. Elgoweini M, Chetty R: Hyalinizing parathyroid adenoma and hyperplasia: report of 3 cases of an unusual histologic variant. *Ann Diagn Pathol* 2011; 15: 329–32.

31. Rosai J, Higa E: Mediastinal endocrine neoplasm of probable thymic origin, related to carcinoid tumor: Clinicopathologic study of eight cases. *Cancer* 1972; 29: 1061–74.

32. Rosai J, Levine G, Weber WR, *et al.*: Carcinoid tumors and oat-cell carcinomas of the thymus. *Pathol Annu* 1976; 11: 201–26.

33. Wick MR, Rosai J: Neuroendocrine neoplasms of the thymus. *Pathol Res Pract* 1988; 183: 188–99.

34. Snover DC, Levine GD, Rosai J: Thymic carcinoma: five distinctive histological variants. *Am J Surg Pathol* 1982; 6: 451–70.

35. Nappi O, Mills SE, Swanson PE, Wick MR: Clear cell tumors of unknown nature and origin: a systematic approach to diagnosis. *Semin Diagn Pathol* 1997; 14: 164–74.

36. Nappi O, Ferrara G, Wick MR: Neoplasms composed of eosinophilic polygonal cells: an overview with consideration of different cytomorphologic patterns. *Semin Diagn Pathol* 1999; 16: 82–90.

37. Murphy MN, Glennon PG, Diocee MS, *et al.*: Nonsecretory parathyroid carcinoma of the mediastinum. *Cancer* 1986; 58: 2468–76.

38. Derreberry T, Yaqub A: Parathyroid FNA and hormone assay. *WV Med J* 2009; 105: 30–4.

39. Lieu D: Cytopathologist-performed ultrasound-guided fine-needle aspiration of parathyroid lesions. *Diagn Cytopathol* 2010; 38: 327–32.

40. Knezevic-Obad A, Tomic-Brzac H, Zarkovic K, Dodig D, Stromar IK: Diagnostic pitfalls in parathyroid gland cytology. *Coll Antropol* 2010; 34: 25–9.

41. Papanicolau-Sengos A, Brumund K, Lin G, Hasteh F: Cytologic findings of a clear cell parathyroid lesion. *Diagn Cytopathol* 2011; December 5 (e-publication).

42. Noussios G, Anagnostis P, Natsis K: Ectopic parathyroid glands and their anatomical, clinical, and surgical implications. *Exp Clin Endocrinol Diabetes* 2012; 120: 604–10.

43. DeLellis RA: Parathyroid carcinoma: an overview. *Adv Anat Pathol* 2005; 12: 53–61.

44. DeLellis RA: Challenging lesions in the differential diagnosis of endocrine tumors: parathyroid carcinoma. *Endocr Pathol* 2008; 19: 221–5.

45. Glenner GG, Grimley PM: Tumors of the extra-adrenal paraganglion system (including chemoreceptors), *In: Atlas of Tumor Pathology, Second Series, Fascicle 9*. Washington, DC, Armed Forces Institute of Pathology, 1974.

46. Wald O, Shapira OM, Murar A, Izhar U: Paraganglioma of the mediastinum: challenges in diagnosis and surgical management. *J Cardiothor Surg* 2010; 5: 19.

47. Lin MW, Chang YL, Lee YC, Huang PM: Non-functional paraganglioma of the posterior mediastinum. *Interact Cardiovasc Thorac Surg* 2009; 9: 540–2.

48. Paul S, Jain SH, Gallegos RP, Aranki SF, Bueno R: Functional paraganglioma of the middle mediastinum. *Ann Thorac Surg* 2007; 83: e14–e16.

49. Ramos R, Moya J, Villalonga R, Morera R, Ferrer G: Mediastinal aortosympathetic paraganglioma: report of two cases. *Asian Cardiovasc Thorac Ann* 2007; 15: e49–e51.

50. Young WF Jr: Paragangliomas: clinical overview. *Ann NY Acad Sci* 2006; 1073: 21–9.

51. Spector JA, Willis DN, Ginsburg HB: Paraganglioma (pheochromocytoma) of the posterior mediastinum: a case report and review of the literature. *J Pediatr Surg* 2003; 38: 1114–16.

52. Andrade CF, Camargo SM, Zanchet M, Felicetti JC, Cardoso PF: Nonfunctioning paraganglioma of the aortopulmonary window. *Ann Thorac Surg* 2003; 75: 1950–1.

53. Isobe T, Oguri T, Yamasaki M, *et al.*: Malignant paraganglioma arising from the posterior mediastinum: a case report and review of the literature. *Hiroshima J Med Sci* 1999; 48: 123–7.

54. Moran CA, Suster S, Fishback N, Koss MN: Mediastinal paragangliomas: a clinicopathologic and immunohistochemical study of 16 cases. *Cancer* 1993; 72: 2358–64.

55. Miller JW: Ein paragangliom des Brustsympathicus. *Zentr Allg Pathol Pathol Anat* 1924; 35: 85–100.

56. Philips B: Intrathoracic pheochromocytoma. *Arch Pathol* 1940; 30: 916–28.

57. Bloom F: Structure and histogenesis of tumors of the aortic bodies in dogs; with a consideration of the morphology of the aortic and carotid bodies. *Arch Pathol* 1943; 36: 1–12.

58. Lattes R: Nonchromaffin paragangliomas of ganglion nodosum, carotid body, and aortic-arch bodies. *Cancer* 1950; 3: 667–94.

59. Olson JL, Salyer WR: Mediastinal paraganglioma (aortic body tumor): A report of four cases and a review of the literature. *Cancer* 1978; 41: 2405–12.

60. Rosai J, Mettler EA: Quimiodectoma de mediastino. *Rev Assoc Med Arg* 1965; 79: 242–6.

61. Lack EE, Stillinger R, Colvin R, *et al.*: Aortico-pulmonary paraganglioma. *Cancer* 1979; 43: 269–78.

62. Odze R, Begin LR: Malignant paraganglioma of the posterior mediastinum. *Cancer* 1990; 65: 564–9.

63. Gallivan MVE, Chun B, Rowden G, *et al.*: Intrathoracic paravertebral malignant paraganglioma. *Arch Pathol Lab Med* 1980; 104: 46–51.

64. Carney JA: The triad of gastric epithelioid leiomyosarcoma, pulmonary chondroma, and functioning extra-adrenal paraganglioma: A five-year review. *Medicine* 1983; 62: 159–69.

65. Spizarny Dl., Rebner M, Gross BH: CT evaluation of enhancing mediastinal masses. *J Comput Assist Tomogr* 1987; 11: 990–3.

66. Ortega PF, Sosa LA, Patel M, Zambrano E: Cystic paraganglioma of the anterior mediastinum. *Ann Diagn Pathol* 2010; 14: 341–6.

67. Capella C, Riva C, Cornaggia M, *et al.*: Histopathology, cytology, and cytochemistry of pheochromocytomas and paragangliomas including chemodectomas. *Pathol Res Pract* 1988; 183: 176–87.

68. Plaza JA, Wakely PE Jr, Moran CA, Fletcher CDM, Suster S: Sclerosing paraganglioma: report of 19 cases of an unusual variant of neuroendocrine tumor that may be mistaken for an aggressive malignant neoplasm. *Am J Surg Pathol* 2006; 30: 7–12.

69. Weinrach DM, Wang KL, Blum MG, Yeldandi AV, Laskin WB: Multifocal presentation of gangliocytic paraganglioma in the mediastinum and esophagus. *Hum Pathol* 2004; 35: 1288–91.

70. Hofmann WJ, Wockel W, Thetter O, Otto HF: Melanotic paraganglioma of

the posterior mediastinum. *Virchows Arch* 1995; 425: 641–6.

71. Wakely PE Jr: Cytopathology-histopathology of the mediastinum. II. Mesenchymal, neural, and neuroendocrine neoplasms. *Ann Diagn Pathol* 2005; 9: 24–32.

72. Varma K, Jain S, Mandal S: Cytomorphologic spectrum in paraganglioma. *Acta Cytol* 2008; 52: 549–56.

73. Brady S, Lechan RM, Schaitzberg SD, *et al.*: Composite pheochromocytoma/ganglioneuroma of the adrenal gland associated with multiple endocrine neoplasia 2A. *Am J Surg Pathol* 1997; 21: 102–8.

74. Lack EE: Pathology of adrenal and extra-adrenal paraganglia. *Major Probl Pathol* 1994; 29: 256–60.

75. Lam KY, Lo CY: Composite pheochromocytoma-ganglioneuroma of the adrenal gland: an uncommon entity with distinctive clinicopathologic features. *Endocr Pathol* 1999; 10: 343–52.

76. Linnoila RI, Keiser HR, Steinberg SM, Lack EE: Histopathology of benign versus malignant sympathoadrenal paragangliomas: clinicopathologic study of 120 cases including unusual histologic features. *Hum Pathol* 1990; 21: 1168–80.

77. Comstock JM, Willmore-Payne C, Holden JA, Coffin CM: Composite pheochromocytoma: a clinicopathologic and molecular comparison with ordinary pheochromocytoma and neuroblastoma. *Am J Clin Pathol* 2009; 132: 69–73.

78. Galazka P, Chrupek M, Kazmirczuk R, *et al.*: Paraganglioma associated with neuroblastoma: rare composite tumor in a 16-year-old girl. *Ann Diagn Paediatr Pathol* 2006; 10: 43–6.

79. Bayley JP, Devilee P, Taschner PE: The SDG mutation database: an online resource for succinate dehydrogenase sequence variants involved in pheochromocytoma, paraganglioma, and mitochondrial complex II deficiency. *BMC Med Genet* 2005; 6: 39.

80. Ghayee HK, Havekes B, Corssmit EP, *et al.*: Mediastinal paragangliomas: association with mutations in the succinate dehydrogenase genes and aggressive behavior. *Endocr Relat Cancer* 2009; 16: 291–9.

81. Ni Y, Zbuk KM, Sadler T, *et al.*: Germline mutations and variants in the succinate dehydrogenase genes in Cowden and Cowden-like syndromes. *Am J Hum Genet* 2008; 83: 261–8.

82. Capen CC, Roth SI: Ultrastructural and functional relationships of normal and pathologic parathyroid cells. *Pathol Annu Decennial* 1975; 10: 267–319.

83. Rode J, Dhillon AP, Doran JF, *et al.*: PGP 9.5, a new marker for human neuroendocrine tumors. *Histopathology* 1985; 9: 147–58.

84. Wick MR, Simpson RW, Niehans GA, *et al.*: Anterior mediastinal tumors: A clinicopathologic study of 100 cases, with emphasis on immunohistochemical analysis. *Prog Surg Pathol* 1990; 11: 79–119.

85. Wilson BS, Lloyd RV: Detection of chromogranin in neuroendocrine cells with a monoclonal antibody. *Am J Pathol* 1984; 115: 458–68.

86. Miettinen M: Synaptophysin and neurofilament protein as markers for neuroendocrine tumors. *Arch Pathol Lab Med* 1987; 111: 813–18.

87. Wick MR: Immunohistology of neuroendocrine and neuroectodermal tumors. *Semin Diagn Pathol* 2000; 17: 194–203.

88. Trojanowski JQ: Neurofilament and glial filament proteins, *In*: Wick MR, Siegal GP (eds): *Monoclonal Antibodies in Diagnostic Immunohistochemistry*. New York, NY, Marcel Dekker, 1988, pp 115–46.

89. Schroder HD, Johannsen L: Demonstration of S100 protein in sustentacular cells of phaeochromocytomas and paragangliomas. *Histopathology* 1986; 10: 1023–33.

90. Ordonez NG, Ibanez ML, Samaan NA, Hickey RC: Immunoperoxidase study of uncommon parathyroid tumors: report of two cases of nonfunctioning parathyroid carcinoma and one intrathyroid parathyroid tumor-producing amyloid. *Am J Surg Pathol* 1983; 7: 535–42.

91. Baker J, Holdaway IM, Jagusch M, *et al.*: Ectopic secretion of ACTH and met-enkephalin from a thymic carcinoid. *J Endocrinol Invest* 1982; 5: 33–8.

92. Pullan PT, Clement-Jones V, Corder R, *et al.*: Ectopic production of methionine-enkephalin and beta-endorphin. *Br Med J* 1980; 280: 758–9.

93. DeLellis RA, Tischler AS, Lee AK, *et al.*: Leu-enkephalin-like immunoreactivity in proliferative lesions of the human adrenal medulla and extra-adrenal paraganglia. *Am J Surg Pathol* 1983; 7: 29–37.

94. Wick MR: Immunohistochemical approaches to the diagnosis of undifferentiated malignant tumors. *Ann Diagn Pathol* 2008; 12: 72–84.

95. Patel SR, Winchester DJ, Benjamin RS: A 15-year experience with chemotherapy of patients with paraganglioma. *Cancer* 1995; 76: 1476–80.

96. Arriaga MA, Myers EN: Ectopic thyroid in the retroesophageal superior mediastinum. *Otolaryngol Head Neck Surg* 1988; 99: 338–40.

97. Zapatero J, Baamonde C, Gonzalez-Argoneses F, *et al.*: Ectopic goiters of the mediastinum: Presentation of two cases and review of the literature. *Jpn J Surg* 1988; 18: 105–9.

98. Dundas P: Intrathoracic aberrant goiter. *Acta Chir Scand* 1964; 128: 729–37.

99. Falor AW, Kelly TR, Jackson JB: Intrathoracic goiter. *Surg Gynecol Obstet* 1963; 117: 604–15.

100. Fish J, Moore RM: Ectopic thyroid tissue and ectopic thyroid carcinoma. *Ann Surg* 1963; 157: 212–22.

101. Wu Y, Wang J: Upper mediastinum invaded by thyroid gland carcinoma: a review of 24 patients. *Zhonghua Wai Ke Za Zhi [Chinese J Surg]* 1996; 34: 238–40.

102. Meissner WA, McManus RG: A comparison of the histologic pattern of benign and malignant thyroid tumors. *J Clin Endocrinol Metab* 1952; 12: 1474–9.

103. Niederle B, Roka R, Fritsch A: Transsternal operations in thyroid cancer. *Surgery* 1985; 98: 1154–61.

104. Woolner LB: Thyroid carcinoma: pathologic classification with data on prognosis. *Semin Nucl Med* 1971; 1: 481–502.

105. Carcangiu ML, Zampi G, Rosai J: Papillary thyroid carcinoma: a study of its many morphologic expressions and clinical correlates. *Pathol Annu* 1985; 20 (Part 1): 1–44.

106. Rosai J: Papillary carcinoma. *Monogr Pathol* 1993; 35: 138–65.

107. Nakashima T, Nakashima A, Murakami D, *et al.*: Follicular carcinoma of the thyroid with massive infiltration into the cervical and mediastinal great veins: our own experience and literature review. *Laryngoscope* 2012; 122: 2855–7.

108. Wang CC, Friedman L, Kennedy GC, *et al.*: A large multicenter correlation study of thyroid nodule cytopathology and histopathology. *Thyroid* 2011; 21: 243–51.

109. Rosai J: Poorly-differentiated thyroid carcinoma: introduction to the issue, its landmarks, and clinical impact. *Endocr Pathol* 2004; 293–6.

110. Tallini G, Carcangiu ML, Rosai J: Oncocytic neoplasms of the thyroid gland. *Acta Pathol Jpn* 1992; 42: 305–15.

111. DeLellis RA: The pathology of medullary thyroid carcinoma and its precursors. *Monogr Pathol* 1993; 35: 72–102.

112. Stanta G, Carcangiu ML, Rosai J: The biochemical and immuohistochemical profile of thyroid neoplasia. *Pathol Annu* 1988; 23(Part 1): 129–57.

113. Rosai J: Immunohistochemical markers of thyroid tumors: significance and diagnostic applications. *Tumori* 2003; 89: 517–19.

114. Chernyavsky VS, Farghani S, Davidov T, *et al.*: Calcitonin-negative neuroendocrine tumor of the thyroid: a distinct clinical entity. *Thyroid* 2011; 21: 193–6.

115. Fiegin GA, Robinson B, Marchevsky AM: Mixed tumor of the mediastinum. *Arch Pathol Lab Med* 1986; 110: 80–1.

116. Steele NP, Wenig BM, Sessions RB: A case of pleomorphic adenoma of the parotid gland metastasizing to a mediastinal lymph node. *Am J Otolaryngol* 2007; 28: 130–3.

117. Marioni G, Marino F, Stramare R, Marchese-Ragona R, Staffieri A. Benign metastasizing pleomorphic adenoma of the parotid gland: a clinicopathologic puzzle. *Head Neck* 2003; 25: 1071–6.

118. Spiro RH, Hajdu SI, Strong EW. Tumors of the submaxillary gland. *Am J Surg* 1976; 132: 463–8.

119. Batsakis JG, Brannon RB, Sciubba JJ. Monomorphic adenomas of major salivary glands: a histologic study of 96 tumors. *Clin Otolaryngol Allied Sci* 1981; 6: 129–43.

120. Haskell HD, Butt KM, Woo WB: Pleomorphic adenoma with extensive lipometaplasia: report of three cases. *Am J Surg Pathol* 2005; 29: 1389–93.

121. Viguer JM, Vicandi B, Jimenez-Heffernan JA, Lopez-Ferrer P, Limeres MA: Fine needle aspiration cytology of pleomorphic adenomoa: an analysis of 212 cases. *Acta Cytol* 1997; 41: 786–94.

122. Chen L, Ray N, He H, Hoschar A: Cytopathologic analysis of stroma-poor salivary gland epithelial/myoepithelial neoplasms on fine needle aspiration. *Acta Cytol* 2012; 56: 25–33.

123. Jo HJ, Ahn HJ, Jung S, Yoon HK: Diagnostic difficulties in fine needle aspiration of benign salivary glandular lesions. *Korean J Pathol* 2012; 46: 569–75.

124. Mori H, Tsukitani K, Ninomiya T, Okada Y: Various expressions of modified myoepithelial cells in salivary pleomorphic adenoma: immunohistochemical studies. *Pathol Res Pract* 1987; 182: 632–46.

125. Alos L, Cardesa A, Bombi JA, Mallofre C, Cuchi A, Traserra J: Myoepithelial tumors of salivary glands: a clinicopathologic, immunohistochemical, ultrastructural, and flow-cytometric study. *Semin Diagn Pathol* 1996; 13: 138–47.

Hematopoietic neoplasms of the mediastinum

Chapter

11

Serhan Alkan, MD

Lymphomas are one of the most common neoplasms encountered in the mediastinum [1]. From a pathologist perspective, when a hematopoietic neoplasm in the mediastinum is suspected, the key points for morphologic investigation are to determine the pattern of infiltrate (nodular versus diffuse), the presence of fibrosis, whether the infiltrate is monomorphic or polymorphic, the size of the cells (small vs intermediate to large size), the nuclear and nucleolar characteristics of the tumor cells, and the number of mitoses (see Fig. 11.1). Histologic evaluation typically starts with an assessment of the growth pattern of the lymphoid cells at a low-power magnification (20× or 40×). If there are nodules present, follicular lymphoma, mantle cell lymphoma, marginal zone lymphoma, and nodular lymphocyte predominance Hodgkin's lymphoma (NLPHL) are the main differential diagnostic entities to explore. If flow cytometric analysis of the lymphoid cells is available, one could easily discern a specific diagnosis of lymphoma with the exception of Hodgkin's lymphoma (HL) [2]. Lack of clonality by flow cytometry (polyclonal light chain expression) favors a reactive process but this impression needs to be correlated with the histologic features of the lesion before a lymphoid malignancy is excluded. Indeed, tissue evaluation is necessary in all lymphoid lesions since HL, including both NLPHL and classical (CHL), cannot be ruled out by flow cytometry. Both classical HL and NLPHL are neoplasms of B-cell; however, the neoplastic cells (Reed-Sternberg cells) are

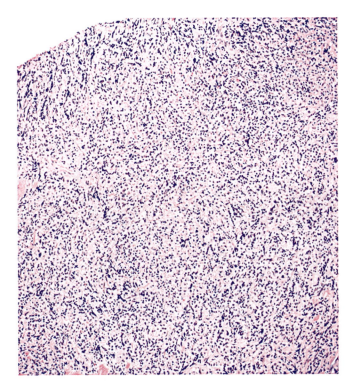 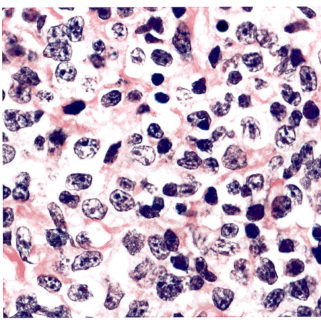

Fig. 11.1 Primary mediastinal large B-cell lymphoma. Low-power magnification (left) is showing marked sclerosis with intermixed lymphocytic infiltrate while high-power magnification illustrates the presence of large cells with ovoid to round nuclei and prominent 1–3 nucleoli and a moderate amount of cytoplasm; fine sclerosis is also noticeable.

Pathology of the Mediastinum, ed. Alberto M. Marchevsky and Mark R. Wick. Published by Cambridge University Press.
© Cambridge University Press 2014.

very rare to analyze by flow cytometry. Although sensitive flow cytometric analysis for diagnosis of HL has been reported, this is still not practical and tissue examination is necessary for the diagnosis of HL. Furthermore, intermediate- to high-grade B-cell lymphomas may also lack surface immunoglobulin light chain expression and require microscopic evaluation [2,3].

Flow cytometric assessment not only aids in diagnosis of lymphoma but it also helps subtyping of low-grade B-cell lymphoproliferative disorders [1,4]. Presence of CD5 is typically seen in small lymphocytic lymphoma (SLL)/chronic lymphocytic leukemia (CLL) and mantle cell lymphoma (MCL), while CD10 is usually (up to 85%) encountered in follicular lymphomas. Although rare, exceptions occur. For example, CD5 may be rarely encountered in marginal zone lymphoma and mantle cell lymphoma may rarely lack expression of CD5 [5]. If CD5 positivity is noted, then CD23 positivity and FMC7 negativity primarily favors SLL/CLL. MCL usually show the opposite findings (CD23: negative, FMC7: positive). Lack of CD5 and CD10 by small-size B-cell lymphoma raises a suspicion of marginal zone lymphoma. However, very frequently pathologists may not have fresh tissue for flow cytometric analysis and may be forced to rely solely on the microscopic analysis of tissue and immunohistochemical markers. Tissue examination is always essential since there may be discrepancy between phenotypic findings and histology [6]. The majority of markers mentioned above for identification of subtype of low-grade B-cell lymphomas can also be studied by immunohistochemical analysis.

Low-grade lymphomas

Small-size lymphocytic process with a predominantly diffuse growth pattern is usually seen in SLL/CLL, MCL, lymphoplasmacytoid lymphoma (LPL), and marginal cell lymphomas (MrCL). However, each subtype may have other subtle histologic patterns including the presence of proliferation centers in SLL/CLL, and of a vaguely nodular pattern with a relatively higher number of histiocytes suggesting MCL. LPL may have a pinkish background due to the presence of a higher number of lymphoplasmacytic cells, and MrCL may have a geographic pattern along with the presence of residual germinal centers. Distinguishing histologic features of SLL include round to oval nuclei with coarse chromatin, the presence of paraimmunoblasts (immunoblast-like cells with a slightly smaller size and prominent central nucleoli) and lymphoplasmacytic cells that have more cytoplasm with eccentric nuclei and occasional Dutcher bodies. Immunohistochemistry easily identifies SLL and MCL by CD5 reactivity and if CD5 is expressed by the lymphoma cells, the infiltrate should be worked up for SLL or MCL. A complete history including a search for peripheral blood lymphocytosis would be useful to investigate for chronic lymphocytic leukemia (CLL). Ancillary studies such as flow cytometry and cytogenetic studies may be useful if mediastinal tissue is scant. The pathologist needs to confirm whether the

B-cell neoplastic process represents mantle cell lymphoma by immunohistochemical examination of Cyclin-D1 expression as CLL/SLL cells are almost always Cyclin-D1 negative. Rarely, mantle cell lymphomas may also lack this marker. Evaluation for SOX11 expression is helpful and this finding is also considered to be specific for diagnosis of mantle cell lymphoma in this context [7].

Lymphoplasmacytic lymphoma show monomorphic lymphoplasmacytic proliferation with Dutcher bodies that lack CD5 and CD10 expression. However, there could be overlapping features with MrZL and clinical information; particularly, observation of very high serum level of IgM (usually >3 gr/dl) favors the diagnosis of LPL [8]. Complete work-up of bone marrow and mucosa-associated lymphoid tissue (MALT) organs is necessary to exclude MrZL and for accurate diagnosis of LPL. Recent studies have shown the presence of frequent LPL mutation involving MYD88 that is very rarely encountered in MrZL and appears to be a promising ancillary assay in this difficult differential diagnosis [9].

One of the most important low-grade B-cell lymphomas in the mediastinum includes primary thymic extranodal MrZL of mucosa-associated lymphoid tissues (MALT) [10]. This lymphoma is believed to be the thymic counterpart of extranodal MrZL that arises from the MALT. Although a diffuse pattern may be encountered, depending on the progression of the disease, the most frequent pattern is the presence of residual follicles that may be misinterpreted as a reactive process. The tumor is composed of monomorphic small B-lymphoid cells with centrocyte-like (small cleaved cells) or monocytoid (moderate to abundant amount of cytoplasm) appearance. Reactive follicles and Hassall corpuscles are usually identified. In fact, due to the presence of these features, differentiation from a reactive process can be challenging in some cases. Therefore, gene rearrangement analysis of the immunoglobulin heavy chain and kappa light chain gene is quite useful since the presence of a monoclonal population supports diagnosis of lymphoma in cases of monocytoid B-cell and centrocytic cell proliferation. These patients typically have a history of autoimmune disorder (such as Sjogren syndrome) and monoclonal gammopathy (IgA, IgG, or IgM) is frequently observed. MALT lymphomas with marked plasmacytic differentiation may be misinterpreted as lymphoplasmacytic lymphoma [8]. However, careful search for centrocyte-like cells and monocytoid B-cells should bring up the possibility of this diagnosis in the work-up.

Primary mediastinal large B-cell lymphoma

This type of lymphoma is only noted to be localized in the mediastinum, and is currently considered as a separate entity and recognized as primary mediastinal large B-cell lymphoma (PMLBL) [11]. PMLBL is one of the most important disorders that should be on the top of the differential diagnostic entity in evaluation of biopsies obtained from the mediastinum, particularly in female adolescents and younger individuals.

Table 11.1. Most common hematopoietic neoplasms considered in differential diagnosis in the mediastinum. The entities listed are based on the determination of the size of the neoplastic cells. Typical morphologic features and ancillary studies that are suggestive of each diagnosis are provided

Small cell infiltrate histology	Ancillary studies
- SLL/CLL: round to oval nuclei, coarse chromatin, proliferation center	CD5+, CD10−, CD23+, FMC7−, cyclin D1−
- MCL: round to oval nuclei, slight irregularity of nuclei	CD5+, CD10−, CD23−, FMC7+, cyclin D1+ [t(11;14)]
- Follicular lymphoma: follicular architecture, centrocytes and centroblasts	CD5−CD10+, bcl6+, bcl2+[t(14;18)]
- Marginal cell lymphoma: monocytoid B-cells, centrocytes, plasma cells, residual follicles	CD5−CD10−, bcl6−, bcl2+, [t(11;18)]
- Lymphoplasmacytoid lymphoma: lymphoplasmacytoid cells, plasma cells	CD5−CD10−, bcl6−, bcl2+, MYD88 (mutated)
- T-lymphoblastic lymphoma: round to oval nuclei with fine chromatin, small nucleoli, high mitosis	CD3, TdT, CD34, other pan T-cell markers variable (CD1a, CD2, CD4, CD5, CD7, CD8)
Intermediate to large cell infiltrate histology	**Ancillary studies**
- BL: small to intermediate size, starry-sky pattern, high mitosis (99%)	CD10+, bcl6+, bcl2−,c-myc+ (most), EBV+/−: C-myc translocated (most)
- DLBCL: large size, mitosis <90%	CD10+/−, bcl6+/−, bcl2+/−, myc+ (minority), EBV-pax5+, oct2/ Bob1+ C-myc translocated (minor)
- B-UNC/BL/DLBCL: may have features in between BL and DLBCL, high mitosis (>90%)	CD10+/−, bcl6+/−, bcl2+/−,c-myc+ (majority) includes double-hit lymphomas, EBV-C-myc translocated (complex c-myc abnormalities)
- MLBCL: large cells, sclerosis	CD10−, CD23+/−, weak CD30+ gain of 9p24, and 2p15
- CHL: mixed population with Reed-Sternberg cells, eosinophils	CD30+, CD15+/−, pax5+(weak), oct2/bob1−/+(variable)
- B-UNC/HL/DLBCL: pleomorphic large cells overlapping features morphologically	Phenotypical overlapping features
- EBV+DLBCL: Age > 50 years old, large cells	EBV+
- Plasmablastic lymphoma: plasmablasts, immunoblasts	CD20−, CD138+, MUM1+, EBV+/−, c-myc+

Abbreviations:
BL: Burkitt lymphoma
DLBCL: Diffuse large B-cell lymphoma
B-UNC/BL/DLBCL: B-cell lymphoma, unclassifiable, with features intermediate between diffuse large B-cell lymphoma and Burkitt lymphoma
MLBCL: Mediastinal large B-cell lymphoma
CHL: Classical Hodgkin's lymphoma
B-UNC/HL/DLBCL: B-cell lymphoma, unclassifiable, with features intermediate between diffuse large B-cell lymphoma and Hodgkin's lymphoma

Diffuse large B-cell lymphoma (DLBCL) may involve the mediastinum secondary to metastasis from other locations or arise primarily from the mediastinum. If DLBCL is not a primary process, the cell of origin of the lymphoma needs to be determined as a germinal center type (GCB) or non-GCB by use of specific markers (see Table 11.1) [12]. In general, GCB-type DLBCL shows a better clinical response to therapy against diffuse large B-cell lymphoma. The great majority of patients with PMLBLs present with a bulky disease in the mediastinum and may require immediate therapeutic intervention, particularly in the presence of superior vena cava syndrome. Since this diagnosis requires exclusion of extrathoracic involvement, clinical correlation for the absence of other organ involvement including peripheral lymph nodes is required. Local extensions to the pleural or pericardial spaces and even to the chest wall may occur. Despite these lymphomas having histological resemblance to other DLBCLs, there has been significant improvement in the understanding of the biology of these disorders, primarily based on the gene expression profiling that shows some overlapping features with classical HL. Intermediate forms in between DLBCL and HL are also observed [13]. Therefore, classification into GCB vs non-GCB is not utilized in this setting.

There is usually prominent fine sclerosis intermixed with large lymphoma cells in PMLBL (Fig. 11.1). However, some cases may not show fibrosis or sclerosis and the presence of this finding is not required for diagnosis. Large cells are usually round to oval and show nucleoli, but immunoblasts are typically not observed. Cases with scattered large cells with a high number of background T-cells or histiocytes are considered to be a variant of DLBCL and are referred to as T-cell rich or histiocyte-rich B-cell lymphoma, respectively [14]. Currently there is no specific immunohistochemical marker to establish diagnosis of PMLBL. However, there are some characteristic features including expression of CD20, CD79a, OCT 2, and BOB-1, while these neoplasms are usually negative for expression of CD10 and immunoglobulin light chains [11]. CD30 expression is variable and heterogeneous and frequently CD23 is positive. Since CD30 is frequently weak positive in PMLBL, this may cause difficulty in distinguishing it from classical HL. Compared to the other diffuse large B-cell lymphomas the prognosis of PMLBL is usually considered to be better or similar to the GCB-type DLBCL. The great majority of these patients respond much better than GCB or non-GCB type DLBCL with standard regimens [11,15].

Hodgkin's lymphoma

The mediastinum is one of the most frequent sites where HL can be seen. Approximately 60% of all mediastinal lymphomas are classified as Classical HL (CHL). Nodular lymphocyte predominant HL (NLPHL) is rare in the mediastinum while the most frequent type of CHL includes nodular sclerosing type up to 80% followed by mixed cellularity type. Broad bands of collagen fibers generating a variable size of nodules containing a mixture of small lymphocytes, plasma cells, histiocytes, and eosinophils and Reed–Sternberg cells are typical features of

nodular sclerosing CHL in contrast to mixed infiltrate lacking sclerosis observed in the mixed cellularity type of CHL (Fig. 11.2). One of the most important histologic features of the nodular sclerosing-type of CHL is the presence of large sclerotic fibrotic bands surrounding the mixed polymorphic cellular infiltrate containing a variable number of Reed-Sternberg cells. The pathologist should search for the correct histologic feature of Reed-Sternberg (RS) cells showing "owl-eyed" eosinophilic prominent nucleoli. Although classical RS-cells are recognized with the presence of two nuclei and eosinophilic nucleoli, this feature may not be observed in all cases of CHL. Furthermore, variant RS-cells can be very difficult to distinguish from the lymphoma cells seen in DLBCL or T-cell lymphoma. Therefore, immunohistochemistry is important for recognition of RS-cells. Fibrotic bands may be also prominent in primary mediastinal large B-cell lymphoma (PMLBL) and eosinophils may not be prominent in some CHL; hence, one should be very careful not to misdiagnose PMLBL as CHL.

The typical immunohistochemical markers to distinguish CHL from diffuse large B-cell lymphoma are the demonstration of CD30 (strong expression) and CD15 (50% of cases positive) while the RS cells typically lack B- or T-cell associated surface markers (CD20, CD79a, CD3) [16]. Since CHLs may rarely show expression of CD20 as well as CD45, the diagnosis of CHL and differentiation from PMLBL may become very difficult in some cases. Although CD20 and CD45 may be observed in up to 15–20% of classical HL, the expression of CD20 and CD45 usually varies in intensity on the RS cells, a very useful clue to distinguish HL from large B-cell lymphoma. In these instances, evaluation of PAX-5 (B-cell transcription factor) as well as other B-cell associated transcription factors such as OCT 2, BOB-1 are quite useful [16,17]. Typically, CHL shows weak PAX-5 expression in RS cells and does not have strong simultaneous expression of OCT 2 and BOB-1, while B-cell lymphomas are

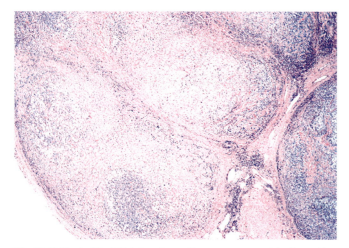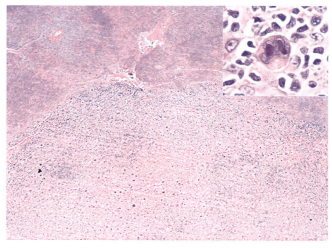

Fig. 11.2 Classical Hodgkin's lymphoma. There are many nodules formed by marked sclerotic bands that contain many lacunar cells as observed by clear spaces . This finding should raise a high suspicion of Hodgkin's lymphoma even at low-power magnification. The lesion on the right lacks clear nodular sclerotic bands and is classified as mixed cellularity type. A typical Reed-Sternberg cell is shown in the inset that could be seen in nodular sclerosing or mixed cellularity type of CHL.

typically strongly positive for both OCT 2 and BOB-1. In addition, CD79a is also negative in the great majority of the CHL cases. In difficult cases, gene rearrangement studies demonstrating a monoclonal B-cell population favors B-cell lymphoma as the RS cells are not usually high enough in number to give rise to a noticeable monoclonal B-cell pattern unless enrichment techniques by microdissection are utilized. The numbers of RS cells vary among the CHL-nodular sclerosing type. Tissues with a very prominent presence of RS cells sheeting out are also referred to as type-2 nodular sclerosing type; however, the prognostic significance of this type is questionable. Histologically, observation of the RS cell rich-variant of nodular sclerosing CHL is very important for differentiating from diffuse large B-cell lymphoma or PMLBL.

If nodular infiltrate is considered to be suspicious for NLPHL, a high-power magnification search for so-called "popcorn-cells" (also known as L&H cells) is necessary. These cells typically show large nuclei with very fine nuclear membrane and prominent membrane associated nucleoli. The diagnostic evaluation for NLPHL requires demonstration of CD20, bcl6, and occasionally EMA expression in L&H cells while lacking other CHL-associated markers (such as CD15 and CD30) [18]. CD20 not only demonstrates larger L&H cells but also a collection of smaller background mantle cells. Although the neoplastic cells are rare, pathologists should also take advantage of assessing the background cells and the architecture of the lesion in order to make the diagnosis of NLPHL when this diagnosis is suspected. The typical L&H cells are surrounded by the T-follicular helper cells (TFH) that are positive for expression of CD4, CD57, CXCL-13, and PD1 [18]. Careful review for rosetting by CD4 cells around the L&H cells is essential for making this diagnosis. Furthermore, CD21 expression also highlights the typical nodular architecture highlighted by increased follicular dendritic cells that is a very characteristic pattern and best appreciated by the use of this marker. Incidentally, T-cell rich B-cell lymphoma (TCRBCL) is one of the most important diagnostic entities which should be considered in the differential diagnosis of NLPHL. Analysis of the background cells allows distinguishing TCRBCL from NLPHL. Typically, the background cells in TCRBCL reveal CD8-predominant T-cell proliferation, as opposed to CD4-positive cells noted in NLPHL [14,18].

Gray zone having intermediate features between classical Hodgkin's lymphoma and large cell non-Hodgkin's lymphoma

One of the greatest difficulties for pathologists examining biopsies from mediastinal lymphomas are cases showing overlapping features of Hodgkin's lymphoma (HL) and diffuse large B-cell lymphoma. These cases are referred to as gray zone having intermediate features between classical HL and large cell non-Hodgkin's lymphoma [19]. In general, there is no single pathognomonic histologic feature. Therefore, constellation of characteristics including histology, immunophenotyping, and molecular findings should be utilized for diagnosis. Some of these cases include lesions with histological appearance similar to CHL while immunophenotypically having features of diffuse large B-cell lymphoma. In contrast, there are some cases which appear to have histologic features of diffuse large B-cell lymphoma but immunophenotypic features of CHL (i.e. CD30, CD15 positive, CD20 negative Reed-Sternberg-like cells that are sheeting out as diffuse large B-cell lymphoma). Interestingly, these cases are still currently difficult diagnostic entities for many of the expert hematopathologists. Furthermore, the gene expression profile analysis also shows significant overlapping gene expression profile and CHL and some of the diffuse large B-cell lymphomas including primary mediastinal large B-cell lymphoma. Gray zone lymphoma is significantly more aggressive compared to CHL, therefore this entity needs to be recognized and distinguished from CHL. Although there is no specific clinical trial to recommend a specific treatment for these patients, a recent study suggests that a hybrid therapy targeting both CHL and diffuse large B-cell lymphoma may have some validity until more studies based on therapy and biology are completed [20].

Burkitt lymphoma

Burkitt lymphoma (BL) needs to be differentiated from other aggressive B-cell lymphomas as it usually responds to therapy despite its aggressive biology of the disease as it also requires CNS prophylaxis. Histologic evaluation reveals a diffuse process that is easily identified as an aggressive process by observation of many increased tingible-body macrophages that are referred to as "starry-sky" pattern. The neoplastic cells are sligthly smaller than centroblasts (small non-cleaved cells) encountered in the germinal centers. They typically reveal a basophilic moderate amount of cytoplasm with squared-off cell borders, round nuclei with finely clumped and dispersed chromatin, and medium-sized paracentral nucleoli (Fig. 11.3). If touch imprints are prepared, the presence of cytoplasmic vacuoles in deep blue cytoplasms should raise this possibility. Although the diagnosis is straightforward in the majority of cases, difficulty can arise in the distinction between BL and DLBCL. In fact, some of the cases may fall into intermediate in between BL and DLBCL as discussed below [21,22]. BL cells arise from the germinal centers and the immunophenotype reflects this biology by the expression of bcl6 and CD10. If B-lymphoblastic lymphoma (B-acute lymphoblastic lymphoma) needs to be excluded, observation of TdT and frequently CD34 are used to support lymphoblastic lymphoma diagnosis, since both of these markers are negative in BL. The most important immunohistochemical stains for the diagnosis of BL are Ki67 and bcl2, as the cells of these neoplasms show high proliferation noted by Ki67 (100%) and lack of bcl2 expression. The demonstration of c-myc translocation by FISH

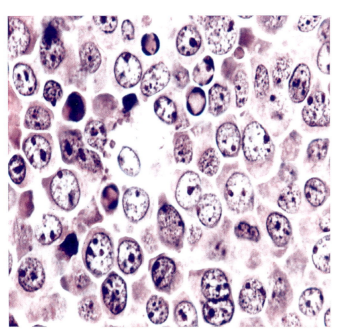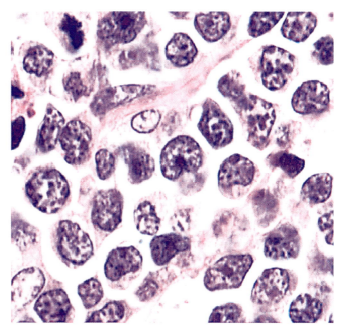

Fig. 11.3 Burkitt lymphoma (left) and double-hit lymphoma (right). Burkitt lymphoma cells reveal a basophilic moderate amount of cytoplasm with squared-off cell borders, round nuclei with finely clumped and dispersed chromatin, and small to medium size paracentral nucleoli. Double-hit lymphoma shown here could be very difficult to distinguish from Burkitt lymphoma as seen here. The cells show slight variation in size. High mitotic rate is seen and this should raise a suspicion of high grade lymphoma. FISH study demonstrated translocations of both c-myc and bcl2 genes; therefore, the lesion was classified as double-hit lymphoma.

assay is also critical for diagnosis as it is observed in 90% of BL cases. Gene expression profiles have been essential in recognizing some of the morphologically challenging cases; however, these ancillary studies are not routinely used. Therefore, histology combined with the above histochemical markers and c-myc FISH analysis are the main elements for diagnostic evaluation of BL. Since double-hit lymphoma (see below) is generally in the differential diagnosis, one may order c-myc, bcl2 and bcl6 FISH assays up front for cases with histologic suggestion of an aggressive B-cell lymphoma.

B-cell lymphoma, unclassifiable, with features intermediate between diffuse large B-cell lymphoma and Burkitt lymphoma (BL)

Recently recognized cases showing features of both diffuse large B-cell lymphoma and Burkitt lymphoma (BL) are now considered to be B-cell lymphoma, unclassifiable, with features intermediate between diffuse large B-cell lymphoma and BL. One of the most important categories of these lymphomas include so-called "double-hit lymphoma"[21,22]. In order to make this diagnosis, analysis of three genes (c-myc, bcl2, and bcl6) are necessary by FISH. Since double-hit lymphomas are usually very resistant to diffuse large B-cell lymphoma and BL treatment protocols in recognition of this entity are very important. Currently, there is not a specific treatment recommended for treatment of these patients. However, it is better to communicate diagnosis as double-hit lymphoma, rather

than putting these cases in the BL category. Presence of two translocations of the above-mentioned oncogenes or three of the oncogenes establishes diagnosis as double-hit or triple-hit lymphoma. Morphologically, these patients typically show a high proliferation rate although it is not as high as those seen in Burkitt lymphoma (Fig. 11.3). Prior to recognition of this entity, some cases used to be most likely classified as Burkitt lymphoma or diffuse large B-cell lymphoma. The Ki-67 proliferation index is usually determined to be high but still slightly lower than 99% positivity encountered in Burkitt lymphomas and c-myc translocation may be absent. Therefore any aggressive lymphoma with Burkitt lymphoma or diffuse large B-cell lymphoma should be investigated for the possibility of double-hit lymphoma. FISH for c-myc translocation or c-myc expression by immunohistochemistry is very useful for investigation of this possibility. Cases with histologic features of BL that do not show the presence of c-myc translocation, do not necessarily suggest the diagnosis of intermediate between diffuse large B-cell lymphoma and BL since up to 10% of typical BL has been shown to lack c-myc translocation.

EBV-positive diffuse large B-cell lymphoma

This entity has been recently recognized and added as a provisional category in the WHO classification. The tumor cells usually show malignant polymorphic or monomorphic large B-cells typically positive for EBV and by definition these patients are older than 50 years old[23]. These patients do not have any defined immunodeficiency or immunosuppression

prior to the diagnosis of lymphoma. Histologically, these cases sometimes may be very difficult to distinguish from diffuse large B-cell lymphoma. Some cases may have Reed-Sternberg-like cells as seen in EBV-associated disease states that may be encountered in infectious mononucleosis cells or methotrexate-associated lymphoproliferative diseases. Therefore one should always perform EBV testing in a patient who is more than 50 years old in order to make this diagnosis. Another important factor in the mediastinum is the consideration of chronic inflammation-associated diffuse large B-cell lymphomas that are typically EBV positive. This lesion usually arises in patients with longstanding chronic pyothorax [24]. The usual sites of involvement include pleural cavity at this location.

Plasmablastic lymphoma

One of the most important lesions to be considered in the differential diagnoses of mediastinal lesions is diffuse large B-cell lymphoma with plasma cell differentiation. Plasmablastic lymphoma was initially recognized in the oral cavity in patients with immunosuppression secondary to HIV infection. However, plasmablastic lymphoma may also be seen in any other locations including the mediastinum. These lymphomas, as the name suggests, show cells with both morphologic and immunophenotypic differentiation of plasmablasts (Fig. 11.4) [25]. This includes expression of CD138 (and CD38 by flow cytometry) as well as lack of or weak expression of B-cell-associated markers (CD79a, CD20, PAX-5). Plasmablastic lymphomas are also positive for MUM-1. Lack of CD20 or other B-cell marker or any T-cell marker along with negativity of CD45 in a

mediastinal tumor should raise the diagnostic possibility of poorly differentiated carcinoma, melanoma, germ cell tumor, and plasmablastic lymphoma. The pathologist should be aware of the latter diagnostic entity and perform immunostains for CD138, MUM-1 in order to make this diagnosis. Since CD138 may also be positive in carcinomas, it may lead to misdiagnosis of epithelial tumor. One of the most characteristic features of plasmablastic lymphoma is the positivity for the EBV in up to 70% of cases. In addition, c-myc translocation is also frequently observed and can be easily detected by FISH analysis. Patients with plasmablastic lymphoma usually have a very poor response to therapy, with a high relapse rate. It is very important to exclude multiple myeloma by clinical history, serum protein electrophoresis, and bone survey since some cases of plasmablastic lymphoma and myeloma have identical histological and immunophenotypical features.

Primary effusion lymphoma

One of the other subtypes of mediastinal diffuse large B-cell lymphoma is primary effusion lymphoma. These lymphomas typically show expression of human herpesvirus 8 (HHV-8) [26]. Any effusion that shows a large number of atypical immunoblastic or plasmablastic cells should be screened for HHV-8 and EBV. All of the cases are HHV-8 positive while EBV is expressed in up to 85% of the cases. The lymphoma cells typically show immunoblastic or plasmablastic proliferation and sometimes anaplastic features. Cytoplasm is abundant and nuclei are large to oval with prominent nucleoli (Fig. 11.5). Patients particularly with prior history of Kaposi

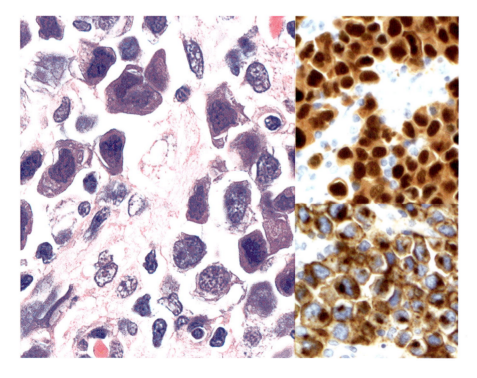

Fig. 11.4 Plasmablastic lymphoma. Clusters of large cells with abundant amphophilic cytoplasm having features of plasmablasts are shown. Membranous expression of CD138 (right upper) or nuclear MUM1 (right lower) demonstrate plasmablastic differentiation. The lesion shown here lacked expression of any B-cell differentiation markers such as CD20, CD79a or pax-5.

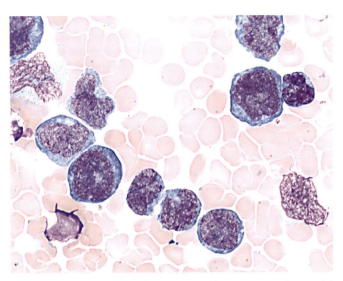

Fig. 11.5 Primary effusion lymphoma (PEL). Wright-Giemsa stained pericardial effusion fluid from an AIDS patient shows many large atypical cells with round to oval nuclei. Based on suspicion of PEL, immunohistochemistry for HHV8 and in situ hybridization for EBV were performed and these studies showed positivity for both viruses.

sarcoma and HIV as well as multicentric Castleman disease are likely to develop primary effusion lymphoma. One of the most important differential diagnoses for primary effusion lymphoma includes pyothorax-associated diffuse large B-cell lymphoma. As mentioned above, prior history of chronic inflammation is very important for making this diagnosis. In addition, immunohistochemical determination of HHV-8 is a characteristic marker of primary effusion lymphoma while it is not seen in pyothorax-associated diffuse large B-cell lymphoma. Patients with diffuse large B-cell lymphoma positive for HHV-8 expression but without primary effusion are considered to be extracavitary primary effusion lymphoma. Patients with DLBCL can also develop pleural effusion secondary to metastasis. Therefore, complete assessment of history, HHV-8, and EBV infections are necessary for accurate classification. The treatment response is very poor for primary effusion lymphomas and patients usually have less than six months of survival. Recent studies have also described unique large B-cell lymphoma in patients with fluid overload that may morphologically show similar features as PEL but are lacking HHV-8 [27]. This study suggests a good outcome to standard therapy against large B-cell lymphoma that is in contrast to PEL.

Lymphoblastic lymphoma

In mediastinal biopsies where the growth pattern of the hematopoietic infiltrate is diffuse, the cell size determination will also allow separation of low-grade lymphomas from high-grade processes. One caveat in lymphomas composed of monomorphic cells is paying particular attention to chromatin pattern and the number of mitotically active cells. Finer chromatin and high mitosis, particularly at this location, brings

lymphoblastic lymphoma as the primary consideration in differential diagnosis. These cases require assessment by additional immunohistochemical markers that are associated with lymphoblastic lymphoma such as TdT, CD34, and CD10 [28]. TdT is a very specific marker for lymphoblastic lymphoma and CD34 is never seen in low-grade lymphoproliferative disorders. T-lymphoblastic lymphoma is one of the most significant lesions that needs to be assessed very carefully in the differential diagnosis of hematopoietic disorders in the mediastinum. Recognition of cortical thymocytes in thymoma or normal thymic tissue is critical as these cells may be mistaken as lymphoblasts. Cells assessed by flow cytometry may lead to observation of cortical thymocytes that may be misinterpreted as lymphoblastic lymphoma. Therefore, one should be very careful in making a diagnosis of T-lymphoblastic lymphoma without histologic evaluation on flow cytometry. Subtle clues on flow cytometry include co-expression of CD4 and CD8 with various maturational stages in cortical thymocytes (normal thymic cells or thymoma cells) [28]. In contrast, lymphoblastic lymphoma cells show very distinct population of CD3 expression along with CD4 or CD8 markers. However, expression of T-cell associated markers vary depending on the differentiation stage (Fig. 11.6). If thymoma is suspected, keratin and p63 stains are quite useful for detecting epithelial cells in tissue sections. Histologic observation of the typical features of thymoma including the presence of thymic epithelial cells is extremely important to assure the diagnosis of thymoma rather than lymphoblastic lymphoma. Rarely, B-lymphoblastic lymphoma may also be encountered and immunohistochemical demonstration of TdT, CD34, and CD10 along with B-cell markers such as PAX-5 and CD19 would be useful for establishing this diagnosis. Only a minority of B-lineage lymphoblastic lymphomas would be CD20 positive and this should be kept in mind if B-lineage lymphoproliferative disease is in consideration. Although rare, extramedullary myeloid neoplasms with similar morphologic features are also encountered in the mediastinum; hence, it should always be considered and excluded by immunohistochemical analysis, and if there is any suspicion of myeloid neoplasms, i.e. prior history of acute myeloid leukemia or chronic myeloproliferative disorder, special markers should be utilized for assessment of myeloid lineage. MPO, CD117, and CD34 are usually positive in myeloid leukemia and CD163 and CD68 in monocytic leukemias [29].

Anaplastic large cell lymphoma

Anaplastic large cell lymphoma (ALCL) rarely occurs in the mediastinal location [30]. One of the most important histologic features is the presence of Hodgkin's-like atypical cells, so-called hallmark cells. These cells typically show kidney-shaped nuclei with broad cytoplasm and an abundant amount of cytoplasm. One of the characteristic features of anaplastic large cell lymphoma is the expression of CD30. This may also rarely lead into misdiagnosis if a full panel of T-cell lymphoma is not

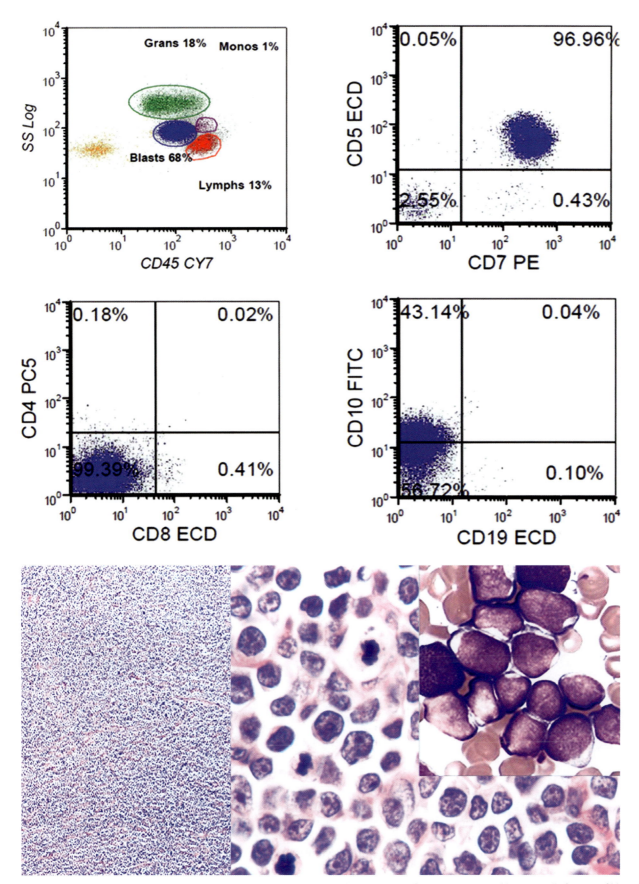

Fig. 11.6 T-cell lymphoblastic lymphoma. Flow cytometric analysis shows moderate intensity of CD45 expression in blasts, typically features of blasts (blue). Blasts are positive for CD5 and CD7 while both CD4 and CD8 are negative; CD10 is partially expressed. The lower panel shows diffuse infiltrate and high-power magnification illustrates rounder nuclei with smooth edges and fine chromatin; occasional small nucleoli are noticeable. High mitotic cells as seen here should always raise a suspicion of lymphoblastic lymphoma. Touch imprint (inset) in this patient reveals typical fine chromatin of blasts.

included. The majority of ALCL do show T-cell associated markers. Anaplastic large cell lymphomas are typically strongly positive for CD30. The lymphoma cells show variable expression of CD4 and in some cases CD8, while CD3 is negative in a minority of cases. One of the most important markers for recognition of this entity is demonstration of anaplastic lymphoma kinase (ALK) in the majority of ALCL [32]. (32) ALK tyrosine kinase maintains the neoplastic cell survival and there are new, promising treatment modalities that target ALK activity in the neoplastic cells. For example, Crizotinib, a drug that is very active in lung carcinoma patients with ALK translocation, also showed activity in anaplastic large cell lymphoma patients with ALK activity.

Peripheral T-cell lymphomas

Peripheral T-cell lymphomas are rare in the mediastinum; however, many patients with mediastinal biopsy should be fully investigated for possible peripheral T-cell lymphoma and the general principles of histologic and phenotypic features also apply at this location [31]. In addition, natural

killer-cell lymphomas are also very rare at this location. Similar to the other biopsy evaluations, one should always perform a pan-T-cell marker such as CD3 in order to potentially lead to further very detailed diagnostic evaluation of cases that may represent peripheral T-cell lymphoma or natural killer-cell lymphoma.

Myeloid sarcoma

Rarely acute myeloid leukemia may present as a primary or secondary process in extramedullary sites, especially in patients with history of acute myeloid leukemia, chronic myeloproliferative disorder, or myelodysplastic syndrome. This lesion was previously known as granulocytic sarcoma (chloroma), extramedullary myeloid tumor and typically presents in large sheets of myeloid blasts. Due to the low frequency myeloid sarcoma in this location, it can pose diagnostic challenges to pathologists. Although rare in the mediastinum, this diagnosis should be considered especially when most lymphoid markers fail in a lesion with histologic resemblance of a hematopoietic neoplasm. Clinical history is essential to

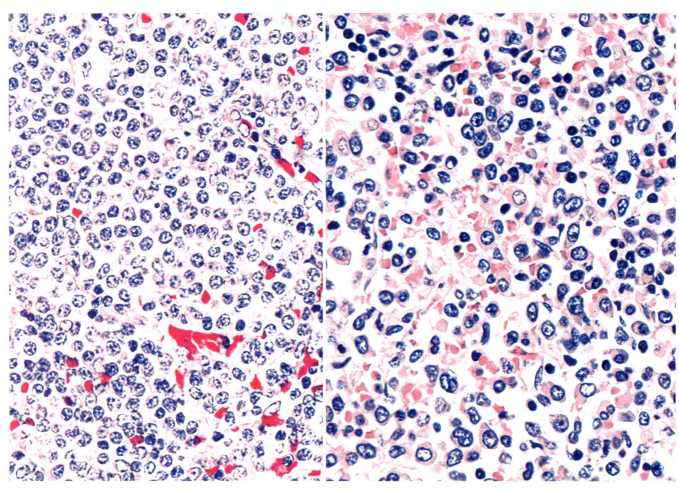

Fig. 11.7 Myeloid sarcoma (extramedullary myeloid tumor). Since the morphology of these lesions may differ depending on the underlying myeloid neoplastic process, two different examples are shown to illustrate this variability. The picture on the left is composed of small to intermediate size cells while the picture on the right shows more pleomorphic larger cells. Both of these lesions could easily be misdiagnosed as lymphoma. However, lack of lymphoid lineage-specific markers led to investigation of myeloid-lineage associated markers such as MPO and diagnosis of extramedullary myeloid tumor were made.

raise this possibility as prior history such as acute myeloid leukemia or chronic myeloproliferative disorder may lead to specific immunohistochemical investigation of this disorder. CD45 (leukocyte common antigen), general hematopoietic lineage marker may show reactivity but could be weak in some cases that may lead to misdiagnosis of the lymphoma. When one is considering a small round blue cell tumor, the possibility of granulocytic sarcoma could be investigated by additional immunohistochemistry. Typically, the leukemic cells are intermediate to large in size and usually show finer chromatin and smaller nucleoli [32]. The leukemic cells usually have thinner nuclear membranes, finer chromatin, and smaller nucleoli that are not typically histologic features seen in lymphoid infiltrates (Fig. 11.7).

CD34 and MPO positivity are the most useful markers in diagnostic evaluation as concurrent positivity for both markers strongly indicates origin of myeloid lineage. However, MPO may not be positive in all cases; therefore, additional stains such as lysozyme, CD43, CD163, and CD68 that are highly sensitive markers but not specific may also be performed. CD33, a very good myeloid marker, is typically observed by flow cytometric evaluation in myeloid disorders also available

by immunohistochemical analysis in paraffin sections. Blastic plasmacytoid dendritic cell neoplasm, important in differential diagnosis, could be distinguished by reactivity of the plasmacytoid dendritic cells with CD4, CD56, CD123, and TCL-1.

Langerhan cell histiocytosis

Langerhan cell histiocytosis (LCH) is an extremely rare tumor to encounter in the mediastinum [33]. Typically the involved tissues show monotonous histiocytic infiltrate composed of histiocytes with abundant eosinophilic cytoplasm and nuclei with coffee bean-shaped nuclei. Many cases also reveal concurrent collections of eosinophils that should raise a suspicion of this neoplasm. Diagnosis could be confirmed by demonstration of LCH-associated markers such as S100, CD1a, and Langerin. Recent studies demonstrated frequent mutation of BRAF V600E and an antibody recognizing mutated BRAF has been utilized for demonstration of this protein in LCH. This finding further supported the notion that LCH is a neoplastic process that is different from the reactive histiocytic infiltrates frequently noted in lung infiltrates [34].

References

1. Hoffman, O.A., et al., Primary mediastinal neoplasms (other than thymoma). *Mayo Clin Proc*, 1993. 68(9): p. 880–91.

2. Kaleem, Z., et al., Lack of expression of surface immunoglobulin light chains in B-cell non-Hodgkin lymphomas. *Am J Clin Pathol*, 2000. 113(3): p. 399–405.

3. Matsushita, H., et al., Clinical and pathological features of B-cell non-Hodgkin lymphomas lacking the surface expression of immunoglobulin light chains. *Clin Chem Lab Med*, 2012. 50(9): p. 1665–70.

4. Schmid, S., et al., Flow cytometry as an accurate tool to complement fine needle aspiration cytology in the diagnosis of low grade malignant lymphomas. *Cytopathology*, 2011. 22(6): p. 397–406.

5. Jevremovic, D., et al., CD5+ B-cell lymphoproliferative disorders: Beyond chronic lymphocytic leukemia and mantle cell lymphoma. *Leuk Res*, 2010. 34(9): p. 1235–8.

6. Nathwani, B.N., et al., The critical role of histology in an era of genomics and proteomics: a commentary and reflection. *Adv Anat Pathol*, 2007. 14(6): p. 375–400.

7. Mozos, A., et al., SOX11 expression is highly specific for mantle cell lymphoma and identifies the cyclin D1-negative subtype. *Haematologica*, 2009. 94(11): p. 1555–62.

8. Lin, P., et al., Lymphoplasmacytic lymphoma and other non-marginal zone lymphomas with plasmacytic differentiation. *Am J Clin Pathol*, 2011. 136(2): p. 195–210.

9. Varettoni, M., et al., Prevalence and clinical significance of the MYD88 (L265P) somatic mutation in Waldenstrom's macroglobulinemia and related lymphoid neoplasms. *Blood*, 2013. 121:2522–8.

10. Shimizu, K., et al., Extranodal marginal zone B-cell lymphoma of mucosa-associated lymphoid tissue (MALT lymphoma) in the thymus: report of four cases. *Jpn J Clin Oncol*, 2005. 35(7): p. 412–16.

11. Pileri, S.A., et al., Pathobiology of primary mediastinal B-cell lymphoma. *Leuk Lymphoma*, 2003. 44 **Suppl 3**: p. S21–6.

12. Visco, C., et al., Comprehensive gene expression profiling and immunohistochemical studies support application of immunophenotypic algorithm for molecular subtype classification in diffuse large B-cell lymphoma: a report from the International DLBCL Rituximab-CHOP Consortium Program Study. *Leukemia*, 2012. 26(9): p. 2103–13.

13. Steidl, C. and R.D. Gascoyne, The molecular pathogenesis of primary mediastinal large B-cell lymphoma. *Blood*, 2011. 118(10): p. 2659–69.

14. Tousseyn, T. and C. De Wolf-Peeters, T cell/histiocyte-rich large B-cell lymphoma: an update on its biology and classification. *Virchows Arch*, 2011. 459(6): p. 557–63.

15. Seidemann, K., et al., Primary mediastinal large B-cell lymphoma with sclerosis in pediatric and adolescent patients: treatment and results from three therapeutic studies of the Berlin-Frankfurt-Munster Group. *J Clin Oncol*, 2003. 21(9): p. 1782–9.

16. Eberle, F.C., H. Mani, and E.S. Jaffe, Histopathology of Hodgkin's lymphoma. *Cancer J*, 2009. 15(2): p. 129–37.

17. Desouki, M.M., et al., PAX-5: a valuable immunohistochemical marker in the differential diagnosis of lymphoid neoplasms. *Clin Med Res*, 2010. 8(2): p. 84–8.

18. Fan, Z., et al., Characterization of variant patterns of nodular lymphocyte predominant hodgkin lymphoma with immunohistologic and clinical correlation. *Am J Surg Pathol*, 2003. 27(10): p. 1346–56.

19. Harris, N.L., Shades of gray between large B-cell lymphomas and Hodgkin

lymphomas: differential diagnosis and biological implications. *Mod Pathol*, 2013. 26 **Suppl 1**: p. S57–70.

20. Dunleavy, K., *et al.*, Gray zone lymphoma: better treated like hodgkin lymphoma or mediastinal large B-cell lymphoma? *Curr Hematol Malig Rep*, 2012. 7(3): p. 241–7.

21. Hasserjian, R.P., *et al.*, Commentary on the WHO classification of tumors of lymphoid tissues (2008): "Gray zone" lymphomas overlapping with Burkitt lymphoma or classical Hodgkin lymphoma. *J Hematop*, 2009. 2(2): p. 89–95.

22. Aukema, S.M., *et al.*, Double-hit B-cell lymphomas. *Blood*, 2011. 117(8): p. 2319–31.

23. Dojcinov, S.D., *et al.*, Age-related EBV-associated lymphoproliferative disorders in the Western population: a spectrum of reactive lymphoid hyperplasia and lymphoma. *Blood*, 2011. 117(18): p. 4726–35.

24. Aozasa, K., T. Takakuwa, and S. Nakatsuka, Pyothorax-associated lymphoma: a lymphoma developing in chronic inflammation. *Adv Anat Pathol*, 2005. 12(6): p. 324–31.

25. Hsi, E.D., *et al.*, Plasmablastic lymphoma and related disorders. *Am J Clin Pathol*, 2011. 136(2): p. 183–94.

26. Chadburn, A., *et al.*, KSHV-positive solid lymphomas represent an extra-cavitary variant of primary effusion lymphoma. *Am J Surg Pathol*, 2004. 28(11): p. 1401–16.

27. Alexanian, S., *et al.*, KSHV/HHV8-negative Effusion-based Lymphoma, a Distinct Entity Associated With Fluid Overload States. *Am J Surg Pathol*, 2013. 37(2): p. 241–9.

28. Patel, J.L., *et al.*, The immunophenotype of T-lymphoblastic lymphoma in children and adolescents: a Children's Oncology Group report. *Br J Haematol*, 2012. 159(4): p. 454–61.

29. Creutzig, U., *et al.*, Diagnosis and management of acute myeloid leukemia in children and adolescents: recommendations from an international expert panel. *Blood*, 2012. 120(16): p. 3187–205.

30. Sevilla, D.W., J.K. Choi, and J.Z. Gong, Mediastinal adenopathy, lung infiltrates, and hemophagocytosis: unusual manifestation of pediatric anaplastic large cell lymphoma: report of two cases. *Am J Clin Pathol*, 2007. 127(3): p. 458–64.

31. Foss, F.M., *et al.*, Peripheral T-cell lymphoma. *Blood*, 2011. 117(25): p. 6756–67.

32. Ramasamy, K., Z. Lim, A. Pagliuca, *et al.*, Acute myeloid leukaemia presenting with mediastinal myeloid sarcoma: report of three cases and review of literature. *Leuk Lymphoma*, 2007. 48(2):p. 290–4.

33. Fahrner, R., B. Hoksch, M. Gugger, *et al.*, Langerhans cell histiocytosis as differential diagnosis of a mediastinal tumor. *Eur J Cardiothorac Surg*, 2008. 33(3): p. 516–17.

34. Sahm, F., *et al.*, BRAFV600E mutant protein is expressed in cells of variable maturation in Langerhans cell histiocytosis. *Blood*, 2012. 120(12): e28–34.

Cystic lesions of the mediastinum

Chapter 12

Mark Wick, MD, and Alberto M. Marchevsky, MD

Even if degenerative change in true neoplasms is considered, intrathoracic cysts are relatively uncommon; most lesions in this category are probably congenital, and they comprise 10–15% of radiographically-detected masses in the mediastinum [1]. Histologically, several tissue types are represented in neoplastic and non-neoplastic mediastinal cysts (Table 12.1), including parathyroid, thymic, bronchogenic, enteric, germinal, lymphoid, pericardial, and metastatic epithelial elements [2,3]. The clinicopathologic attributes of such lesions are considered in this chapter.

Congenital cystic lesions
Embryologic information

To understand the likely origins of most cysts in the mediastinum, it is appropriate to consider selected details of thoracic embryologic development [4]. Specifically, these concern the pharyngeal pouches, the respiratory diverticulum, the primitive gut, and the pleuropericardial membranes.

The thymus and parathyroid

During the fifth week of human fetal growth, the third and fourth pharyngeal pouches begin to differentiate. They are paired anlages with dorsal and ventral "wings"; the inferior parathyroid glands take origin from the dorsal aspects of the third pouches, and the ventral portions of those tissues are the progenitors of the thymus (Fig. 12.1). The superior parathyroids derive from the dorsal fourth pharyngeal pouches, and a portion of the "temporary" thymus may also do so [4]. The parathyroid glands and thymus migrate ventrally and caudally at the sixth week of fetal development, and at that point they lose contact with the remainder of the pharynx. Their subsequent descent traverses tissues behind the thyroid gland and sternocleidomastoid muscles. Thus, one can easily anticipate that tissue from the developing parathyroids and thymus may be implanted in those locations. Postmortem analyses of that phenomenon have shown that cervical thymic rests are found in 20% of adults and 33% of infants [5,6].

Table 12.1. Mediastinal cysts and other cystic lesions

Congenital cystic lesions

Parathyroid cyst

Unilocular thymic cyst

Bronchogenic cyst

Enteric cyst

Pericardial cyst

Meningocele

Acquired cystic lesions

Infectious cysts
  Echinococcus granulosus

Multilocular and secondary thymic cysts
  Proliferating multilocular thymic cyst

Mullerian cyst of the posterior mediastinum

Primary cystic lesions

Lymphangioma ("cystic hygroma")

Multiloculated cystic adenomatoid tumor

Multicystic mesothelial proliferation of borderline malignancy

Mature cystic teratoma

Cystic change in mediastinal neoplasms

Thymoma

Seminoma

Thymic neuroendocrine carcinoma

Thymic carcinoma

Posterior mediastinal neurilemmomas

Metastatic well-differentiated serous carcinoma of the ovary

Respiratory organs

Approximately three weeks into fetal development, the respiratory system arises from the foregut as a diverticular structure. The pulmonary anlage grow caudally and develop into two

Pathology of the Mediastinum, ed. Alberto M. Marchevsky and Mark R. Wick. Published by Cambridge University Press.
© Cambridge University Press 2014.

lateral branches – the lung buds – which subsequently become the large conducting airways and the pulmonary parenchyma (Fig. 12.2). Small portions of the respiratory diverticulum may be left behind near the foregut, and fragments of the lung buds may likewise be split off inside the thorax as maturation occurs. Such embryonic rests are most commonly found near the intersection of the right mainstem bronchus and the trachea, or beneath the carina. Mesenchymal induction around ectopic lung tissue yields investments of smooth muscle and cartilage, just as in the eutopic bronchial tree.

Foregut

In the first two weeks of fetal growth, the foregut is represented by a solid cylinder of tissue that subsequently develops internal vacuolar change to yield a hollow tube. In that evolution, microcystic rests may be misplaced in the wall of the developing gut, and they then grow as blind sacs which contain alimentary epithelium. It is columnar during early embryonic development, but later converts partially to a squamous lining [2]. Mesenchymal induction around the epithelium once more produces a muscular investment.

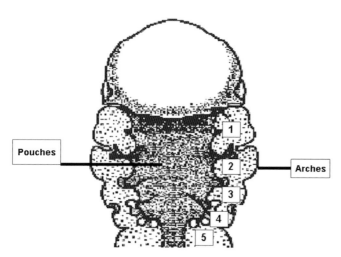

Fig. 12.1 Diagram of the embryological relationship between pharyngeal pouches and arches in the developing human fetus. The third and fourth pouches give rise to the parathyroids and thymus, and displaced remnants of such fetal structures may yield the later development of congenital mediastinal cysts.

Pleuropericardial membranes

The thoracic cavity is subdivided into the pleural and pericardial spaces by the pleuropericardial membranes. These begin as small horizontal ridges in the ventrolateral portions of the embryo, and they invaginate during gestational week three to join one another and intersect the midline mesocardium and lung roots. In that process, diverticular structures may form in the ventral-parietal recesses of the pericardium [7]. These have particular relevance to the development of pericardial cysts.

Specific pathologic entities
Parathyroid cysts and unilocular thymic cysts

Based on the foregoing discussion, one might well expect that thymic and parathyroid cysts can be encountered in cervical and mediastinal locations. Those that are bounded by a thin cortex of parathyroid tissue and unaccompanied by clinical hypercalcemia are uncommon in cervical sites and rare in the mediastinum. Such lesions usually present as asymptomatic masses [8]. They also may contain identifiable thymic tissue [9], reflecting the common developmental origin of the two glands. If neither parathyroid nor thymic elements predominate microscopically, one may use the term "third pharyngeal pouch cyst" diagnostically.

Unilocular thymic cysts (UTCs) are more often seen in the anterosuperior mediastinum than in retrosternocleidomastoid soft tissue [10]. It was once thought that they were postinflammatory lesions that were formed by degeneration of Hassall's corpuscles [11]. Nevertheless, the inclusion of parathyroid tissue (or salivary glandular rests) in some thymic cysts casts doubt on that premise [12]. Along with Leong [9], we believe that UTCs are usually congenital in nature.

Intrathoracic UTCs occur predominantly between the ages of 20 and 50 years, usually in asymptomatic patients [9–13]. Uncommonly, they come to clinical attention because of secondary infection and rapid enlargement [14]. In imaging studies, these lesions appear as smooth, circumscribed masses in the anterior-superior mediastinum, and rare examples may be massive. UTCs are typically uniform in radiographic density and may contain "rim" calcification [9]. Computed tomography (CT) demonstrates that the cyst contents approximate the attenuation of water in most instances (Fig. 12.3) [15].

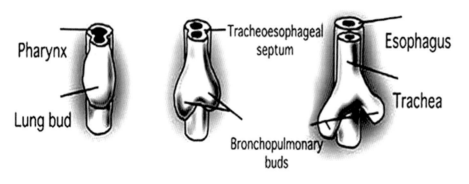

Fig. 12.2 Diagram of the developing lung buds in the human embryo, and their relationship to other intrathoracic structures.

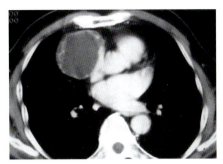

Fig. 12.3 Computed tomogram showing a unilocular thymic cyst in the anterior mediastinum, the internal consistency of which is above that of water in this case.

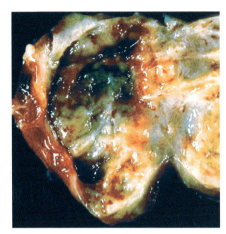

Fig. 12.4 Gross photograph of excised unilocular thymic cyst, showing a somewhat "shaggy" internal lining.

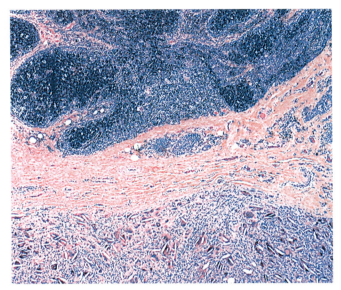

Fig. 12.5 Cholesterol granulomas and thymic tissue are present in the wall of this unilocular thymic cyst (H&E 160X).

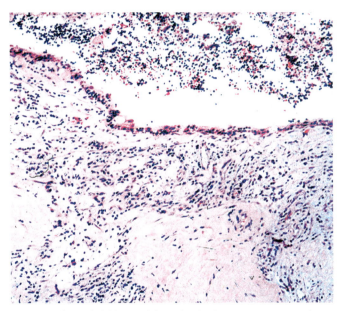

Fig. 12.6 The epithelial lining of this unilocular thymic cyst is squamoid (H&E 250X).

The sizes of UTCs range from 1 to > 20 cm [16], with a generally smooth exterior fibrous capsule. The fluid cyst contents vary from clear and watery to turbid or hemorrhagic, and internal surfaces are either smooth or "shaggy" (Fig. 12.4).

Histologic examination shows the inconstant presence of an epithelial lining, and many lesions comprise only degenerating cellular debris, cholesterol, granulation tissue, and foreign-body granulomas [9,16]. Indeed, the presence of prominent cholesterol granulomas (Fig. 12.5) constitutes good supportive evidence for the thymic nature of any anterior mediastinal cyst; that tissue response is uncommon in other cystic lesions. If epithelium is present, it may be squamous, simple cuboidal, or columnar (Fig. 12.6), and all of those cell types may be admixed in the same cyst [17]. Smooth muscle and cartilage are absent, but one may see mural remnants of thymic tissue, including lymphoid aggregates and Hassall's corpuscles, in roughly 50% of cases. Epithelial proliferation in thymic cysts merits special mention; it is most often seen in variants of *multilocular* thymic cysts [18] (see below), but uncommonly may also be observed in association with UTC.

Cervical UTCs that contain only a simple epithelial lining and sparse fibrovascular stroma are difficult to confirm as thymic in nature. In particular, the alternative possibility of a branchial origin is often considered for such lesions [19]. In some instances, one may need to make a descriptive diagnosis only, leaving the line of differentiation open to question.

Well-documented examples of carcinomatous evolution in thymic cysts are relatively rare [20,21], especially so in particular reference to UTC. Most of the malignant tumors in this setting have had the image of basaloid squamous cell carcinoma, but other thymic carcinoma variants also may be encountered. In the majority of reported cases the malignant neoplasms associated with thymic cysts have behaved surprisingly favorably. Sugio *et al.* also have documented a case where a thymoma arose in the wall of a UTC [22].

(a)

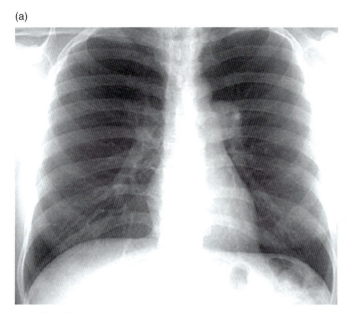

(b)

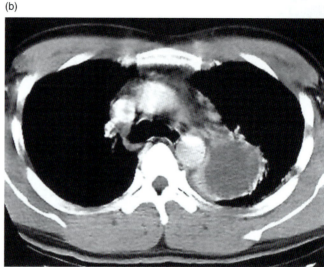

Fig. 12.7 Chest radiograph **(a)** and computed tomogram **(b)** showing a left-sided bronchogenic cyst. The lesion communicates with the left-sided airways and is unilocular.

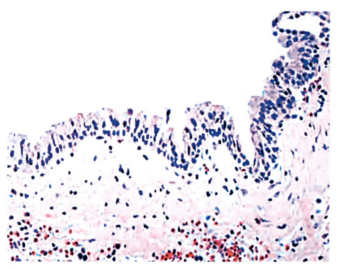

Fig. 12.9 Bronchial-type epithelium, smooth muscle, and cartilage are present in the wall of this bronchogenic cyst (H&E 200X).

Fig. 12.8 The epithelium in this bronchogenic cyst comprises ciliated columnar cells, as true in virtually all cases (H&E 250X).

Bronchogenic cysts

Bronchogenic cysts are thought to derive from supernumerary lung buds, as mentioned earlier in this discussion. They are most commonly situated in the middle or anterior mediastinum, or within the pulmonary parenchyma, but other intrathoracic locations may be observed as well [2,23–25]. Patients with bronchogenic cysts may be of any age, and there is no sex predilection. Intrapulmonary cysts sometimes demonstrate a communication with the tracheobronchial tree, and they may present with symptoms and signs of bacterial superinfection [26]. On the other hand, mediastinal lesions are characteristically asymptomatic and are usually detected on screening chest radiographs [25,27].

The radiological image of a bronchogenic cyst (BC) is that of a round or oval mass (Fig. 12.7) that molds itself to surrounding structures. As true of thymic cysts, BCs are uniformly dense and may exhibit a rim of calcification. Angiographic studies demonstrate an independent systemic arterial vascular supply to the cysts in some instances [26].

BCs can be macroscopically unilocular or septated and they may be multiple [26]. These lesions have thin fibrous walls and are filled with milky, mucoid, or gelatinous material [3].

Microscopically, a bronchial-type epithelial lining is virtually always apparent, comprising pseudostratified, often-ciliated columnar cells. In addition, smooth muscle or islands of cartilage are seen in the cyst wall in 70% to 80% of cases (Figs. 12.8 and 12.9). Cholesterol granulomas are absent, as are adjacent thymic remnants.

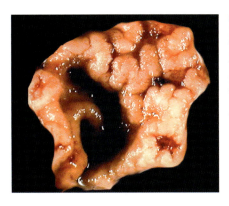

Fig. 12.10 Gross photograph of excised gastroenteric cyst of the posterior mediastinum. The cuff of tissue surrounding the "mouth" of the cyst has the macroscopic appearance of gastric mucosa.

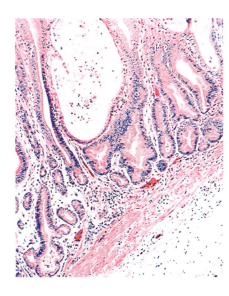

Fig. 12.11 This photomicrograph of an excised gastroenteric cyst demonstrates a specialized gastric-type epithelial mucosal lining (H&E 200X).

Surgical excision is curative in the vast majority of BC cases. Exceptionally, these lesions may be complicated by the development of associated sarcomas (usually of the smooth-muscle type) or carcinomas, but those possibilities are reflected only by anecdotal reports [25,28–32].

Enteric cysts

Esophageal and gastroenteric cysts of the mediastinum probably evolve from misplaced rests of the developing foregut [2], and are seen typically in children under the age of 15. Esophageal cysts may present with dysphagia or subnormal weight gain, but gastroenteric cysts (GECs) are associated with a broader array of symptoms including cough, vomiting, fever, and pneumonia or empyema [33–40]. GECs also may be linked to bony anomalies including hemivertebrae and spina bifida [37,39].

Radiographically, intrathoracic enteric cysts are usually rounded or irregularly shaped posterior mediastinal masses that are uniform in density or loculated. In cases where the cyst contents have leaked into surrounding tissues, pleural effusions or pulmonary consolidation may be seen as well [38,40].

Enteric cysts have thick fibromuscular walls and smooth or "corrugated" mucosal linings (Fig. 12.10). They range in size from 2 to 10 cm, may be unilocular or multichambered, and are sometimes associated with pericystic fibrous adhesions [2,3,40].

Microscopically, both esophageal cysts and GECs feature a double layer of smooth muscle. Esophageal cysts can have either a columnar or a squamous epithelial lining, whereas GECs contain specialized gastric glandular mucosa – sometimes complete with chief and parietal cells – or intestinal epithelium (Fig. 12.11) [2,40].

Gastric acid secretion by such lesions may lead to erosion of the cyst wall and perforation [41]. A number of fatalities have occurred due to the latter complication [40,41], but enteric cysts are typically relatively innocuous and are cured by simple excision. Malignant transformation has occurred extraordinarily rarely, as reviewed by Lee *et al.* [42].

Pericardial cysts

Mediastinal pericardial cysts virtually always are located in the cardiophrenic angle, probably as remnants of the ventral-parietal recesses of the pleuropericardial membranes. These lesions are seen in patients of all ages, usually as asymptomatic abnormalities on chest roentgenograms [2,7,43,44]. Rare cases have presented with dyspnea or substernal chest pain [7].

Radiologically, pericardial cysts are irregularly rounded masses that abut the cardiac contours but are clearly separated from the soft tissues of the chest wall (Fig. 12.12) [44]. They may be seen in the anterior, middle, or posterior mediastinal compartments. Computed tomograms or magnetic resonance images demonstrate a thin cyst wall and water-isodense fluid contents [15].

The gross image of pericardial cysts is unimpressive, represented by delicate fibrovascular walls with a smooth internal lining and resembling common hernia sacs. Histologically, one observes an external layer of laminated fibrous tissue mantled by cytologically bland mesothelial cells (Fig. 12.13) [2,3]. These are usually present as a single layer, but focal mesothelial hyperplasia may be apparent as well. Cartilage, smooth muscle, cholesterolotic granulomas, and specialized glandular epithelial elements are all absent in pericardial cysts.

Surgery is curative in all cases. There have been no reports of malignant change in pericardial cysts.

Meningocele

Meningoceles – i.e., herniations of the dura mater – occasionally present in the posterior mediastinum as cystic masses, in both children and adults [45–47]. They may produce no symptoms whatsoever or be associated with neurological deficits. Radiographic studies show a unilocular thin-walled cystic mass with the internal density of water, closely apposed to the spinal column. Vertebral defects in the vertebral bodies are often visible as well on magnetic resonance images. Excised meningoceles have thin fibrovascular walls that are mantled by an attenuated layer of meningothelial cells; psammomatous microcalcifications may be present as well.

(a)

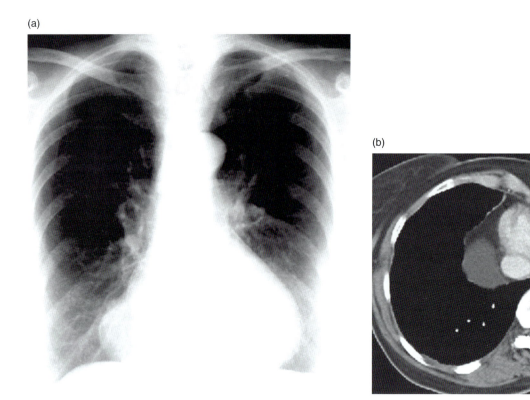

(b)

Fig. 12.12 Chest radiograph **(a)** and computed tomogram **(b)** showing a pericardial cyst of the anterior mediastinum, projecting into the right hemithorax. The lesion abuts the cardiac contours.

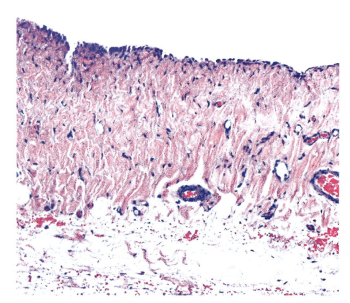

Fig. 12.13 Microscopically, this pericardial cyst shows a flattened mesothelial lining and an attenuated fibroadipose tissue wall (H&E 160X).

Acquired mediastinal cystic lesions

Infectious and post-inflammatory cystic lesions

Intramediastinal abscesses represent a complication of primary or secondary suppurative mediastinitis. They can be seen in patients of any age and in any of the mediastinal compartments. Most of these lesions are caused by bacterial infections, and the clinical context makes their pathologic diagnosis straightforward [48–50].

A more unusual infectious mediastinal cyst has been documented by Karnak and colleagues. They described a four-year-old boy with an isolated mass in the posterior mediastinum; excision showed a hydatid cyst caused by infection with *Echinococcus granulosus* [51].

Rarely, patients with pancreatitis and pancreatic pseudocysts will manifest the latter lesions via transdiaphragmatic herniation and secondary involvement of the posterior mediastinum [52–54]. Again, the clinical setting typically makes the diagnosis obvious; therefore, pathologists are rarely presented with pseudocysts as surgical specimens.

Multilocular thymic cysts and secondary thymic cysts

Contrary to the formerly-held generalization that all thymic cysts were congenital, there are well-defined circumstances in which such lesions are clearly acquired in nature. The most well-known of these situations concern multilocular thymic cysts (MTCs) and secondary formation of thymic cysts in lesions of mediastinal lymphoma. Another reported, but less certain, cause of acquired thymic cysts is that of surgical trauma to the thymus gland. Jaramillo *et al.* have documented three cases in which thymic cysts were seen in patients who had undergone previous thoracic surgery [55].

MTC was first defined as an entity by Suster and Rosai in 1991 [56], and those authors posited that it represented an

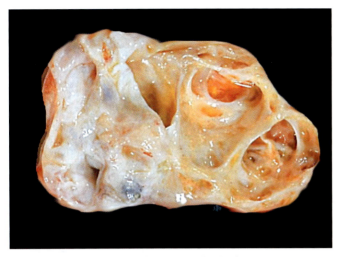

Fig. 12.14 Gross photograph of excised multilocular thymic cyst, demonstrating several internal septations.

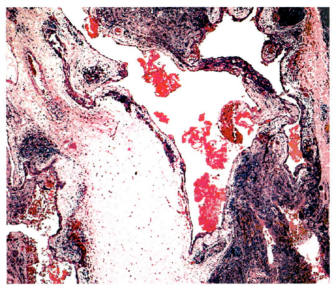

Fig. 12.15 The septa in this multilocular thymic cyst are variably invested by lymphoid tissue, some of which demonstrates incipient formation of germinal centers. Most of them have no epithelial lining (H&E 100X).

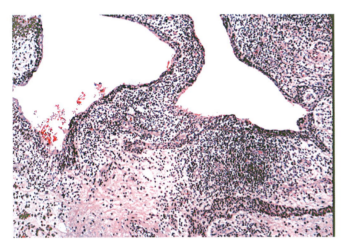

Fig. 12.16 The septa in another multilocular thymic cyst show attenuated squamoid epithelial surfaces (H&E 200X).

acquired process rather than a congenital abnormality. Support for that contention has steadily accrued subsequently, in the form of an association between MTC and various intrathoracic neoplasms (including thymoma, seminoma, thymic carcinoma, teratoma, and Langerhans' cell histiocytosis [57–63]; autoimmune disorders such as Sjogren's syndrome [64]; and infection with the human immunodeficiency virus [65–68]). The last of those scenarios is reminiscent of parotid cysts that are seen in the context of the acquired immunodeficiency syndrome [68].

Multilocular cysts are usually seen in adults, although occasional pediatric cases have been reported [56,57]. Most patients are typically asymptomatic and their lesions are found incidentally on screening radiographs. However, some individuals present with chest discomfort or dyspnea. Imaging studies of the thorax often – but not invariably – show the internal fibrous septation that is characteristic of MTC, and soft tissue attenuation also may be seen in the walls of such lesions [69]. Accordingly, cystic neoplasms are potentially included in the radiographic differential diagnosis of MTC.

Pathologically, one observes loculated spaces in MTC of varying sizes and shapes, bounded by fibrovascular tissue (Fig. 12.14). The capsule is typically intact, but it may be adherent to adjacent structures in the chest. Cyst contents may be watery, mucoid, or milky. The epithelial cells in the lining of MTC are cytologically-bland; they can be squamoid, cuboidal, or columnar [56]. Small nests of non-neoplastic thymic epithelium – sometimes with the image of Hassall's corpuscles – are present in the cyst septations or capsule. Degenerative cellular debris, focal hemorrhage, lymphoid follicles with germinal centers, cholesterol granulomas, and stromal fibrovascular proliferation are additional common findings in MTC (Figs. 12.15 and 12.16) [56]. Chetty and Reddi reported an unusual example of this lesion in which rhabdomyoma-like elements were also seen [70].

"Proliferating" MTC is a distinctive variant of this pathologic entity [18]. In that subtype, interconnecting and pseudoinvasive cords of modestly-atypical thymic epithelium project away from the central cystic cavities (Fig. 12.17). The epithelial cells have nucleoli and demonstrate mitotic activity, causing potential concern over possible malignancy. However, on scanning microscopy, proliferating MTCs show a circumscription that would not be expected in thymic carcinomas – with a "pushing" front to the proliferative elements – supporting their benign nature. This variation from the usual histologic image of MTC appears to have no prognostic significance whatsoever.

As mentioned earlier, the possibility does indeed exist that a true neoplasm will be associated with MTC. Hence, thorough histological sampling is indicated in each case. In particular, several reports have been made of treated mediastinal Hodgkin and non-Hodgkin lymphoma (HL) being associated with intrathoracic masses that have the appearance of MTCs [71–81]. Initially, it was thought that such cysts always represented a

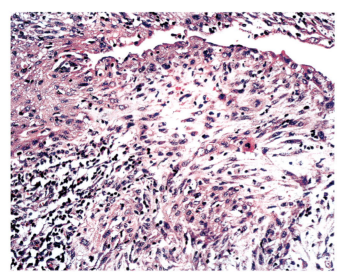

Fig. 12.17 Striking pseudoepitheliomatous hyperplasia is present in the wall of this "proliferating" multilocular thymic cyst (H&E 300X).

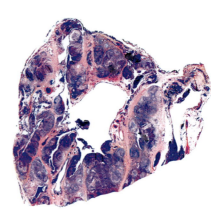

Fig. 12.18 The formation of a cyst lined by thymic epithelium is visible in the center of this mass of excised mediastinal Hodgkin lymphoma (H&E 75X).

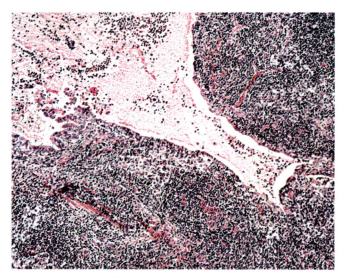

Fig. 12.19 A microcyst lined by thymic epithelium is present within this intramediastinal lymphomatous mass (H&E 200X).

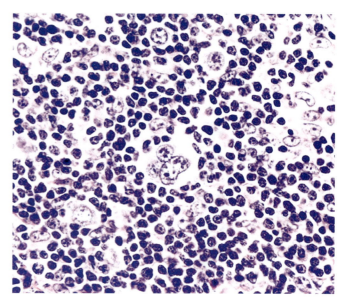

Fig. 12.20 The walls of the cyst show the typical appearance of classical Hodgkin lymphoma (H&E 300X).

byproduct of irradiation or chemotherapy. However, examples of HL have also been well-documented in which cystic lesions clearly predated such treatments [75,76]. Small epithelial cysts in HL appear to be centered on dilated and degenerating Hassall's corpuscles. Therefore, we believe that the lymphomatous infiltrate probably compromises the structure of the epithelial nests, leading to secondary cyst formation (Figs. 12.18–12.20). *"Ex vacuo"* enlargement of these microcysts probably takes place after therapeutic ablation of the surrounding malignant tissue.

Mullerian cysts of the posterior mediastinum

In 2005, Hattori [82] reported a posterior mediastinal cyst in an adult woman, the epithelial lining of which resembled that of endosalpingiosis in the abdomen. Since then, several other examples of "Hattori cysts" have been documented [83,84]. These lesions have a paravertebral location and are typically unilocular with fluid contents. Their epithelial lining is ciliated and mirrors the appearance of a Fallopian tube (Fig. 12.21). Immunohistochemical evaluation has demonstrated reactivity for CA-125, estrogen receptor protein, and progesterone receptor protein in Hattori cysts. Simple excision is curative.

Primary cystic neoplasms of the mediastinum

Three lineages of primary neoplasms in the mediastinum – vascular, mesothelial, and teratoid – may yield *de novo* cystic masses.

Vascular lesions

Lymphangiomas ("cystic hygromas") and hemangiomas have been encountered in all three mediastinal compartments as thin-walled cystic masses [85–89]. Lymphangiomas may

(a)

(b)

(c)

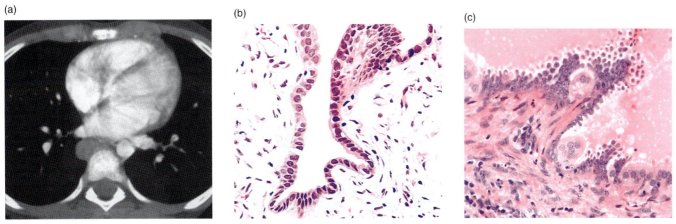

Fig. 12.21 This paravertebral cyst of the posterior mediastinum, as seen in a computed tomogram **(a)**, is lined by columnar epithelial cells, some of which are ciliated **(b and c)**. The appearance is synonymous with that of cystic endosalpingiosis of the abdomen.

(a)

(b)

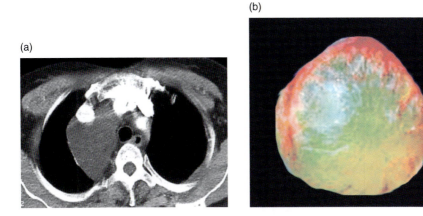

Fig. 12.22 Computed tomographic **(a)** and gross **(b)** images of anterior mediastinal lymphangioma, showing a nondescript fluid-filled spherical mass with a thin fibrous wall.

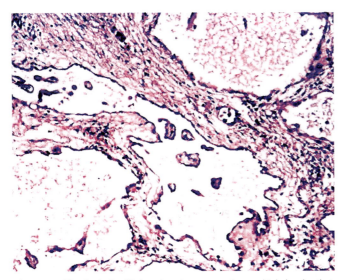

Fig. 12.23 Histologically, this lymphangioma comprises multiple locules that are lined by plump lymphatic endothelial cells. Their contents are principally represented by a cellular proteinaceous fluid (H&E 200X).

be either unilocular or multilocular on imaging studies, whereas cystic hemangiomas usually show internal septations [89,90]. Their vascular nature is easily demonstrated with the use of "dynamic" radiographic techniques that employ contrast agents, or by angiography. These lesions predominate in children, but some present for the first time in adulthood. Pathologically, lymphangiomas are thin-walled collapsible cysts that contain watery serous fluid, comprising relatively large chambers lined by an inconspicuous layer of flattened endothelium (Figs. 12.22 and 12.23). Lymphorrhagia is common in the lesional stromal tissue, and vascular channels may contain numerous lymphocytes as well. Hemangiomas show a more complex internal substructure, with more numerous and closely apposed vascular channels, and these tumors contain many more erythrocytes than lymphangiomas do. A recently developed monoclonal antibody – "D2–40"– has been touted as a selective endothelial marker which can be used to identify lymphangiogenic neoplasms objectively by immunohistology [93].

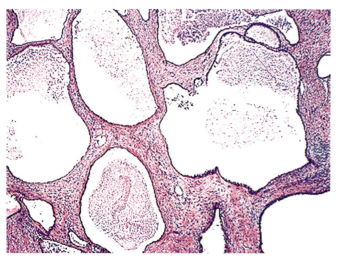

Fig. 12.24 Multicystic mesothelial proliferation of borderline malignancy, arising in the anterior mediastinum. This lesion is composed of multiple chambers lined by plump, slightly atypical mesothelial cells (H&E 100X).

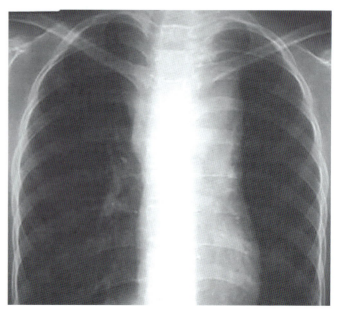

Fig. 12.25 Chest radiograph showing a mature cystic teratoma of the anterosuperior mediastinum. The lesion contains delicate mural calcification.

(a)

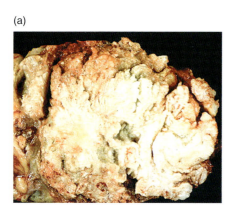

(b)

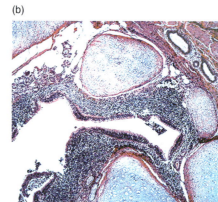

Fig. 12.26 Gross photograph **(a)** of an excised mature cystic mediastinal teratoma. Its contents are dominated by "cheesy" keratinous material. Other histologic components include cartilage and respiratory epithelium **(b)**, potentially leading to diagnostic confusion with bronchogenic cyst (H&E 100X).

Mesothelial neoplasms

Two types of cystic mesothelial neoplasm have been described in the mediastinum. Plaza *et al.* [94] documented a multiloculated cystic adenomatoid tumor in the anterior mediastinum of an adult woman who presented with chest pain. That benign neoplasm showed a striking histological similarity to adenomatoid tumors of the gynecologic and testicular adnexae, which are familiar to all surgical pathologists. Two reports have also concerned cystic lesions in the anterior mediastinum with structural homology to a tumor more commonly seen in the pelvic peritoneum; namely, multicystic mesothelial proliferation of borderline malignancy (MMPBM; "multiple mesothelial inclusion cysts"; "multicystic mesothelioma") (Fig. 12.24) [95,96]. The tumor cells lining the loculated chambers in MMPBM usually have a "hobnail" epithelioid character; they are immunoreactive for keratin, calretinin, mesothelin, HMBE-1 antigen, and WT-1. Internal septations are composed of hypocellular fibrous tissue.

Cystic germ cell tumors

Although germ cell tumors of the mediastinum are rare in general, the most frequently-seen representative of that group is benign cystic teratoma (BCT) of the thymic region [43,44,97–100]. This tumor is typically observed during adolescence or young adulthood, usually in asymptomatic patients, and with a striking predilection for males. It presents as an anterosuperior mediastinal mass on thoracic imaging studies, often with peripheral "eggshell" calcification (Fig. 12.25) [45,104]. Pathologic evaluation shows cellular constituents that reflect at least two of the three embryonic lineages, principally represented by cytologically-bland, mature,

(b)

(a)

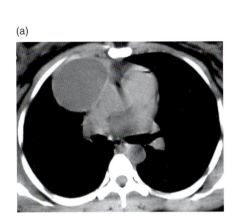

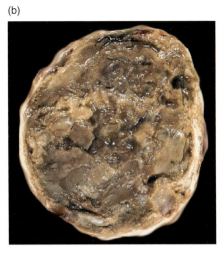

Fig. 12.27 (a) CT and (b) macroscopic photograph of an excised thymoma demonstrating near-total cystification. This change may be caused by infarctive-type ischemic necrosis, and has no adverse biological implications.

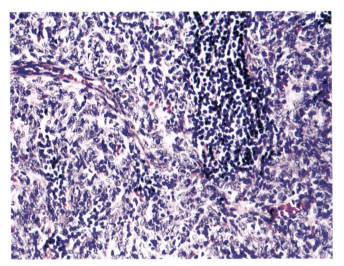

Fig. 12.28 Remnants of a typical thymoma are seen here, in the wall of a cystic thymoma (H&E 300X).

architecturally-abnormal tissues which do not include primitive neuroepithelial elements. Cysts in BCTs are usually mantled by squamous or respiratory-type epithelium, and keratinous debris is commonly seen in the cystic cavities (Fig. 12.26) [43,44]. Unlike the situation pertaining to cystic teratomas of the testis, there is no malignant potential associated with anterior mediastinal BCT, and excision is curative.

Cystic change in predominantly "solid" mediastinal neoplasms

In general, the vast majority of tumors of the mediastinum are solid masses at a radiographic and macroscopic level. However, a distinctive subset of them may undergo substantial degenerative change and cystification, potentially simulating the images of the other lesions described thus far in this discussion.

Probably the best example of this phenomenon is represented by effete changes in thymoma. Suster and Rosai [105]

described ten examples of that neoplasm in which extensive cystic alteration had taken place, sufficient to confuse them with non-neoplastic thymic cysts. These tumors were characterized by multiple large cystic cavities and serosanguinous or grumous contents (Fig. 12.27). Some tissue surrounding the cystic spaces had typical features of thymoma – at least focally – including an epithelial cell constituency (Fig. 12.28), permeation by lymphocytes, and perivascular serum lakes. However, many of the internal septa were devoid of an epithelial covering. The authors of that study suggested that cystification in thymoma is an extreme outcome of the microcyst formation that is so common in that neoplasm [105]. Notably, they also found secondary fibroinflammatory changes around the cystic lesions, often causing them to adhere to adjacent intrathoracic structures. That observation should not lead one to a diagnosis of malignancy, because it does not reflect true tumoral invasion. Indeed, all of the patients in the series of Suster and Rosai had favorable outcomes.

Moran and Suster [106] extended these observations in a further series of thymomas that showed extreme hemorrhagic change and even internal necrosis, again yielding cystification. Such alterations were felt to have a degenerative vasoocclusive-infarctive etiology, rather than reflecting tumor necrosis as seen in malignancies. That premise was supported by outcomes data in the study, which showed no tumor-related deaths.

Prominent cystic change has likewise been reported in thymic seminoma (Fig. 12.29), thymic neuroendocrine tumors (Fig. 12.30), non-endocrine primary thymic carcinomas, and posterior mediastinal neurilemmomas [107–110]. Aside from producing potential diagnostic confusion at radiographic and pathologic levels of examination, that alteration again does not appear to affect tumor behavior or prognosis in such cases.

Finally, Moran et al. [111] have recently described three examples of well-differentiated ovarian serous carcinoma that selectively metastasized to the anterior mediastinum. All of the

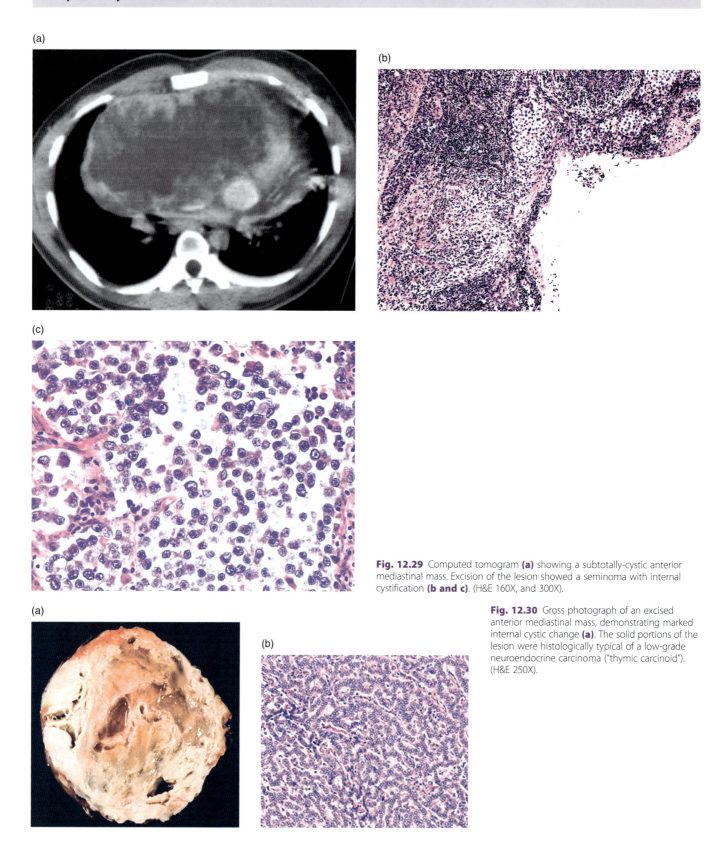

(a)

(b)

(c)

Fig. 12.29 Computed tomogram **(a)** showing a subtotally-cystic anterior mediastinal mass. Excision of the lesion showed a seminoma with internal cystification **(b and c)**. (H&E 160X, and 300X).

(a)

(b)

Fig. 12.30 Gross photograph of an excised anterior mediastinal mass, demonstrating marked internal cystic change **(a)**. The solid portions of the lesion were histologically typical of a low-grade neuroendocrine carcinoma ("thymic carcinoid"). (H&E 250X).

patients in that series had presented with stage III disease but had no other extra-abdominal tumor implants other than those in the mediastinum. Pathologic examination of the excised intrathoracic lesions demonstrated a histologic image which was remarkably similar to that of MTC, except for the focal presence of an atypical papillary epithelial proliferation. The latter component was immunoreactive for MOC-31 and CA-125, establishing its identity as metastatic Mullerian-type carcinoma.

References

1. Kirwan WO, Walbaum PR, McCormack RM: Cystic intrathoracic derivatives of the foregut and their complications. *Thorax* 1973; 28: 424–8.

2. Salyer DC, Salyer WR, Eggleston JC: Benign developmental cysts of the mediastinum. *Arch Pathol Lab Med* 1977; 101:136–9.

3. Marchevsky AM: Mediastinal tumor-like conditions and tumors that can simulate thymic neoplasms, *In*: Givel J-C (Ed): *Surgery of the Thymus.* Berlin, Springer-Verlag, 1990; pp. 151–62.

4. Langman J: *Medical Embryology.* Baltimore, Williams & Wilkins, 1969; pp. 183–280.

5. Wenglowski R: Uber die Halsfisteln und Cysten. *Langenbecks Arch Klin Chir* 1912; 100: 789–892.

6. Gilmour JR: The embryology of the parathyroid glands, the thymus, and certain associated rudiments. *J Pathol Bacteriol* 1937; 45: 507–22.

7. Lillie WI, McDonald JR, Clagett OT: Pericardial celomic cysts and pericardial diverticula: A concept of etiology and report of cases. *J Thorac Surg* 1950; 20: 494–504.

8. Clark OH: Mediastinal parathyroid tumors. *Arch Surg* 1988; 123:1096–1100.

9. Leong ASY: Thymic cysts, *In*: Givel J-C (Ed): *Surgery of the Thymus.* Berlin, Springer-Verlag, 1990; pp. 71–7.

10. Indeglia RA, Shea MA, Grage TB: Congenital cysts of the thymus gland. *Arch Surg* 1967; 94: 149–52.

11. Krech WG, Storey CF, Umiker WC: Thymic cysts: A review of the literature and report of two cases. *J Thorac Cardiovasc Surg* 1954; 27: 477–93.

12. Breckler IA, Johnston DG: Choristoma of the thymus. *Am J Dis Child* 1956; 92: 175–8.

13. Ovrum E, Birkeland S: Mediastinal tumors and cysts: A review of 91 cases. *Scand J Thorac Cardiovasc Surg* 1979; 13: 161–8.

14. Youngson GG, Ein SH, Geddie WR, *et al.*: Infected thymic cyst. *Pediatr Pulmonol* 1987; 3: 276–9.

15. Schnyder P, Gamsu G: Computed tomography and magnetic resonance imaging, *In*: Givel J-C (Ed): *Surgery of the Thymus.* Berlin, Springer-Verlag, 1990; pp. 217–25.

16. Bieger RC, McAdams AJ: Thymic cysts. *Arch Pathol* 1966; 82: 535–41.

17. Guba AM, Adam AE, Jaques DA, *et al.*: Cervical presentation of thymic cysts. *Am J Surg* 1978; 136: 430–6.

18. Suster S, Barbuto D, Carlson G, Rosai J: Multilocular thymic cysts with pseudoepitheliomatous hyperplasia. *Hum Pathol* 1991; 22: 455–60.

19. Lyons TJ, Dickson JAS, Variend S: Cervical thymic cysts. *J Pediatr Surg* 1989; 24: 241–3.

20. Leong ASY, Brown JH: Malignant transformation in a thymic cyst. *Am J Surg Pathol* 1984; 8: 471–5.

21. Chalabreysse L, Etienne-Mastroianni B, Adeleine P, *et al.*: Thymic carcinoma: a clinicopathological and immunohistological study of 19 cases. *Histopathology* 2004; 44: 367–74.

22. Sugio K, Ondo K, Yamaguchi M, *et al.*: Thymoma arising in a thymic cyst. *Ann Thorac Cardiovasc Surg* 2000; 6: 329–31.

23. Ramenofsky ML, Leape LL, McCauley RGK: Bronchogenic cyst. *J Pediatr Surg* 1979; 14: 219–24.

24. Maier HC: Bronchogenic cysts of the mediastinum. *Ann Surg* 1948; 127: 476–502.

25. Cuypers P, DeLevn P, Cappelle L, *et al.*: Bronchogenic cysts: a review of 20 cases. *Eur J Cardiothorac Surg* 1996; 10: 393–6.

26. Agha FP, Master K, Kaplan S, *et al.*: Multiple bronchogenic cysts in the mediastinum. *Br J Radiol* 1975; 48: 54–7.

27. Robbins LL: The roentgenologic appearance of "bronchiogenic" cysts. *Am J Roentgenol* 1943; 50: 321–33.

28. Bernheim J, Griffel B, Versano S, *et al.*: Mediastinal leiomyosarcoma in the wall of a bronchial cyst. *Arch Pathol Lab Med* 1980; 104: 221.

29. Endo C, Imai T, Nakagawa H, Ebina A, Kaimori M: Bronchioloalveolar carcinoma arising in a bronchogenic cyst. *Ann Thorac Surg* 2000; 69: 933–5.

30. Okada Y, Mori H, Maeda T, *et al.*: Congenital mediastinal bronchogenic cyst with malignant transformation: an autopsy report. *Pathol Int* 1996; 46: 594–600.

31. Miralles-Lozano F, Gonzalez-Martinez B, Luna-More S, Valencia-Rodriguez A: Carcinoma arising in a calcified

bronchogenic cyst. *Respiration* 1981; 42: 135–7.

32. Ashizawa K, Okimoto T, Shirafuji T, *et al.*: Anterior mediastinal bronchogenic cyst: demonstration of complicating malignancy by CT and MRI. *Br J Radiol* 2001; 74: 959–61.

33. Ladd WE, Scott HW Jr: Esophageal duplications or mediastinal cysts of enteric origin. *Surgery* 1944; 16: 815–35.

34. Black RA, Benjamin EL: Enterogenous abnormalities: cysts and diverticula. *Am J Dis Child* 1936; 51: 1126–37.

35. Poncher HG, Milles F: Cysts and diverticula of intestinal origin. *Am J Dis Child* 1933; 45: 1064–78.

36. Veeneklaas GMH: Pathogenesis of intrathoracic gastrogenic cysts. *Am J Dis Child* 1952; 83: 500–7.

37. Fallon M, Gordon ARG, Lendrum AC: Mediastinal cysts of foregut origin associated with vertebral abnormalities. *Br J Surg* 1954; 41: 520–33.

38. Sabiston D, Scott HW: Primary neoplasms and cysts of the mediastinum. *Ann Surg* 1961; 136: 777–97.

39. Crispin RH, Logan WD Jr, Abbott OA: Mediastinal gastroenteric cyst with vertebral anomaly. *Dis Chest* 1965; 47: 346–7.

40. Chitale AR: Gastric cyst of the mediastinum: A distinct clinicopathological entity. *J Pediatr* 1969; 75:104–10.

41. Spock A, Schneider S, Baylin J: Mediastinal gastric cysts. *Am Rev Respir Dis* 1966; 94: 97–110.

42. Lee MY, Jensen E, Kwak S, Larson RA: Metastatic adenocarcinoma arising in a congenital foregut cyst of the esophagus: a case report with review of the literature. *Am J Clin Oncol* 1998; 21: 64–6.

43. Abell MR: Mediastinal cysts. *Arch Pathol* 1956; 61: 360–71.

44. Morrison IM: Tumors and cysts of the mediastinum. *Thorax* 1958; 13: 294–307.

45. Jeung MY, Gasser B, Gangi A, *et al.*: Imaging of cystic masses of the mediastinum. *Radiographics* 2002; 22 (Suppl): S79–S93.

46. Maldonado RG, Extremera BG, Alegre V, Vara-Thorbeck R: Intrathoracic meningocele presenting as a mediastinal mass lesion: case report. *Zentralbl Neurochir* 1992; 53: 11–14.

47. Wilhelm E: Meningocele of the thoracic cavity: contribution to differential diagnosis of tumors of the posterior mediastinum. *Thoraxchirurgie* 1954; 2: 147–55.

48. Hirai T, Kimura S, Mori N: Head and neck infections caused by *Streptococcus milleri* group: an analysis of 17 cases. *Auris Nasus Larynx* 2005; 32: 55–8.

49. Novellas S, Kechabtia K, Chevallier P, Sedat J, Bruneton JN: Descending necrotizing mediastinitis: a rare pathology to keep in mind. *Clin Imaging* 2005; 29: 138–40.

50. Mihos P, Potaris K, Gakidis I, Papadakis D, Rallis G: Management of descending necrotizing mediastinitis. *J Oral Maxillofac Surg* 2004; 62: 966–72.

51. Karnak I, Ciftci AO, Tanyel FC: Hydatid cyst: an unusual etiology for a cystic lesion of the posterior mediastinum. *J Pediatr Surg* 1998; 33: 759–60.

52. Landreneau RJ, Johnson JA, Keenan RJ, *et al.*: "Spontaneous" mediastinal pancreatic pseudocyst fistulization to the esophagus. *Ann Thorac Surg* 1994; 57: 208–10.

53. Johnston RH Jr, Owensby LC, Vargas GM, Garcia-Rinaldi R: Pancreatic pseudocyst of the mediastinum. *Ann Thorac Surg* 1986; 41: 210–12.

54. Banks PA, McLellan PA, Gerzof SG, *et al.*: Mediastinal pancreatic pseudocyst. *Dig Dis Sci* 1984; 29: 664–8.

55. Jaramillo P, Perez-Atayde A, Griscom NT: Apparent association between thymic cysts and prior thoracotomy. *Radiology* 1989; 172: 207–9.

56. Suster S, Rosai J: Multilocular thymic cyst: an acquired reactive process. Study of 18 cases. *Am J Surg Pathol* 1991; 15: 388–98.

57. Rakheja D, Weinberg AG: Multilocular thymic cyst associated with mature mediastinal teratoma: a report of 2 cases. *Arch Pathol Lab Med* 2004; 128: 227–8.

58. Hattori H: High-grade thymic carcinoma other than basaloid or mucoepidermoid type could be associated with multilocular thymic cyst: report of two cases. *Histopathology* 2003; 43: 501–2.

59. Wakely PE Jr, Suster S: Langerhans' cell histiocytosis of the thymus associated with multilocular thymic cyst. *Hum Pathol* 2000; 31: 1532–5.

60. Kawashima O, Kamiyoshihara M, Sakata S, *et al.*: Basaloid carcinoma of the thymus. *Ann Thorac Surg* 1999; 68: 1863–5.

61. Silverman JF, Olson PR, Dabbs DJ, Landreneau R: Fine-needle aspiration cytology of a mediastinal seminoma associated with multilocular thymic cyst. *Diagn Cytopathol* 1999; 20: 224–8.

62. Liang SB, Ohtsuki Y, Sonobe H, *et al.*: Multilocular thymic cysts associated with thymoma: a case report. *Pathol Res Pract* 1996; 192: 1283–7.

63. Iezzoni JC, Nass LB: Thymic basaloid carcinoma: a case report and review of the literature. *Mod Pathol* 1996; 9: 21–5.

64. Kondo K, Mihoshi T, Sakiyama S, Shimosato Y, Monden Y: Multilocular thymic cyst associated with Sjogren's syndrome. *Ann Thorac Surg* 2001; 72: 1367–9.

65. Chieng DC, Demaria S, Yee HT, Yang GC: Multilocular thymic cyst with follicular lymphoid hyperplasia in a male infected with HIV: a case report with fine needle aspiration cytology. *Acta Cytol* 1999; 43: 1119–23.

66. Kontny HU, Sleasman JW, Kingma DW, *et al.*: Multilocular thymic cysts in children with human immunodeficiency virus infection: clinical and pathologic aspects. *J Pediatr* 1997; 131: 264–70.

67. Avila NA, Mueller BU, Carrasquillo JA, *et al.*: Multilocular thymic cysts: imaging features in children with human immunodeficiency virus infection. *Radiology* 1996; 201: 130–4.

68. Leonidas JC, Berdon WE, Valderrama E, *et al.*: Human immunodeficiency virus infection and multilocular thymic cysts. *Radiology* 1996; 198: 377–9.

69. Choi YW, McAdams HP, Jeon SC, *et al.*: Idiopathic multilocular thymic cyst: CT features with clinical and histopathologic correlation. *Am J Roentgenol* 2001; 177: 881–5.

70. Chetty R, Reddi A: Rhabdomyomatous multilocular thymic cyst. *Am J Clin Pathol* 2003; 119: 816–21.

71. Katz M, Peikarski JD, Bayle-Weisgerber C, *et al.*: Residual mediastinal mass following radiation therapy for Hodgkin's disease. *Ann Radiol* 1977; 20: 667–72.

72. Baron RL, Sagel SS, Baglan RJ: Thymic cysts following radiation therapy for Hodgkin's disease. *Radiology* 1981; 141: 593–7.

73. Murray JA, Parker AC: Mediastinal Hodgkin's disease and thymic cysts. *Acta Haematol* 1984; 71: 282–4.

74. Kin HC, Nosher J, Haas A, *et al.*: Cystic degeneration of thymic Hodgkin's disease following radiation therapy. *Cancer* 1985; 55: 354–6.

75. Kaesberg PR, Foley DB, Pellett J, *et al.*: Concurrent development of a thymic cyst and mediastinal Hodgkin's disease. *Med Pediatr Oncol* 1988; 16: 293–4.

76. Lewis CR, Manoharan A: Benign thymic cysts in Hodgkin's disease: Report of a case and review of published cases. *Thorax* 1987; 42: 633–4.

77. Gadomski A, Wagiel K: Cyst of lower mediastinum in a 14 year old boy with tumor of mediastinum in the course of Hodgkin's disease. *Wiad Lek [Pol J Med]* 1998; 51 (Suppl): 331–3.

78. Kamiya N, Yokoi K, Mori K, Tominaga K, Miyazawa N: Thymic Hodgkin's disease with cystic variants: a case report. *Nihon Kyobu Shikkan Gakkai Zasshi [Jpn J Thorac Dis]* 1995; 33: 999–1002.

79. Takeshita K, Terashima T, Urano T, *et al.*: Hodgkin's disease with a giant thymic cyst. *Nihon Kyobu Shikkan Gakkai Zasshi [Jpn J Thorac Dis]* 1994; 32: 680–4.

80. Borgna-Pignatti C, Andreis IB, Rugolotto S, Balter R, Bontempini L: Thymic cyst appearing after treatment of mediastinal non-Hodgkin lymphoma. *Med Pediatr Oncol* 1994; 22: 70–2.

81. Veeze-Kuijpers B, Van Andel JG, Stiegelis WF, Boldewijn JK: Benign thymic cyst following mantle radiotherapy for Hodgkin's disease. *Clin Radiol* 1987; 38: 289–90.

82. Hattori H: Ciliated cyst of probable Mullerian origin arising in the posterior mediastinum. *Virchows Arch* 2005; 446: 82–4.

83. Thomas-de-Montpreville V, Dulmet E: Cysts of the posterior mediastinum showing Mullerian differentiation (Hattori cysts). *Ann Diagn Pathol* 2007; 11: 417–20.

84. Batt RE, Mhawech-Fauceglia P, Odunsi K, Yeh J: Pathogenesis of mediastinal paravertebral Mullerian cysts of Hattori: developmental endosalpingiosis – Mullerianosis. *Int J Gynecol Pathol* 2010; 29: 546–51.

85. Povraz AS, Kilic D, Hatipoglu A, *et al.*: Cystic lymphangioma confined to mediastinum in an adult. *Jpn J Thorac Cardiovasc Surg* 2004; 52: 567–79.

86. Daya SK, Gowda RM, Gowda MR, Khan IA: Thoracic cystic lymphangioma (cystic hygroma): a chest pain syndrome – a case report. *Angiology* 2004; 55: 561–4.

87. Shetty RC, Aggarwal BK, Kamath SG, *et al.*: Giant cystic lymphangioma of the middle mediastinum. *Indian J Chest Dis Allied Sci* 2003; 45: 125–9.

88. Marc K, Kabiri H, Caidi M, *et al.*: Cystic lymphangioma of the mediastinum: seven cases. *Rev Pneumonol Clin* 2002; 58: 214–18.

89. Oshikiri T, Morikawa T, Jinushi E, Kawakami Y, Katoh H: Five cases of lymphangioma of the mediastinum in adults. *Ann Thorac Cardiovasc Surg* 2001; 7: 103–5.

90. Charruau L, Parrens M, Jougon J, *et al.*: Mediastinal lymphangioma in adults: CT and MR imaging features. *Eur Radiol* 2000; 10: 1310–14.

91. Riquet M, Briere J, LePimpec-Barthes F, Puvo P: Lymphangiohemangioma of the mediastinum. *Ann Thorac Surg* 1997; 64: 1476–8.

92. Wright CC, Cohen DM, Vegunta RK, Davis JT, King DR: Intrathoracic cystic hygroma: a report of three cases. *J Pediatr Surg* 1996; 31: 1430–2.

93. Fukunaga M: Expression of D2-40 in lymphatic endothelium of normal tissues and in vascular tumors. *Histopathology* 2005; 46: 396–402.

94. Plaza JA, Dominguez F, Suster S: Cystic adenomatoid tumor of the mediastinum. *Am J Surg Pathol* 2004; 28: 132–8.

95. Drut R, Quijano G: Multilocular mesothelial inclusion cysts (so-called benign multicystic mesothelioma) of pericardium. *Histopathology* 1999; 34: 472–4.

96. Sasaki H, Yano M, Kiriyama M, *et al.*: Multicystic mesothelial cyst of mediastinum: report of a case. *Surg Today* 2003; 33: 199–201.

97. Kim JH, Goo JM, Lee HJ, *et al.*: Cystic tumors in the anterior mediastinum: radiologic-pathologic correlation. *J Comput Assist Tomogr* 2003; 27: 714–23.

98. Wakely PE Jr: Cytopathology-histopathology of the mediastinum: epithelial, lymphoproliferative, and germ cell neoplasms. *Ann Diagn Pathol* 2002; 6: 30–43.

99. Takeda S, Miyoshi S, Ohta M, *et al.*: Primary germ cell tumors in the mediastinum: a 50-year experience at a single Japanese institution. *Cancer* 2003; 97: 367–76.

100. Weidner N: Germ cell tumors of the mediastinum. *Semin Diagn Pathol* 1999; 16: 42–50.

101. Moran CA, Suster S: Primary germ cell tumors of the mediastinum: I. Analysis of 322 cases with special emphasis on teratomatous lesions and a proposal for histopathologic classification and clinical staging. *Cancer* 1997; 80: 681–90.

102. Verhaeghe W, Meysman M, Noppen M, *et al.*: Benign cystic teratoma: an uncommon cause of anterior mediastinal mass. *Acta Clin Belg* 1995; 50: 126–9.

103. Dulmet EM, Macchiarini P, Suc B, Verley JM: Germ cell tumors of the mediastinum: a 30-year experience. *Cancer* 1993; 72: 1894–1901.

104. Wu TT, Wang HC, Chang YC, *et al.*: Mature mediastinal teratoma: sonographic imaging patterns and pathologic correlation. *J Ultrasound Med* 2002; 21: 759–65.

105. Suster S, Rosai J: Cystic thymomas: a clinicopathologic study of ten cases. *Cancer* 1992; 69: 92–7.

106. Moran CA, Suster S: Thymoma with prominent cystic and hemorrhagic changes and areas of necrosis and infarction: a clinicopathologic study of 25 cases. *Am J Surg Pathol* 2001; 25: 1086–90.

107. Moran CA, Suster S: Mediastinal seminomas with prominent cystic changes: a clinicopathologic study of 10 cases. *Am J Surg Pathol* 1995; 19: 1047–53.

108. Takeda S, Hirano H, Maeda H, *et al.*: Thymic carcinoma with a large cystic lesion. *Jpn J Thorac Cardiovasc Surg* 2004; 52: 574–6.

109. Moran CA, Suster S: Angiomatoid neuroendocrine carcinoma of the thymus: report of a distinctive morphological variant of neuroendocrine tumor of the thymus resembling a vascular neoplasm. *Hum Pathol* 1999; 30: 635–9.

110. Petkar M, Vaideeswar P, Deshpande JR: Surgical pathology of cystic lesions of the mediastinum. *J Postgrad Med* 2001; 47: 235–9.

111. Moran CA, Suster S, Silva EG: Low-grade serous carcinoma of the ovary metastatic to the anterior mediastinum simulating multilocular thymic cysts: a clinicopathologic and immunohistochemical study of 3 cases. *Am J Surg Pathol* 2005; 29: 496–9.

Mesenchymal tumors of the mediastinum

Bonnie Balzer, MD, Mark R. Wick, MD, and Susan Parson, MD

Background

In some respects, a review of mediastinal soft tissue neoplasia is a daunting task, because virtually any lesion of somatic soft tissues may arise in this location. The full spectrum of these tumors was first adequately depicted by Pachter and Lattes [1,2,3], and has been summarized in detail on only a few occasions since then [4,5,6,7]. The important contributions of the past years have been not in descriptions of "new" entities, but instead, much of the pertinent literature has dealt with well-characterized tumors and tumor-like processes that were previously unrecognized in the mediastinum. Even so, apart from tumors of nerve sheath, neuroectoderm, adipose tissue, and lymphatic vessels, the majority of intrathoracic soft tissue tumors arise not in mediastinal tissues, but in the visceral structures that they support. Accordingly, most of the neoplasms and pseudoneoplastic processes to be described herein are rather uncommon.

Tumors of peripheral nerve sheath differentiation

Schwannoma (neurilemmoma)

The most common of mediastinal peripheral nerve sheath tumors, schwannomas, are characteristically symmetric lobulated masses in the posterior mediastinum [8]. These lesions, because of their location, may assume a large size before causing symptoms. Indeed, presentation with tracheal, esophageal, or spinal nerve root compression [9] is not common compared with incidental roentgenographic detection [10,11].

Most patients are young adults, although schwannomas may arise at virtually any age [12,13]. Multiple lesions may be observed in unusual instances, particularly in patients with neurofibromatosis, although their presence is not pathognomonic of that disorder [14,15].

The gross pathologic appearance of most such tumors is that of an encapsulated mass that is sharply demarcated from adjacent soft tissues (Fig. 13.1a). In general, the lesion is intimately associated with a large nerve, and may appear to be intraneural in the early stages of its development.

Histologically, the characteristic feature of schwannoma is the juxtaposition of cellular foci (Antoni A) with areas of myxoid degenerative change (Antoni B). The former of these patterns is composed of fusiform cells with elongated, wavy nuclei, and finely fibrillar eosinophilic cytoplasm. They are arranged in compact fascicles that interdigitate or form neurotactoids. Nuclear palisades and Verocay bodies are frequently encountered. Less commonly, cells in Antoni A foci are more loosely arranged. In Antoni B areas, greater variation in cellular size and shape may be observed (Fig. 13.1). Cystification of a myxoid stroma may be prominent. Hyalinized small arteries and arterioles may be noted. On rare occasions, glandular foci may be seen [15,16].

The immunohistochemical hallmark of nerve sheath neoplasms is the expression of Sl00 protein, although not all lesions are reactive [17,18]. Vimentin expression may be accompanied by glial fibrillary acidic protein [19], but staining for cytokeratins and desmin is unexpected [20]. Other neural markers may label these tumors, including CD56 and CD57 [21], and antibodies to myelin basic protein and nerve growth factor receptor [22,23].

Ultrastructurally, schwannomas resemble normal Schwann cells, with numerous interdigitating cell [24] processes extending from elongate or fusiform cells. Cell junctions are seen at sites of apposition, and a continuous basal lamina is present [25]. In some examples, processes envelop collagen bundles in a manner analogous to the mesaxon of peripheral nerve [26]. In occasional examples of schwannoma, striking cellular pleomorphism and nuclear atypia may be seen. The latter features, although cytologically worrisome, are not accompanied by mitotic activity, but instead represent degenerative changes. Such lesions have been referred to as "ancient" schwannomas.

For practical purposes, the granular cell tumor (GCT) represents another variant of schwannoma [27]. Among mediastinal tumors, GCT is uncommon, and has been described only anecdotally [28]. A malignant GCT of the mediastinum has also been reported [29].

Pathology of the Mediastinum, ed. Alberto M. Marchevsky and Mark R. Wick. Published by Cambridge University Press.
© Cambridge University Press 2014.

(a)

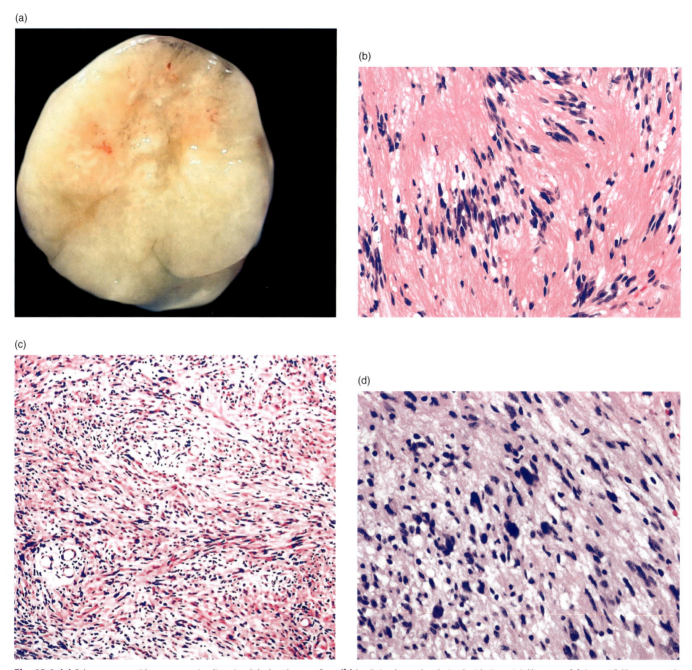

(b)

(c)

(d)

Fig. 13.1 (a) Schwannoma with macroscopic glistening lobulated cut surface; **(b)** hyalinized vessels admixed with Antoni A-like areas; **(c)** Antoni B-like areas with admixed small lymphocytes; **(d)** Ancient change.

Two other histologic variants of schwannoma merit brief discussion. The first is the melanotic schwannoma [30]. Most arise in the posterior mediastinum, and are similar in most respects to other schwannomas (Fig. 13.2) [31]. The pigment is largely due to the presence of melanosomes. Unlike non-pigmented nerve sheath tumors, these melanotic neoplasms may occasionally express melanocytic antigens (e.g., HMB45; Melan-A; PNL2; tyrosinase).

A peculiar variation on this theme has been described recently by Carney, in which melanotic epithelioid and spindle cell lesions of intramediastinal spinal roots were found to contain psammoma bodies [32]. Over half of the patients with "psammomatous melanotic schwannomas" also present with the familial complex of myxomas, spotty pigmentation, and endocrine overactivity. Seven of 31 patients in Carney's original study died with disease, three apparently from metastases.

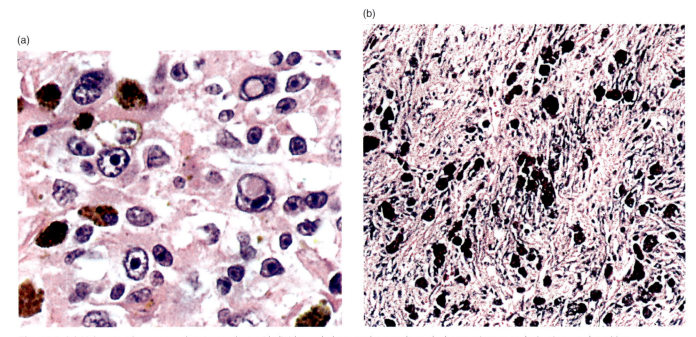

Fig. 13.2 (a) Melanotic schwannoma showing nuclear epithelioid morphology, nucleomegaly, nucleolar prominence, melanin pigment deposition and nuclear inclusions; **(b)** Lower power appearance with pigment deposition and spindled cells in whorls and fascicles.

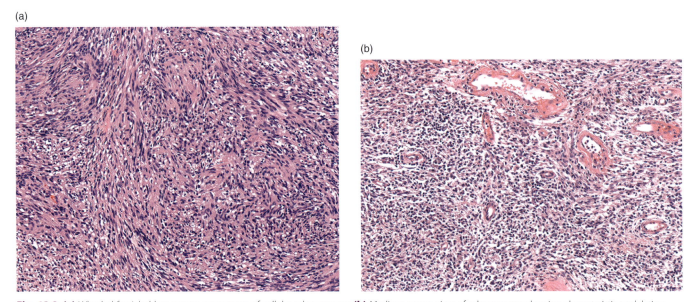

Fig. 13.3 (a) Whorled fascicled low-power appearance of cellular schwannoma; **(b)** Medium-power view of schwannoma showing characteristic undulating nuclei and hyalinized vessels.

Finally, a distinctive peripheral nerve sheath tumor has been described that is dominated by cellular foci of fusiform cells arranged in neurotactoid, fascicular, herringbone, or storiform patterns. Termed "cellular schwannomas"[33], these lesions may lack characteristic Antoni A and Antoni B areas (Fig. 13.3). They are further distinguished by variable cytologic atypia and mitotic activity, often with peripheral aggregates of lymphocytes within or adjacent to the capsule[34]. These encapsulated tumors are most often seen in the mediastinum, retroperitoneum, and paravertebral tissues. Despite initial concerns that cellular schwannomas were low-grade malignancies of peripheral nerve sheath, subsequent clinicopathologic analyses have confirmed their indolent behavior[35]. Local recurrence is variable (5–40%) and may be higher than conventional schwannomas; however, behavior may be due at least in part to the anatomic constraints of complete resectability posed by their location in deep anatomic regions[36]. These lesions show the ultrastructural appearance of Schwann cells; there is disagreement over whether they are as often positive for S100 protein as other forms of schwannoma.

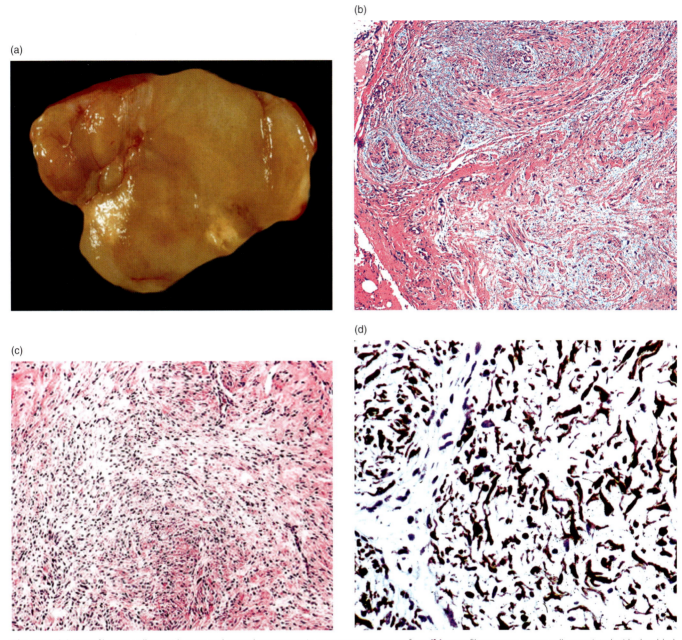

Fig. 13.4 **(a)** Neurofibroma, yellow, with even and smooth macroscopic appearance on cut surface; **(b)** neurofibromatous tumor cells associated with shredded carrot like collagen fibrils and myxoid stroma; **(c)** neurofibroma with hyalinized and stroma and **(d)** S100 positivity.

With the exception of some familial melanotic variants, as noted above, complete surgical resection is considered curative for schwannoma, regardless of histologic type.

Neurofibroma

Neurofibromas (NFs) are the second most common mediastinal nerve sheath tumor, and generally present as solitary lesions in the posterior compartment. There is no obvious gender predilection. Most NFs are asymptomatic, but may cause a spectrum of neural deficits. The most important aspect of NF in the mediastinum or other sites is their association with neurofibromatosis [37]. The presence of multiple mediastinal NFs or single deep plexiform lesions is pathognomonic of this disorder [38–40]. The latter most commonly involve the vagus nerve or the sympathetic chain [41].

Grossly, NF is circumscribed but non-encapsulated, and is centered on, or grows within, a nerve. Most NFs are firm and gray-white, but some may be mucoid, due to accumulation of stromal mucins (Fig. 13.4a). NFs differ from schwannomas histologically, in that NFs are composed of a uniform spindle cell population without obvious palisading. Areas of compact growth, neurotactoid-like structures, and even a storiform pattern may be seen (Fig. 13.4b and c).

(a)

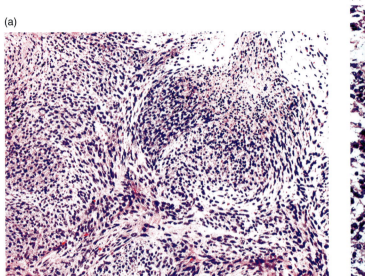

(b)

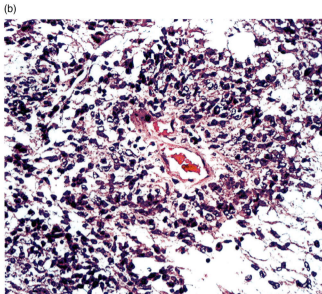

Fig. 13.5 MPNST with **(a)** storiform and fascicled appearance and **(b)** perivascular hypercellularity.

Areas resembling Antoni B changes are lacking; when myxoid changes exist, they are usually diffuse in nature. An admixture of fibroblast-like perineurial cells may be seen, and mast cells may be conspicuous. Nuclear pleomorphism is slight, and mitotic activity should be absent. Areas of atypia or mitotic activity warrant careful examination for the presence of malignant change.

The immunohistochemical profile of NF is essentially identical to that of schwannoma, although S100 protein (Fig. 13.4d), CD56, and CD57 are less commonly detected. An admixture of epithelial membrane antigen-reactive cells, presumably exhibiting perineurial differentiation, may be seen. Ultrastructural analysis reveals an admixture of perineurial, fibroblastic, and schwannian elements.

Unless they attain a large size, entrap nerves, or impinge on thoracic viscera, NFs are cured by surgical excision. Solitary lesions recur infrequently, and are uncommonly associated with malignant degeneration. In contrast, multiple or plexiform lesions in neurofibromatosis recur more often, and may undergo malignant transformation in approximately 1–3% of cases.

Malignant peripheral nerve sheath tumors

Among sarcomas, malignant peripheral nerve sheath tumors (MPNST) are relatively common, yet they are infrequently reported in the mediastinum [42,43]. They occur in one of three settings [44]: in neurofibromatosis, sporadically [45], and as a consequence of prior radiation [46]. These lesions tend to occur in young adults; by comparison, mediastinal MPNST is extremely uncommon in childhood [47].

Most MPNST are posterior mediastinal lesions; some appear to arise in a large nerve or a nerve trunk. Not all lesions share this attribute, but with a history of neurofibromatosis, the diagnosis of MPNST is relatively secure.

Clinical associations are often critical in the accurate diagnosis of MPNST, because there are few histologic features of these tumors that are pathognomonic. Many cases are dominated by a spindled or pleomorphic cell population arranged in a storiform pattern, like that of malignant fibrous histiocytoma. Fewer than one third of MPNST show nuclear palisading, Verocay bodies, or attempts at neurotactoid differentiation (Fig. 13.5). The diagnosis may be complicated by the presence of pigmented elements, or the presence of a predominantly epithelioid-cell population, which may have clear cytoplasm in some cases. In each of these instances, an alternative diagnosis of malignant melanoma may mistakenly be considered [48].

In 10% to 20% of cases, divergent mesenchymal or epithelial elements may be present. These include rhabdomyoblastic [49], angiosarcomatous, chondro-osseous, and glandular patterns (Fig. 13.6) [50]. None of these elements appears to impact the prognosis of MPNST, but their presence may help to identify the neurogenic nature of the tumor [51,52].

The most diagnostically useful immunostaining pattern is exhibited by the dominant spindled and pleomorphic or epithelioid cell population. These cells stain for S100 protein, CD56, or CD57 in two thirds of cases, but not with keratins. Podoplanin is seen in the majority of epithelioid MPNST but is rarely positive in spindle cell/conventional MPNST [53]. The occasional detection of myogenic markers, including desmin or muscle-specific actin, and the occasional detection of cytokeratins [54] – even in lesions lacking overt epithelial differentiation [55]– may complicate the immunohistologic diagnosis of MPNST [56]. In such cases, the presence of neural features on electron microscopy is useful [57–59].

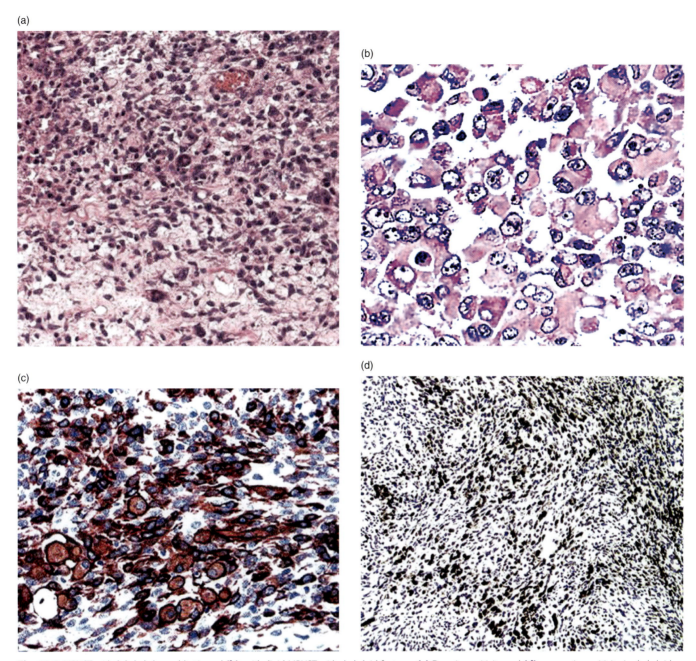

Fig. 13.6 MPNST with **(a)** rhabdomyoblastic and **(b)** epithelioid MPNST with rhabdoid features; **(c)** Desmin positivity and **(d)** myogenin positivity in rhabdoid elements of a malignant Triton tumor.

The overall outlook for patients with mediastinal MPNST is adverse, and it is especially so in the context of neurofibromatosis. Behavior is worsened by a large tumor size and intraneurial spread of such lesions, both of which complicate attempts at surgical resection.

Tumors of neuroectodermal tissue

Neuroblastoma

Neuroblastoma (NB) and its variants – the differentiating neuroblastoma and ganglioneuroblastoma – are part of a morphologic and functional spectrum [60]. Intrathoracic NB comprise less than 20% of all such lesions, and only rarely represent metastases from an adrenal source [61]. The average age at diagnosis for mediastinal NB is four to eight years, but a number of these tumors are detected before one year of age [62]. They may attain a large size, and bony erosion or visceral displacement may be pronounced. Nonetheless, most are encapsulated, and are amenable to surgical extirpation [63]. As in retroperitoneal sites, mediastinal NB are more aggressive in older children [64–66].

Grossly, NB is firm and grayish in appearance, and contains areas of calcification in up to 25% of cases. The cut surface shows areas of degeneration or tumoral hemorrhage.

(a)

(b)

(c)

(d)

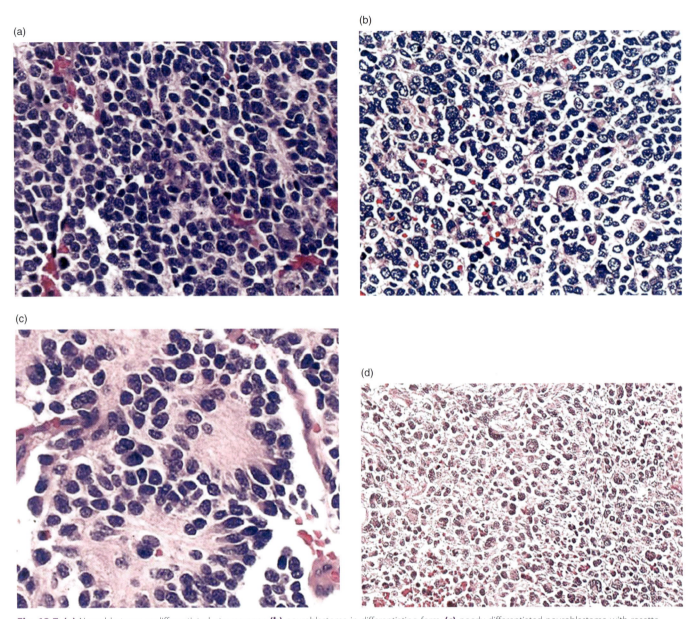

Fig. 13.7 **(a)** Neuroblastoma undifferentiated, stroma poor; **(b)** neuroblastoma in differentiating form; **(c)** poorly differentiated neuroblastoma with rosette formation; **(d)** maturing neuroblastoma with ganglionic differentiation (ganglioneuroblastoma).

The presence of a distinct nodule in an otherwise uniform lesion may indicate a neuroblastic clonal evolution (as seen in the so-called composite ganglioneuroblastoma), a feature that often equates with an unfavorable prognosis [67].

In contrast to adrenal lesions, mediastinal NB usually manifests a recognizable degree of neuritic cellular differentiation and may contain abundant neurofibrillary matrix or gangliocytic elements [68]. In ganglioneuroblastoma, a neurofibromatous stroma may predominate. The basic cellular element in all histologic variants is the neuroblast, a small round cell with little cytoplasm and a round, hyperchromatic nucleus. These cells form sheets or clusters that are interrupted by a delicately vascular stroma. Homer-Wright pseudorosettes or perivascular condensations of cells can be present (Fig. 13.7).

Clinically, mediastinal NB has a comparatively better prognosis than NB reported in other sites [69]. Although resectability has long been suspected as the main factor in this difference, recent data have shown that 60–65% of mediastinal NB present at an early stage (I, II), compared with 38% of other NBs. In addition, 100% of NB tested showed favorable histology based upon the Shimada classification, compared with 85% of NB in other locations. Finally, N-myc amplification in all tested mediastinal NBs had an N-copy number of less than 10 copies, compared with an N-myc amplification of > 10 copies (12%) in the other NBs. These findings suggest that the favorable prognosis is more closely linked to biological prognostic factors rather than the degree of the surgical resection [70,71].

Ganglioneuroma

The ganglioneuroma (GN) represents the most common neuroectodermal tumor of thoracic sympathetic nerves. It is uncommon before one year of age, but most often presents in the first two decades [72]. GN is typically asymptomatic; it is more common in males, well encapsulated, and usually situated near the midline. It may assume a dumb-bell configuration, like some examples of schwannian tumors. Bony erosion is not frequently noted. Regardless of the size or extent of the tumor, very few, if any, GN are fatal [73].

This tumor is firm, and the cut surface may appear whorled or mucoid. Histologically, GN is composed of nests of mature ganglion cells supported by a fibrillar or neurofibroma-like matrix [74,75]. Because gangliocytes may be sparse in some examples, careful histologic examination of all "neurofibromas" in the posterior mediastinum is recommended in young patients. Intratumoral lymphocytes should not be mistaken for collections of neuroblastic elements. Neuroblasts indicate that the lesion is in fact a well-differentiated ganglioneuroblastoma, although the clinical behavior of such tumors does not differ appreciably from that of GN.

Ewing sarcoma family of tumors (ESFT) / extraskeletal Ewing sarcoma (EES) / primitive neuroectodermal tumor (PNET)

The Ewing sarcoma family of tumors (ESFT) constitutes a morphologically heterogeneous group of tumors defined by non-random chromosomal translocations involving the EWS gene and one of a growing number of fusion partners. The ESFT are considerably less common than NB in the mediastinal soft tissues. Separation of NB and ESFT on histologic or ultrastructural grounds is usually readily accomplished [76], especially through the use of cytogenetic or molecular analyses. ESFT lack N-*myc* [77] amplification and instead show a characteristic t(11;22) [78] chromosomal translocation that is not seen in NB [79].

Like undifferentiated or poorly differentiated NB, ESFTs are examples of the small round blue cell tumor group. Histologically, the ESFT is composed of diffuse or pseudolobulated sheets of small undifferentiated cells with high nuclear to cytoplasmic ratio. The cytoplasm is scant but when seen is amphophilic or eosinophilic (Fig. 13.8a and b). A periodic acid Schiff stain will demonstrate intracytoplasmic glycogen which digests with diastase. Occasionally, the tumor can be myxoid or show rosette formation, but neurofibrillary stroma or other matrix type production does not occur. Frequently, ESFT undergoes extensive spontaneous tumor cell necrosis, and the small amount of residual viable tumor may be concentrated in a "peritheliomatous" or a perivascular distribution. Some examples of pleomorphic ESFT with nucleomegaly and nucleolar prominence have been reported.

The typical immunohistochemical profile of *both* NB and ESFT also includes potential reactivity for neuron specific enolase, CD56, CD57, and synaptophysin [80]. Sporadic positivity for cytokeratin, epithelial membrane antigen, and carcinoembryonic antigen in PNET has been reported. Because some examples may also express myogenic determinants, we consider such lesions to be primitive mesenchymal neoplasms with the capacity for divergent differentiation [81–84]. The ability of ESFT to express class I histocompatibility antigens, CD99, and FLI-1 is an additional source of its diagnostic distinction from NB (Fig. 13.8c and d). Based on those data, it is evident that PNET are synonymous biologically with osseous ESFT [85].

The pathogenesis of ESFT is mediated by chromosomal translocation derived fusion oncogenes [86]. Although ~85% of EFT harbor the FLI1-EWSR1 t(11;22)(q24;q12) fusion, an increasing number of fusion partners have been discovered. The second most common translocation found is t(21;22)(q22; q12) ERG-EWSR1, which accounts for 5–15% of EFT. The remainder of translocations account for less than 1% and involve chromosomes 7, 17, 2, 20, 6, 4, 22, 1, 2, and 16 with fusion partners ETV1, E1AF, FEV, NFATC2, POU5F1, SMARCA5, ZSG, ZNF278, SP3, and FUS. Both FISH and PCR can be used to detect these translocations [87].

More frequently one sees ESFT arising in the chest wall or pleuropulmonary tissues ("Askin tumors"). ESFT are distinguished from NB by their clinical features; they tend to occur in adolescents or young adults rather than in young children [88]. ESFT have no cholinergic activity, and they lack overt neural differentiation. Stage for stage, ESFT is a more aggressive neoplasm than NB, and surgical extirpation alone is rarely curative. Current therapy for patients with ESFT consists of chemotherapy and surgery with or without radiation therapy. Despite advancements in therapy, the most reliable prognostic factor in ESFT is whether the disease is localized or metastatic. Combined treatment modalities yield prolonged disease-free survival in no more than 50% of patients [89,90].

Among other neuroectodermal tumors, rare examples of melanotic neuroectodermal tumor of infancy ("progonoma") have been reported [91]. The lack of teratomatous elements in those lesions militate against the alternate diagnosis of teratoid germ cell tumor with neuroectodermal or ependymal differentiation [92].

Ependymoma

Extracranial and extraspinal ependymomas are unusual [93–95]. Only eight cases have been described in the mediastinum, all in the posterior compartment [96] and all in females aged 35 to 71 [97]. Clinically, they are mostly asymptomatic although symptoms secondary to mass effect have been described. Grossly and radiologically they appear circumscribed and show a size range of 5–10 cm.

Histologically, mediastinal ependymomas show identical morphology to that of these tumors in their more common locations. Perivascular pseudorosettes and true ependymal rosette formation is present. Myxopapillary variants of ependymoma have also been described in the mediastinum [98].

(a)

(b)

(c)

(d)

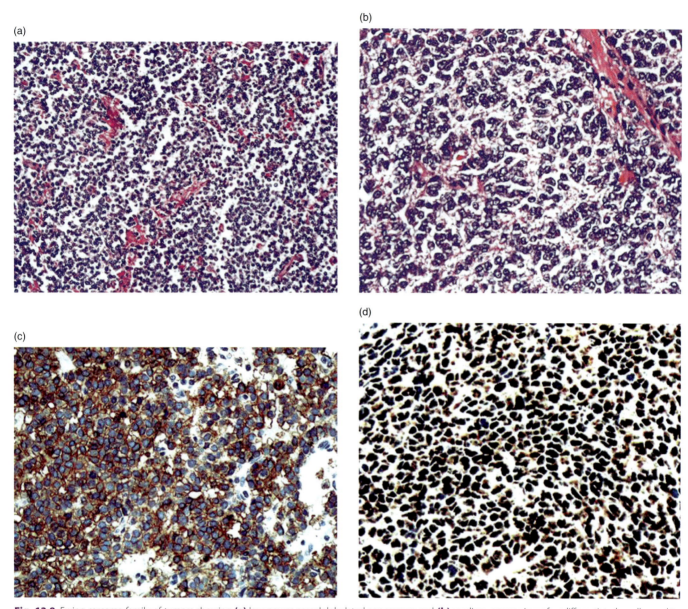

Fig. 13.8 Ewing sarcoma family of tumors showing **(a)** low-power pseudolobulated appearance and **(b)** medium-power view of undifferentiated small round to ovoid tumor cells with indistinct cytoplasmic borders and high N:C ratio; **(c)** membranous strong CD99 reactivity; **(d)** Fli-1 nuclear reactivity in Ewing sarcoma.

By immunohistochemistry tumor cells are positive for glial fibrillary acidic protein and epithelial membrane antigen. Ultrastructural studies demonstrate intracytoplasmic lumina containing microvilli, occasional cytoplasmic basal bodies, and apical cilia. Clinical behavior is indolent and complete resection is considered optimal therapy. Lymph node metastasis has been reported [99].

Lymphatic/vascular tumors

Tumors of endothelium, as a group, comprise approximately one-half of all non-neurogenic mediastinal neoplasms. Most are lesions of lymphatic vessels, and the overwhelming majority are clinically benign.

Lymphangiomas

Lymphangiomas are benign multicystic or cavernous proliferations of lymphatic endothelium and associated mesenchyme. Primary mediastinal lymphangiomas are relatively uncommon, compared with lesions in other somatic sites; nevertheless, they are the single most common vascular tumor encountered in this region [100]. Most lymphangiomas are asymptomatic anterior or anterosuperior lesions, and are usually discovered during adulthood [101].

Despite the relative frequency of primary mediastinal lesions, *secondary* involvement of intrathoracic structures by cervical lymphangiomas ("cystic hygromas") is an even more common phenomenon [102–104]. Those tumors generally occur in

(a)

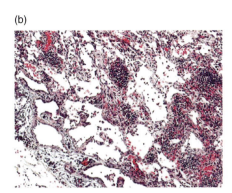

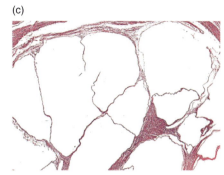

Fig. 13.9 (a) Gross appearance of cystic lymphangioma; **(b)** lymphangioma (deep type) with lymphoid aggregates interspersed among lymphatic channels; **(c)** microscopic example of lymphangioma with ectatic lymphatic channels.

very young children; owing to their size and locally infiltrative nature, they present with considerable disfigurement and vascular or tracheal compression [105,106]. Complete surgical resection of markedly infiltrative lesions is often impossible, and local recurrence may result [107,108].

Some lymphangiomas may regress in response to radiotherapy [109]. However, this approach to the management of unresectable lesions is not recommended, because malignant transformation has been described in this setting [110].

Lymphangiomas are soft, gray and white sponge-like masses that, when incised, exude chylous fluid (Fig. 13.9a). Histologically, irregularly anastomosing channels are lined by flattened endothelium (Fig. 13.9c). These spaces are often intimately associated with lymphoid tissue (Fig. 13.9b). The lymphatic nature of lymphangiomas can be demonstrated by immunoreactivity for podoplanin, recognized by antibody D2–40; that marker does not label non-lymphatic endothelia.

In unusual cases, multiple lymphangiomas may arise in somatic and visceral sites. Such examples of "lymphangiomatosis" [111,112] usually affect children. Mediastinal involvement is often accompanied by chylothoraxt, a finding that implies an adverse prognosis [113]. Because of their multiplicity and their tendency to show a diffuse infiltrative growth pattern, with extension into adjacent pulmonary parenchyma, multifocal lymphangiomas are rarely resectable. Finally, as noted above, malignant transformation may rarely occur in mediastinal lymphangiomas if they are irradiated.

Hemangiomas

Compared with tumors of lymphatic vessels, mediastinal hemangiomas are uncommon; most examples are encountered in the superior mediastinum [114]. There is no gender predilection, and, in contrast to patients with primary lymphangiomas, most individuals present with cough, stridor, hoarseness, dysphagia, or vena caval obstruction. Neurological impingement in the superoanterior compartment may result in Horner's

syndrome, whereas posterior extension and spinal involvement can lead to sensorimotor deficits. Multiple hemangiomas in the mediastinum are seen uncommonly.

Hemangiomas are variably-solid and -cystic, reddish masses that are bloody when incised (Fig. 13.10a). As in other sites, they are composed of anastomosing capillary channels or cavernous endothelially lined spaces [115]; cavernous lesions are more common in children (Fig. 13.10b) [116]. Grossly infiltrative margins are a worrisome feature that often predict recurrence [117]. The constituent cells are cytologically bland, and mitotic activity is sparse or absent. Stromal edema or myxoid changes may be conspicuous, intervascular stromal cells are fusiform or stellate.

Surgical excision is usually curative if it is complete. Occasionally, however, either its large size or juxtaposition to other mediastinal structures impedes total removal of mediastinal hemangiomas.

Immunohistochemical identification of hemangiomas is rarely necessary, but those which have a markedly cellular composition may sometimes simulate other lesions morphologically. In such cases, reactivity for CD31, CD34, GLUT-1, and FLI-1 will serve to establish the endothelial nature of the tumors.

Borderline and malignant vascular tumors

Vascular lesions with borderline or overtly malignant behavior are infrequently encountered in the mediastinum. The first group of them comprises vasoformative lesions that are composed of randomly disposed epithelioid or spindle cells, a proportion of which contain intracytoplasmic lumina.

Epithelioid hemangioendothelioma

The first authors to use the term "epithelioid hemangioendothelioma" (EH) were Enzinger and Weiss [118]. This tumor may arise in the lungs, liver, bones, skin, and soft tissue.

(a)

(b)

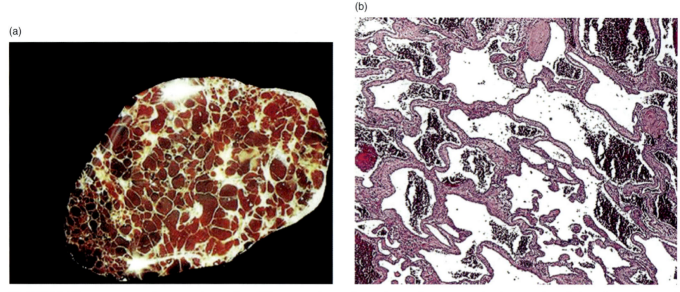

Fig 13.10 (a) Gross appearance of cavernous hemangioma; **(b)** cavernous hemangioma, microscopic appearance showing muscular walled ectatic irregular spaced venous channels containing erythrocytes.

(b)

(a)

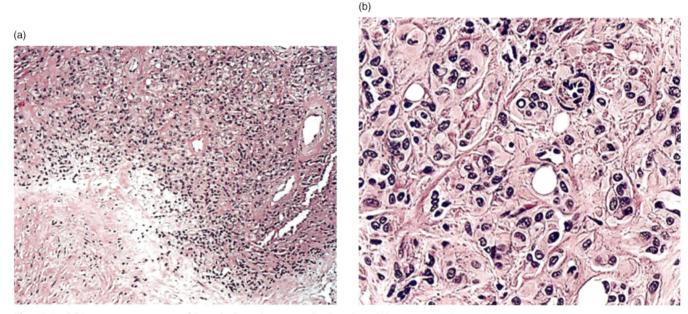

Fig. 13.11 (a) Low power appearance of EH in the lung, showing small cells with cord-like growth and foci of hyaline necrosis; **(b)** medium-power view of lobulated and nested EH tumor cells, some with a distinct intracytoplasmic lumen.

Mediastinal examples have been documented in both the antero-superior and posterior compartments [119,120,121].

As in other sites, mediastinal EH may be relatively circum-scribed but unencapsulated [122]. It comprises round to oval cells that are dispersed in a collagenous, or sometimes-pseudocartilaginous stroma (Fig. 13.11). Alternately, the neo-plastic cells form nests in which intracytoplasmic lumina are apparent. Nuclei are generally small and bland, and cytoplasm is eosinophilic or amphophilic. Mitotic activity is generally not pronounced in EH, and tumoral necrosis is absent.

An unusual example of EH was reported by Lamovec *et al.*, in which osteoclast-like giant cells were admixed with other-wise typical endothelial elements [123]. The vascular nature of the epithelioid cells in EH can be confirmed by the ultrastructural presence of cytoplasmic Weibel-Palade bodies and active pino-cytosis. Histochemical binding of *Ulex europaeus* I agglutinin is also typical, as is immunohistochemical reactivity for CD31, CD34, and FLI-1 [124].

EH generally pursues a prolonged clinical course of growth. Even so, the potential for local recurrence, and metastatic disease in as many as 20% of lesions, justifies its designation as a low-grade ("borderline") malignancy [125].

Kaposiform hemangioendothelioma

Another hemangioendothelioma morphotype that may be encountered in the mediastinum is "kaposiform" hemangioen-dothelioma (KHE) [126]. It is predominantly seen in children, and mediastinal localization is far less common than a cutane-ous one. A peculiarity of this neoplasm – especially when it attains a large size – is the presence of the Kasabach-Merritt phenomenon, wherein platelets become trapped in the tumor and the patient develops secondary thrombocytopenia [127].

Microscopically, KHE manifests an image that combines elements of capillary hemangioma and Kaposi sarcoma. Hence, one sees small-caliber tubular blood vessels punctuat-ing a multi-micronodular spindle-cell proliferation, with extravasated erythrocytes in the background. Mitotic activity is modest, as is nuclear atypia. Peripheral aspects of KHE are indistinct, blending with the adjacent soft tissue.

Whereas Kaposi sarcoma cells are usually immunoreactive for *Herpesvirus* 8-latent nuclear antigen 1 (HHV8LNA1; see below), that marker is lacking in KHE [128]. Positivity for CD31, CD34, GLUT-1, FLI-1, and Proxil [129] is typical.

The behavior of KHE is again that of a "borderline" malig-nancy, principally reflected by a tendency for recurrence. Only rare metastasizing lesions of this type have been seen. The presence of the Kasabach-Merritt phenomenon is itself an adverse finding, because of the profound consumption coagu-lopathy that it produces.

Kaposi sarcoma

Kaposi sarcoma (KS) is best-known as a cutaneous malig-nancy, nowadays most often seen in the context of systemic infection with the human immunodeficiency virus (HIV). Nevertheless, this tumor also has the ability to arise in various viscera and in the deep soft tissue. Mediastinal lesions are typically centered in intrathoracic lymph nodes, but we have also seen occasional examples of KS in the mediastinal soft tissue in HIV-infected individuals. Because of its association with that virus, mediastinal KS occurs in patients who are young to middle-aged adults. Concurrent tumoral involve-ment of the great vessels, pericardium, pleura, and lungs causes cardiorespiratory insufficiency in such cases. Some patients also have Castleman disease or effusion-related non-Hodgkin lymphoma, both of which, like KS, are also related causally to *Herpesvirus* 8.

Grossly, KS is typified by a multinodular, reddish-violet lesion with indistinct borders. Its cut surfaces are fleshy and violaceous, but frank bloodiness is not a typical feature.

Microscopically, deep KS usually is a dense spindle-cell proliferation in which a proportion of the lesional cells contain cytoplasmic vacuoles. Extravasation of erythrocytes through-out the tumor is frequent. Nuclear atypia in the lesional cells varies considerably, and, in its extreme form, one may have difficulty with a diagnostic separation from spindle-cell

angiosarcoma. Other potential KS morphotypes include a lymphangioma-like form and a sclerotic variant.

Immunohistological studies demonstrate only variable reactivity in KS for CD31, CD34, and FLI-1, but podoplanin is consistently detectable [130]. In addition, immunostains or *in-situ* hybridization studies for HHV8LNA1 are positive in approximately 85% of cases [131].

The prognosis of mediastinal KS is difficult to judge with certainty, because of the considerable comorbidities which patients with that tumor have. If the tumor is clinically judged to be the cause of significant organ dysfunction, irradiation or chemotherapy are indicated.

Angiosarcoma

Less than 1% of mediastinal malignancies represent angiosar-coma (AS) [132]; those examples are more common in young patients, unlike the population that typically develops *cutane-ous* AS [133]. This neoplasm is aggressive; it may assume a very large size, and exhibits obviously infiltrative growth.

Overt histological vasogenesis, which is typical of AS in non-mediastinal sites, is also manifest in the thorax. Tumor cells with large, hyperchromatic, pleomorphic nuclei form interanastomosing channels that "dissect" through the sup-porting stroma (Fig. 13.12). Lesional borders are indistinct. AS of the epithelioid type is also more common in deep soft tissue sites such as the mediastinum (Fig. 13.13a). Vascular spaces in that lesion can be relatively inconspicuous, and diagnostic confusion with other epithelioid neoplasms may consequently occur. As mentioned earlier, the spindle-cell variant of AS has some resemblance to Kaposi sarcoma and it may imitate other spindle-cell malignancies as well (Fig. 13.13b).

Immunoreactivity for CD31, CD34, FLI-1, or podoplanin is typical of AS (Fig. 13.14). Epithelioid variants may also aberrantly express keratin and CA72.4, but other epithelial markers such as epithelial membrane antigen and p63 are lacking in such tumors. Myogenous and neural determinants are likewise absent.

Fibroblastic, myofibroblastic and "fibrohistiocytic" tumors
Desmoid-type fibromatosis

Fibroblastic-myofibroblastic tumors such as "desmoid"-type (aggressive) fibromatosis (DTF) are encountered in virtually all soft tissue sites. When they occur in the mediastinum, these neoplasms may arise in either the posterior or anterior compartments, and are most often seen in children and young adults [134–138]. Because of the relative infrequency of infantile (myo)fibromatosis in the mediastinum, it will not be discussed here.

DTF is typified macroscopically by a deceptively circum-scribed appearance, with a fascicular white-tan cut surface (Fig. 13.15a). No necrosis or hemorrhage is present.

(a)

(b)

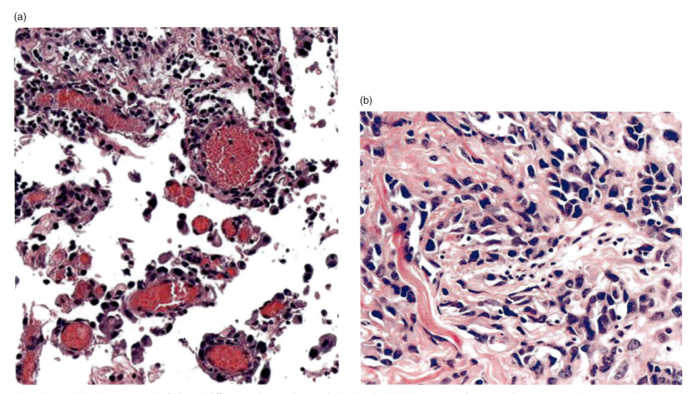

Fig. 13.12 (a) Angiosarcoma with fairly well-differentiated areas showing hobnail endothelioid tumor cells forming rudimentary vascular channels with discohesion; **(b)** cellular area of angiosarcoma with high-grade cytology and a rare cell with a poorly formed intracytoplasmic lumen.

(a)

(b)

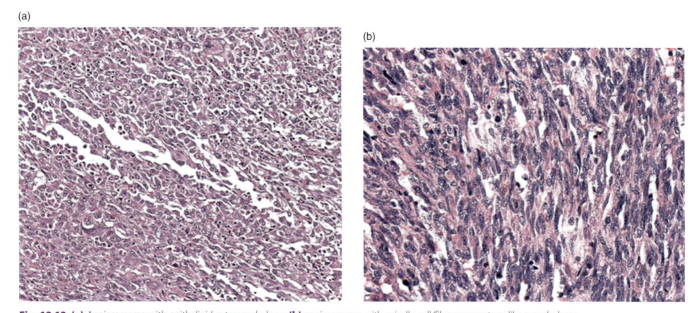

Fig. 13.13 (a) Angiosarcoma with epithelioid cytomorphology; **(b)** angiosarcoma with spindle cell/fibrosarcomatous-like morphology.

Histologically, one sees interweaving and sparsely-cellular bundles of cytologically-bland fusiform cells, set in a myxofibrous stroma (Fig. 13.15b). Few if any mitoses are present in DTF, and if one sees more than one per several high-power microscopic fields, the alternative diagnosis of low-grade fibrosarcoma should seriously be considered.

Supporting stromal vessels have a small caliber but show surprisingly thick walls. The lesion tends to "shade-off" into surrounding connective tissue at a histological level, and therefore has indistinct borders. Invasion of other anatomic structures, such as large blood vessels and nerves, is a potential finding [139].

(a)

(b)

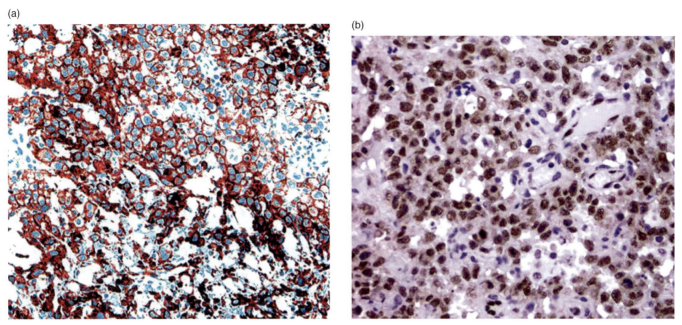

Fig. 13.14 (a) CD31 positivity in angiosarcoma with membranous circumferential positivity; **(b)** Fli-1 nuclear positivity in angiosarcoma.

(a)

(b)

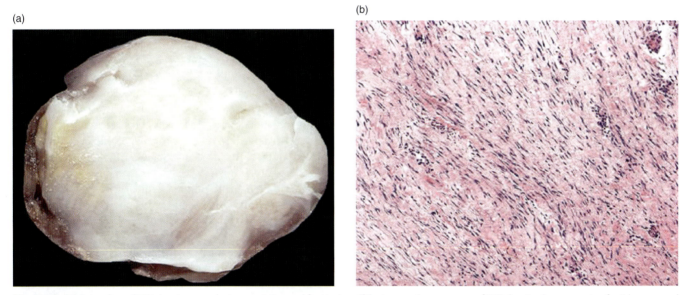

Fig. 13.15 (a) Cut surface of DTF showing pseudocircumscription and firm texture; **(b)** microscopic appearance of DTF showing long sweeping fascicles arranged in a regular intersecting pattern among parallel thin vascular channels with slight perivascular lymphocytic infiltrates.

Immunophenotypically, DTF shows a myoid phenotype, being potentially reactive for vimentin, various actin isoforms, desmin, caldesmon, and calponin. A distinctive feature of this lesion, however, is the presence of intranuclear beta-catenin, which tends to separate DTF from other bland spindle-cell proliferations.

If desmoid tumors can be completely resected [140,141] successfully, surgical cure is possible. Recurrences are common, however, and these are likewise best managed operatively. Irradiation has been used to treat extremely large and infiltrative examples of DTF, with mixed results. Chemotherapy is increasingly used in treating fibromatosis, and has shown promise in controlling growth of unresectable tumors and in delaying recurrence in previously marginally resected tumors.

Fibrosarcoma and related lesions

Historically, adult-type mediastinal fibrosarcomas (FS) were regarded as relatively common neoplasms [142–148]. However, in recent years, many lesions classified as such have been shown to actually represent other malignancies or various sarcoma subtypes. These include pleomorphic undifferentiated sarcoma (malignant fibrous histiocytoma; MFH), myxofibrosarcoma, low-grade fibromyxoid sarcoma of Evans, leiomyosarcoma, malignant peripheral nerve sheath tumor, synovial sarcoma, and sarcomatoid carcinoma or mesothelioma, all of which may occur in the anterior or posterior mediastinum [149]. Hence, the true incidence of FS in general at those locations is low, but mediastinal fibrosarcomas are rare. As mentioned earlier, its diagnostic distinction from DTF rests on the cytological atypia of the spindle cell population, and the presence of mitotic activity.

Grossly, FS has a cut surface resembling "fish flesh", and may contain areas of hemorrhage and necrosis. Histological images in this tumor vary somewhat, and a classical "herringbone" growth pattern is by no means present uniformly. Likewise, the amount of stromal collagen associated with the tumor cells is variable. Mitotic activity and nuclear pleomorphism comprise a spectrum in FS, and these factors obviously affect the grading of such lesions.

The immunohistochemical diagnosis of FS is one of ultimate exclusion. If a comprehensive panel of myogenous, epithelial, and neural markers is negative, and no distinctive cytogenetic indicators of other tumors exist (e.g., t(7;16) or t (X;18) chromosomal translocations), the diagnosis of FS may be considered. It should be assigned to a vimentin-positive neoplasm that is cytologically malignant and completely constituted by spindle-cells.

The prognosis of mediastinal FS depends principally on its grade, size, and surgical resectability. Those tumors with a high histological grade respond more consistently to irradiation and chemotherapy, but have a greater risk of metastasis compared with those of lower grade, which have a propensity for locally aggressive behavior.

Pleomorphic undifferentiated sarcoma (previously included under malignant fibrous histiocytoma (MFH))

Although it is the most common histologic morphotype of soft tissue sarcoma, pleomorphic undifferentiated sarcoma or MFH is not often seen in the mediastinum. Under 100 cases have been reported, the bulk of which have arisen in the posterior mediastinum [150-152]. As in other sites, these tumors are aggressive. An apparent exception to that statement, as described by Yellin et al., concerned a patient who died of tumor after 16 years of disease-free survival [153]. That particular lesion had initially been interpreted as a neurofibroma, and the possibility that it represented a "dedifferentiated" neurogenic tumor cannot be excluded.

The gross appearance of MFH is variable, depending on the cellularity of the lesion, the presence of myxoid stroma, and the extent of tumoral necrosis.

Histologically, most tumors are composed of atypical spindled and pleomorphic cells which are often arranged in a storiform pattern. Bizarre multinucleated tumor cells are not uncommon, and many pathologically-shaped mitotic figures can be seen as well (Fig. 13.16).

As is true of fibrosarcoma, the immunophenotype of MFH is one that lacks specialized epithelial, myogenous, and neural markers. Some cases can be labeled for alpha-isoform actin, but that particular determinant is not restricted to myogenic cells. The differential diagnosis includes other potentially-pleomorphic sarcomas such as rhabdomyosarcoma, liposarcoma, MPNST, and "dedifferentiated" liposarcoma. The probability of a primary undifferentiated sarcoma occurring in the mediastinum and visceral organs, particularly the lung, is extremely low, compared to a primary sarcomatoid carcinoma or metastasis. A clear clinical history should resolve the possibility of metastasis. However, on biopsies or small samples, sarcomatoid carcinoma may be indistinguishable from an undifferentiated sarcoma despite the use of immunohistochemistry, unless defining carcinomatous components are present.

Congenital infantile fibrosarcoma

Congenital infantile fibrosarcoma has rarely been reported in the mediastinum as the subject of case reports [154]. It is a malignant neoplasm, which is essentially confined to patients under ten years of age. Historically it has been described under the names desmoplastic fibrosarcoma of infancy, medullary fibromatosis of infancy, and juvenile fibrosarcoma.

Histologically the tumor is composed of uniform, spindled fibroblasts or myofibroblasts exhibiting elongated nuclei with hyperchromatic granular chromatin nucleolar prominence, and scanty cytoplasm. Architecturally, the tumor cells are arranged in cellular or hypercellular patterns of fascicles intersecting at acute angles. There is an intimate mixture of inflammatory cells mostly consisting of small lymphocytes. Frequent mitotic figures often with abnormal forms are present. Other features include a variably myxoid stroma, hemangiopericytic vasculature, and round cell transformation (Fig. 13.17).

Immunohistochemical studies definitionally lack evidence of any specific lineage although actin may be variably positive in a myofibroblastic pattern. Other markers including cytokeratin, desmin, S100 protein, CD34, epithelial membrane antigen, and CD117 are negative.

Cytogenetically, the following reproducible translocation t(12;15)(p13;26) defines the neoplasm [155]. This translocation involves the NTRK3 tyrosine kinase receptor [156]. This translocation is shared also with congenital mesoblastic nephroma [157].

Clinically, the vast majority of tumors occur under the age of two years with a small subset of diagnoses reported between the ages of two and ten years, and must be confirmed by cytogenetic analysis [158]. There is an approximate 25% recurrence rate and 10% metastatic disease under the age of 5. The differential diagnosis includes infantile fibromatosis (lipofibromatosis), fibrous hamartoma of infancy, desmoids

(a)

(b)

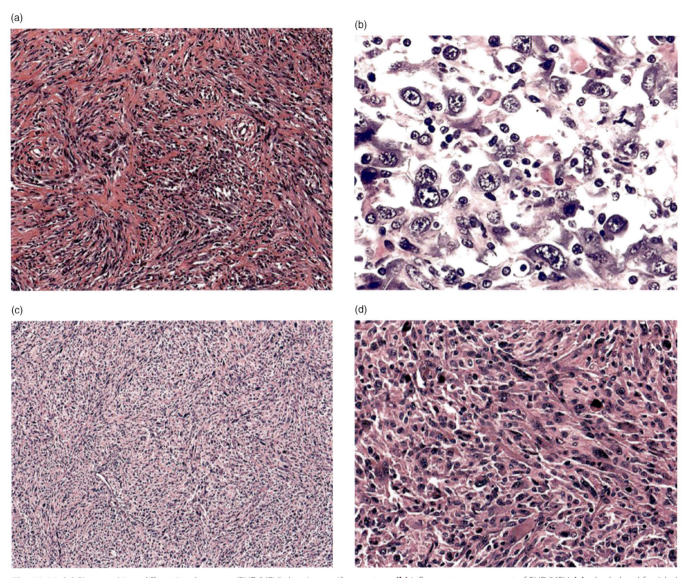

(c)

(d)

Fig. 13.16 (a) Pleomorphic undifferentiated sarcoma (PUD/MFH) showing storiform pattern; **(b)** inflammatory component of PUD/MFH; **(c)** whorled and fascicled appearance of PUD/MFH; **(d)** high-power view of cytologic pleomorphism, nuclear hyperchromasia, and variably spindled appearance.

(a)

(b)

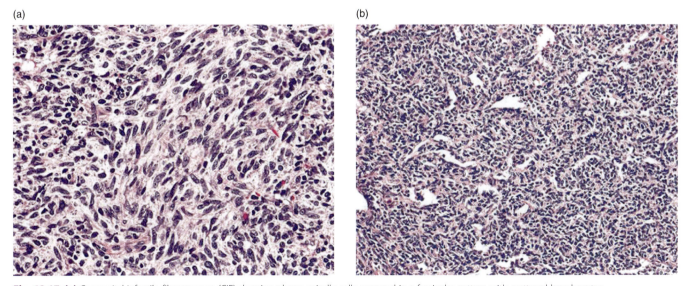

Fig. 13.17 (a) Congenital infantile fibrosarcoma (CIF) showing plump spindle cells arranged in a fascicular pattern with scattered lymphocytes.
(b) Hemangiopericytic pattern in CIF.

(a)

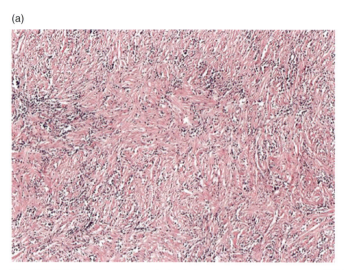

(b)

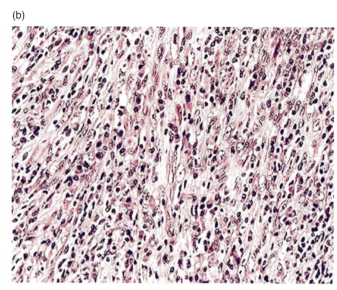

Fig. 13.18 (a) Low-power view of whorled somewhat storiform pattern of IMT with small indistinct spindled myofibroblasts embedded in hyalinized stroma; **(b)** medium-power view of IMT with interspersed inflammatory cells.

type fibromatosis, synovial sarcoma, and embryonal rhabdomyosarcoma [159,160].

Inflammatory myofibroblastic tumor

"Inflammatory myofibroblastic tumors" (IMTs) are a group of neoplasms which were first documented in the lung and have since been reported in many extrapulmonary sites and, uncommonly, in the mediastinum [161–163]. Inflammatory myofibroblastic tumor has been described under a variety of names (plasma cell granuloma, plasma cell pseudotumor, inflammatory myofibroblastic proliferation, myxoid hamartoma) implying an IMT is a non-neoplastic entity [164]. In 1994 and 1995 the first cases of IMT with clonal rearrangements were described. In 1999 a 2p23 rearrangement was described in two cases.

Inflammatory myofibroblastic tumor has a predilection for children and young adults with over 50% occurring in children and less than 10% in adults. In general, the WHO has classified IMT as a tumor of intermediate biologic behavior, in which a significant minority of tumors demonstrate local recurrence (~25% if extrapulmonary, ~<2% if pulmonary) [165]. Metastasis has been documented in ~5% of cases to lung, liver, brain, and bone, although controversy still exists as to whether or not these are multifocal rather than true metastasis, at least in some cases.

Histologic features are not tightly correlated to biologic behavior in IMT. Characteristically, IMTs are variably cellular, usually forming loose fascicles of relatively uniform elongated spindle cells with vesicular nuclei. Within the proliferation there are admixed stellate-shaped and ganglion-like cells. A distinctive and mixed inflammatory cell infiltrate is uniformly prominent and composed predominantly of lymphocytes, plasma cells, but infrequently eosinophils and histiocytes (Fig. 13.18). A myxoid stroma, occasionally alternating with hyalinized fibrous stroma is present. Foci of necrosis may be present [166].

Some examples of IMT do exhibit cytologic atypia in the form of marked nuclear hyperchromasia, pleomorphism, and nucleomegaly. Mitotic figures can be found, but are typically not abundant and abnormal forms are absent. Recurrent IMTs may exhibit histologic atypia and transformation to "round cell" morphology, higher cellularity, and an increased mitotic index, which correlate more reliably to aggressive clinical behavior [167].

Immunohistochemically, IMT is positive for smooth muscle actin. Keratin is typically weak if reactive and commonly found within bladder IMT, but typically negative in lung and mediastinal IMT. Other lineage markers, including S100 protein, vascular markers, and skeletal muscle markers, are negative. By immunohistochemistry ALK-1 is positive in ~50% of cases (Fig. 13.19), most commonly in IMTs occurring in younger age groups [168].

Cytogenetic studies demonstrate involvement of 2p23. Activation of the ALK receptor tyrosine kinase is accomplished by chromosomal fusion with TPM3 and 4(19p13.1), TPM3 (1q22.23), ATIC, and SEC31L1. Fusion of the ALK receptor with partner RAN-BP2 has been shown to correlate with aggressive clinical behavior, but has not been reported in IMT of the mediastinum.

Tumors of adipose tissue
Lipoma variants

Lipomas are infrequently encountered in the mediastinal tissues [169,170]. Most are asymptomatic solitary lesions in adults, which may be mistaken for intrathoracic fluid collections in plain-film radiographs [171]. Computed tomography, in contrast, generally shows the sharp circumscription of these uniformly hypodense masses. Surgical excision is generally undertaken only for those lesions that cause symptoms due to encroachment upon other structures.

(a)

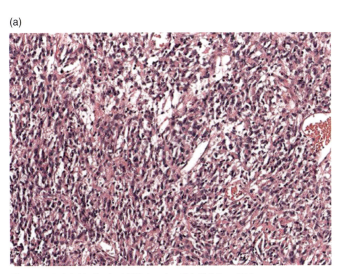

(b)

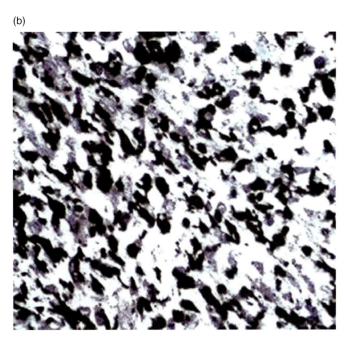

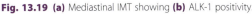

Fig. 13.19 (a) Mediastinal IMT showing **(b)** ALK-1 positivity.

Grossly, lipomas are encapsulated yellow to white tumors that variably resemble mature fat. Histologically, most lesions are entirely composed of mature adipose cells. However, in some instances, spindle cells may be interspersed or vasoformative foci may be encountered, defining the variants known as "spindle-cell lipoma" and "angiolipoma," respectively. All lipomas are cytologically bland, without mitoses.

On occasion, the mediastinum may be widened diffusely by unencapsulated mature fat. Such instances of "lipomatosis" [172–174] are often associated with elevated blood levels of endogenous or exogenous steroids [175,176].

Hibernomas

Hibernomas are benign neoplasms composed of fetal brown adipose tissue which have rarely been described in the mediastinum. Clinically they present with a mass effect and are typically seen in the left mediastinum in patients younger than 50 years of age [177]. Imaging studies may reveal a tumor with well defined edges and non-homogeneous density or characterized by numerous lobules divided by well vascularized connective tissue [178]. The tumor cells are round or polygonal, multivacuolated with centrally placed nuclei, with some resemblance to lipoblasts (Fig. 13.20). Cytogenetically, although involvement of 11q13 [179] region has been described, fluorescence in situ hybridization reveals a more complex rearrangement. Excision is considered curative [180].

Lipoblastoma

Lipoblastomas, which are almost exclusively encountered in young children, represent lobular proliferations of immature but biologically benign lipoblastic elements [181]. When they are clearly encapsulated, solitary lesions with that constituency are termed "lipoblastomas", whereas diffuse or multifocal infiltration of soft tissue characterizes the histologically-similar process known as "lipoblastomatosis". [182] The former tumor type is usually found in peripheral superficial soft tissues; lipoblastomatosis often involves truncal, paravertebral, axillary, or mediastinal soft tissues. Because of its infiltrative nature, lipoblastomatosis is more prone to be symptomatic at presentation and is also more likely to recur after surgical resection. In some cases lipoblastomas can undergo maturation and have an identical histologic appearance to lipomas. Therefore with large, deeply located tumors with lipomatous differentiation in pediatric patients, a diagnosis of mature lipoblastoma should always be considered.

Histologically, lipoblastomas are composed of irregular lobules of immature fat with mature adipocytic elements that are more centrally placed. The lobules are separated by fibrous septa. The stroma may be myxoid in nature, but the delicate "chicken-wire" vascular pattern of myxoid liposarcoma is not seen. Lipoblasts are present, as the name "lipoblastoma" implies; they may be univacuolated or multivacuolated (Fig. 13.21). However, unlike those in well-differentiated liposarcomas or myxoid liposarcoma, the lipoblasts do not show any nuclear atypia or mitotic activity, and they are not concentrated near fibrous septa.

Whether it is solitary or multifocal, lipoblastoma has no capacity for metastasis. The likelihood of regrowth depends on the success of efforts at complete surgical removal [183]. A characteristic cytogenetic feature is a rearrangement of 8q11–13.

(a)

(b)

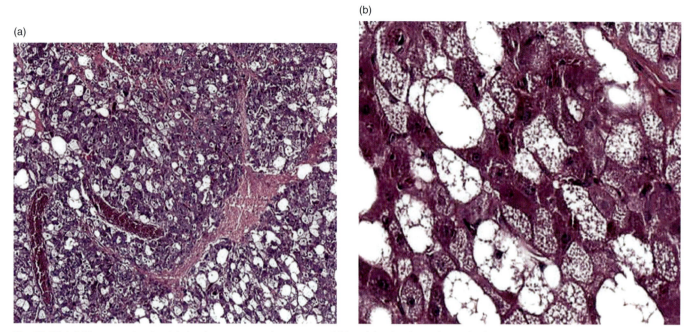

Fig. 13.20 (a) Hibernoma showing lobulated appearance at low power and **(b)** multiloculated cytoplasm at high power.

(a)

(b)

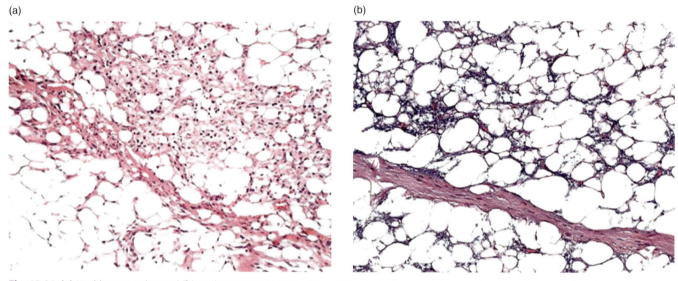

Fig. 13.21 (a) Lipoblastoma at low and **(b)** medium power demonstrating variably sized adipocytes, interspersed septa, and mature adipocytes.

Myelolipomas

A subset of the rare extra-adrenal myelolipomas arise in the mediastinum, predominantly in the posterior compartment. They have been the subject of case reports and total less than ten reported cases in the literature. They may be symptomatic similar to other mass lesions of the mediastinum or asymptomatic and incidentally discovered. Histologically, myelolipomas may have a predominance of either the hematopoietic or fatty component, and may have a conspicuous lymphocyte population. Clinically, they are considered benign and cured by excision.

Liposarcomas

Among non-neurogenous mediastinal neoplasms, liposarcoma (LS) is relatively common. Most examples have been discovered in adults [184–189], with only anecdotal cases in children [190–192]. In one unusual case, a young man infected with human immuno-deficiency virus (HIV) developed a mediastinal LS that subsequently "dedifferentiated" and metastasized to the lungs, pleura, and pericardium [193].

Most intrathoracic LS arise in the mediastinal soft tissue in the anterior or posterior compartments and present with symptoms of airway compression or chest pain [194].

(a)

(b)

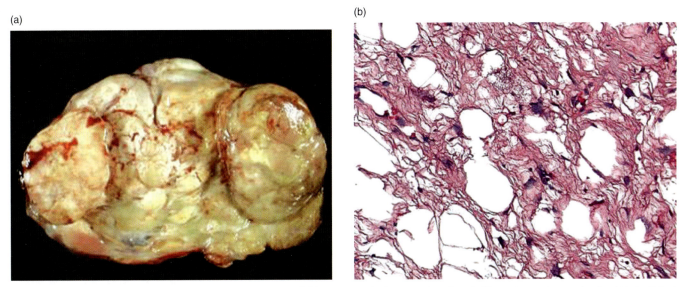

Fig. 13.22 (a) Liposarcoma of the mediastinum, gross appearance and **(b)** microscopic high-power view of atypical hyperchromatic stromal cells within hyalinized septa admixed with variably sized adipocytes.

(a)

(b)

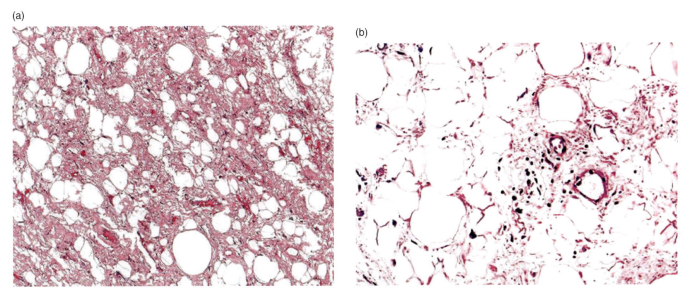

Fig. 13.23 (a) Well-differentiated liposarcoma (WDL), dedifferentiated liposarcoma showing adipocyte variation and easily found atypical hyperchromatic stromal cells; **(b)** lipoma-like variant with scant atypical hyperchromatic stromal cells embedded in between adipocytes rather than in fibrous septa.

Macroscopically, LS is an unencapsulated, lobulated yellow-white mass that peripherally infiltrates adjacent soft tissue and may invade viscera (Fig. 13.22a) [195].

All variants of liposarcoma have been reported in the mediastinum, including well differentiated (Fig. 13.22b and Fig. 13.23b) and dedifferentiated liposarcoma, low-grade myxoid/high-grade round cell (Fig. 13.24), pleomorphic liposarcoma, and unclassified liposarcoma. Not uncommonly, the fat-predominant "lipoma-like" variant of well-differentiated liposarcoma can mimic a lipoma, and the key diagnostic atypical hyperchromatic stromal cells or pleomorphic cells may be rarely seen and can be concealed among the adipocytes and within the septa (Fig. 13.23).

"Dedifferentiation"– which is actually the development of new clonal evolution within the neoplasm, is a distinctive phenomenon linked to well-differentiated liposarcoma that commonly heralds aggressive clinical behavior in LS. Histologically, dedifferentiation is typified by a sharply-demarcated highly cellular secondary non-lipogenic neoplastic component that often has the morphology of pleomorphic undifferentiated sarcoma/MFH. In some cases, paradoxical heterologous sarcomatous subtypes, including osteosarcoma, chondrosarcoma, fibrosarcoma, rhabdomyosarcoma, or angiosarcoma, are reported and account for ~5% of the overall patterns [196]. Apparently no clinical significance of prognostic difference has been shown in association with these patterns compared to the

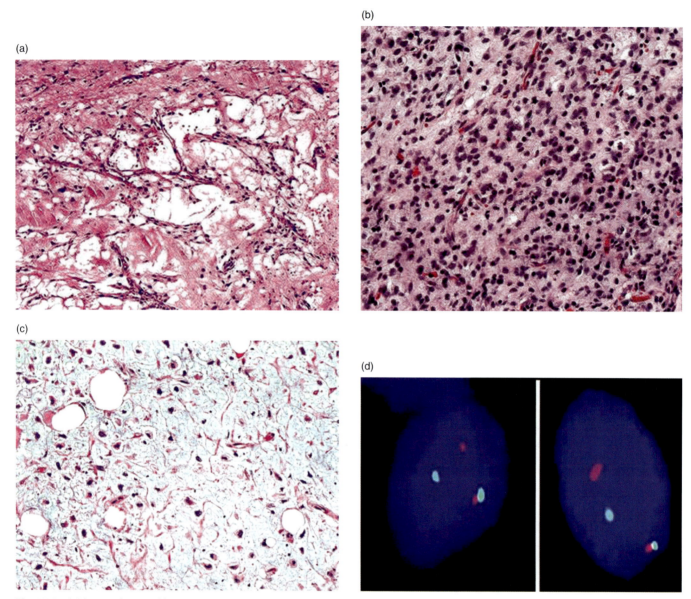

Fig. 13.24 (a) Low-grade myxoid liposarcoma; **(b)** round cell transformation to high-grade liposarcoma showing a lack of lipogenic differentiation; **(c)** low-grade myxoid liposarcoma myxoid matrix and hyalinized areas resembling well-differentiated liposarcoma; **(d)** FUS DDIT break apart probes demonstrating positive results in myxoid liposarcoma.

more common undifferentiated sarcomatous component. In addition, distinctive subtype of dedifferentiation – so called "meningothelial-like whorls" – is described as a characteristic pattern of dedifferentiation in liposarcomas. [197]

Lineage-related immunohistochemical markers are not particularly useful for the diagnosis of LS, although the presence of vimentin and S100 protein (in lipoblastic elements) characterizes these tumors. It is more helpful to undertake cytogenetic and molecular analyses for MDM2 or CDK4 gene amplification to confirm well-differentiated or dedifferentiated LS. A distinctive cytogenetic translocation is present in myxoid/round cell liposarcoma, t(12;16)(q13;p11), which can be identified by fluorescence in situ hybridization and PCR as well as by routine cytogenetic studies. Pleomorphic liposarcoma often has a complex karyotype but no reproducible distinctive cytogenetic abnormalities.

Surgical resection is the treatment of choice for all variants of LS. Although it may result in the cure of well-differentiated tumors as well as a subset of myxoid LS, it is rarely curative in large, infiltrative, or poorly-differentiated neoplasms. In these cases, multimodality therapy including debulking surgery with neoadjuvant or adjuvant radiation and chemotherapy is usually required to achieve any benefit.

Myogenic neoplasms

Rhabdomyosarcoma

Rhabdomyosarcomas (RMS) may present at any age; however, most tumors of this type occur in children during the first decade of life, and they usually arise in peripheral soft tissues

(a)

(b)

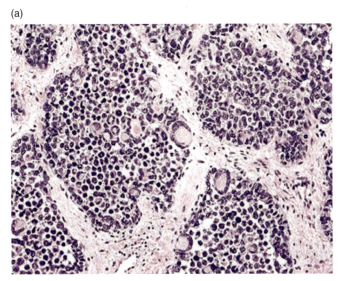
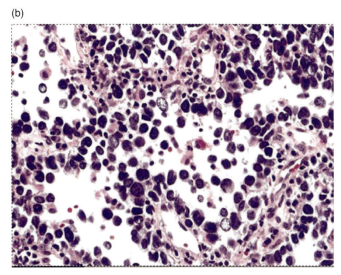

Fig. 13.25 (a) Alveolav RMS (ARMS), low-power view showing alveolar architecture with tumor nodules bounded by fibrous septa; **(b)** ARMS, higher-power view showing cell discohesion within the tumor nodules.

of the extremities, head and neck, or pelvis. The majority of RMS of the mediastinum arises from primary mediastinal germ cell tumors. Mediastinal primary RMS is distinctly rare. [198]

The gross appearance of RMS depends on its location; tumors growing within skeletal muscle or soft tissue may have ill-defined borders, whereas those arising in association with mucosal surfaces are better circumscribed and may appear lobulated or polypoid. Cut surfaces show a variable appearance, and some may be distinctly myxoid.

All of the variants of RMS have been described in mediastinal tissues, corresponding to the subtypes seen in somatic soft tissue and the more common anatomic sites. Subclassification of RMS is histologically based but at least four classification schemes exist [199]. Common to all is the division of rhabdomyosarcoma into prognostic categories. In general, RMS can be classified into embryonal, botryoid (previously a variant of embryonal), alveolar, and pleomorphic (adult type). Spindle cell RMS is recognized as a variant of embryonal type.

The embryonal form of RMS is the most common; it comprises moderately pleomorphic small- to medium-sized round cells with scant eosinophilic cytoplasm, round to oval hyperchromatic nuclei, and inconspicuous nucleoli. Occasionally, maturing rhabdomyoblasts are prominent, demonstrating distinctly eosinophilic cytoplasm. It should be remembered that such cells are also seen in "malignant Triton tumor", a subtype of MPNST. Indeed, a rhabdomyoblast-containing neoplasm in the mediastinum of an adult is probably most likely to be neurogenic rather than a true RMS.

Alveolar RMS differs from embryonal lesions in several respects, the most obvious being its alveolar appearance and tumor cell discohesion. This feature results in large rounded atypical cells "floating free" in spaces that are bounded by vascular septa. Large, atypical, and multinucleated cells with

dense abundant eosinophilic cytoplasm are also more common in alveolar RMS (Fig. 13.25).

Tumors composed predominantly of spindle cells (Fig. 13.26a) or large pleomorphic cells (Fig. 13.26b) are more commonly present in the adult population. These tumors tend to lack the primitive appearance of embryonal and alveolar RMS.

The diagnosis of RMS often relies on immunohistochemical and ultrastructural evaluation. The former of those studies typically show reactivity in all rhabdomyosarcomas for muscle-specific actin, desmin, myogenin, Myo-D1, and other antigens associated with the contractile myogenous apparatus. [200–202] By electron microscopy, the juxtaposition of cytoplasmic thick and thin filaments, with variably well-formed Z-bands or complete sarcomeric units, is diagnostic. In very primitive tumors, these features may be difficult to appreciate.

The behavior of RMS varies with histologic appearance, location, and stage of the primary lesion.

Patients in whom tumors can be completely resected, or with only microscopic residual disease, have an overall five-year survival of >70% when adjuvant chemotherapy is also employed. Alveolar RMS generally has a worse prognosis, although this distinction is less clear in examples of mediastinal RMS. Local recurrence or metastasis, regardless of histologic type, portends an unfavorable outcome; fewer than 20% of patients with those findings enjoy long-term survival.

Cytogenetic abnormalities are distinctive in RMS [203]. In embryonal RMS complex karyotypes are generally present but there is consistent loss of heterozygosity of 11p15 in most cases. Other aberrations include additional copies of chromosomes 2, 8 and 13, and rearrangements of chromosome 1. Alveolar rhabdomyosarcoma is characterized by a distinctive t(2;13)(q35;q14) translocation, which can be detected by FISH

247

(a)

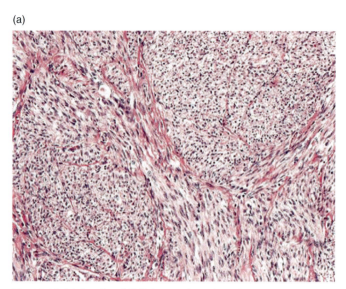

(b)

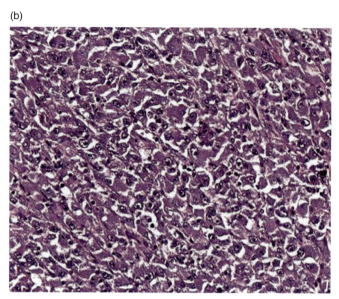

Fig. 13.26 **(a)** Spindle cell RMS showing fascicular architecture and some resemblance in pattern to leiomyosarcoma; **(b)** highly cellular area of pleomorphic RMS.

or RT-PCR. Transcription factors are encoded by the genes involved which are the PAX3 gene on 2q35 and the FKHR gene on 13q14. A variant translocation has been described, t(1;13)(p36;q14), fusing the PAX7 gene on 1p36 with FKHR. The PAX7-FKHR fusion transcript containing tumors appear to have a better prognosis. Pleomorphic rhabdomyosarcomas have a highly complex karyotype lacking any reproducible cytogenetic characteristics.

Rhabdomyoma variants

Though rare case reports exist, for all practical purposes, benign rhabdomyogenic tumors (rhabdomyomas) do not occur in the extravisceral mediastinal soft tissues.[204]

Smooth muscle tumors

The recognition of true smooth muscle differentiation is largely presumptive when based solely on routine histologic evaluation. Although the classical histological features are generally sufficient to suggest the diagnosis, ancillary techniques are generally required to confirm it.

These comments notwithstanding, the diagnosis of smooth muscle tumors in the mediastinum is unusual[205]. Examples of vascular, tracheal, or esophageal leiomyomas may bulge into the mediastinum, but lesions that are primary in the mediastinal soft tissue are rare[206–208]. In particular, leiomyosarcomas (LMS) are characteristically associated with mediastinal viscera such as the esophagus[209–215].

The gross appearances of leiomyoma and LMS in the thorax are similar to those seen in other somatic soft tissues and the same diagnostic criteria for determining malignancy apply. Macroscopically, leiomyosarcomas differ from leiomyomas principally by the larger size of LMS and the tendency for it to show a softer, more fleshy consistency on cut surfaces,

potentially with foci of necrosis and hemorrhage. Both have a whorled pattern macroscopically, but only LMS exhibits tumoral hemorrhage or necrosis.

Histologically, each is usually a tumor of spindle cells (Fig. 13.27), although epithelioid variants are well-recognized as well. The so-called degenerative/ancient changes primarily described in gynecologic leiomyosarcomas as "symplastic" leiomyomas are not well documented in extra-gynecologic sites and such findings should raise suspicion for a leiomyosarcoma. Mitotic indices usually exceed 2 mitotic figures per 10 high-power microscopic fields. LMS often exhibits the fascicular, irregular growth of cytologically-atypical spindle cells, and it commonly invades adjacent soft tissue.

Ultrastructurally, smooth muscle cells contain abundant thin cytoplasmic filaments that are interrupted at intervals by dense bodies. Subplasmalemmal plaques, pinocytosis, and an incomplete basal lamina are usually seen. Immunohistochemically, smooth muscle tumors show similarities to neoplasms of striated muscle, in that desmin and muscle-specific actin are commonly expressed. However, those two classes of myogenous neoplasms do differ because only smooth muscle lesions express caldesmon and calponin. The occasional presence of S100 protein, CD56, and CD57 in smooth muscle tumors may cause some diagnostic confusion with histologically-similar peripheral nerve sheath tumors[216].

Because it is intimately associated with visceral or vascular structures, the size and infiltrative nature of LMS may preclude surgical extirpation. Adjuvant radiotherapy may be beneficial in such instances.

Tumors with osteochondroid differentiation

As a group, primary mediastinal tumors showing cartilaginous or osteogenic patterns of differentiation are rare in their frequency.

(a)

(b)

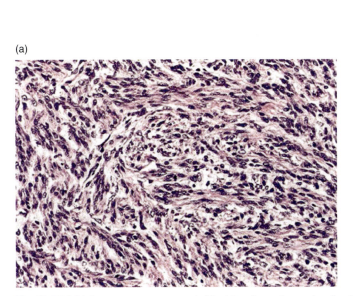
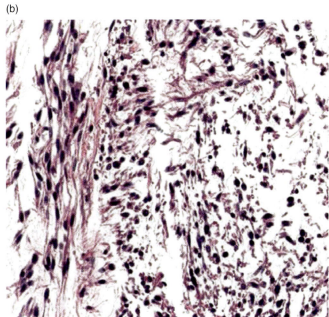

Fig. 13.27 (a) Leiomyosarcoma composed of fascicles of smooth muscle cells with fusiform nuclei and perinuclear clearing arranged in fascicles with a somewhat hyalinized stroma; **(b)** myxoid or edematous change in a leiomyosarcoma can produce a deceptively paucicellular appearance.

(a)

(b)

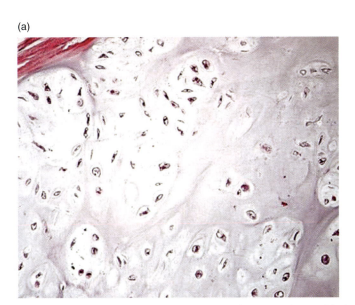
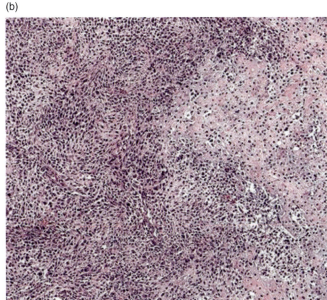

Fig. 13.28 (a) Hyaline-type well-differentiated chondrosarcoma showing lobules composed of lacunae containing chondrocytes and a bluish chondroid matrix; **(b)** dedifferentiated chondrosarcoma with progression from cartilaginous-forming chondrocytes (left) to undifferentiated PUD/MFH-like areas (right).

To date, the bulk of conventional hyaline type cartilaginous neoplasms, including chondrosarcomas involving the mediastinum have arisen in, or have been associated with the tracheobronchial tree [217] or the thoracic vertebrae [218]. Occasionally, however, a purely mediastinal localization is seen [219]. They have the identical histological features as their primary skeletal counterparts and range from well differentiated to poorly differentiated (Grade 1–3) and show dedifferentiation on occasion (Fig. 13.28).

Extraskeletal mesenchymal chondrosarcoma

Primary extraskeletal mesenchymal chondrosarcoma of the mediastinum is exceedingly rare with only anecdotal cases reported [220]. Mesenchymal chondrosarcoma may occur near the spinal cord, also known as a parameningeal presentation. Patients with tumors in such a location can present with diffuse pain or even paralysis due to compression of the spinal cord by the tumor.

(a)

(b)

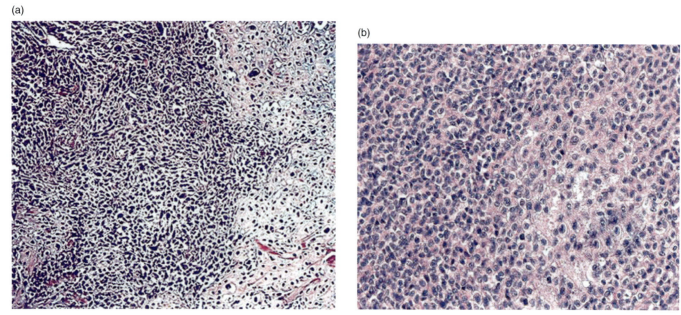

Fig. 13.29 (a) Extraskeletal mesenchymal chondrosarcoma showing juxtaposition of cartilaginous differentiation and high-grade round cell areas; **(b)** round cell predominance in extraskeletal mesenchymal chondrosarcoma.

Mesenchymal chondrosarcoma has a biphasic histological appearance. Microscopically, it is a biphasic tumor composed of both highly cellular areas composed of small round cells arranged in a distinctive hemangiopericytic pattern admixed with foci of well-differentiated cartilage (Fig. 13.29). The differential diagnosis includes other small round cell tumors, notably, poorly differentiated synovial sarcoma, Ewing sarcoma, rhabdomyosarcoma and small cell osteosarcoma, if primary in the bone. In addition to the admixture of matrix and morphologic appearance, immunohistochemistry and molecular or FISH studies to exclude the EWSR1 and SYT translocations will aid in arriving at the correct diagnosis among these possibilities.

Surgical resection is the optimal first treatment. In the mediastinum extraskeletal mesenchymal chondrosarcoma has a similar prognosis to the tumor in other locations. In the large pathologic review conducted at the Mayo Clinic, the overall prognosis for this tumor was poor with ~75% of the 23 patients dead of disease between six months and 23 years after initial diagnosis.

Extraskeletal myxoid chondrosarcoma (EMC)

Primary EMC of the mediastinum is extraordinarily rare with only a single case reported near the spinal cord, which behaved aggressively showing bilateral lung metastases. The vast majority of mediastinal EMC cases are metastases. Morphologically, primary mediastinal EMC is indistinguishable from its soft tissue counterpart in that it has a multinodular architecture in which the lobules are formed by interanastomosing cords and strands and occasionally nests of epithelioid, ovoid, or spindled cells with eosinophilic cytoplasm and hyperchromatic nuclei. There is a prominent myxoid chondroid matrix.

Immunohistochemically, EMC frequently expresses S100 protein and EMA, but may be negative for these and all lineage markers, including keratins and myoid markers. A recent study has shown that neuroendocrine markers may be positive. Ultrastructurally, extraskeletal myxoid chondrosarcoma was characterized by distinct cords of cells immersed in a glycosaminoglycan-rich matrix. The cells were rich in mitochondria, had well-developed Golgi apparatus and there were numerous smooth vesicles. EMC is characterized by a recurrent t(9;22)(q22;q12) translocation fusing the EWS gene on chromosome 22 with a novel orphan nuclear receptor gene CHN on chromosome 9.

The major differential diagnostic considerations of EMC in the mediastinum include metastasis of a primary soft tissue EMC, a myoepithelioma/myoepithelial carcinoma, neuroendocrine neoplasms, melanoma, and the recently described primary pulmonary myxoid sarcoma (PPS) with EWSR1-CREB1 fusion [221].

Immunostains can be used to separate all but the latter consideration. PPS can be histologically and immunophenotypically indistinguishable from EMC. However, though both EMC and PPS harbor EWSR1 containing translocations, the fusion partners are mutually exclusive: CHN and CREB1 respectively.

Extraosseous osteosarcoma (EOS)

Extraosseous osteosarcomas (EOS) of the mediastinum occur infrequently [222–224]. Reported lesions in this category have generally assumed an osteoblastic appearance, with deposits of eosinophilic osteoid material that has been elaborated by cytologically malignant polygonal or spindle cells (Fig. 13.30) [225]. Pleomorphic and multinucleated giant cells

(a)

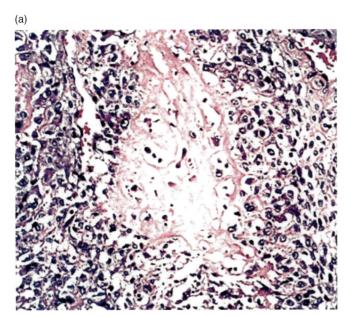

(b)

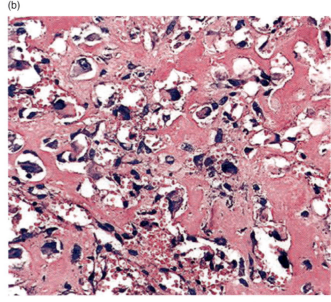

Fig. 13.30 **(a)** Posterior mediastinal osteosarcoma, composed of epithelioid cells with distinct cytoplasmic borders and high-grade cytologic features in an area devoid of osteoid production; **(b)** distinct osteoid matrix deposition admixed with high-grade epithelioid cells in a posterior mediastinal osteosarcoma.

can also be seen. Rather surprisingly, an association between mediastinal EOS and the vertebrae or ribs has been observed only rarely. As discussed in a study by Bane *et al.*, EOS usually is an aggressive neoplasm, with a tendency for pulmonary, osseous, and soft tissue metastases [226]. Post-radiation osteosarcoma is also described in this location [227].

The presence of an osteoid-forming tumor in the mediastinum, because of its rarity as a primary tumor, raises a differential diagnosis of a metastatic extramediastinal osteosarcoma, a sarcomatoid carcinoma, and a dedifferentiated liposarcoma with heterologous elements. Before accepting a primary osteosarcoma of the mediastinum these other considerations, which are more probable, must be excluded.

Other mediastinal soft tissue neoplasms

Solitary fibrous tumor-hemangiopericytoma

"Solitary fibrous tumor" and "hemangiopericytoma" have now been merged nosologically into one group. Such lesions in the thorax are most often seen in the pleura, but primary mediastinal examples are now well-documented [228–230]. These lesions may occur anywhere in the mediastinum, and tend to be seen in older individuals. Solitary fibrous tumors (SFTs) are borderline malignancies and may be locally aggressive; tumor-related deaths have been reported.

Histologically, SFTs are composed of spindle cells with a variable degree of nuclear atypicality, arranged haphazardly in a collagenous stroma. Areas of marked stromal sclerosis may punctuate such masses, and myxoid change is also possible. Some foci in SFTs clearly resemble the morphotype of "hemangiopericytoma" (Fig. 13.31). These are typified by

bluntly-fusiform tumor cell nests which are invested by reticulin and punctuated regularly by "staghorn-" or "moose antler-" like blood vessels. Thymomas may present exactly the same morphotype, and, therefore, one must first consider that possibility when "hemangiopericytoma"-like tumors are encountered in the anterior mediastinum.

Densely cellular foci in SFTs may contain elements with pleomorphism and overt nuclear atypia (Fig. 13.32). In the same areas, mitotic activity is often brisk, and tumoral hemorrhage and necrosis may be present. Such findings have been used by some authors to define overt malignancy in SFT; however, it should be noted that in this grouping of neoplasms, biologic behavior may not be tightly correlated to histological parameters.

The immunophenotypic hallmark of this neoplasm is its consistent expression of CD34 (Fig. 13.33) [231]. Subsequent studies have shown that in addition to CD34, co-expression of CD99 and *bcl*-2 protein are consistently expressed to such a degree that two of these three markers are seen in over 90% of cases [232]. Solitary fibrous tumor is reactive for vimentin, and the vast majority do not express keratin. In addition, p63, epithelial membrane antigen, and S100 protein are negative. Those characteristics differ from those of most other non-vascular mesenchymal tumors in the mediastinum. Frankly malignant SFT has also been reported to label immunohistologically focally for keratin and for mutant p53 protein.

Ultrastructurally, SFT comprises fibroblast-like cells, with no evidence of myogenous, epithelial, or neural differentiation [233]. This technique, however, will not serve to separate SFT from other fibroblastic neoplasms or proliferations.

Until recently, SFT has not been shown to have a distinctive cytogenetic profile. However, a recurrent NAB2-STAT6

(a)

(b)

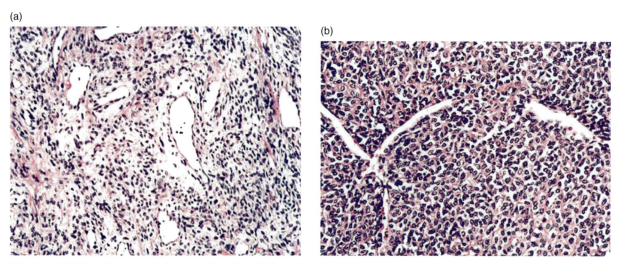

Fig. 13.31 (a) Solitary fibrous tumor showing traditional spindled morphology and hyalinized staghorn vessels; **(b)** more cellular areas resembling hemangiopericytoma.

(a)

(b)

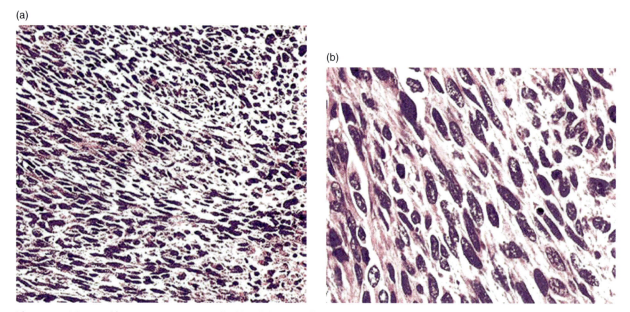

Fig. 13.32 (a) Atypical features in SFT consisting of highly cellular areas in fascicles and nuclear pleomorphism with hyperchromasia; **(b)** cytologic features of atypia in SFT.

(b)

(a)

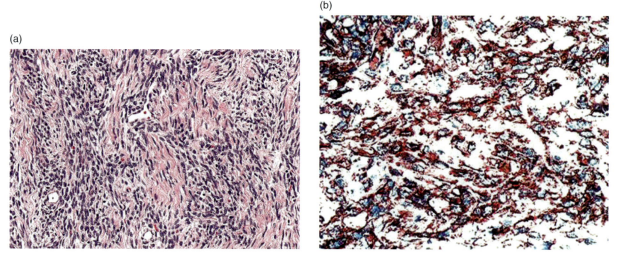

Fig. 13.33 (a) Solitary fibrous tumor showing classical histology; **(b)** CD34 positivity in SFT.

(a)

(b)

(c)

(d)

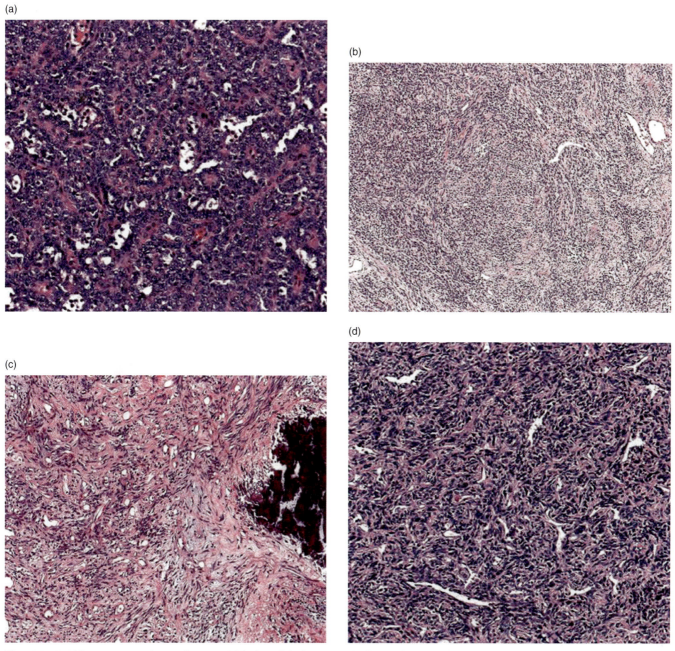

Fig. 13.34 Variable appearances of synovial sarcoma **(a)** high-grade biphasic epithelioid synovial sarcoma showing pseudoglandular formation lined by enlarged, markedly atypical epithelioid cells showing classical histology; **(b)** monophasic synovial sarcoma showing fascicles of uniform cells with hemangiopericytic vasculature; **(c)** myxoid and partially calcified areas of synovial sarcoma; **(d)** classical features of synovial sarcoma showing hemangiopericytic vasculature with intermediate nuclear atypia and hyalinized stroma.

fusion has been reported in 55% (29) of 53 of SFTs tested by whole exome sequencing [234].

Synovial sarcoma

Although it is characteristically a neoplasm seen in the somatic soft tissues of the extremities or the head and neck, synovial sarcoma (SS) may occasionally arise in anterior or posterior mediastinal tissues [235]. It is potentially seen throughout

adult life and has a slight male predominance. As in other sites, mediastinal SS typically follows an aggressive clinical course.

Histologically, SS is classically a biphasic neoplasm, consisting of sheets and fascicles of plump spindle cells that show a transition to, or abrupt separation from, an epithelioid component. The latter element may show overt glandular or even papillary differentiation, form irregularly sized cellular nests, or line intratumoral spaces. The stroma of SS is often vascular,

(a)

(b)

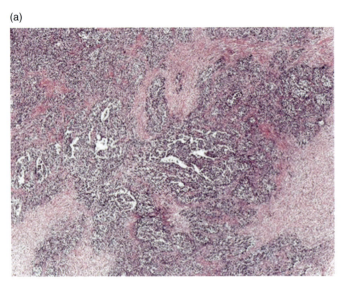
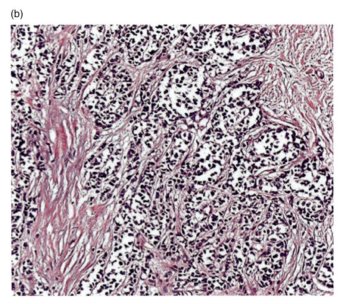

Fig. 13.35 **(a)** Desmoplastic small round cell tumor showing infiltrative nests and diffuse sheets of **(b)** undifferentiated small round-to-angulated tumor cells embedded in a desmoplastic stroma.

and a hemangiopericytoma-like appearance may again obtain in such cases. A myxoid variant of this tumor exists, and another subtype shows prominent collagenization of the stroma in likeness to SFT. Indeed, those two lesions may be very difficult to separate from one another without the aid of adjunct studies.

Immunohistochemical analysis reveals reactivity for keratin and epithelial membrane antigen in epithelioid, transitional, and spindle-cell foci in SS in the majority of cases. CD99 and *bcl*-2 protein are also commonly present, but CD34 is unexpected. S100 protein, CD56, and CD57 are apparent in a small proportion of tumors. An antibody directed toward transducer-like enhancer of split 1 (TLE-1) has been shown to be positive in the majority of synovial sarcomas and in a spindle-cell malignancy is particularly helpful in suggesting the diagnosis of SS. However, it has also been demonstrated in other spindle cell malignancies within the differential diagnosis, particularly nerve sheath tumors [236]. The most specific adjunct test remains *in-situ* hybridization studies or molecular assessments for the characteristic t(X;18) chromosomal translocation of synovial sarcoma [237].

Desmoplastic small round cell tumor

Desmoplastic small round cell tumor (DSRCT) is a distinctive type of small round blue cell tumor with a predilection for serosal surfaces, such as the peritoneum, that predominantly affects males in the second or third decade of life. It has rarely been reported in the mediastinum [238] but primary intra-abdominal DSRCT may secondarily involve mediastinal lymph nodes and tissues [239].

On microscopic examination, the tumor cells exhibit round, ovoid, or spindled hyperchromatic nuclei with condensed chromatin and form angulated nodules, cords, nests

or sheets embedded in a collagenous "desmoplastic" stroma (Fig. 13.35). Mitotic figures are common. The differential diagnosis includes other small round blue cell tumors, most commonly Ewing family tumors, rhabdomyosarcoma, poorly differentiated synovial sarcoma, and neuroblastoma as well as lymphoblastic lymphoma.

Immunohistochemistry demonstrates a polyphenotypic pattern of antigens related to different cell lineages, including cytokeratin, epithelial membrane antigen, and desmin in a characteristic Golgi pattern. Neuron-specific enolase, synaptophysin, and CD99 are also reported positive in a subset of tumors. WT1 protein directed against the carboxy-terminus consistently demonstrates nuclear positivity [240]. Myogenin and MyoD1 is negative. The molecular hallmark of DSCRT is the EWS-WT1 reciprocal translocation gene fusion that can be detected by FISH and RT-PCR.

DSRCT is a very aggressive malignancy with a five-year survival rate of less than 15%. Treatment options include surgery, radiotherapy, and chemotherapy with or without stem cell transplantation [241]. More recently molecularly targeted therapies have been introduced [242].

Alveolar soft part sarcoma

Primary alveolar soft part sarcoma (ASPS) is rare with the largest series consisting of two cases, one in the posterior and one in the anterior mediastinum in male patients of 22 and 23 years of age [243]. Pulmonary metastases were present at the time of diagnosis. Histologically, ASPS is invariate in its morphology and demonstrates the characteristic nested aggregates of large polygonal cells with round to oval nuclei, prominent nucleoli, and moderate amounts of eosinophilic cytoplasm (Fig. 13.36). Special studies include periodic acid–Schiff (PAS)

(a)

(b)

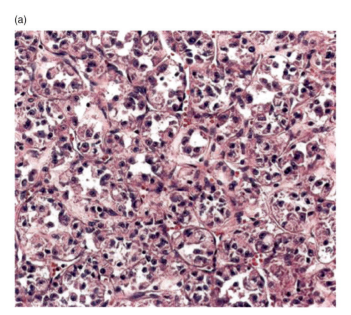
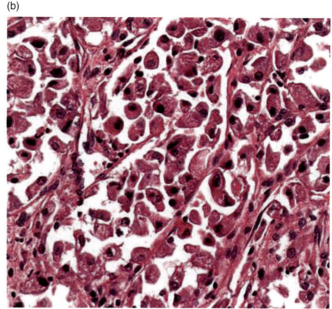

Fig. 13.36 **(a)** Nested appearance of alveolar soft part sarcoma divided by fibrovascular septa; **(b)** nests of enlarged discohesive tumor cells with epithelioid nuclei and eosinophilic eccentrically placed cytoplasm.

stains which highlight the definitional diastase-resistant intracytoplasmic crystals.

Immunohistochemical analysis demonstrates a lack of differentiation, in that epithelial, myoid, neuroectodermal, and neuroendocrine lineage markers are negative. Aberrant consistent cytoplasmic positivity is often present for MyoD1. A marker for transcription factor E3 (TFE3) is available and demonstrates crisp uniform and diffuse nuclear immunoreactivity.

Ultrastructurally, neoplastic cells of ASPS have abundant mitochondria, a prominent smooth endoplasmic reticulum, and a well-developed Golgi apparatus. Intracytoplasmic rhomboid crystals with sparse electron-dense secretory granules are present.

Cytogenetically, ASPS is characterized by a non-reciprocal chromosomal translocation fusing the *TFE3* (transcription factor binding to immunoglobulin heavy constant μ enhancer 3) with the ASPL gene at 17q25 resulting in der(17)t(X;17)(p11;25). The chromosomal abnormality can be detected by FISH and RT-PCR.

The biologic behavior of ASPS is relentless showing up to a 75% metastatic rate mostly to the lungs and brain, although metastasis to bone and soft tissue is also not uncommon. Primary resection remains the primary therapy, but disease-free intervals, some more than a decade long, can be achieved and metastatectomy and chemotherapy and radiation therapy have some benefit in advanced disease.

Chordoma

Chordoma typically involves the soft tissue adjacent to bones in the lumbosacral and cervical spine or skull base. However, paravertebral tumors of this type in the posterior mediastinum

occasionally occur as well [244–246]. Those lesions are typified by a variegated white-gray chondroid or mucoid gross appearance, and a variably cellular histologic pattern in which numerous large, multivacuolated "physaliferous" cells are encountered. Intralesional necrosis and hemorrhage may be conspicuous (Fig. 13.37).

Chordoma is another neoplasm in which "dedifferentiation" may be seen. That phenomenon yields a sharply dimorphic appearance, in which conventional chordoma is abruptly juxtaposed to a high-grade pleomorphic sarcoma histologically.

Immunohistochemical studies of chordomas show reactivity for keratin and S100 protein; epithelial membrane antigen, CD56, and HBME-1 are often present as well (Fig. 13.38). Specialized markers of glandular epithelial differentiation, such as MOC31, Ber-EP4, and carcinoembryonic antigen, are absent.

If complete surgical excision is possible, an operative cure of chordoma may be secured. However, many lesions do not lend themselves to that therapy, and those require irradiation or chemotherapy or both.

Melanocytic and myomelanocytic tumors
Lymphangiomyoma/PEComa/angiomyolipoma

Perivascular epithelioid cell tumor (PEComa) is the name given to a group of neoplasms which share distinctive morphologic, immunophenotypic, and genetic features. Simply put, PEComa shows co-differentiation towards perilymphatic smooth muscle and melanocytes [247,248]. Genetically, PEComas are associated with the tuberous sclerosis complex (TSC) [249]

(b)

(a)

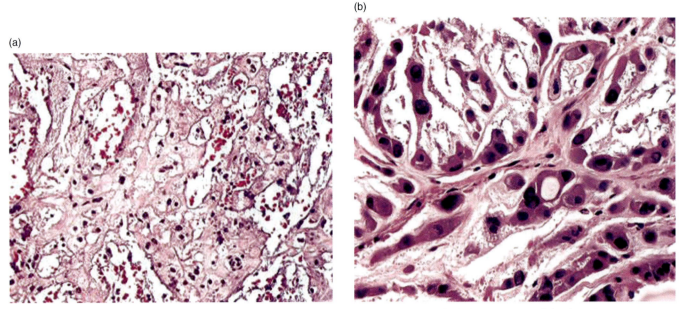

Fig. 13.37 (a) Physaliferous cells of chordoma with myxoid stroma and lightly eosinophilic cytoplasm; **(b)** higher-power view of chordoma demonstrating nests and cords of ovoid tumor cells with eosinophilic cytoplasm admixed with classical physaliferous cells.

(a)

(b)

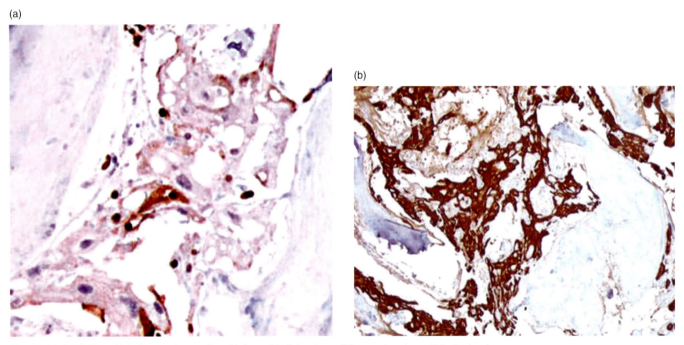

Fig. 13.38 (a) S100 positivity in cytoplasm and weakly in nuclei of chordoma; **(b)** strong keratin positivity in chordoma.

which results from loss of TSC1 (9q34) or TSC2 (16p13.3) genes [250]. Both sporadic and TSC-associated PEComas have been shown to exhibit similar alterations of the TSC genes. PEComas have been reported in the lung, mediastinal and retroperitoneal lymph nodes, kidney/liver (angiomyolipoma), blood vessel walls, somatic soft tissue and bone. PEComas of the lung include lymphangioleiomyomatosis (LAM) and clear cell "sugar" tumor

(CCST) [251]. Clinically, LAM has been described predominantly in premenopausal women and is called "lymphangiomyoma" when solitary, and "lymphangiomyomatosis" (LAM) in its multiplex form [252].

Macroscopically, LAM is a lobulated, red-gray mass. Histologically, it comprises bundles of fusiform cells that may be intimately associated with lymphatic channels. Admixed adipose tissue elements, prominent large blood vessels, clear cell

(a)

(b)

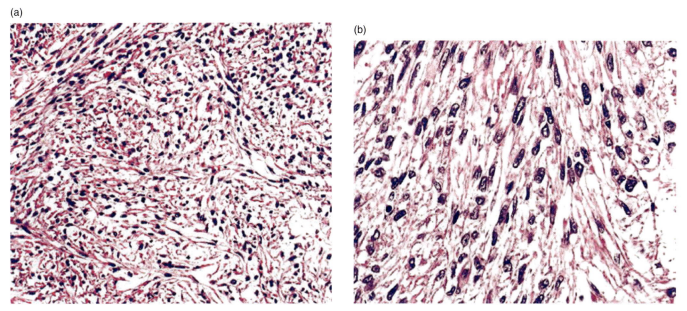

Fig. 13.39 (a) Clear cell pattern of histologically typical PEComa; **(b)** fascicle formation and myxoid appearance in PEComa.

change, epithelioid morphology, and potentially-clear cytoplasm are all part of the microscopic spectrum of such lesions. In the lung, tumor-cell fascicles (Fig. 13.39) may form, mimicking a purely myoid tumor. Characteristically, in at least some areas these cells encircle or entrap small interalveolar vessels, resulting in septal widening and, ultimately, small airway obstruction. Collections of lymphocytes may be seen, and vascular damage results in hemorrhage and hemosiderin deposition.

Owing to their unusual pattern of differentiation, the lesional cells of LAM demonstrate conjoint immunoreactivity for myoid and melanocytic markers. Classically, and most commonly, the definitional markers have been smooth muscle actin and HMB-45. However, muscle-specific actin, desmin, caldesmon or other muscle markers, including calponin, can be immunoreactive. Skeletal muscle markers, including myogenin and MyoD1, are not described in PEComa. Variations exist in the reactivity patterns of the melanocytic markers, and Melan-A, microphthalmia transcription factor and tyrosinase have all been reported as positive in PEComa, but less frequently than HMB-45. S100-protein is uncommon, but described. Of note, transcription factor E3 (TFE-3), which is positive in ASPS, is positive in ~60% of PEComas.

Biologically, despite their usually bland microscopic appearance, PEComas in the mediastinum may present with symptomatic airway obstruction, accumulation of a chylous effusion, or direct pulmonary involvement. Patients with multifocal pulmonary disease are less amenable to surgical therapy short of lung transplantation, and are therefore at greater risk for fatal progression [253]. For managerial purposes PEComas are classified into benign, uncertain, and malignant categories, based on histologic criteria [254].

Clear cell sarcoma of soft tissue

Primary clear cell sarcoma of soft tissue (malignant melanoma of soft parts) has been reported rarely in the mediastinum and presents with symptoms caused by mass effect due to advanced size at discovery.

Clear cell sarcoma of soft tissue (CCST) generally presents in younger adults although it has been described primarily in patients older than 50 years of age. In a subset of cases association with tendons is present [255,256].

Histologically the tumor has an infiltrative appearance and is composed of medium-sized angulated nests and fascicles of primarily spindled or fusiform cells with clear to amphophilic cytoplasm, and ovoid vesicular nuclei with prominent nucleoli. Classically, intermixed multinucleated tumor giant cells with a wreath-like appearance are found. Variable histologic features include myxoid changes and epithelioid cells.

Immunohistochemical studies of CCST demonstrate expression of antigens associated with melanin synthesis including cytoplasmic HMB-45 and Melan-A, nuclear and cytoplasmic immunoreactivity to S100 protein, and nuclear reactivity with microphthalmia transcription factor. Other specific lineage markers are negative. Electron microscopy reveals pigmented and non-pigmented melanosomes in various developmental phases.

Cytogenetic studies have consistently demonstrated a reciprocal chromosome translocation, t(12;22)(q13;q12) in CCST, which fuses the 3′ portion of the Ewing sarcoma (*EWSR1*) oncogene on chromosome 22q with the 3′ portion of the activating transcription factor 1 (*ATF1*) oncogene on chromosome 12q, resulting in a *EWSR1/ATF1* chimeric transcript that has become the molecular hallmark of this tumor [257]. In addition to the diagnostic t(12;22), polysomy of chromosome 8 has been observed as a secondary abnormality in many cases of CCST.

The major differential diagnostic considerations of CCST in the mediastinum, once melanocytic differentiation has been established, includes metastatic melanoma, pigmented melanotic schwannoma, and PEComa. In general these can be separated on the basis of morphology. Judicious use of immunohistochemistry will reveal positivity for myoid markers consistently in PEComas, which is absent in the other tumors. Melanotic schwannoma is diffusely and heavily pigmented unlike clear cell sarcoma. Finally, a careful history often but not always reveals a primary melanoma; however, in select cases detection of the defining reciprocal translocation may be required and can be accomplished by FISH or RT-PCR analysis.

Clinically CCS is an aggressive sarcoma with a five-year survival rate of ~50% with excision, which is considered the mainstay of therapy. In some cases, long disease free intervals (10–20 years) can be attained. Like melanoma it may metastasize to regional lymph nodes which is a poor prognostic indicator.

Sarcomatoid malignant melanoma

Primary mediastinal melanoma has not been described unequivocally. However, asymptomatic metastatic lesions are occasionally seen in that location, some of which have a sarcoma-like appearance histologically [258]. The potential for diagnostic confusion with benign and malignant pigmented (melanotic) peripheral nerve sheath tumors, CCST, and pigmented neuroectodermal tumor of infancy must be considered in cases of sarcomatoid melanoma.

Unfortunately, the immunophenotypic features in many of these lesions may overlap. With the exception of CCST, most of the latter neoplasms typically exhibit immunoreactivity for specialized melanocytic markers such as Melan-A, HMB-45, tyrosinase, and PNL2, and express only S100 protein. Nonetheless, the strength and *pattern* of S100-reactivity can be helpful, because in spindle cell tumors diffuse labeling of virtually every tumor cell is characteristic of melanoma and CCST but not MPNST. However, epithelioid MPNST can have diffuse strong S100 positivity.

Sarcoma arising in germ cell neoplasms

Although rare, sarcomas may develop within mediastinal teratomas or mixed germ cell neoplasms. Areas of chondrosarcoma, osteosarcoma, rhabdomyosarcoma (Fig. 13.40), leiomyosarcoma, and angiosarcoma have been encountered. Those elements are important diagnostically, because treatments aimed at mesenchymal malignancies must be added to the therapeutic regimens designed for germ cell tumors. The overall outlook for patients with these "composite" neoplasms is poor.

Other mediastinal lesions

A variety of other benign non-epithelial mediastinal lesions has been reported anecdotally. These include meningocele [259,260], meningioma [261], and myxoma [262]. Though neoplasms with multiple lines of mesenchymal differentiation have been described under the heading of "mesenchymoma" [263,264], the terminology itself is disputed and it is probable that these neoplasms represent various differentiated and undifferentiated mesenchymal lesions which range from hamartomas to sarcomas. Of the above mentioned entities, meningoceles are probably the most common (Fig. 13.41); their presence in paravertebral mediastinal tissues is potentially associated with neurofibromatosis.

(a)

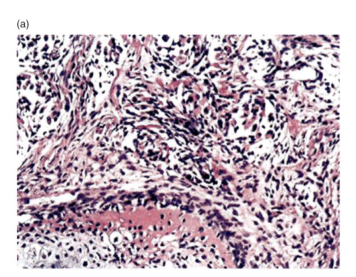

(b)

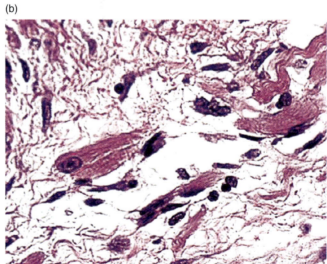

Fig. 13.40 (a) Rhabdomyosarcomatous transformation in germ cell tumor, showing cartilaginous teratomatous elements; **(b)** high-power view of rhabdomyoblasts.

Soft tissue neoplasms of the thymus
Thymolipoma

In contrast to other benign fatty neoplasms of mediastinal soft tissue, thymolipoma (TL) is a lesion comprising intimately-admixed and histologically banal thymic tissue and fat, contained by the thymic capsule. TL is clearly not merely a lipoma involving the thymus; the quantity of thymic tissue seen therein is always in excess of that of the normal thymus. Furthermore, unlike the situation with mediastinal lipomas, several paraneoplastic conditions that are usually associated with thymoma may also be seen in conjunction with TL, including pure red cell aplasia, hypogammaglobulinemia, aplastic anemia, and myasthenia gravis, among others [265].

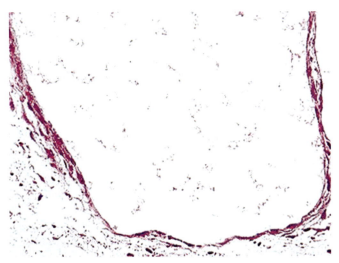

Fig. 13.41 Meningocele consisting of cystic cavity with paucicellular and myxoid change of the peripheral stroma.

Most of these tumors occur in young adults, although all age groups have been represented in the literature. TLs usually are asymptomatic, and they are found incidentally on routine screening chest roentgenograms. However, as many as 10% of patients present with symptoms of tracheal compression or with the aforementioned paraneoplastic conditions. Interestingly, the latter tend to remit after the tumor is removed.

TL is an encapsulated, lobulated yellow mass composed predominantly of mature adipose tissue. Histologic variants showing thymic epithelial proliferation in cellular cords ("proliferating thymolipoma") or with prominent intralesional vascularity have been described (Fig. 13.42). Simple excision is generally curative.

Thymoliposarcoma

The distinction between thymolipoma and its very rare malignant counterpart, the so-called "thymoliposarcoma" (TLS), is based principally on the histologic appearances of the tumors [266]. Gross infiltration of adjacent soft tissue or regional metastasis by TLS also provide overt evidence of malignancy.

The microscopic features of TLS are variable, but they are predicated on a low-power microscopic appearance which generally simulates that of TL. In contrast to that lesion, admixed foci of thymic tissue are separated by tumoral areas that are potentially indistinguishable from well-differentiated liposarcoma, with scattered cytologically-atypical adipocytes dispersed in a background of relatively uniform adipocytic tumor cells (Fig. 13.43). Areas with increased cellularity, rosette-like structures, and spindle-cell or pleomorphic cellular foci also have been documented. The latter elements pose a challenge in differential diagnosis of this tumor, because they may resemble sarcomatoid thymic carcinoma or spindle-cell thymoma.

(a)

(b)

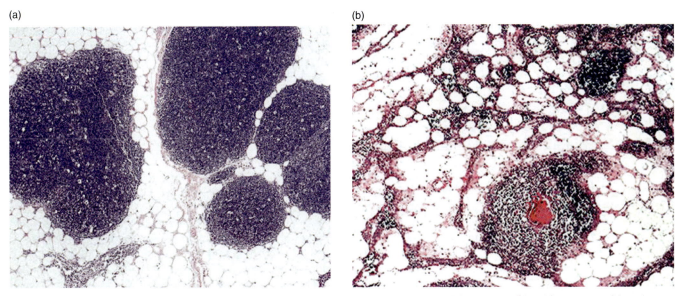

Fig. 13.42 (a) Conventional thymolipoma showing lobules of mature adipocytes arranged among residual thymic tissue; **(b)** proliferating type of thymolipoma.

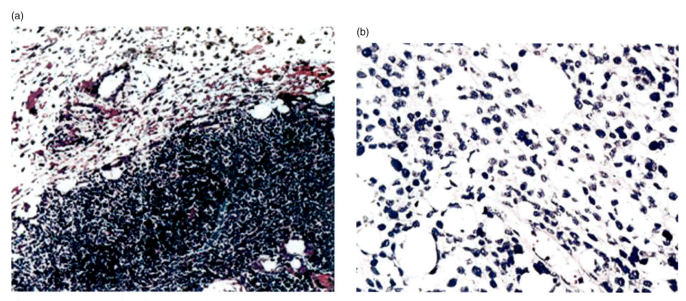

Fig. 13.43 (a) Atypia in thymoliposarcoma admixed within well-defined thymus; **(b)** hypercellularity and atypia in thymoliposarcoma.

The sarcomatous elements in TLS lack epithelial differentiation on immunohistochemical analysis. To date, no molecular analyses of TLS have been conducted, and it is not known whether this neoplasm shows abnormalities in the MDM2, CDK4, *FUS*, or *DDIT* genes, as seen in *de novo* liposarcomas. Nonetheless, the presence of admixed benign thymic tissue in TLS is sufficient to exclude the alternate diagnosis of mediastinal liposarcoma.

Other thymic mesenchymal neoplasms

A unique malignant neoplasm with tumoral osteoid production, which arose in an ectopic hamartomatous thymus, has been reported [267]. Secondary mediastinal involvement was apparent with progression of that lesion.

Rosai has also discussed a thymic large-cell mesenchymal neoplasm that exhibited the histologic features of malignant rhabdoid tumor (MRT) [268]. A histologically similar neoplasm was reported by Lemos and Hamoudi, using the diagnostic term of "malignant histiocytoma." Rare examples of MRT in the posterior mediastinal paravertebral soft tissue also have been described [269,270].

Differential diagnostic considerations and use of immunohistochemistry

Although the differential diagnosis of mesenchymal tumors could be an exhaustive topic, the major clinically relevant categories involve separating 1) benign from malignant tumors, 2) carcinoma from melanoma, mesothelioma, and sarcoma, and 3) primary from metastatic mediastinal neoplasms. Although subtyping of sarcomas is becoming increasingly important, in general only high-grade sarcomas receive adjuvant therapy and similar regimens among the different high-grade sarcoma subtypes are still utilized. Adjuvant radiation therapy depends upon respectability.

Some general immunohistochemical panels are tabulated below for common morphologic patterns. Although immunohistochemistry is useful it is subject to technical issues and interpretative errors. In addition, these general panels are best modified on the basis of the histological features of the tumor and the clinical presentation.

Spindle cell tumors pose some of the most difficult diagnostic problems, in part due to the increasing use of core biopsies for diagnosis. Although sarcomatoid carcinoma does show keratin positivity it may be weak and focal and entirely negative on the biopsy. In short, distinguishing sarcomatoid carcinoma from a sarcoma, particularly an undifferentiated sarcoma on a biopsy may not be possible if the keratin immunostains are negative.

Large epithelioid cell tumors are a heterogenous group and often demonstrate characteristic cytologic features or architecture. Neuroendocrine neoplasms are relatively common in the thorax and span a spectrum from low to high grade with variable degrees of keratin positivity. It should be distinguished from paraganglioma on the basis of differential expression of keratin and S100. Alveolar soft part sarcoma has a distinctive morphology but lacks positivity by lineage and screening immunohistochemical marker. It is sufficiently rare in the mediastinum that it warrants more sophisticated immunostaining for TFE3 and FISH for the translocation to confirm the diagnosis.

In summary, immunohistochemistry is an adjunct tool that should be used as a complement and adjunctive tool in conjunction with morphology, clinical, and radiologic information. Antibody selection must be based on the histological differential diagnosis and although panels can be used as described above they should be interpreted with the knowledge

Table 13.1. Spindle cell tumors

	Cytokeratin	S100	Calretinin	Desmin	CD34	Actin	EMA
S carcinoma	+	−	−	−	−	+/−	+
Mesothelioma	+	−	+	−	−	−	+
SS	+	+/− f	−	−	−	−	+
LMS	−	−	−	+	−	+	−
SFT	−	−	−	−	+	+	−
Melanoma	−	+	−	−	−	+/− f	−
IMT	−/+ f, w	−	−	−/+ w	−	+	−

S. carcinoma: sarcomatoid; SS: synovial sarcoma; LMS: leiomyosarcoma; SFT: solitary fibrous tumor; f: focal; w: weak

Table 13.2. Epithelioid large cell tumors

	CK	S100	HMB45	Desmin	CD138	CD34	Actin	CD30	Syn
Carcinoma	+	−	−	−	−	−	+/−	−	−
PEComa	+	−	+	−/+	−	−	+	−	−
PC neoplasm	−	−	−	−	+	−	−	−	−
Melanoma	−	+	+	−	−	−	−	−	−
ALCL	−	−	−	−	−	−	−	+	−
NEN	+	−	−	−	−	−	−	−	+
LMS	−	−	−	+	−	−	+	−	−
RMS	−	−/+ f	−	+	−	−	+/−	−	−
ASPS	−	−	−	−	−	−	−	−	−
Angiosarcoma	−/+	−	−	−	−	+	−	−	−
Chordoma	+	+	−	−	−	−	−	−	−
Myoepithelioma	+	+/−	−	−	−	−	+	−/+	−
Paraganglioma	−	+ (SC)	−	−	−	−	−	−	+
Seminoma/GCT	−/+	−	−	−	−	−	−	−/+	−

PC: plasma cell; ALCL: anaplastic large cell lymphoma; NEN: neuroendocrine neoplasm; LMS: leiomyosarcoma; RMS: rhabdomyosarcoma; ASPS: alveolar soft part sarcoma; f: focal; SC: sustentacular cells; GCT: germ cell tumor (embryonal carcinoma, choriocarcinoma); CK: cytokeratin; Syn: synaptophysin.

Table 13.3. Small round cell tumors

	CK	S100	LCA	Desmin	CD99	Fli−1	TdT	NSE	Syn
Carcinoma/NECA	+	−	−	−	−	−	+/−	−	+
RMS	−	−	−	+	−	−	−	−	−
ESFT/PNET	−	−	−	−	+	+	−	−	−
Lymphoma	−	−	+	−	−	+/−	+	−	−
Melanoma	−	+	−	−	−	−	−	−	−
NB	−	−/−+(G)	−	−	−	−	−	+	+

NECA: neuroendocrine carcinoma; RMS: rhabdomyosarcoma; ESFT/PNET: Ewing sarcoma family of tumors/primitive neuroectodermal tumor; NB: neuroblastsma; G: gangliocytic cells

Table 13.4. Pleomorphic undifferentiated tumors

	CK	S100	Desmin	Actin	CD30
Carcinoma	+	−	−	+/−	−
Melanoma	+	−	−/+	+	−
ALCL	−	−	−	−	−
Undiff. sarcoma	−	−	−	+/− w	−
Seminoma/EC	−/+	−	−	−	−/+

ALCL: anaplastic large cell lymphoma; EC: GCT: germ cell tumor (embryonal carcinoma, choriocarcinoma); CK: cytokeratin.

that sensitivity and specificity or aberrant immunoreactivity can lead to pitfalls in diagnosis.

Common pitfalls include interpretation of tumor cell positivity for myoid markers with entrapped or atrophic muscle cells, aberrant cytokeratin expression in melanoma or leiomyosarcoma, and CD31 positivity in macrophages. The pattern of reactivity of any given marker is important, for example, nuclear versus cytoplasmic, membranous and focal versus diffuse. Non-specific background reactivity is a common occurrence in immunohistochemistry and if internal control tissue is present, attention to its pattern of reactivity is helpful in distinguishing this effect.

References

1. Pachter MR, Lattes R: Mesenchymal tumors of the mediastinum. I. Tumors of fibrous tissue, adipose tissue, smooth muscle and striated muscle. *Cancer* 16:74–94, 1963

2. Pachter MR, Lattes R: Mesenchymal tumors of the mediastinum. II. Tumors of blood vascular origin. *Cancer* 16:95–107, 1963

3. Pachter MR, Lattes R: Mesenchymal tumors of the mediastinum. III. Tumors of lymph vascular origin. *Cancer* 16:108–17, 1963

4. Besnayak I, Szende B, Lapis K: *Mediastinal Tumors and Pseudotumors. Diagnosis, Pathology and Surgical Treatment*. New York, NY, Karger, 1984

5. Benjamin SP, McCormack U, Effler DB, et al.: Primary tumors of the mediastinum. *Chest* 62:297–303, 1972

6. Conkle DM, Adkins RB Jr: Primary malignant tumors of the mediastinum. *Ann Thorac Surg* 14:553–67, 1972

7. Marchevsky AM, Kaneko M: *Surgical Pathology of the Mediastinum*. New York, NY, Raven, 1984

8. Davidson KG, Walbaum PR, McCormack RJM: Intrathoracic neural tumors. *Thorax* 33:359–67, 1978

9. Mathew BG, Jones RM, Campbell MJ: Horner's syndrome due to superior-mediastinal schwannoma. *J Neurol Neurosurg Psychiatr* 51:1460–1, 1988 (letter)

10. Chaves Espinosa JI, Chaves Fernandez JA, Hoyer OH, et al.: Endothoracic neurogenic neoplasms, analysis of 30 cases. *Rev Interam Radiol* 5:49–54, 1980

11. Ecker RR, Timmes LJ, Miscall L: Neurogenic tumors of the intrathoracic vagus nerve. *Arch Surg* 86:222–9, 1963

12. Enzinger FM, Weiss SW: *Soft Tissue Tumors* (ed 2). St Louis, MO, Mosby, 1989

13. Gale AW, Jelihovsky T, Grant AF, et al.: Neurogenic tumors of the mediastinum. *Ann Thorac Surg* 17:434–43, 1974

14. Strickland B, Wolverson MK: Intrathoracic vagus nerve tumors. *Thorax* 29:215–22, 1974

15. Dehner LP: *Pediatric Surgical Pathology* (ed 2). New York, NY, Williams & Wilkins, 1987

16. Woodruff JM: Peripheral nerve tumors showing glandular differentiation (glandular schwannoma). *Cancer* 37:2399–413, 1976

17. Nakazato Y, Ishizeki J. Takahashi K, et al.: Immunohistochemical localization of S-100 protein in granular cell myoblastoma. *Cancer* 49: 1624–8, 1982

18. Steffansson K, Wollmann R, Jerkovic M: SlOO protein in soft tissue tumors derived from Schwann cells and melanocytes. *Am J Pathol* 106:261–8, 1982

19. Wick MR, Manivel JC, Swanson PE: Contributions of immunohistochemical analysis to the diagnosis of soft tissue tumors: A review. *Prog Surg Pathol* 8: 197–249, 1988

20. Wick MR, Swanson PE, Manivel JC: Immunohistochemical analysis of soft tissue sarcomas. Comparisons with electron microscopy. *Appl Pathol* 16:169–96, 1980

21. Swanson PE, Manivel JC, Wick MR: Immunoreactivity for Leu 7 in neurofibrosarcoma and other spindle-cell soft tissue sarcomas. *Am J Pathol* 126:546–60, 1987

22. Johnson MD, Glick AD, Davis BW: Immunohistochemical evaluation of Leu-7, myelin basic protein, S-100 protein, glial fibrillary acidic protein, and LN3 immunoreactivity in nerve sheath tumors and sarcomas. *Arch Pathol Lab Med* 112: 155–60, 1988

23. Thompson SJ, Schatteman GC, Gown AM, et al.: A monoclonal antibody against nerve growth factor receptor. Immunohistochemical analysis of normal and neoplastic human tissue. *Am J Clin Pathol* 92:415–23, 1989

24. Lassmann H, Jurecka W, Lassmann G, et al.: Different types of benign nerve sheath tumors: Light microscopy, electron microscopy and autoradiography. *Virchows Arch [A]* 375:197–210, 1977

25. Sian CS, Ryan SF: The ultrastructure of neurilemmoma with emphasis on Antoni B tissue. *Hum Pathol* 12: 145–60, 1981

26. Wick MR, Swanson PE, Manivel JC: Immunohistochemical analysis of soft tissue sarcomas. Comparisons with electron microscopy. *Appl Pathol* 16:169–96, 1980

27. Robinson JM, Knoll R, Henry DA: Intrathoracic granular cell myoblastoma. *South Med J* 81:1453–7, 1988

28. Rosenbloom PM, Barrows GH, Kmetz DR, et al.: Granular cell myoblastoma arising from the thoracic sympathetic nerve chain. *J Pediatr Surg* 10:819–22, 1975

29. Harrier KWV, Patchefsky AS: Malignant granular cell myoblastoma of the posterior mediastinum. *Chest* 61:95–6, 1972

30. Mandybur TI: Melanotic nerve sheath tumours. *J Neurosurg* 41:187–92, 1974

31. Paris F, Cabanes J, Munoz C, *et al.*: Melanotic spinothoracic schwannoma. *Thorax* 34:243–6. 1979

32. Carney JA: Psammomatous melanotic schwannoma. A distinctive, heritable tumor with special associations, including cardiac myxoma and the Cushing syndrome. *Am J Surg Pathol* 14:206–22, 1990

33. Fletcher CDM, Davies SE, McKee PH: Cellular schwannoma: A distinct pseudosarcomatous entity. *Histopathol* 11:21–35, 1987

34. Woodruff JM, Goodwin TA, Erlandson RA, *et al.*: Cellular schwannoma. A variety of schwannoma sometimes mistaken for a malignant tumor. *Am J Surg Pathol* 5:733–44, 1981

35. Lodding P, Kindblom L-G, Angervall L, *et al.*: Cellular schwannoma. A clinicopathologic study of 29 cases. *Virchows Arch [A]* 410:237–48, 1990

36. White W, Rosenblum M, Woodruff J: Cellular schwannoma: A clinicopathologic study of 57 cases. *Mod Pathol* 3:106A, 1990 (abstr)

37. Bourgouin PM, Shepard JO, Moore EH, *et al.*: Plexiform neurofibromatosis of the mediastinum: CT appearance. *Am J Radiol* 151:461–3, 1988

38. Chalmers AH, Armstrong P: Plexiform mediastinal neurofibromas. A report of two cases. *Br J Radiol* 50:215–17, 1977

39. Zorbas JA. Kreatsas GK: Neurofibroma of the intrathoracic vagus nerve in a man with Recklinghausen's disease. Case report. *Milit Med* 142:384–5, 1977

40. Dines DE, Payne WS, Howard PH Jr: Von Recklinghausen's neurofibromatosis with plexiform mediastinal involvement. Report of a case. *Dis Chest* 50:437–9, 1966

41. Sarin CL, Bennett MH, Jackson JW: Intrathoracic neurofibroma of the vagus nerve. *Br J Dis Chest* 68:46–50, 1974

42. Dines DE, Payne WS, Howard PH Jr: Von Recklinghausen's neurofibromatosis with plexiform mediastinal involvement. Report of a case. *Dis Chest* 50:437–9, 1966

43. Storm FK, Eilber FR, Mirra J, *et al.*: Neurofibrosarcoma. *Cancer* 45:126–9, 1980

44. Guccion JG, Enzinger FM: Malignant schwannoma associated with von Recklinghausen's neurofibromatosis. *Virchows Arch [A]* 383:43–57, 1979

45. D'Agostino AN, Soule EH, Miller RH: Primary malignant neoplasms of nerves (malignant neurilemmomas) in patients without manifestations of multiple neurofibromatosis (von Recklinghausen's disease). *Cancer* 16:1003–14, 1963

46. Ducatman BS, Scheithauer BW: Postirradiation neurofibrosarcoma. *Cancer* 51:1028–33, 1983

47. Stout AP: The malignant tumors of the peripheral nerves. *Am J Cancer* 25:1–36, 1935

48. Ducatman BS, Scheithauer BW, Piepgras DG, *et al.*: Malignant peripheral nerve sheath tumors. A clinicopathologic study of 120 cases. *Cancer* 57:2006–21, 1986

49. Woodruff JM, Chernik NL, Smith MC, *et al.*: Peripheral nerve tumors with rhabdomyosarcomatous differentiation (malignant "triton" tumors). *Cancer* 32:426–39, 1973

50. Ducatman BS, Scheithauer BW: Malignant peripheral nerve sheath tumors with divergent differentiation. *Cancer* 54:1049–57, 1984

51. Ghosh BC, Ghosh L, Huvos AG, *et al.*: Malignant schwannoma. A clinicopathologic study. *Cancer* 31:184–90, 1973

52. Krumerman MS, Stingle W: Synchronous malignant glandular schwannomas in congenital neurofibromatosis. *Cancer* 41:2444–51, 1978

53. Wick MR, Swanson PE, Scheithauer BW, *et al.*: Malignant peripheral nerve sheath tumor. An immunohistochemical study of 62 cases. *Am J Clin Pathol* 87:425–33, 1987

54. Nakajima T, Watanabe S, Sa to Y, *et al.*: An immunoperoxidase study of S-100 protein distribution in normal and neoplastic tissues. *Am J Surg Pathol* 6:715–27, 1982

55. Miettinen M: Immunohistochemistry of peripheral nerve sheath sarcomas. *Mod Pathol* 3:67 A, 1990 (abstr)

56. Tsuneyoshi M, Enjoji M: Primary malignant peripheral nerve tumors (malignant schwannomas): A clinicopathologic and electron microscopic study. *Acta Pathol Jpn* 29:363–75, 1979

57. Erlandson RA, Woodruff JM: Peripheral nerve sheath tumors: An electron microscopic study of 43 cases. *Cancer* 49:273–87, 1982

58. Grieger TA, Carl M, Liebert HP, *et al.*: Mediastinal liposarcoma in a patient infected with the human immunodeficiency virus. *Am J Med* 84:366, 1988 (letter)

59. Chitale AR, Dickersin GR: Electron microscopy in the diagnosis of malignant schwannomas. A report of six cases. *Cancer* 51:1448–61, 1983

60. de Lorimier AA, Bragg KU, Linden G: Neuroblastoma in childhood. *Am J Dis Child* 118:441–50, 1969

61. Bar-Ziv J, Nogrady MB: Mediastinal neuroblastoma and ganglioneuroma. The differentiation between primary and secondary involvement on the chest roentgenogram. *AJR* 125:380–90, 1975

62. Carachi R, Campbell PE, Kent M: Thoracic neural crest tumors. A clinical review. *Cancer* 51:949–54, 1983

63. Evans AE, Chatten J, D'Angio GJ, *et al.*: A review of 17 IVS neuroblastoma patients at the Children's Hospital of Philadelphia. *Cancer* 45:833–9, 1980

64. Fortner J, Nicastri A, Murphy ML: Neuroblastoma: Natural history and results of treating 133 cases. *Ann Surg* 167:132–42, 1968

65. King RM, Telander RL, Smithson WA, *et al.*: Primary mediastinal tumors in children. *J Pediatr Surg* 17:512–20, 1982

66. Perez CA, Vietti T, Ackerman LV, *et al.*: Tumors of the sympathetic nervous system in children. An appraisal of treatment and results. *Radiology* 88:750–60, 1967

67. Adam A, Hochholzer L: Ganglioneuroblastoma of the posterior mediastinum: A clinicopathologic review of 80 cases. *Cancer* 47:373–81, 1981

68. Alterman K, Schueller EF: Maturation of neuroblastoma to ganglioneuroma. *Am J Dis Child* 120:217–22, 1970

69. Schmidt ML, Lal A, Seeger RC, Maris JM, Shimada H, O'Leary M, Gerbing RB, Matthay KK: Favorable prognosis for patients 12 to 18 months of age with stage 4 non-amplified MYCN neuroblastoma: a Children's Cancer Group Study. *Clin Oncol*, 23: 6474–80, 2005. Epub 2005 Aug 22.

70. Gutierrez JC, Fischer AC, Sola JE, *et al.*: Markedly improving survival of neuroblastoma: a 30-year analysis of 1,646 patients. *Pediatr Surg Int.* 23:637–46, 2007

71. Gutierrez JC, Fischer AC, Sola JE, Perez EA, Koniaris LG: *Eur J Pediatr Surg* 10: 353–9, 2000

72. Hamilton JP, Koop CE: Ganglioneuromas in children. *Surg Gynecol Obstet* 121:803–12, 1965

73. Young DG: Thoracic neuroblastoma/ganglioneuroma. *J Pediatr Surg* 18:37–41, 1983

74. Bender BL, Ghatak NR: Light and electron microscopic observations on a ganglioneuroma. *Acta Neuropathol* 42:7–10, 1978

75. Yokoyama M, Okada K, Tokue A, et al.: Ultrastructural and biochemical study of benign ganglioneuroma. *Virchows Arch [A]* 361:195–209, 1973

76. Henderson DW, Leppard PJ, Brennan JS, et al.: Primitive neuroepithelial tumours of soft tissue and of bone: further ultrastructural and immunocytochemical clarification of 'Ewing's sarcoma', including freeze fracture analysis. *J Submicrosc Cytol Pathol* 21:35–57, 1989

77. Triche TJ, Cavazzana AO, Navarro S, et al.: N-myc protein expression in small round cell tumors. *Prog Clin Biol Res* 271:475–85, 1988

78. McKeon C, Thiele CJ, Ross MA, et al.: Indistinguishable patterns of protooncogene expression in two distinct but closely related tumors: Ewing's sarcoma and neuroepithelioma. *Cancer Res* 49:4307–11, 1988

79. Thiele CJ, McKeon C, Triche TJ, et al.: Differential pro; to-oncogene expression characterizes histopathologically indistinguishable tumors of the peripheral nervous system. *J Clin Invest* 80:804–11, 1987

80. Cavazanna AO, Miser JS, Jefferson J, et al.: Experimental evidence for a neural origin of Ewing's sarcoma of bone. *Am J Pathol* 127:507–18, 1987

81. Hachitanda Y, Tsuneyoshi M, Enjoji M, et al.: Congenital primitive neuroectodermal tumor with epithelial and glial differentiation. An ultrastructural and immunohistochemical study. *Arch Pathol Lab Med* 114:101–5, 1990

82. Moll R, Lee I, Gould V, et al.: Immunocytochemical analysis of Ewing's tumors. Patterns of expression of intermediate filaments and desmosomal proteins indicate cell type heterogeneity and pluripotential differentiation. *Am J Pathol* 127:288–304, 1987

83. Shinoda M, Tsutsumi Y, Hata J-I, et al.: Peripheral neuroepithelioma in childhood. Immunohistochemical demonstration of epithelial differentiation. *Arch Pathol Lab Med* 112:1155–8, 1988

84. Swanson PE, Dehner LP, Wick MR: Polyphenotypic small cell tumors of childhood. *Lab Invest* 58:9P, 1988

85. Fujii Y, Hongo T, Nakagawa Y, et al.: Cell culture of small round cell tumor originating in the thoracopulmonary region. Evidence for derivation from a primitive pluripotential cell. *Cancer* 64:43–51, 1989

86. Turc-Carel C, Aurias A, Mugneret F, et al.: Chromosomes in Ewing's sarcoma. I. An evaluation of 85 cases of remarkable consistency oft(II;22) (q24; q 12). *Cancer Genet Cytogenet* 32:229–38, 1988

87. Blau O. Molecular investigation of Ewing sarcoma: about detecting translocations. *Olga Blau EMBO Mol Med* 4: 449–50, 2012

88. Marina NM, Etcubanas E, Parham DM, et al.: Peripheral primitive neuroectodermal tumor (peripheral neuroepithelioma) in children. A review of the St. Jude experience and controversies in diagnosis and management. *Cancer* 64:1952–60, 1989

89. Marina NM, Etcubanas E, Parham DM, et al.: Peripheral primitive neuroectodermal tumor (peripheral neuroepithelioma) in children. A review of the St. Jude experience and controversies in diagnosis and management. *Cancer* 64:1952–60, 1989

90. Crist WM, Raney RB, Newton W, et al.: Intrathoracic soft tissue sarcomas in children. *Cancer* 50:598–604, 1982

91. Misugi K, Okajima H, Newton WA, et al.: Mediastinal origin of a melanotic progonoma or retinal anlage tumor. Ultrastructural evidence for neural crest origin. *Cancer* 18:477–84, 1965

92. D'Abrera VSE, Burfitt-Williams W: Melanotic neuroectodermal neoplasm of the posterior mediastinum. *J Pathol* III:165–72, 1973

93. Doglioni C, Bontempini L, Iuzzolino P, et al.: Ependymoma of the mediastinum. *Arch Pathol Lab Med* 112:194–6, 1988

94. Mori T, Nomori H, Yoshioka M, Ikeda K, Shibata H, Ohba Y, Yoshimoto K, Iyama K: A case of primary mediastinal ependymoma. *Ann Thorac Cardiovasc Surg* 15:332–5, 2009

95. Doglione C, Bontempini L, Iuzzolino P, Furlan G, Rosai J: Ependymoma of the mediastinum. *Arch Pathol Lab Med* 112:194–6, 1988

96. Maeda S, Takahashi S, Koike K, Sato M: Primary ependymoma in the posterior mediastinum. *Ann Thorac Cardiovasc Surg* 17:494–7, 2011. Epub 2011, Jul 13.

97. Wilson RW, Moran CA: Primary ependymoma of the mediastinum: a clinicopathologic study of three cases. *Ann Diagn Pathol* 2:293–300, 1998

98. Estrozi B, Queiroga E, Bacchi CE, Faria Soares de Almeida V, Lucas de Carvalho J, Lageman GM, Rosado-de-Christenson M, Suster S: Myxopapillary ependymoma of the posterior mediastinum. *Ann Diagn Pathol* 10:283–7, 2006

99. Wilson RW, Moran CA: Primary ependymoma of the mediastinum: a clinicopathologic study of three cases. *Ann Diagn Pathol* 2:293–300, 1998

100. Brown LR, Reiman HM, Rosenow EC III, et al.: Intrathoracic lymphangioma. *Mayo Clin Proc* 61:882–92, 1986

101. Feng YF, Masterson JB, Riddell RH: Lymphangioma of the middle mediastinum as an incidental finding on a chest radiograph. *Thorax* 35:955–6, 1980

102. Bratu M, Brown M, Carter M, et al.: Cystic hygroma of the mediastinum in children. *Am J Dis Child* 119:348–51, 1970

103. Curley SA, Ablin DS, Kosloske AM: Giant cystic hygroma of the posterior mediastinum. *J Pediatr Surg* 24:398–400, 1989

104. Perkes EA, Haller JO, Kassner EG, et al.: Mediastinal cystic hygroma in infants. Two cases with no extension into the neck. *Clin Pediatr* 18:168–70, 1979

105. Scholefield JH, Angwin R: Posterior mediastinal lymphangioma presenting with thoracic inlet compression. *Br J Hosp Med* 41:183–4, 1989

106. Sumner TE, Volberg FM, Kiser PE, et al.: Mediastinal cystic hygroma in children. *Pediatr Radiol* II:160–2, 1981

107. Hall ER Jr, Blades B: Lymphangioma of mediastinum. Report of 2 cases. *Dis Chest* 32:207–13, 1957

108. Feutz EP, Yune HY, Mandelbaum I, et al.: Intrathoracic cystic hygroma. A report of three cases. *Radiology* 108:61–6, 1973

109. Ionescu GO, Tuleasca I, Gavrilita N, et al.: Infantile giant mediastinal cystic hygroma. *J Pediatr Surg* II:469–70, 1976

110. King DT, Duffy DM, Hirose FM, et al.: Lymphangiosarcoma arising from lymphangioma circumscriptum. *Arch Dermatol* 115:969–72, 1979

111. Gilsanz V, Yeh He, Baron MG: Multiple lymphangiomas of the neck, axilla, mediastinum and bones in an adult. *Radiology* 120:161–2, 1976

112. Watts MA, Gibbons JA, Aaron BL: Mediastinal and osseous lymphangiomatosis, case report and review. *Ann Thorac Surg* 34:324–8, 1982

113. Berberich FR, Bernstain ID, Ochs HD, et al.: Lymphangiomatosis with chylothorax. *J Pediatr* 87:941–3, 1975

114. Gindhart TD, Tucker WY, Choy SH: Cavernous hemangioma of the superior mediastinum. Report of a case with electron microscopy and computerized tomography. *Am J Surg Pathol* 3: 353–61, 1979

115. Kings GLM: Multifocal hemangiomatous malformation: A case. *Thorax* 30:485–8, 1975

116. Kalicinski ZH, Joszt W, Perdzynski W, et al.: Hemangioma of the superior caval vein. *J Pediatr Surg* 17:178–9, 1982

117. Davis JM, Mark GJ, Greene R: Benign blood vascular tumors of the mediastinum. Report of four cases and review of the literature. *Radiology* 126:581–7, 1978

118. Weiss SW, Enzinger FM: Epithelioid hemangioendothelioma. A vascular tumor often mistaken for carcinoma. *Cancer* 50:970–81, 1982

119. Suster S, Moran CA, Koss MN. Epithelioid hemangioendothelioma of the anterior mediastinum. Clinicopathologic, immunohistochemical, and ultrastructural analysis of 12 cases. *Am J Surg Pathol*.1994 Sep;18(9):871–81.

120. Awotwi JD, Zusman J, Waring WW, et al.: Benign hemangioendothelioma:A rare type of posterior mediastinal mass in children. *J Pediatr Surg* 18:581–4, 1983

121. Rosai J, Gold J, Landy R: The histiocytoid hemangiomas. A unifying concept embracing several previously described entities of skin, soft tissue, large vessels, bone and heart. *Hum Pathol I*:707–30, 1979

122. Moreno A, Canada MA, Minguella J, et al.: Histiocytoid hemangioma of the innominate vein. *Pathol Res Pract* 183:785–8, 1988

123. Gibbs AR, Johnson NF, Giddings JC, et al.: Primary angiosarcoma of the mediastinum: Light and electron microscopic demonstration off actor VIII-related antigen in neoplastic cells. *Hum Pathol* 15:687–91, 1984

124. Wychulis AR, Payne WS, Clagett OT, et al.: Surgical treatment of mediastinal tumors. A forty year experience. *J Thorac Cardiovasc Surg* 62:379–92, 1971

125. Iwami D, Shimaoka S, Mochizuki I, Sakuma T. Kaposiform hemangioendothelioma of the mediastinum in a 7-month-old boy: a case report. *J Pediatr Surg.* 2006 Aug;41 (8):1486–8.

126. Croteau SE, Liang MG, Kozakewich HP, Alomari AI, Fishman SJ, Mulliken JB, Trenor CC. Kaposiform hemangioendothelioma: atypical features and risks of Kasabach-Merritt phenomenon in 107 referrals. *J. Pediatr.* 2013 Jan;162(1):142–7.

127. Lyons LL, North PE, Mac-Moune Lai F, Stoler MH, Folpe AL, Weiss SW. Kaposiform hemangioendothelioma: a study of 33 cases emphasizing its pathologic, immunophenotypic, and biologic uniqueness from juvenile hemangioma. *Am J Surg Pathol.* 2004 May;28(5):559–68.

128. Miettinen M, Wang ZF. Prox1 transcription factor as a marker for vascular tumors-evaluation of 314 vascular endothelial and 1086 nonvascular tumors. *Am J. Surg Pathol.* 2012 Mar;36(3):351–9.

129. Gibbs AR, Johnson NF, Giddings JC, et al.: Primary angiosarcoma of the mediastinum: Light and electron microscopic demonstration off actor VIII-related antigen in neoplastic cells. *Hum Pathol* 15:687–91, 1984

130. Rosado FG, Itani DM, Coffin CM, Cates JM. Utility of immunohistochemical staining with FLI1, D2–40, CD31, and CD34 in the diagnosis of acquired immunodeficiency syndrome-related and non-acquired immunodeficiency syndrome-related Kaposi sarcoma. *Arch Pathol Lab Med.* 2012 Mar;136(3):301–4.

131. Weissferdt A, Kalhor N, Suster S, Moran CA. Primary angiosarcomas of the anterior mediastinum: a clinicopathologic and immunohistochemical study of 9 cases. *Hum Pathol.* 2010 Dec;41 (12):1711–17.

132. Deyrup AT, Miettinen M, North PE, Khoury JD, Tighiouart M, Spunt SL, Parham D, Weiss SW, Shehata BM. Angiosarcomas arising in the viscera and soft tissue of children and young adults: a clinicopathologic study of 15 cases. *Am J Surg Pathol.* 2009 Feb;33(2):264–9.

133. Dosios TJ, Angouras DC, Floros DG. Primary desmoid tumor of the posterior mediastinum. *Ann Thorac Surg.* 1998 Dec;66(6):2098–9.

134. Kocak Z, Adli M, Erdir O, Erekul S, Cakmak A. Intrathoracic desmoid tumor of the posterior mediastinum with transdiaphragmatic extension. Report of a case. *Tumori.* 2000 Nov–Dec;86(6):489–91.

135. Ko SF, Ng SH, Hsiao CC, Hsieh CS, Lin JW, Huang CC, Shih TY. Juvenile fibromatosis of the posterior mediastinum with intraspinal extension. *AJNR Am J Neuroradiol.* 1996 Mar;17(3):522–4.

136. Black WC, Armstrong P, Daniel TM, Cooper PH. Computed tomography of aggressive fibromatosis in the posterior mediastinum. *J Comput Assist Tomogr.* 1987 Jan–Feb;11(1):153–5.

137. Tam CG, Broome DR, Shannon RL. Desmoid tumor of the anterior mediastinum: CT and radiologic features. *J Comput Assist Tomogr.* 1994 May–Jun;18(3):499–501.

138. Borzellino G, Minicozzi AM, Giovinazzo F, Faggian G, Iuzzolino P, Cordiano C Cardoso PF, da Silva LC, Bonamigo TP, Geyer G. Intrathoracic desmoid tumor with invasion of the great vessels. *Eur J Cardiothorac Surg.* 2002 Dec;22(6):1017–19.

139. Borzellino G, Minicozzi AM, Giovinazzo F, Faggian G, Iuzzolino P, Cordiano C. Intra-thoracic desmoid tumour in a patient with a previous aortocoronary bypass. *World J Surg Oncol.* 2006 Jul 10;4:43

140. Bouchikh M, Arame A, Riquet M, Le Pimpec-Barthes F. Cardiac failure due to a giant desmoid tumour of the posterior mediastinum. *Eur J Cardiothorac Surg.* 2013, May; 3; doi: 10.1093/ejcts/ezt214

141. Puleo S, Di Cataldo A, Li Destri G, *et al.*: Radiohyperthermia for subcutaneous metastasis of hemangiopericytoma of the mediastinum: Case report. *Tumori* 74:485–8, 1988

142. Arisi C, Colombo L: Betrachung zu den Fibrosarkomen in Mediastinum (kasuistischer Beitrag). *Ref Prax Pneumol* 22:404, 1968

143. Baldwin RS: Hypoglycemia associated with fibrosarcoma of the mediastinum. Review of Doege's patient. *Ann Surg* 160:975–7, 1964

144. Barua NR, Patel AR, Takita H, *et al.*: Fibrosarcoma of the mediastinum. *J Surg Oncol* 12: 11–17, 1979

145. Ringertz N, Lindholm SO: Mediastinal tumors and cysts. *J Thorac Surg* 31: 458–87, 1956

146. Walsh CH, Wright AD, Coore HG: Hypoglycemia associated with an intrathoracic fibrosarcoma. *Clin Endocrinol* 4:393–8, 1975

147. Watanabe Y: Long term survival of a patient with fibrosarcoma of the mediastinum. *Jpn J Thorac Surg* 26:507–12, 1973

148. Bahrami A, Folpe AL. Adult-type fibrosarcoma: A reevaluation of 163 putative cases diagnosed at a single institution over a 48-year period. *Am J Surg Pathol.* 2010 Oct;34(10):1504–13.

149. Chen W, Chan CW, Mok CK: Malignant fibrous histiocytoma of the mediastinum. *Cancer* 50:797–800, 1982

150. Mills SA, Breyer RH, Johnston FR, *et al.*: Malignant fibrous histiocytoma of the mediastinum and lung. A report of three cases. *J Thorac Cardiovasc Surg* 84:367–72, 1982

151. Morshius WJ, Cox AL, Lacquet LK, *et al.*: Primary malignant fibrous histiocytoma of the mediastinum. *Thorax* 45:154–5, 1990

152. Yellin A, Herczeg E, Tichler TE, *et al.*: Malignant fibrous histiocytoma of the anterior mediastinum: A rare case with 19 years survival. *Respir Med* 83:369–73, 1989

153. Kogon B, Shehata B, Katzenstein H, Samai C, Mahle W, Maher K, Olson T. Primary congenital infantile fibrosarcoma of the heart: the first confirmed case *Ann Thorac Surg.* 2011 Apr;91(4):1276–80.

154. Strehl S, Ladenstein R, Wrba F, Salzer-Kuntschik M, Gadner H, Ambros PF. Translocation (12;13) in a case of infantile fibrosarcoma. *Cancer Genet Cytogenet.* 1993 Nov;71(1):94–6.

155. Bourgeois JM, Knezevich SR, Mathers JA, Sorensen PH. Molecular detection of the ETV6-NTRK3 gene fusion differentiates congenital fibrosarcoma from other childhood spindle cell tumors. *Am J Surg Pathol.* 2000 Jul;24(7):937–46.

156. Sandberg AA, Bridge JA. Updates on the cytogenetics and molecular genetics of bone and soft tissue tumors: congenital (infantile) fibrosarcoma and mesoblastic nephroma. *Cancer Genet Cytogenet.* 2002 Jan 1;132(1):1–13.

157. Coffin CM, Jaszcz W, O'Shea PA, Dehner LP. So-called congenital-infantile fibrosarcoma: does it exist and what is it? *Pediatr Pathol.* 1994 Jan–Feb;14(1):133–50.

158. Coffin CM, Dehner LP. Fibroblastic-myofibroblastic tumors in children and adolescents: a clinicopathologic study of 108 examples in 103 patients. *Pediatr Pathol.* 1991 Jul–Aug;11(4):569–88.

159. Sheng WQ, Hisaoka M, Okamoto S, Tanaka A, Meis-Kindblom JM, Kindblom LG, Ishida T, Nojima T, Hashimoto H. Congenital-infantile fibrosarcoma. A clinicopathologic study of 10 cases and molecular detection of the ETV6-NTRK3 fusion transcripts using paraffin-embedded tissues. *Am J Clin Pathol.* 2001 Mar;115(3):348–55.

160. Sugiyama K, Nakajima Y. Inflammatory myofibroblastic tumor in the mediastinum mimicking a malignant tumor. *Diagn Interv Radiol.* 2008 Dec;14(4):197–9.

161. Chen CH, Lin RL, Liu HC, Chen CH, Hung TT, Huang WC. Inflammatory myofibroblastic tumor mimicking anterior mediastinal malignancy. *Ann Thorac Surg.* 2008 Oct;86(4):1362–4.

162. Makimoto Y, Nabeshima K, Iwasaki H, Ishiguro A, Miyoshi T, Shiraishi T, Iwasaki A, Shirakusa T. Inflammatory myofibroblastic tumor of the posterior mediastinum: an older adult case with anaplastic lymphoma kinase abnormalities determined using immunohistochemistry and fluorescence in situ hybridization. *Virchows Arch.* 2005 Apr;446(4):451–5.

163. Makimoto Y, Nabeshima K, Iwasaki H, Ishiguro A, Miyoshi T, Shiraishi T, Iwasaki A, Shirakusa T. Inflammatory myofibroblastic tumor of the posterior mediastinum: an older adult case with anaplastic lymphoma kinase abnormalities determined using immunohistochemistry and fluorescence in situ hybridization. *Virchows Arch.* 2005 Apr;446(4):451–5.

164. Corneli G, Alifano M, Forti Parri S, Lacava N, Boaron M. Invasive inflammatory pseudo-tumor involving the lung and the mediastinum. *Thorac Cardiovasc Surg.* 2001 Apr;49(2):124–6.

165. Coffin CM, Hornick JL, Fletcher CD. Inflammatory myofibroblastic tumor: comparison of clinicopathologic, histologic, and immunohistochemical features including ALK expression in atypical and aggressive cases. *Am J Surg Pathol.* 2007 Apr;31(4):509–20.

166. Mariño-Enríquez A, Wang WL, Roy A, Lopez-Terrada D, Lazar AJ, Fletcher CD, Coffin CM, Hornick JL. Epithelioid inflammatory myofibroblastic sarcoma: An aggressive intra-abdominal variant of inflammatory myofibroblastic tumor with nuclear membrane or perinuclear ALK. *Am J Surg Pathol.* 2011 Jan;35(1):135–44.

167. Sigel JE, Smith TA, Reith JD, Goldblum JR. Immunohistochemical analysis of anaplastic lymphoma kinase expression in deep soft tissue calcifying fibrous pseudotumor: evidence of a late sclerosing stage of inflammatory myofibroblastic tumor? *Ann Diagn Pathol.* 2001 Feb;5(1):10–14.

168. Politis J, Funahasi A, Gehlsen JA, *et al.*: Intrathoracic lipomas. Report of three cases and review of the literature with emphasis on endobronchial lipoma. *J Thorac Cardiovasc Surg* 77: 550–6, 1979

169. Sarama RF, DiGiacomo WA, Safirstein BH: Primary mediastinal lipoma. *J Med Soc NJ* 78:901–2, 1981

170. Homer MJ, Wechsler RJ, Carter BL: Mediastinal lipomatosis. CT confirmation of a normal variant. *Radiology* 128:657–61, 1978

171. Lee WJ, Fattal G: Mediastinal lipomatosis in simple obesity. *Chest* 70:308–9, 1976

172. Chong GC, Cooper T, Payne WS: Steroid induced mediastinal lipomatosis. *Minn Med* 4:597–8, 1973

173. Tabrisky J, Rowe JH, Cristie SG, *et al.*: Benign mediastinal lipoblastomatosis. *J Pediatr Surg* 9:399–401, 1974.

174. Koerner HJ, Sun KDC: Mediastinal lipomatosis secondary to steroid therapy. *AJR* 98:461–75, 1966

175. Shukla LW, Katz JA, Wagner ML: Mediastinal lipomatosis: A complication of high dose steroid therapy in children. *Pediatr Radiol* 19:57–8, 1988

176. Udwadia ZF, Kumar N, Bhaduri AS. Mediastinal hibernoma. *Eur J Cardiothorac Surg.* 1999 Apr;15 (4):533–5.

177. A Baldi, M Santini, P Mellone, V Esposito, AM Groeger, M Caputi, and F Baldi. Mediastinal hibernoma: a case report. *J Clin Pathol.* 2004 September; 57(9): 993–4.

178. Turaga KK, Edibaldo S, Sanger WG, Nelson M, Hunter WI, Miettinen M, Gatalica Z. A (9;11)(q34;q13) translocation in a hibernoma. *Cancer Genetics and Cytogenetics* Volume 170, Issue 2, 15 October, 2006; pp. 163–6.

179. Furlong M, Fanburg-Smith J, Miettinen M. The Morphologic Spectrum of Hibernoma: A Clinicopathologic Study of 170 Cases. *American Journal of Surgical Pathology*: June 2001, 25(6):809–14.

180. Vellios F, Baez J, Schumacker HB: Lipoblastomatosis: a tumor of fetal fat different from hibernoma. Report of a case with observations on the embryogenesis of human adipose tissue. *Am J Pathol* 34:1140–59, 1958

181. Dudgeon DL, Haller JA Jr: Pediatric lipoblastomatosis. Two unusual cases. *Surgery* 95:371–3, 1984

182. Tabrisky J, Rowe JH, Cristie SG, *et al.*: Benign mediastinal lipoblastomatosis. *J Pediatr Surg* 9:399–401, 1974

183. Ganzel BL, Mavroudis C, Gray LA Jr: A mediastinal liposarcoma: An illustrative approach to mediastinal tumors. *J Ky Med Assoc* 87:459–62, 1989

184. Mclean TR, Almassi GH, Hackbarth DA, *et al.*: Mediastinal involvement by myxoid liposarcoma. *Ann Thorac Surg* 47:920–1, 1989

185. Prohm P, Winter J, Ulatowski L: Liposarcoma of the mediastinum: Case report and review of the literature. *Thorac Cardiovasc Surg* 29: 119–21, 1981

186. Schwietzer DL, Aguam AS: Primary liposarcoma of the mediastinum. Report of a case and review of the literature. *J Thorac Cardiovasc Surg* 74:83–97, 1977

187. Standerfer RJ, Armistead SH, Paneth M: Liposarcoma of the mediastinum. Report of two cases and review of the literature. *Thorax* 36:693–4, 1981

188. Dogan R, Ayrancioglu K, Aksu O: Primary mediastinal liposarcoma. A report of a case and review of the literature. *Eur J Cardiothorac Surg* 3:367–70, 1989

189. Kauffman SL, Stout AP: Lipoblastic tumors of children. *Cancer* 12:912–25, 1959

190. Plukker JTM, Joosten HJM, Rensing M, *et al.*: Primary liposarcoma of the mediastinum in a child. *J Surg Oncol* 37:257–63, 1988

191. Wilson JR, Bartley TD: Liposarcoma of the mediastinum. Report of a case in a child and review of the literature. *J Thorac Cardiovasc Surg* 48:486–90, 1964

192. Grieger TA, Carl M, Liebert HP, *et al.*: Mediastinal liposarcoma in a patient infected with the human immunodeficiency virus. *Am J Med* 84:366, 1988 (letter)

193. Enzinger FM, Winslow DJ: Liposarcoma. A study of 103 cases. *Virchows Arch [A]* 335:367–88, 1962.

194. Mendez G Jr, Isikoff MB, Isikoff SK, *et al.*: Fatty tumors of the thorax demonstrated by CT. *Am J Radiol* 133:207–12, 1979.

195. McCormick D, Mentzel T, Beham A, Fletcher CD. Dedifferentiated liposarcoma. Clinicopathologic analysis of 32 cases suggesting a better prognostic subgroup among pleomorphic sarcomas. *Am J Surg Pathol* 18: 1213–23, 1994

196. Fanburg-Smith JC, Miettinen M: Liposarcoma with meningothelial-like whorls: a study of 17 cases of a distinctive histological pattern associated with dedifferentiated liposarcoma. *Histopathology* 33 (5): 414–24, November 1998.

197. Suster S, Moran CA, Koss MN: Rhabdomyosarcomas of the anterior mediastinum: report of four cases unassociated with germ cell, teratomatous, or thymic carcinomatous components. *Hum Pathol.* Apr;25(4):349–56, 1994

198. Parham DM. Pathologic Classification of Rhabdomyosarcomas and Correlations with Molecular Studies. *Mod Pathol*;14(5):506–14, 2001

199. Altmannsberger M, Weber K, Droste R, *et al.*: Desmin is a specific marker for rhabdomyosarcoma of human and rat origin. *Am J Pathol* I 18:85–95, 1985

200. Seidal T, Kindblom L-G, Angervall L: Myoglobin, desmin and vimentin in ultrastructurally proven rhabdomyomas and rhabdomyosarcomas. An immunohistochemical study utilizing a series of monoclonal and polyclonal antibodies. *Appl Pathol* 5:201–19, 1987

201. Tsukuda T, McNutt MA, Ross R, *et al.*: HHF35, a muscle actin-specific monoclonal antibody. 11. Reactivity in normal, reactive, and neoplastic human tissues. *Am J Pathol* 127:389–402, 1987

202. Xia SJ, Pressey JG Barr FG; Molecular pathogenesis of rhabdomyosarcoma; *Cancer Biol Ther.* Mar-Apr;1(2):97–104, 2002

203. Miller R, Kurtz SM, Powers JM: Mediastinal rhabdomyoma. *Cancer* 42: 1983–8, 1978

204. Sunderrajan EV, Luger AM, Rosenholtz MJ, *et al.*: Leiomyosarcoma in the mediastinum presenting as superior vena cava syndrome. *Cancer* 53:2553–6, 1984

205. Baumgartner WA, Mark D: Esophageal leiomyoma first seen as a mediastinal mass. *Arch Surg* 115:94–6, 1980

206. Griff LE, Cooper J: Leiomyoma of the esophagus presenting as a mediastinal mass. *AJR* 101:472–81, 1967

207. Seremetis MG, de Guzman VC, Lyons WS, *et al.*: Leiomyoma of the esophagus. *Ann Thorac Surg* 16:308–16, 1973

208. Sunderrajan EV, Luger AM, Rosenholtz MJ, *et al.*: Leiomyosarcoma in the mediastinum presenting as superior vena cava syndrome. *Cancer* 53:2553–6, 1984

209. Henrichs KJ, Wenisch HJC, Hofmann W, *et al.*: Leiomyosarcoma of the pulmonary artery. A light and electron microscopic study. *Virchows Arch [A]* 383:207–16, 1979

210. Davis GL, Bergmann M, O'Kane H: Leiomyosarcoma of the superior vena cava. A first case with resection. *J Thorac Cardiovasc Surg* 72:408–12, 1976

211. Rasaretnam R, Panabokke RG: Leiomyosarcoma of the mediastinum. *Br J Dis Chest* 69:63–9, 1975

212. Wang NS, Seemayer TA, Ahmed MN, *et al.*: Pulmonary leiomyosarcoma associated with an arteriovenous fistula. *Arch Pathol* 98: 100–5, 1974

213. Bernheim J, Griffel B, Versano S, *et al.*: Mediastinal leiomyosarcoma in the wall of a bronchial cyst. *Arch Pathol Lab Med* 104:221, 1980 (letter)

214. Hayes WL, Farha SJ, Brown RL: Primary leiomyosarcoma of the pulmonary artery. *Am J Cardiol* 34:615–17, 1974

215. Swanson PE, Stanley MW, Scheithauer BW, *et al.*: Primary cutaneous leiomyosarcoma. A histologic and immunohistochemical study of nine cases, with ultrastructural correlation. *J Cutan Pathol* 15:129–41, 1988

216. Daniels AC, Conner GH, Straus FH: Primary chondrosarcoma of the tracheobronchial tree. Report of a unique case and brief review. *Arch Pathol* 84:615–24, 1967

217. Daroczi G: Radikal operiertes Chondrom des hinteren Mediastinums. *Zentralb1 Chir* 81:1245–8, 1956

218. Widdowson DJ, Lewis-Jones HG: A large soft-tissue chondroma arising from the posterior mediastinum. *Clin Radiol* 39: 333–5, 1988

219. Chetty R: Extraskeletal mesenchymal chondrosarcoma of the mediastinum. *Histopathology* 17:261–78, 1990

220. Thway K, Nicholson AG, Lawson K, Gonzalez D, Rice A, Balzer BL, Swansbury J, Min T, Thompson L, Adu-Poku K, Campbell A, Fisher C. Primary pulmonary myxoid sarcoma with EWSR1-CREB1 fusion: a new tumor entity. *Am J Surg Pathol.* 2011;35:1722–32.

221. Greenwood SM, Meschter SC: Extraske1etal osteogenic sarcoma of the mediastinum. *Arch Pathol Lab Med* 113:430–3, 1989

222. Tarr RW, Kerner T, McCook B, *et al.*: Primary extraosseous osteogenic sarcoma of the mediastinum: Clinical, pathologic, and radiologic correlation. *South Med J* 81:1317–19, 1988

223. Wilson H: Extraskeletal ossifying tumors. *Ann Surg* 113:95–112, 1941

224. Ikeda T, Ishihara T, Yoshimatsu H, *et al.*: Primary osteogenic sarcoma of the mediastinum. *Thorax* 29:582–8, 1974

225. Bane BL, Evans HL, Ro JY, *et al.*: Extraskeletal osteosarcoma. A clinicopathologic review of 26 cases. *Cancer* 66:2762–70, 1990

226. Catanese J, Dutcher JP, Dorfman HD, *et al.*: Mediastinal osteosarcoma with extension to lungs in a patient treated for Hodgkin's disease. *Cancer* 62:2252–7, 1988

227. Witkin GB, Rosai J: Solitary fibrous tumor of the mediastinum. A report of 14 cases. *Am J Surg Pathol* 13:547–557, 1989

228. Suehisa H, Yamashita M, Komori E, Sawada S, Teramoto N. Solitary fibrous tumor of the mediastinum. *Gen Thorac Cardiovasc Surg.* 2010 Apr;58(4):205–8.

229. Gannon BR, O'Hara CD, Reid K, Isotalo PA. Solitary fibrous tumor of the anterior mediastinum: a rare extrapleural neoplasm. *Tumori.* 2007 Sep–Oct;93(5):508–10.

230. van de Rijn M, Lombard CM, Rouse RV: Expression of CD34 by solitary fibrous tumors of the pleura. *Mediastinum, and Lung Am J Surg Pathol.* 18(8):814–20, August 1994

231. Rao N, Colby TV, Falconieri G, Cohen H, Moran CA, Suster S: Intrapulmonary solitary fibrous tumors: clinicopathologic and immunohistochemical study of 24 cases. *Am J Surg Pathol.* 2013 Feb;37 (2):155–66.

232. Rodríguez-Gil Y, González MA, Carcavilla CB, Santamaría JS: Lines of cell differentiation in solitary fibrous tumor: an ultrastructural and immunohistochemical study of 10 cases. *Ultrastruct Pathol.* 2009; 33:274–85.

233. Chmielecki J, Crago AM, Rosenberg M, O'Connor R, Walker SR, Ambrogio L, Auclair D, McKenna A, Heinrich MC, Frank DA, Meyerson M: Whole-exome sequencing identifies a recurrent NAB2-STAT6 fusion in solitary fibrous tumors. *Nat Genet.* 2013 Feb;45 (2):131–2.

234. Witkin GB, Miettinen M, Rosai J: A biphasic tumor of the mediastinum with features of synovial sarcoma. A report of four cases. *Am J Surg Pathol* 13:490–9, 1989

235. Kosemehmetoglu K, Vrana JA, Folpe AL: TLE1 expression is not specific for synovial sarcoma: a whole section study of 163 soft tissue and bone neoplasms. *Mod Pathol.* 2009;22:872–8.

236. Suster S, Moran CA. Primary synovial sarcomas of the mediastinum: a clinicopathologic, immunohistochemical, and ultrastructural study of 15 cases. *Am J Surg Pathol.* 2005 May;29(5):569–78.

237. Nayak, HK, Vangipuram DR, Ujjwal S, Premashish K, Kumar, N, Kapoor N: Mediastinal mass-a rare presentation of desmoplastic small round cell tumour. *BMJ Case Reports* 2011; doi:10.1136/bcr.10.2011.5042.

238. Saab R, Khoury JD, Krasin M, Davidoff AM, Navid F. Desmoplastic small round cell tumor in childhood: the St. Jude Children's Research Hospital experience. *Pediatr Blood Cancer.* 2007 Sep;49(3):274–9.

239. Hill AD *et al.*: WT1 staining reliably differentiates desmoplastic small round cell tumor from Ewing sarcoma/primitive neuroectodermal tumor. An immunohistochemical and molecular diagnostic study. *Am J Clin Pathol* 2000;114: 345–53.

240. Kushner BH, LaQuaglia MP, Wollner N, Meyers PA, Lindsley KL, Ghavimi F, Merchant TE, Boulad F, Cheung NK, Bonilla MA, Crouch G, Kelleher JF Jr, Steinherz PG, Gerald WL: Desmoplastic small round-cell tumor: prolonged progression-free survival with aggressive multimodality therapy. *J Clin Oncol.* 1996 May;14(5):1526–31.

241. Chao J, Budd GT, Chu P, Frankel P, Garcia D, Junqueira M, Loera S, Somlo G, Sato J, Chow WA. Phase II clinical trial of imatinib mesylate in therapy of KIT and/or PDGFRalpha-expressing Ewing sarcoma family of tumors and desmoplastic small round cell tumors. *Anticancer Res.* 2010 Feb;30(2):547–52.

242. Flieder DB, Moran CA, Suster SA: Primary alveolar soft part sarcoma of the mediastinum. A clinical and immunohistochemical study of two cases. *Histopathology.* 1997 Nov;31 (5):469–73.

243. Gregorius FK, Batzdorf U: Removal of thoracic chordoma by staged laminectomy and thoracotomy: Case report. *Am Surg* 45:535–7, 1979

244. Castellano GC, Johnston HW: Intrathoracic chordoma presenting as a posterior mediastinal tumor. *South Med J* 68:109–112, 1975

245. Clemons RL, Blank RH, Hutcheson JB, *et al.*: Chordoma presenting as a posterior mediastinal mass.

A choristoma. *J Thorac Cardiovasc Surg* 63:922–6, 1972

246. Vasquez JJ, Fernandez-Cuervo L, Fidalgo B: Lymphangiomyomatosis. Morphometric study and ultrastructural confirmation of the histogenesis of the lung lesion. *Cancer* 37:2321–8, 1976

247. Wolff M: Lymphangiomyoma: Clinicopathological study and ultrastructural confirmation of its histogenesis. *Cancer 31*:988–1007, 1973

248. Lack EE, Dolan MF, Finisio J, *et al.*: Pulmonary and extrapulmonary lymphangioleiomyomatosis. Report of a case with bilateral renal angiomyolipomas, multifocal lymphangioleiomyomatosis, and a glial polyp of the endocervix. *Am J Surg Pathol* 10:650–7, 1986

249. Guido Martignoni, Maurizio Pea, Daniela Reghellin, Giuseppe Zamboni, and Franco Bonetti. PEComas: the past, the present and the future. *Virchows Arch.* 2008 February; 452(2): 119–132.

250. Gaffey MJ, Mills SE, Askin FB, Ross GW, Sale GE, Kulander BG, Visscher DW, Yousem SA, Colby TV. Clear cell tumor of the lung. A clinicopathologic, immunohistochemical, and ultrastructural study of eight cases. *Am J Surg Pathol* 14:248–59, 1990

251. Flieder DB, Travis WD. Clear cell 'sugar' tumor of the lung: association with lymphangioleiomyomatosis and multifocal micronodular pneumocyte hyperplasia in a patient with tuberous sclerosis. *Am J Surg Pathol* 21:1242–7, 1997

252. Stovin PG: Pulmonary lymphangiomyomatosis syndrome. *J Pathol* 109:7–10, 1973

253. Watts MA, Gibbons JA, Aaron BL. Mediastinal and osseous lymphangiomatosis, case report and review. *Ann Thorac Surg* 34:324–8, 1982

254. Folpe AL, Mentzel T, Lehr HA, Fisher C, Balzer BL, Weiss SW: Perivascular epithelioid cell neoplasms of soft tissue and gynecologic origin: a clinicopathologic study of 26 cases and review of the literature. *Am J Surg Pathol* 29:1558–1575, 2005

255. Rocco G, Rosaria de Chiara A, Fazioli F, Scognamiglio F, La Rocca A, Apice G, Riva C. Primary Giant Clear cell Sarcoma (Soft Tissue Malignant Melanoma) of the Sternum. *Annals of Thoracic Surgery.* 2009 Jun;87:1927–8.

256. Tirabosco R, Lang-Lazdunski L, Diss TC, Amary MFC, Rodriguez-Justo M, Landau D, Lorenzi W, Flanagan AM: Clear cell sarcoma of the mediastinum. *Annals of Diagnostic Pathology.*2009, June; 13:197–200.

257. Dim DC, Cooley LD, Miranda RN: Clear Cell Sarcoma of Tendons and Aponeuroses. A Review. *Arch Pathol Lab Med.* 2007 Jan;131(1): 152–6.

258. Feldman L, Kricun ME: Malignant melanoma presenting as a mediastinal mass. *JAMA* 241:396–7, 1979

259. Jeong JW, Park KY, Yoon SM, Choe du W, Kim CH, Lee JC. A large intrathoracic meningocele in a patient with neurofibromatosis-1. *Korean J Intern Med.* 2010 Jun;25(2):221–3.

260. Strollo DC, Rosado-de-Christenson ML, Jett JR. Primary mediastinal tumors: part II. Tumors of the middle and posterior mediastinum. *Chest.* 1997 Nov 5;112(5):1344–57.

261. Wilson AJ, Ratliff JL, Lagios MD, et al: Mediastinal meningioma. *Am J Surg Pathol.* 3:557–62, 1979

262. Jaituni S, Arkee MSK, Caterine JM: Mediastinal myxoma: A case report. *J Iowa Med Soc* 64:107–10, 1974

263. Hawley RG, Murthy MSN: Malignant mesenchymoma of the mediastinum: Report of a case. *Ohio State Med J* 69:617–24, 1973

264. Patil SS, Deshmukh VV: Malignant mesenchymoma of the mediastinum. A case report. *J Dis Chest* 15:315–19, 1973

265. Otto HF, Loening TH, Lachenmayer L, *et al*: Thymolipoma in association with myasthenia gravis. *Cancer* 50:1623–8, 1982

266. Havlicek F, Rosai J: A sarcoma of thymic stroma with features of liposarcoma. *Am J Clin Pathol* 82:217–24, 1984

267. Valderrama E, Kahn LB, Wind E: Extraskeletal osteosarcoma arising in an ectopic hamartomatous thymus. Report of a case and review of the literature. *Cancer* 51:11132–7, 1983

268. Rosai J: The pathology of thymic neoplasia, in Berard CW, Dorfman RF, Kaufman N (eds): *Malignant Lymphoma (Monographs in Pathology).* Baltimore, MD, Williams & Wilkins, 1987, pp 161–83.

269. Lemos LB, Hamoudi AB: Malignant thymic tumor in an infant (malignant histiocytoma). *Arch Pathol Lab Med* 102:84–9, 1978

270. Lynch HT, Shurin SB, Dahms BB, *et al.*: Paravertebral malignant rhabdoid tumor in infancy. *Cancer* 52:290–6, 1983

269

Tell me what you need, so I'll know what to say

Frank C. Detterbeck, MD

Introduction

This chapter addresses the question: "What information do thoracic surgeons and oncologists need from pathologists in diagnosing mediastinal tumors?" Mediastinal tumors represent a difficult topic. This is in part due to the rarity of these lesions, as well as the number of different entities that are encountered. Most clinicians struggle to have a "routine" in how they approach the evaluation and diagnosis of such tumors. The treatment varies dramatically depending on the diagnosis, thus there is a lot riding on the pathologic diagnosis. However, the same issues (rarity, spectrum of disease) also confront the pathologist.

Part of the reason why mediastinal tumors are difficult is because of the discrepancy between the clinical problem and the available literature. The clinician is faced with an unknown diagnosis in a patient of a specific age, gender, and presentation. The literature is replete with series involving a known specific diagnosis, and then reports on average age, gender distribution, and percentage of these patients that have particular features. This discrepancy is a major factor for why most clinicians feel they are struggling until a definitive diagnosis is reached.

Making a clinical diagnosis is tremendously important, however, or at least narrowing the spectrum down to lesions that are strongly suspected. This allows those involved to structure their approach and process of evaluation. In particular, whether a tissue biopsy is needed, and what sort of biopsy is influenced by what is suspected. Furthermore, the processing of the tissues is influenced by this as well. Finally, interpretation and discussion are greatly improved by having an understanding of which entities are clinically most plausible.

This chapter will focus only on anterior mediastinal tumors. These account for the majority of mediastinal tumors [1,2]. Middle and posterior mediastinal tumors are beyond the scope of what can be addressed here.

Strategy to approach to anterior mediastinal tumors
Making a clinical diagnosis

A sophisticated approach to mediastinal tumors demands first making a clinical diagnosis. It is best to start with the general incidence of mediastinal tumors and then to hone this with the addition of more specific findings to strengthen or weaken the initial assessment. Although there are a few very specific "pathognomonic" findings, using this as a starting point only works in a small minority of cases and invites delays and confusion for the majority. Starting with a first pass clinical diagnosis allows specific findings to be addressed in a directed fashion in more well-defined patients. Factors that help make the initial clinical diagnosis include age and gender of the patient, the radiographic appearance, and the clinical presentation.

The majority of anterior mediastinal masses in men and women over 40 years of age are thymomas (Fig. 14.1a and, b). The probability of a thymoma becomes very high once substernal goiters are excluded, which are almost invariably easily identified on a CT scan. This serves as a useful starting point in structuring a clinical approach. It should be noted however that about 10–20% of patients have one of a number of rare tumors (grouped together as "miscellaneous").

For women between 10 and 40 years of age, the greatest proportion of anterior mediastinal masses are lymphomas (either Hodgkin's disease [HD] or mediastinal large cell non-Hodgkin's lymphoma [MLC-NHL]). Benign teratomas and thymomas comprise a significant minority (Fig. 14.2a). Other tumors are fairly uncommon but do occur frequently enough to be kept in mind.

In men between 10 and 40 years of age, however, there is no dominant tumor type that can narrow the diagnosis based on age and gender alone (Fig. 14.2b). A useful clinical approach is to consider the duration of symptoms. A rapid development of

Pathology of the Mediastinum, ed. Alberto M. Marchevsky and Mark R. Wick. Published by Cambridge University Press.
© Cambridge University Press 2014.

(a)

Anterior mediastinal tumors in women > 40 years old

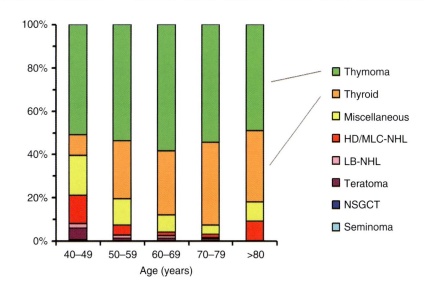

Fig. 14.1 Anterior mediastinal tumors in patients over 40 years of age.
Proportion of tumor types by decades of age [14-38] in **(a)** women; **(b)** men.
HD/MLC-NHL: Hodgkin's disease/mediastinal large cell non-Hodgkin's lymphoma; LB-NHL: lymphoblastic non-Hodgkin's lymphoma; NSGCT: non-seminomatous germ cell tumor.

(b)

Anterior mediastinal tumors in men > 40 years old

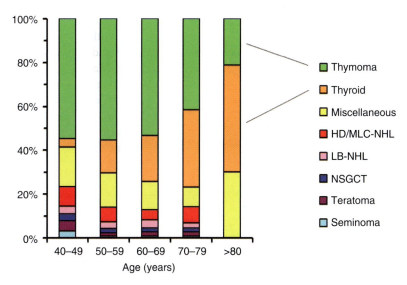

symptoms is highly suggestive of a non-seminomatous germ cell tumor (NSGCT) or a lymphoblastic lymphoma. An intermediate course suggests a mediastinal lymphoma (HD or MLC-NHL) or a seminoma. An indolent course or a lack of symptoms suggests a thymoma (especially in the older cohorts) or a teratoma (especially in the younger cohorts).

Certain specific findings can be tremendously helpful when present. The presence of myasthenia gravis (or another parathymic syndrome such as red cell aplasia or hypogammaglobulinemia) clearly identifies an anterior mediastinal mass as a thymoma. Markedly elevated serum α-fetoprotein or human chorionic globulin (β-HCG) levels are pathognomonic for a NSGCT. These findings are so specific that a biopsy is not needed. The presence of fat density, or more rarely a fragment of a bone or tooth strongly points to a teratoma, while fevers

and night sweats suggest a mediastinal lymphoma. Other radiographic features can be helpful, but generally provide only a softer suggestion of a particular diagnosis. At any rate, while information about the clinical presentation is readily available to the clinician, it is not necessarily available or communicated to the pathologist.

A sophisticated approach involves narrowing down the possibilities based on age and gender, and then adding information about the clinical presentation and radiographic features to generate a clinical diagnosis. Occasionally this can be corroborated by specific clinical findings, radiographic characteristics, or laboratory tests, and this can obviate the need for a biopsy. If a biopsy is needed after such a sophisticated clinical approach, it generally involves a limited differential diagnosis, although in some instances discordant aspects of the

(a)
Anterior mediastinal tumors in women aged 10–39 years

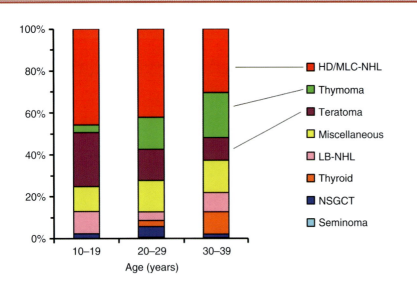

Legend:
- HD/MLC-NHL
- Thymoma
- Teratoma
- Miscellaneous
- LB-NHL
- Thyroid
- NSGCT
- Seminoma

Age (years): 10–19, 20–29, 30–39

(b)
Anterior mediastinal tumors in men aged 10–39 years

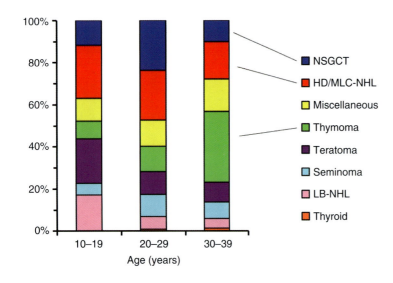

Legend:
- NSGCT
- HD/MLC-NHL
- Miscellaneous
- Thymoma
- Teratoma
- Seminoma
- LB-NHL
- Thyroid

Age (years): 10–19, 20–29, 30–39

Fig. 14.2 Anterior mediastinal tumors in patients aged 10–39 years. Proportion of tumor types by decades of age [14–38] in: **(a)** women; **(b)** men. HD/MLC-NHL: Hodgkin's disease/mediastinal large cell non-Hodgkin's lymphoma; LB-NHL: lymphoblastic non-Hodgkin's lymphoma; NSGCT: non-seminomatous germ cell tumor.

presentation may leave considerable uncertainty. Unfortunately, because these tumors are rare, they are often evaluated by clinicians who have dealt with only a limited volume of mediastinal tumors. The differential diagnosis may be influenced somewhat by a radiologist's assessment of the imaging, but this is often generated without knowing the clinical context – with the result that the entities considered may in reality be very unlikely given the age or clinical context. This makes the task of the pathologist more difficult.

When is a biopsy needed?

From the previous discussion, it is clear that in a large proportion of patients over the age of 40 an anterior mediastinal mass can be quite reliably diagnosed as a thymic malignancy on

clinical grounds. A biopsy is not necessarily needed to confirm this unless preoperative chemotherapy is the planned treatment strategy (i.e. it is invasive into adjacent mediastinal structures/organs). A biopsy to establish a diagnosis is needed in a minority of patients with a presentation that does not fit well for a thymic malignancy. While this may represent an unusual presentation of a usual disease (i.e. thymoma or lymphoma) in this setting a large variety of possible rare tumors must be considered.

In women aged 10–40 years old a biopsy to confirm a clinical diagnosis of lymphoma and to identify the subtype is needed even when the clinical diagnosis of lymphoma is quite certain. If a clinical diagnosis of thymoma or teratoma is highly likely, a biopsy is not necessary. In the vast majority of remaining cases however, a biopsy will be necessary to distinguish between a variety of possible lesions. In men aged 10–40 years old, serum markers can diagnose a NSGCT in a substantial minority of cases. However, in the vast majority of cases, a biopsy will be needed to differentiate between a large variety of possible lesions.

Specific differential diagnoses

Easy situations

A clinical diagnosis of thymoma can often be made very reliably, and a biopsy is often not needed if resection is the planned treatment. One should be very cautious about using a frozen section to confirm the diagnosis at the time of resection however, because this can be notoriously difficult [3]. An initial biopsy is needed if preoperative chemotherapy is planned. In this situation it is generally quite clear that the tumor is a thymoma: it is only confirmation thereof that is needed. It is not necessary to define the type of thymoma, because the treatment will be determined by the degree of invasion (i.e. stage) and not the WHO type [4]. In fact, even the differentiation between thymic carcinoma and thymoma has little impact on the clinical management strategy [4].

The well-known existence of tumor heterogeneity in thymomas and the need to examine multiple sections should raise concern about the ability to determine the subtype on a limited biopsy specimen [5]. Furthermore, the ability to reliably identify the subtype from a limited (e.g. core needle) biopsy is questionable [6]. There is variability in the definition of the subtype when examining resected specimens [7-9], and no data exists regarding correlation of the subtype identified on a limited biopsy with that determined at subsequent resection. However, as noted above, determination of the subtype of thymoma is of little importance in determining treatment, and it is recommended that subtyping be avoided on the basis of cytologic specimens, and be considered only suggestive (not definitive) on core needle specimens [6].

In many patients a clinical diagnosis of lymphoma is highly likely based on the clinical presentation, and the issue is confirmation of this and identification of the lymphoma type in order to guide treatment. In contrast to thymoma, the subtype of lymphoma is very important in determining the therapy to be used. Lymphoblastic lymphoma has characteristic cytologic features and can usually be clearly diagnosed on the basis of cytology (e.g. a pleural effusion or bone marrow aspirate) [10]. This type of lymphoma is usually strongly suspected on clinical grounds based on the presentation (younger patients, rapid onset, presence of pleural effusion etc.) [11]. Other mediastinal lymphomas (HD or MLC-NHL) sometimes present a challenge in obtaining sufficient tissue in biopsy samples. Because these tumors often have prominent sclerosis, cytologic samples are often insufficient for a definitive *de novo* diagnosis (as opposed to diagnosis of a recurrence of a previously identified lymphoma) [11]. A core needle biopsy or a surgical biopsy is usually necessary. An initial assessment of the adequacy of

tissue is useful (at the time of obtaining the samples). Given adequate tissue, there is usually little difficulty in confirming lymphoma and classifying the subtype; differentiating these lesions from other mediastinal tumors is not an issue.

Confirmation of a NSGCT is usually not necessary, given the characteristic marked elevation of serum markers and their specificity for this tumor [2,12]. Subtyping of NSGCT does not impact therapy and is not needed at diagnosis. In experienced centers, treatment is begun on the basis of serum markers and the clinical presentation. A biopsy may occasionally be needed if the presentation is unusual or in less experienced centers; however the diagnosis is generally easily established from a needle biopsy.

More difficult situations

Differentiation between a benign thymic cyst and a cystic thymoma or other neoplasm may be difficult. Given the need to examine such a lesion extensively after resection, it is questionable how reliably these diagnoses can be established on a limited biopsy [3,13]. Resection may be required to be certain. Distinguishing a thymoma from thymic hyperplasia is a relevant clinical issue, which may be difficult based on a limited tissue sample; given adequate tissue this is straightforward. A frequent clinical issue is to differentiate a thymoma from a lymphoma. Once again, this can be very difficult based on a limited tissue sample, but should be possible to accomplish readily given a large enough biopsy.

From the discussion in the section on "When is a biopsy necessary", there remains a substantial minority of cases in which it is hard to differentiate clinically between a variety of rare mediastinal tumors. This presents a challenge for pathologists as well. Some things may be easier – identification of a thymoma or lymphoma with unusual presentation/radiographic appearance, or a seminoma, parathyroid adenoma etc. However more rare tumors are a challenge because of lack of experience, a lack of extensive literature, and a lack of well-defined criteria to define these neoplasms.

These more difficult situations require a collaborative effort. The clinicians, radiologists, and pathologists should discuss and weigh the various pieces of information available and use collaborative judgment in order to reach a diagnosis. This should be viewed as an iterative process. Ideally, cases in which a highly reliable clinical diagnosis cannot be reached should be discussed *prior* to a biopsy with these specialties, as this may influence the type of biopsy that is obtained and details of how the tissue is processed. Recognition of the fact that achieving a diagnosis may be difficult should also set the stage for a possible repeat biopsy, perhaps using a different technique and involving a larger sample. The need for further tissue sampling should not necessarily be viewed as a failure of the initial biopsy if it is part of a thoughtful approach.

In atypical cases or cases with unusual features, consultation with a larger center should be pursued. Usually, people interpret this to mean that the slides are sent out for external review. However, the optimal process of establishing a diagnosis involves a multidisciplinary effort, using clinical, radiographic, and histologic information. Sending only the tissue for an outside review provides information on only one aspect of the case. It may be desirable to have the case reviewed by a multidisciplinary tumor board at a larger center or to have the patient seen in such a center. When a case appears to be a rare, unusual, or difficult case, there should be little argument against seeking further input.

Conclusion

Establishing a clinical diagnosis, or at least narrowing it down to a few likely possibilities, should be the first step in approaching a patient with an anterior mediastinal mass.

Good communication between the clinician, pathologist (and radiologist) is essential. In many instances the diagnosis is already quite certain, and only confirmation is needed prior to initiating treatment. In the case of thymoma, further subtyping is unnecessary and fraught with uncertainty from a limited biopsy. In the case of a lymphoma, subtyping is essential to guide treatment, and mandates that a sufficiently large biopsy is available. For the minority of cases in which a likely clinical diagnosis cannot be achieved, a multidisciplinary discussion is best to plan the strategy for biopsy and tissue handling. Consultation with a larger center should be sought when dealing with more rare types of mediastinal tumors in order to plan a diagnostic and therapeutic approach.

References

1. Davis RJ, Oldham HN Jr, Sabiston DC. Primary cysts and neoplasms of the mediastinum: Recent changes in clinical presentation, methods of diagnosis, management, and results. *Ann Thorac Surg.* 1987;44:229–37.

2. Detterbeck F. Clinical Approach to Mediastinal Masses. In: Kuzdzal JML, Muller M, Papagiannopoulos K, Detterbeck F, Van Raemdonck D, Thomas P, Rocco G, Venuta F, eds. *ESTS Textbook of Thoracic Surgery.* Exeter, UK: European Society of Thoracic Surgeons 2013.

3. Detterbeck F, Moran C, Huang J, Suster S, Walsh G, Kaiser L, *et al.* Which Way is Up? Policies and procedures for surgeons and pathologists regarding resection specimens of thymic malignancy. *J Thorac Oncol.* 2011;6: S1730–S8.

4. NCCN. NCCN Clinical Practice Guidelines in Oncology (NCCN Guidelines). Thymomas and Thymic Carcinomas. 2012 [cited February 20, 2013]; Version 2.2013

5. Moran CA, Suster S. On the histologic heterogeneity of thymic epithelial neoplasms. Impact of sampling in subtyping and classification of thymomas. *Am J Clin Pathol.* 2000;114:760–6.

6. Marchevsky A, Marx A, Strobel P, Suster S, Veuta F, Marino M, *et al.* Policies and reporting guidelines for small biopsy specimens of mediastinal masses. *J Thorac Oncol.* 2011;6:S1724–S9.

7. Dawson A, Ibrahim NBN, Gibbs AR. Observer variation in the histopathological classification of thymoma: Correlation with prognosis. *J Clin Pathol.* 1994;47:519–23.

8. Verghese E, den Bakker M, Campbell A, Hussein A, Nicholson A, Rice A, *et al.* Interobserver variation in the classification of thymic tumours–a multicentre study using the WHO classification system. *Histopathology.* 2008;53:218–23.

9. Detterbeck FC. Clinical value of the WHO classification system of thymoma. *Ann Thorac Surg.* 2006;81:2328–34.

10. Bartlett N, Wagner N. Lymphoma of the mediastinum. In: Pearson F, Cooper J, Deslauriers J, Ginsberg RJ, Hiebert C, Patterson G, *et al.*, eds. *Thoracic Surgery.* 2nd ed. New York: Churchill Livingstone 2002:1720–32.

11. Detterbeck F. Mediastinal Lymphomas. In: Kuzdzal JML, Muller M, Papagiannopoulos K, Detterbeck F, Van Raemdonck D, Thomas P, Rocco G, Venuta F, eds. *ESTS Textbook of Thoracic Surgery.* Exeter, UK: European Society of Thoracic Surgeons 2013.

12. Bokemeyer C, Nichols CR, Droz JP, Schmoll HJ, Horwich A, Gerl A, *et al.* Extragonadal germ cell tumors of the mediastinum and retroperitoneum: results from an international analysis. *J Clin Oncol.* 2002;20:1864–73.

13. den Bakker M, Oosterhuis JW. Tumours and tumour-like conditions of the thymus other than thymoma; a practical approach. *Histopathology.* 2009;54:69–89.

14. Davis RD Jr, Oldham HN Jr, Sabiston DC Jr. Primary cysts and neoplasms of the mediastinum: recent changes in clinical presentation, methods of diagnosis, management, and results. *Ann Thorac Surg.* 1987;44:229–37.

15. Levasseur P, Kaswin R, Rojas-Miranda A, N'Guimbous JF, Merlier M, Le Brigand H. Profile of surgical tumors of the mediastinum. Apropos of a series of 742 operated patients. *Nouv Presse Med.* 1976;5:2857–9.

16. Cohen AJ, Thompson L, Edwards FH, Bellamy RF. Primary cysts and tumors of the mediastinum. *Ann Thorac Surg.* 1991;51:378–84; discussion 85–6.

17. Rubush JL, Gardner IR, Boyd WC, Ehrenhaft JL. Mediastinal tumors. Review of 186 cases. *J Thorac Cardiovasc Surg.* 1973 Feb;65:216–22.

18. Wychulis AR, Payne WS, Clagett OT, Woolner LB. Surgical treatment of mediastinal tumors: a 40 year experience. *J Thorac Cardiovasc Surg.* 1971 Sep;62:379–92.

19. Mullen B, Richardson JD. Primary anterior mediastinal tumors in children and adults. *Ann Thorac Surg.* 1986 Sep;42:338–45.

20. Takeda S, Miyoshi S, Minami M, Ohta M, Okumura M, Kusafuka T, *et al.* Clinical spectrum of primary mediastinal tumors: A comparison of adult and pediatric populations (Abstract). *Chest.* October 2000;118(4 (Suppl)):S206.

21. Whooley BP, Urschel JD, Antkowiak JG, Takita H. Primary tumors of the mediastinum. *J Surg Oncol.* 1999 Feb;70:95–9.

22. Azarow KS, Pearl RH, Zurcher R, Edwards FH, Cohen AJ. Primary

mediastinal masses. A comparison of adult and pediatric populations. *J Thorac Cardiovasc Surg.* 1993 Jul;106:67–72.

23. Luosto R, Koikkalainen K, Jyrala A, Franssila K. Mediastinal tumours. A follow-up study of 208 patients. *Scand J Thorac Cardiovasc Surg.* 1978;12:253–9.

24. Yousem SA, Weiss LM, Warnke RA. Primary mediastinal non-Hodgkin's lymphomas: a morphologic and immunologic study of 19 cases. *Am J Clin Pathol.* 1985 Jun;83:676–80.

25. Lamarre L, Jacobson JO, Aisenberg AC, Harris NL. Primary large cell lymphoma of the mediastinum. A histologic and immunophenotypic study of 29 cases. *Am J Surg Pathol.* 1989 Sep;13:730–9.

26. Trump DL, Mann RB. Diffuse large cell and undifferentiated lymphomas with prominent mediastinal involvement. *Cancer.* 1982 Jul 15;50:277–82.

27. Todeschini G, Ambrosetti A, Meneghini V, Pizzolo G, Menestrina F, Chilosi M, *et al.* Mediastinal large-B-cell lymphoma with sclerosis: a clinical study of 21 patients. *J Clin Oncol.* 1990 May;8:804–8.

28. al-Sharabati M, Chittal S, Duga-Neulat I, Laurent G, Mazerolles C, al-Saati T, *et al.* Primary anterior mediastinal B-cell lymphoma. A clinicopathologic and immunohistochemical study of 16 cases. *Cancer.* 1991 May 15;67:2579–87.

29. Kadin ME, Glatstein E, Dorfman RF. Clinicopathologic studies of 117 untreated patients subjected to laparotomy for the staging of Hodgkin's disease. *Cancer.* 1971 Jun;27:1277–94.

30. Nathwani BN, Diamond LW, Winberg CD, Kim H, Bearman RM, Glick JH, *et al.* Lymphoblastic lymphoma: a clinicopathologic study of 95 patients. *Cancer.* 1981 Dec 1;48:2347–57.

31. Moran CA, Suster S. Primary germ cell tumors of the mediastinum: I. Analysis of 322 cases with special emphasis on teratomatous lesions and a proposal for histopathologic classification and clinical staging. *Cancer.* 1997 Aug 15;80:681–90.

32. Wax MK, Briant TD. Management of substernal goitre. *J Otolaryngol.* 1992 Jun;21:165–70.

33. Detterbeck FC, Parsons AM. Thymic tumors. *Ann Thorac Surg.* 2004 May;77:1860–9.

34. Lewis JE, Wick MR, Scheithauer BW, Bernatz PE, Taylor WF. Thymoma: A clinicopathologic review. *Cancer.* 1987;60:2727–43.

35. Verley JM, Hollmann KH. Thymoma: A comparative study of clinical stages, histologic features, and survival in 200 cases. *Cancer.* 1985;55:1074–86.

36. Gamondès JP, Balawi A, Greenland T, Adleine P, Mornex JF, Zhang J, *et al.* Seventeen years of surgical treatment of thymoma: Factors influencing survival. *Eur J Cardio-thorac Surg.* 1991;5:124–31.

37. Batata M, Martini N, Huvos AG, Aguilar R, Beattie EJ. Thymomas: Clinicopathologic features, therapy, and prognosis. *Cancer.* 1974;34:389–96.

38. Wilkins EJ. Thymus: Myasthenia gravis and thymoma. In: Grillo H, Austen WG, Wilkins E Jr, Mathisen DJ, Vlahakes G, eds. *Current Therapy in Cardiothracic Surgery.* Philadelphia: B C Decker Inc. 1989:117–21.

Chapter 15

Clinical pathology of disorders of the mediastinum

Kent Lewandrowski, MD

Introduction

Disorders of the mediastinum include immune and inflammatory conditions, mediastinal cysts, ectopic thyroid/goiter, cardiovascular disorders, and tumors which may be either benign or malignant (Table 15.1). In some cases laboratory testing is essential for determining a correct diagnosis whereas, in others, laboratory studies may be useful to assess the overall condition of the patient prior to determining appropriate therapy. This chapter will focus on the role of the clinical laboratory in the diagnosis and management of mediastinal disorders. General laboratory studies not specifically related to diagnosis will not be discussed.

Myasthenia gravis: Myasthenia gravis (MG) is an autoimmune disorder characterized by muscle weakness and easy fatigability of the cranial muscles (especially the extraocular muscles and eyelids) often associated with generalized weakness. MG is associated with thymoma in approximately 15% of cases and with thymic hyperplasia in up to 65% of cases [1]. Additional associations include other autoimmune disorders and extrathymic malignancies.

The etiology of MG is an autoimmune mediated decrease in acetylcholinesterase receptors (AChRs) at the postsynaptic neuromuscular junction. The decrease in AChRs is caused by anti-AChR antibodies that either: 1) block the receptor, 2) accelerate destruction of the receptor, or 3) damage the postsynaptic membrane [1,2]. Occasionally MG is caused by an autoantibody to muscle specific receptor tyrosine kinase antigen (MuSK). Anti-AChR antibodies are found in approximately 90% of patients with MG [3]. A variety of autoantibody tests are available to evaluate patients with suspected MG. In selecting the appropriate test(s) it is important to consider the context of the patient;

1. Isolated MG.
2. MG associated with thymoma.
3. MG associated with other autoimmune disorders.
4. Inherited MG syndromes resulting from genetic mutations of elements of the neuromuscular junction.
5. Differentiating MG from Lambert–Eaton syndrome (LES).

Table 15.1. Disorders of the mediastinum

Immune: myasthenia gravis

Inflammatory/infectious: thymitis, mediastinitis

Mediastinal cysts

Ectopic thyroid/goiter

Tumors: thymoma, parathyroid tumors, neuroendocrine tumors, neurogenic tumors, lymphoma, Hodgkin lymphoma, germ cell tumors

Cardiac disease: coronary artery disease and acute coronary syndromes, congestive heart failure, myocarditis, cardiac transplant rejection, hypertrophic cardiomyopathy, pericarditis and pericardial effusion, endocarditis

In most cases hospital laboratories send blood testing for MG to outside reference laboratories rather than performing the testing in-house. This reflects the relatively low volume of requests for MG testing and a lack of in-house expertise to assist in interpretation of the test results. Most reference laboratories offer MG test panels comprised of different combinations of autoantibodies tailored to the specific clinical setting. Some reference laboratories have established reflex testing algorithms based on the results of the test panel and the levels of the autoantibody titers. The panels offered by one reference laboratory are described below. For further details the reader is referred to reference 3 from which the following text was partially derived.

Adult MG panel

- Anti-AChR binding antibody: Specimens with a positive anti-AChR binding antibody test are confirmed by re-testing with radiolabelled alpha-bungarotoxin without the presence of acetylcholine receptors to detect false positive anti-AChR results (see methodologic considerations below).
- Anti-AChR modulating antibodies.
- Anti-striational antibodies.

Pathology of the Mediastinum, ed. Alberto M. Marchevsky and Mark R. Wick. Published by Cambridge University Press.
© Cambridge University Press 2014.

Comments: The autoantibodies in this panel may be positive in conditions other than MG such as Lambert–Eaton syndrome (see below) and in patients with malignancies in the absence of MG. In patients with MG, the antibody titers may be negative for many months after onset of symptoms. Serial antibody titers can be used to monitor therapy. High autoantibody titers do not strongly correlate with disease severity. High titers of anti-AChR modulating antibodies coupled with a positive anti-striational antibody strongly suggests thymoma. Postive anti-striational antibodies may also be observed in patients with autoimmune liver disease and in a minority of patients with LES. If clinical suspicion for MG is high in a patient with otherwise negative autoantibody titers, consideration should be given to testing for MuSK autoantibody.

Pediatric MG panel

- Anti-AChR binding antibody.
- Anti-AChR modulating antibodies.

Comments: MG in children may reflect an acquired auto-immune disorder or a seronegative inherited disease resulting from genetic mutations of elements of the neuromuscular junction. Positive titers may be observed in conditions other than MG as described above and in graft versus host disease.

Thymoma MG panel

- Same as adult panel plus:
- CRMP-5-IgG by Western blot (Collapsin response-mediator protein-5).
- Anti-AChR ganglionic neuronal antibody.
- Neuronal (VG) K+ channel autoantibody.
- GAD65 antibody (Glutamic acid decarboxylase).

Comments: These additional autoantibodies are often positive in patients with thymoma.

MG/Lambert–Eaton syndrome panel

- Same as adult panel plus:
- N-type calcium channel antibody.
- P/Q-type voltage gated calcium channel antibody.

Comments: LES is an autoimmune disorder of the neuromuscular junction presumably resulting from autoantibodies that bind to presynaptic motor nerve voltage-gated P/Q-type calcium channels. In the majority of patients this reflects a paraneoplastic syndrome most often associated with small cell lung cancer [1]. However, LES can occur in patients without malignancy. Distinguishing MG from LES is sometimes difficult based on clinical and electromyelographic findings. Hence the above panel is intended to diagnose and distinguish either MG or LES based on the observed pattern of autoantibodies. The N-type calcium channel antibody is more commonly associated with small cell lung cancer than P/Q-type calcium channel antibody. Positive antibody titers are not conclusively diagnostic of either MG or LES as positive results can be observed in other disorders and in patients with malignancy without neuromuscular disease.

Methodologic considerations: Testing for anti-AChR antibodies is typically performed by radioimmunoassay methods. Labeled alpha-bungarotoxin (derived from snake venom) firmly binds AChR but not at the same site as anti-AChR antibody [4,5]. The alpha-bungarotoxin is first mixed with AChR and allowed to bind. Then the patient's serum sample is added. If anti-AChR are present they will bind to the alpha-bungarotoxin-AChR complexes. The resulting triple complex of alpha-bungarotoxin-AChR-anti-AChR antibody is then precipitated with antihuman immunoglobulin and the precipitate counted. The amount of radioactivity is proportional to the titer of anti-AChR antibody. The basic assay can also be modified to detect either blocking or modulating antibodies [5].

Mediastinal germ cell tumors: Primary germ cell tumors (GCT) of the mediastinum include benign mature teratomas, pure seminomas, mixed seminomatous/non-seminomatous tumors and non-seminomatous germ cell tumors (NSGCT). Mature teratomas may be asymptomatic or present with findings resulting from a mass effect. There are no distinguishing clinical laboratory findings. Occasionally patients have presented with a pleural effusion (transudate) due to rupture of the teratoma into the pleural space [6]. Clinical laboratory findings in seminomas may include elevations in beta-human chorionic gonadotropin (b-hCG) and plasma lactate dehydrogenase (LDH). Elevated levels of b-hCG in the context of appropriate clinical and radiologic findings are very useful to establish the initial diagnosis of a mediastinal seminoma. In one study, 43% of seminomas exhibited an elevated b-hCG (median value 8.5 MIU/ml, range 1–89) and 43% an elevation in LDH (median 523 IU/L, range 160–2019) [7]. When elevated initially, serial b-hCG levels may be used to monitor therapy and to follow patients after completion of therapy for recurrent or residual disease.

It is important to understand the difference in the use of b-hCG for the diagnosis of pregnancy versus the use of this test as a tumor marker. In the case of GCT, assays for b-hCG should detect both the intact b-hCG molecule and free beta subunits because the free beta subunits may be produced in excess of the intact molecule. Most hospitals send tumor marker samples for b-hCG to outside reference laboratories that use assays specifically designed for this purpose. The assays should also have excellent accuracy and reproducibility (precision) at the upper range of the normal cut-off value. This is particularly important when monitoring patients for residual/recurrent disease as even slight changes in the b-hCG value will have significant clinical implications. b-hCG assays from various manufacturers may produce different values when measured on the same specimen. For this reason it is important to use the same assay when following patients over time. False positive b-hCG results may be observed due to interference from heterophile antibodies. In most cases this can be resolved by blocking the antibodies and then retesting the sample.

In the case of NSGCT, clinical laboratory findings may include elevations in b-hCG and/or alpha fetoprotein (AFP) and LDH. In a study by Bokemeyer et al. [8], 74% of NSGCT showed elevations in AFP (median 2,548 ng/ml, range 1–500,000), 38% in b-hCG (median 5 MIU/ml, range 1–3,138,122) and 52% in LDH (median 489 IU/L, range 90–3,427). Most hospitals send tumor marker testing for AFP to outside reference laboratories. These laboratories offer AFP tests that have been specifically designed and validated for use as a tumor marker as opposed to AFP assays used for prenatal screening. In the case of NSGCT that initially exhibit elevations in either AFP and/or b-hCG, these markers are useful to assist in both diagnosis and in monitoring therapy/recurrence. It is important to note that AFP levels may be elevated in conditions other than NSGCT such as hepatocellular carcinoma, other malignancies, and non-neoplastic diseases.

AFP, b-hCG, and LDH are also important prognostic markers in patients with NSGCT. In a landmark study, the International Germ Cell Cancer Collaborative Group studied prognostic factors on 5,202 patients with NSGCT and 660 patients with seminoma [8]. A subgroup of these represented primary mediastinal tumors. For seminoma the only adverse prognostic factor identified was the presence of non-pulmonary visceral metastases. However, for NSGCT all three blood markers were of prognostic significance as shown in Table 15.2 [8].

Thymic neuroendocrine tumors: Neuroendocrine tumors of the thymus are rare, are typically aggressive, and are associated with endocrinopathies in 50% of cases including Cushing syndrome (33–40%) and multiple endocrine neoplasia (19–25%) [9]. Only rarely do patients present with carcinoid syndrome. Occasionally they may present with LES [9]. Presumably some of these tumors would exhibit a positive serum chromogranin A tumor marker test (a serum neuroendocrine tumor marker) or serum non-specific enolase (NSE) albeit, due to the rarity of these tumors, there is no information on this in the literature. For tumors that present with Cushing syndrome the laboratory evaluation mirrors that of the work-up of Cushing syndrome more generally. Cushing syndrome may result from adrenal cortical tumors, pituitary ACTH-producing adenomas, or from ectopic ACTH production by tumors. Various laboratory-based approaches to the diagnosis of Cushing syndrome have been published. Most strategies rely on screening for Cushing syndrome followed by confirmatory testing. One such approach is shown in Fig. 15.1. Initial screening tests may include testing for salivary cortisol at its diurnal nadir between 11 pm–12 midnight (elevated in Cushing syndrome) or the 1 mg overnight dexamethasone (DMS) suppression test. Screening using isolated serum cortisol testing is of limited value because cortisol levels exhibit a wide diurnal range and may be elevated in many conditions including stress. Measurement of serum cortisol between 11 pm and 12 midnight is

Table 15.2. Laboratory marker prognostic factors in non-seminomatous germ cell tumors identified by the International Germ Cell Cancer Collaborative Group

Good prognosis

LDH < 1.5 times the upper limit of normal (ULN), and
b-hCG < 5000 IU/L, and
AFP < 1000 ng/ml
All three criteria must be satisfied
5-year survival 92%

Intermediate prognosis

LDH $\geq$ 1.5 and $\leq$ 10 times the upper limit of normal, or
b-hCG $\geq$ 5000 and $\leq$ 50,000 IU/L, or
AFP $\geq$ 1000 and $\leq$ 10,000 ng/ml
5-year survival 80%

Poor prognosis

LDH > 10 times the upper limit of normal, or
b-hCG > 50,000 IU/L, or
AFP > 10,000 ng/ml
5-year survival 48%

Key: LDH: lactate dehydrogenase; AFP: alpha-fetoprotein; b-hCG: beta human chorionic gonadotropin

impractical. Normally a patient's serum cortisol will suppress overnight following administration of 1 mg of DMS. Failure to suppress may reflect Cushing syndrome or other conditions such as stress. Confirmatory testing may include a 24 hour urine free cortisol level or suppression testing using 2 mg of DMS (so-called low dose DMS test). Either an elevated urinary cortisol level or failure to suppress the serum cortisol overnight following 2 mg of DMS confirms the diagnosis of Cushing syndrome. It then remains to determine the cause of the Cushing syndrome (adrenal, pituitary, or ectopic ACTH). In the case of ectopic ACTH production the ACTH level will be elevated and the patient's serum cortisol will not suppress even with the high dose DMS suppression test as shown in Fig. 15.1.

Ectopic parathyroid adenoma: Parathyroid adenoma is the most common cause (85%) of primary hyperparathyroidism (pHPT). In approximately 10% of cases the adenoma occurs in an ectopic location including the mediastinum. Ectopic adenomas are a common cause of recurrent or persisting pHPT and may present a significant challenge in localization and surgical excision [10,11,12]. However, from the perspective of the clinical laboratory, ectopic parathyroid tumors are no different than the typical parathyroid adenomas arising in the juxta-thyroidal tissues of the neck. Laboratory studies will usually show hypercalcemia (elevated total and/or ionized calcium), a normal or low phosphate level (due to a parathyroid hormone (PTH) driven increase in renal phosphate excretion), an elevated parathyroid hormone, and an

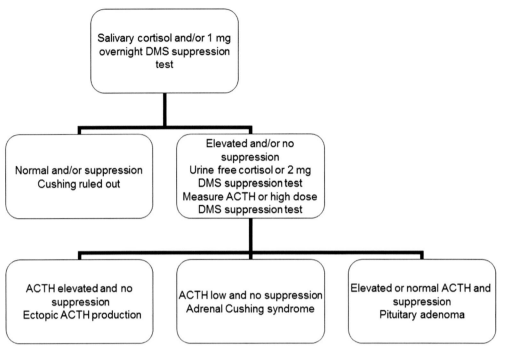

Fig. 15.1 Laboratory approach to Cushing syndrome.
DMS: dexamethasone; ACTH: adrenocorticotropic hormone.

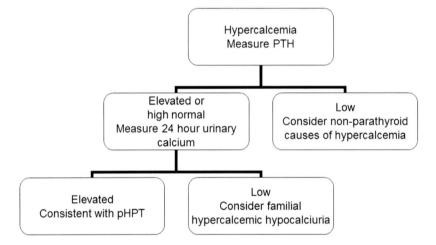

Fig. 15.2 Approach to differentiating primary hyperparathyroidism from other causes of hypercalcemia. PTH: parathyroid hormone; pHPT: primary hyperparathyroidism.

elevated urinary calcium level (greater than 200 mg/24 hours resulting from an increase in the renal filtered load of calcium). However, initially most patients will present simply with hypercalcemia (including total and ionized calcium). Hypercalcemia may be caused by pHPT, familial syndromes (familial hypercalcemic hypocalciuria), secondary HPT, hypercalcemia of malignancy, granulomatous disorders, various drugs (e.g. thiazide diuretics, lithium) or intoxication with vitamin D, A, or excessive calcium intake in the setting of kidney disease or milk alkali syndrome. Given the diverse etiologies of hypercalcemia it is useful to have a systematic approach as shown in Fig. 15.2. The evaluation of non-hyperparathyroid hypercalcemia will not be discussed beyond what is shown in Fig. 15.2. The first step in

evaluating hypercalcemia without an obvious underlying cause is to measure PTH. If the hypercalcemia was first detected using a total plasma calcium some authorities prefer to confirm the hypercalcemia with an ionized calcium level. If the PTH level is elevated or in the high normal range (inappropriately normal for the elevated calcium level) then a 24 hour urinary calcium value should be obtained. An elevated urinary calcium level confirms the diagnosis of hyperparathyroidism.

Ectopic mediastinal thyroid: Ectopic thyroid tissue producing a mediastinal mass is relatively rare comprising 1% of mediastinal tumors [13]. Most patients are asymptomatic although symptoms resulting from a mass effect may occur. In the vast majority of cases the patients exhibit normal

Table 15.3. Blood cardiac markers for myocardial necrosis

Marker	Kinetics	Comment(s)
Myoglobin	May be detected in as little as 1 hour following myocardial infarction	Sensitive for myocardial necrosis but suffers from poor specificity
Creatine kinase (CPK) and its isoenzyme CK-MB	Appears in blood within 4–6 hours following myocardial infarction, peaks within 24 hours and returns to baseline within 2–3 days	Troponin has replaced CPK/CK-MB in most institutions
Troponin-I and T	Appears in blood within 4–6 hours following myocardial infarction, peaks at 1–2 days and returns to baseline after 7–10 days	Gold standard marker for myocardial necrosis. May be elevated in myocardial infarction and other causes of myocyte injury such as myocarditis, myocardial contusion and transplant rejection

thyroid tests [13]. Occasional cases associated with Graves disease have been reported which may result in failure to cure hyperthyroidism following treatment of the normally-located gland [14]. The clinical laboratory findings are the same as in typical Graves disease patients without mediastinal thyroid tissue including elevated total and free thyroid hormones (T4/T3), an elevated thyroid stimulating hormone (TSH) and, if measured, elevated thyroid stimulating immunoglobulin (TSI).

Heart disease: With the development of new and improved laboratory tests the clinical laboratory has become increasingly important in the evaluation of cardiovascular disease. Specific comments on the more important tests and their clinical applications follows below.

Acute coronary syndromes (ACS): Atherosclerotic coronary artery disease may be asymptomatic or present as stable angina, unstable angina, or acute myocardial infarction. The later two conditions are collectively referred to as the acute coronary syndromes. Acute myocardial infarction (AMI) includes patients who present with ST-segment elevation (STEMI), the majority of whom develop a typical Q-wave AMI, and those without ST-segment elevation (NSTEMI). In patients presenting with STEMI, cardiac markers are not required for diagnosis although they are usually ordered as part of the routine evaluation of the patient and to assist in infarct sizing. In patients with NSTEMI the presence or absence of an elevation in cardiac markers is the major criteria to differentiate those with unstable angina versus true non-ST-segment elevation acute myocardial infarction. Over the years a number of laboratory tests have been used to assess patients for myocardial necrosis including aspartate aminotransferase (AST or SGOT), lactate dehydrogenase (LDH) and its isoenzymes 1 and 2, creatine kinase (CPK) and its isoenzyme creatine kinase MB (CK-MB), myoglobin and the cardiac troponins I and T (cTnI and cTnT). The use of AST/SGOT and LDH fell out of favor two decades ago. Current tests that are still in use include myoglobin, CPK and CK-MB, and troponin (Table 15.3). Troponin I and T, myoglobin, and CK-MB are measured using immunoassays producing "mass" units (e.g. ng/ml) whereas CPK is measured using an enzymatic assay producing units per liter. The recent development of new so-called "high sensitivity" troponin assays are rapidly changing

the laboratory approach to ACS and will soon supplant all other markers. Currently most hospitals perform serial testing for cardiac markers at baseline, at 4–6 hours following presentation to the emergency department, and at 12–18 hours. Accelerated rule-out multi-marker protocols have been reported using serial values over shorter time intervals. In myocardial infarction a typical rise and fall pattern in cardiac markers will be observed unlike some other causes of myocardial injury (e.g. myocarditis, cardiac transplant rejection) where the markers may remain persistently elevated. A rise and fall pattern will also be observed following cardiac contusion and cardiac surgery. Myoglobin is used by only a minority of hospitals in the United States. Elevated levels are highly sensitive for myocardial necrosis albeit the test suffers from poor specificity due to frequent elevations observed with even modest degrees of skeletal muscle injury. The principal advantage of myoglobin is that, because it is a relatively small protein, elevated blood levels can be detected in as little as one hour following myocardial injury. Thus myoglobin is considered an early marker of myocardial necrosis. Both CPK/CK-MB and troponin can be detected in blood within 4–6 hours following acute myocardial infarction. However, troponin stays elevated for considerably longer than CPK/CK-MB and remains positive for up to a week or more following AMI. Although CK-MB is present in the myocardium, small amounts of CK-MB are also found in skeletal muscle. Therefore CPK and CK-MB will be elevated following either myocardial or skeletal muscle injury. The traditional approach to differentiating cardiac from skeletal muscle injury has relied on calculating the percent CK-MB of the total CPK (so-called percent CK-MB or "relative index" when immunoassays producing mass units are used). However, both troponin I and troponin T are cardiac specific and have essentially replaced CPK/CK-MB in most institutions. The remainder of this discussion shall therefore focus only on troponin I and T.

Current consensus guidelines for the classification and diagnosis of AMI and the use of blood biomarkers have recently been reviewed [15]. The diagnosis of AMI requires detection of a rise (and/or fall) of a cardiac biomarker with at least one value above the 99th percentile upper reference limit (see below) with at least one other criteria including:

1. Characteristic symptoms.
2. Characteristic electrocardiographic changes (see reference 15).
3. Imaging or angiographic evidence of AMI (see reference 15).

According to current guidelines, the normal range for cardiac troponin should be established as the 99th percentile of a normal reference population. Therefore, by definition, 1% of presumptively healthy individuals will have a troponin value above the upper reference limit. Ideally the assay will exhibit an imprecision (coefficient of variation) of less than 10% at the cut-off value. Many assays currently on the market do not fully meet these guidelines. It is important to note that an elevated troponin value is not diagnostic of AMI. Rather it is the typical rise and fall pattern of troponin in the appropriate clinical context that is used to establish the diagnosis. Troponin values can be elevated in conditions other than AMI such as cardiac surgery and procedures, myocarditis, sepsis and other critical illnesses, pulmonary embolism, and a variety of other causes [16]. Finally, cardiac troponin values can be used to risk stratify patients with unstable angina (UA). Patients with UA with detectable troponin values that are below the 99th percentile cut-off exhibit a significantly greater risk for future adverse events than patients with UA with an undetectable troponin value [17,18].

In recent years manufacturers have been developing so-called "high sensitivity" troponin assays that are able to detect troponin levels nearly a log value below (pg/ml rather than ng/ml) the conventional troponin assays. As of this writing some of these assays are available in Europe but none have yet been approved by the food and drug administration for use in the United States. This will likely change in the near future. With higher analytical sensitivity, it has become apparent that patients presenting with signs and symptoms of ACS can probably be ruled in or out in a much shorter time interval than is possible with current assays. These strategies rely on serial troponin testing over a short 4–6-hour time frame. However, the improvement in sensitivity is partially offset with a decrease in specificity as more patients without AMI will exhibit detectable levels of troponin with these new assays. The optimal clinical use of the new high sensitivity troponin assays is rapidly evolving (see reference 19 for a review).

Congestive heart failure: Heart failure is usually classified by the New York Heart Association Classification that divides heart failure into four classes based on severity (normal and classes I–IV). Patients with class IV heart failure are symptomatic at rest with markedly abnormal left ventricular function despite therapy. Class I heart failure is essentially asymptomatic with or without exercise. Patients exhibit mildly abnormal left ventricular function. Classes II and III represent intermediate grades of increasing severity. Heart failure (HF) can be diagnosed based on history and clinical findings but even in the hands of experienced cardiologists many cases of mild to moderate heart failure are missed. Cardiac ultrasound is very useful for the diagnosis of HF but it is expensive, requires an expert to interpret, and is not always readily available. In recent years blood markers for heart failure (brain natriuretic peptide (BNP) and its inactive N-terminal fragment NT-proBNP) have become commercially available resulting in a significant improvement in the ability of physicians to reliably diagnose HF [20]. Studies have shown that testing for B-type natriuretic peptides is superior to clinical judgment alone for the diagnosis of heart failure and the combination of testing with clinical findings produced the highest sensitivity and specificity [20]. A number of potential biomarkers for use in the diagnosis and management of heart failure have been studied but most are not available for routine clinical practice (see reference 21 for a comprehensive review). BNP arises from a pre-prohormone that is synthesized by cardiac myocytes and cleaved to prohormone-BNP. The prohormone is released into the circulation in response to left ventricular stress and is cleaved into the active hormone, BNP, and the inactive NT-proBNP fragment. Immunoassays are available for BNP and NT-proBNP. Both markers appear equally useful for clinical purposes albeit there are minor differences between the two (e.g. BNP has a shorter half life than NT-proBNP). The physiologic actions of BNP include diuresis, natriuresis, and vasodilatation, all of which are an appropriate physiological response in patients with HF.

The value of natriuretic hormone testing has been evaluated in a number of clinical situations. The most firmly established applications are for the diagnosis of HF and the differential diagnosis of dypsnea. Identifying the cause of dyspnea can be clinically challenging. The differential diagnosis includes HF, pneumonia, exacerbation of chronic obstructive pulmonary disease, asthma, and other causes. In the case of HF, both BNP and NT-proBNP will be elevated in the majority of patients and the degree of elevation correlates with the severity of HF. The use of natriuretic peptide testing permits a rapid diagnosis and early institution of appropriate therapy. The use of this test has been shown to result in a decrease in hospital length-of-stay, reduced cost, and a reduction in re-admission and mortality following hospitalization.

Serial testing for BNP/NT-proBNP has been used to monitor therapy after the patient has been admitted to the hospital with HF. Falling levels of the marker correlate with improvement in the patient's clinical condition. There is no consensus as to how frequently testing should be performed in the hospital. One protocol in use at the Massachusetts General Hospital utilizes NT-proBNP testing on admission, once during the course of emergent therapy and, finally, one test at discharge to re-establish the patient's new baseline. Testing for BNP/NT-proBNP is also being evaluated in the outpatient setting to assist in monitoring patients with previously diagnosed heart failure. A rising level of natriuretic peptide from baseline signals the need for more aggressive therapy. Presumably outpatient monitoring will, in addition to improving treatment, prevent re-hospitalization for acute decompensated HF.

Table 15.4. Applications of natriuretic hormone testing (see reference 21 for further details)

Clinical application	Comment
Diagnosis of heart failure	More sensitive and specific than clinical judgment alone. Facilitates rapid early diagnosis of heart failure with institution of appropriate therapy.
Differential diagnosis of dyspnea	Allows clinician to rule-in or -out heart failure in patients with dyspnea
Prognosis in acute and chronic heart failure	Levels of natriuretic peptides correlate with severity of heart failure and adverse outcomes
Prognosis in patients with acute coronary syndromes	Levels of natriuretic peptides correlate with short- and long-term prognosis in acute coronary syndromes
Management of heart failure	Serial values on inpatients and outpatients may be useful to manage therapy of heart failure and prevent re-hospitalization
Screening asymptomatic patients at risk for heart failure	

Natriuretic peptide testing is also useful as a prognostic indicator in patients with HF and in patients with acute coronary syndromes (Table 15.4). The higher the natriuretic peptide level the worse the prognosis over both short- and long-term time periods.

Other markers in heart failure: Galectin-3 and ST2 are two new recently food and drug administration-approved markers with potential utility in patients with heart failure. ST2 is a member of the interleukin receptor family that occurs in both a trans-membrane form and a soluble form in blood. The soluble form is up-regulated in response to myocyte stretch and therefore becomes elevated in patients with heart failure. The main application of ST2 measurement is as a prognostic marker. Patients with dyspnea both with and without HF exhibit a significantly higher risk of mortality. Presumably these patients would be candidates for more aggressive therapy. Galectin-3 is a member of the galectin family of proteins that bind beta-galactosides. Galectin-3 is produced by activated macrophages [21] and plays a role in various intracellular pathways and in promotion of fibrosis. In patients with heart failure an elevated galectin-3 has been associated with an increased risk of mortality and with increased risk of re-hospitalization. Therefore this marker may be useful in identifying patients with a high risk for re-hospitalization who may benefit from more aggressive therapy.

Mediastinitis: Mediastinitis is a life-threatening condition that may occur following mediastinal spread of various infectious diseases but most often occurs following cardiovascular surgery [22]. Other causes include chest trauma and esophageal perforation. The most common microbiological agents are gram positive cocci (Staphlococcus aureus and epidermidis) although other organisms may also be observed. The typical laboratory findings reflect a severe infection with or without sepsis including an elevated white blood cell count and disseminated intravascular coagulation. If surgical drainage is present the fluid should be sent for Gram stain and culture. Blood cultures may also be positive in patients with bacteremia (see reference 22 for a review).

Genetic testing in cardiomyopathy: Cardiomyopathies (also called "heart muscle diseases") are typically classified into one of four types:

- Dilated cardiomyopathy.
- Hypertrophic cardiomyopathy.
- Restrictive cardiomyopathy.
- Arrhythmogenic right ventricular cardiomyopathy.

A recently recognized additional type has been identified: left ventricular non-compaction cardiomyopathy (LVNC).

Although many cases of cardiomyopathy are truly idiopathic, recent research has shown that a number of cases are due to genetic causes affecting energy metabolism, or structural and contractile proteins [23]. Up to 90% of cases of hypertrophic cardiomyopathy (HCM) are familial (autosomal dominant) with most of the remaining cases being sporadic mutations [24]. In the case of HCM, the genetic mutations occur in genes coding for sarcomeric contractile proteins. Other causes of HCM include Friedrich ataxia, Fabry disease, and Noonan syndrome. Current consensus practice is to screen all first degree relatives of patients with adult-onset HCM with electrocardiograms (ECG) and echocardiography at regular intervals [24]. In the case of dilated cardiomyopathy about 30–50% of cases appear to have a genetic basis, although many non-genetic causes are well known [23]. Inheritance is usually autosomal dominant but can be X linked or autosomal recessive. The genetic mutations mostly occur in cytoskeletal proteins although some mutations occur in sarcomere proteins. Again screening of first degree relatives is recommended [23]. In the case of arrhythmogenic right ventricular cardiomyopathy (ARVCM), many cases are familial including the related syndrome, Naxos syndrome, which is caused by mutations in gamma-catenin (plakoglobin), an intracellular adhesion protein [23]. First degree relatives of patients with ARVCM should be screened with ECG, echocardiograms, and Holter monitoring [24]. At least some cases of restrictive cardiomyopathy appear to have a genetic basis.

Genetic testing for CM is available from a limited number of laboratories. While in many cases such testing may elucidate the genetic cause of the cardiomyopathy, the clinical treatment

of the patient is usually not altered. Some exceptions to this statement exist such as ARVCM. However, genetic testing may be very useful for relatives of an affected patient as a negative test rules out the presence of the gene.

Most laboratories offer testing for individual known genetic mutations and broad-based panels covering a number of different possible mutations. For example, one laboratory offers test panels for (at the time of this writing) hypertrophic cardiomyopathy (18 genes), dilated cardiomyopathy (27 genes), arrhythmogenic right ventricular cardiomyopathy (8 genes), and left ventricular noncompaction syndrome (10 genes) (see Partners Center for Personalized Medicine: Laboratory for Molecular Medicine website: http://pcpgm.partners.org/lmm/tests/cardiomyopathy).

Catecholaminergic polymorphic ventricular tachycardia (CPVT): CPVT is characterized by syncope during exercise or acute emotion resulting from tachycardia [25]. There is no known underlying structural cardiac pathology. The diagnosis can be achieved by provocative testing and treated effectively with beta-blockers. At present two gene mutations have been identified (RYR2 which is autosomal dominant and CASQ2 which is autosomal recessive). Genetic screening of first degree relatives is recommended if the genetic mutation is known as the disorder will be frequently fatal if untreated [25].

Genetic testing in congenital heart disease (CHD): In some cases congenital heart diseases are caused by genetic mutations including mutations in elastin, gata-binding protein, jagged 1 and NK2 transcription factor related locus 5. Genetic testing may be indicated in patients and their relatives to establish the presence of the genetic defect or to rule out a genetic cause for the CHD. A detailed discussion of this topic is beyond the scope of this chapter. An excellent review of the subject may be found at the Partners Center for Personalized Genetic Medicine: Laboratory for Molecular Medicine website: http://pcpgm.partners.org/lmm/tests/cardiomyopathy).

References

1. Douglas A, Frosch M, Girolami U. Peripheral nerve and skeletal muscle. In: Kumar V, Abbas A, Fausto N (eds). *Robbins and Cotran Pathologic Basis of Disease* (7th edn), 2004, chapter 27, pp. 1325–46. Philadelphia, PA. Elsevier Saunders.

2. Drachman D. Myasthenia gravis and other diseases of the neuromuscular junction. In: Hauser S (ed). *Harrison's Neurology in Clinical Medicine* (1st edn), chapter 36, pp. 527–36. 2006. New York, NY. McGraw Hill.

3. *Mayo Clinic Medical Laboratories Interpretive Handbook.* 2009–2010. pp. 461–5. Rochester, MN. Mayo Medical Laboratories.

4. Rose J, McFarlin D. Myasthenia gravis. In: Frank M, Austen K, Claman H (eds). *Samters Immunologic Diseases* (5th edn), 1995. Vol II, p. 1061. Boston, MA. Little Brown and Co.

5. Bylund D, Nakamura R. Organ specific autoimmune diseases. In: McPhersom R, Pincu M (eds). *Henry's Clinical Diagnosis and Management by Laboratory Methods* (21st edn), 2007. pp. 945–60. Philadelphia, PA. Saunders

6. Takeda S, Miyoshi S, Ohta M, Minami M, Masaoka A, Matsuda H. Primary germ cell tumors of the mediastinum. *Cancer* 2003;97:367–76

7. Bokemeyer C, Nichols C, Droz J Schmoll H, Horwich A, Gerl A, Fossa S, Beyer J, Pont J, Kanz L, Einhorn L, Hartmann J. Extragonadal germ cell tumors of the mediastinum and retroperitoneum: results from an international analysis. *J Clin Oncol* 2002;20:1863–4

8. The International Germ Cell Cancer Collaborative Group. International germ cell consensus classification: a prognostic factor-based staging system for metastatic germ cell cancers. *J Clin Oncol* 1997;15:594–603

9. Chaer R, Massad M, Evans A, Snow N, Geha A. Primary neuroendocrine tumors of the thymus. *Ann Thorac Surg* 2002;74:1733–40

10. Abbas F, Raziuddin B, Amanullah M, Jamsheer T. Mediastinal parathyroid adenoma causing primary hyperparathyroidism. *J Pak Med Assoc* 2007;57:93–5

11. Uludag M, Isgor A, Yetkin G, Murat A, Adut K, Ismail A. Supernumary ectopic parathyroid glands. Persistent hyperparathyroidism due to mediastinal parathyroid adenoma localized by preoperative single photon emission computed tomography and intraoperative gamma probe application. *Hormones* 2009;8:144–9

12. Douza C, Bhagavan K, Gopalakrishnan R. Ectopic parathyroid adenoma. *Thyroid Res Pract* 2012;9:68–70

13. Barbetakis N, Chnaris A, Papoulidis P, Siobolas P, Kostopoulos G. Ectopic medistinal thyroid tissue-a case report and review of the literature. *Hospital Chronicles* 2010;5:99–102

14. Papalambros E, Griniatsos J, Vassiliki S, Dimitris H, Evangelos F, Frangiska S, Margarita A, Christos B, Elias B. A hyperthyroid patient with ectopic mediastinal thyroid goiter affected by Graves disease. *Endocrinologist* 2005;15:292–4

15. Thygesan K, Alpert J, Jaffe A, Simons M, Chaitman B, White D. Third universal definition of myocardial infarction. *Circulation* 2012;126:2021–33

16. Kelley K, Januzzi J, Christenson R. Increases in cardiac troponin in conditions other than acute coronary syndrome and heart failure. *Clin Chem* 2009;55:2098–112

17. Lindahl B, Venge P, Wallentin L. Relation between troponin T and the risk of subsequent cardiac events in unstable coronary artery disease. *Circulation* 1996;94:1651–7

18. Kavsak P, Newman A, Lustig V, MacRae A, Palomake G, Ko D, Tu J, Jaffe A. Long-term health outcomes associated with detectable troponin I concentrations. *Clin Chem* 2007;53:220–7

19. Mohammed A, Januzzi J. Clinical applications of highly sensitive troponin assays. *Cardiology in Review* 2010;18:12–19

20. Januzzi J, Carmargo C, Anwaruddin S, Chen A, Krauser D, Cameron R, Nagurney J, Jones D, Brown D, Melanson S, Sluss P, Lewandrowski E,

Lewandrowski K. The N-terminal Pro-BNP investigation of dyspnea in the emergency department (PRIDE) study. *Am J cardiol* 2005;95:948–54

21. Braunwald E. Biomarkers in heart failure. *NEJM* 2008;358:2148–59

22. Mueller D, Mancini M. *Mediastinitis. Medscape Drugs, Diseases and*

Procedures. http://emedicine.medscape.com/article/425308-overview. Updated Jan 19, 2012

23. Schoen F. The heart. In: Kumar V, Abbas A, Fausto N (eds). *Robbins and Cotran Pathologic Basis of Disease* (7th edn), 2004 chapter 12, pp. 555–617. Elsevier Saunders, Philadelphia, PA.

24. Murphy R, Starling R. Genetics and cardiomyopathy: where are we now? *Cleveland J Med* 2005;72:465–83

25. Napolitano C, Priori S, Bloise R. Catecholaminergic polymorphic ventricular tachycardia. *Gene Reviews.* www.ncbi.nlm.nih.gov/pubmed/20301466. Updated Feb 16, 2012

Surgical pathology of the heart

Gregory A. Fishbein, MD, Atsuko Seki, MD, and Michael C. Fishbein, MD

Endomyocardial biopsy

Introduction

Sakakibara and Konno in Japan were the first to employ large-scale use of endomyocardial biopsy for the surgical pathology diagnosis of cardiac conditions [1]. Caves is credited for modifications of the procedure that is most widely used now, primarily for the monitoring of cardiac allograft rejection [2]. Evaluation of endomyocardial biopsies (EMB) may be critical in a number of diagnostic scenarios including evaluation of allograft rejection, myocarditis, cardiomyopathy, drug toxicity, and cardiac tumors. Furthermore, EMB has utility in guiding therapy and prognostication. The pathologist therefore plays an important role in collaboration with cardiologists and surgeons in determining appropriate diagnostic and treatment strategies.

Pathologic assessment of EMB may be complex; standard protocols should be observed [3]. The pathologist must be cognizant of the clinical scenario to ensure the necessary techniques are used in ascertaining and handling of diagnostic material. Optimal EMB consist of at least three fragments of endomyocardium, 1–2 mm in greatest dimension, immediately fixed in 10% buffered formalin at room temperature. If focal lesions are anticipated, additional sampling may be prudent. Under specific circumstances, molecular studies and special stains may require that one or two fragments of diagnostic tissue be snap-frozen in liquid nitrogen and kept at -80°C. Additionally, under certain circumstances one fragment of tissue should be fixed in 2.5% Karnovsky solution or glutaraldehyde for electron microscopy (EM). Peripheral blood sample collected in ethylenediaminetetraacetate (EDTA) or citrate may be required when viral or genomic studies are indicated. In rare instances when EMB is used to evaluate cardiac tumors, tissue collected in Roswell Park Memorial Institute medium (RPMI) solution will facilitate cytogenetic, fluorescence in situ hybridization (FISH), and flow cytometric studies. Table 16.1 lists the various entities herein discussed, their histologic features, and appropriate ancillary studies.

Routine evaluation of EMB includes light microscopy on formalin-fixed, paraffin-embedded tissue. Multiple sections should be stained with hematoxylin and eosin (H&E). Additional sections for histochemical and/or immunohistochemical staining may be indicated.

Myocarditis

Myocarditis describes a variety of inflammatory conditions involving the myocardium. These may be secondary immunologic phenomena, infection, or may simply be idiopathic. Idiopathic myocarditis is usually attributed to viral infection. However, documentation of viral infection of the heart through culture of tissue, electron microscopy, or other morphologic methods is exceedingly rare. Myocarditis is a disease that is both chronic and acute. Severe presentations, so-called "fulminant" myocarditis, include acute heart failure, arrhythmias, and sudden death. EMB is essential in determining management and diagnosis of myocarditis in both chronic and acute settings.

The diagnosis of myocarditis by EMB is made by the identification of inflammatory infiltrates and/or fibrosis, in accordance with the Dallas Criteria [4] (Table 16.2). The Dallas Criteria defines idiopathic myocarditis as, "an inflammatory infiltrate of the myocardium with necrosis and/or degeneration of adjacent myocytes not typical of the ischemic damage associated with coronary artery disease." Of note, the "necrosis" present in myocarditis is usually not typical coagulative necrosis unless the patient is in shock. More often the injury takes the form of myocytolysis, with clearing or dropout of the sarcoplasm, rather than the hypereosinophilia of ischemic necrosis. In evaluating the EMB, the pathologist should note the distribution of inflammation (focal, confluent, diffuse), the extent of inflammation (mild, moderate, severe), and the type of inflammation (lymphocytic, eosinophilic, granulomatous, giant cell, neutrophilic, mixed) (Fig. 16.1). Similarly, the pathologist should evaluate the EMB for fibrosis, identifying the distribution (endocardial, interstitial), extent (mild, moderate, severe), and type (perivascular, interstitial, replacement).

Pathology of the Mediastinum, ed. Alberto M. Marchevsky and Mark R. Wick. Published by Cambridge University Press.
© Cambridge University Press 2014.

Table 16.1. Endomyocardial biopsy: pathology and ancillary studies

Differential diagnosis	Histologic findings	Ancillary studies
Myocarditis	Inflammation (lymphocytic, neutrophilic, eosinophilic, giant cell, granulomatous) with or without associated myocyte damage and necrosis	Viral molecular studies (tissue and peripheral blood)
Hypertrophic cardiomyopathy	Myocyte hypertrophy, interstitial and/or replacement fibrosis, myocyte disarray, thickening of small vessels	Molecular genetic testing (sarcomeric genes)
Arrhythmogenic right ventricular cardiomyopathy	Fibrofatty replacement of myocardium, myocardial atrophy	Molecular genetic testing (mostly involving desmosomal proteins)
Idiopathic dilated cardiomyopathy	Myocyte hypertrophy, hyperchromatic "boxcar" nuclei, perinuclear halo, interstitial fibrosis	Molecular analyses show mutated genes in ~30% of cases (e.g. titin)
Idiopathic restrictive cardiomyopathy	Non-specific	Clinical diagnostic studies demonstrating restrictive heart failure
Dystrophin cardiomyopathy	Non-specific	Genetic testing. Decreased or absent IHC/IF staining for dystrophin
Desmin cardiomyopathy	Non-specific	EM showing granulofilamentous aggregates in myocyte cytoplasm
Lamin associated cardiomyopathy	Interstitial and/or replacement fibrosis, myocyte hypertrophy, myocyte vacuolization, enlarged/irregular nuclei	IHC/IF staining for lamin. Molecular genetic testing for LMNA mutations
Mitochondrial cardiomyopathies	Enlarged myocytes, cytoplasmic vacuolization	EM showing morphologic alterations of mitochondria. Molecular mutation analyses (myocardial tissue and/or peripheral blood)
Cardiac sarcoidosis	Non-necrotizing granulomatous inflammation	Histochemical staining to exclude AFB and fungal organisms
Endomyocardial fibrosis/ Löffler endocarditis	Acute phase: inflammation with numerous and degranulating eosinophils, endocardial thrombosis. Chronic phase: endocardial fibrosis and thickening	
Iron overload	Intracellular iron in macrophages and cardiac myocytes	Histochemical staining for iron
Cardiac amyloidosis	Amyloid deposits in myocardium and/or vascular walls	Histochemical staining for amyloid (Congo Red, sulfate Alcian blue, S/T thioflavin). IHC (transthyretin, κ and λ light chains, amyloid A, apolipoprotein), IF, immunoelectron microscopy, protein sequencing, mass spectrometry to subtype amyloid
Storage diseases	Variable: intracellular glycogen, vacuolated hypertrophic cardiac myocytes, non-specific changes	EM. PAS with and without diastase, Alcian blue
Allograft rejection	ACR: interstitial and/or perivascular inflammation with varying degrees of myocyte injury. AMR: endothelial swelling, intravascular macrophages, interstitial edema, hemorrhage, myocyte necrosis	IHC staining for CD3, CD20, CD68 (ACR). IHC/IF staining for C4d or C3d (AMR)
Drug toxicity/ hypersensitivity	Variable: myocardial necrosis, prominent contraction bands, foci of cellular injury of different ages, myocarditis, non-specific fibrosis	Drug serology
Cardiac tumors	Variable: myxoma, sarcoma, fibroma, rhabdomyoma, lipomatous hypertrophy, etc...	IHC for tumor classification, RPMI for cytogenetic/FISH studies and/or flow cytometry, molecular mutation analyses

EM = electron microscopy; IHC = immunohistochemistry; IF = immunofluorescence; PAS = periodic acid–Schiff; ACR = acute cellular rejection; AMR = antibody-mediated rejection; AFB = acid-fast bacilli, FISH = fluorescence in situ hybridization, RPMI = Roswell Park Memorial Institute medium; LM/NA = lamin & sodium-calcium exchanger protein; S/T-thioflavin = Thioflavin-T.

Table 16.2. The Dallas Criteria for EMB diagnosis of myocarditis

Classification

First biopsy
  Myocarditis with or without fibrosis
  Borderline myocarditis (second biopsy may be indicated)
  No myocarditis
Subsequent biopsies
  Ongoing (persistent) myocarditis with or without fibrosis
  Resolving (healing) myocarditis with or without fibrosis
  Resolved (healed) myocarditis with or without fibrosis

Descriptors		
	Inflammatory infiltrate	*Fibrosis*
Distribution	Focal, confluent, diffuse	Endocardial, interstitial
Extent	Mild, moderate, severe	Mild, moderate, severe
Type	Lymphocytic, eosinophilic, granulomatous, giant cell, neutrophilic, mixed	Perivascular, replacement

Numerous infectious organisms have been associated with myocarditis; the most common pathogens include viruses, bacteria, and parasites. Enteroviruses (e.g. *Coxsackie B*), erythroviruses (e.g. *Parvovirus B19*), adenoviruses, and herpes viruses comprise the most frequent causes in the developed world [5]. However, bacteria (e.g. *Corynebacterium diphtheriae, Borrelia burgdorferi, Ehrlichia* species) and parasites (e.g. *Trypanosoma cruzi, Babesia*) contribute to the global burden of disease.

EMB detection of giant cell myocarditis is extremely important. Histologically, giant cell myocarditis shows profound inflammatory infiltrate consisting of lymphocytes, macrophages, multinucleated giant cells, and eosinophils. Myocyte injury and necrosis are diffuse. The disease may present as acute heart failure or even cardiogenic shock. While giant cell myocarditis may have the most ominous clinical findings, if patients can be supported by intra-aortic balloon or ventricular assist devices, full recovery is not uncommon [6].

Several systemic immunologic disorders may produce a secondary myocarditis. These include collagen vascular diseases, such as systemic lupus erythematosus (SLE), dermatopolymyositis, rheumatoid arthritis, ankylosing spondylitis, and scleroderma [7]. Vasculitides such as Churg–Strauss disease, granulomatosis with polyangiitis, Takayasu arteritis, and inflammatory bowel disease may affect the heart. In these cases, myocarditis may or may not accompany vasculitis on EMB [8].

The potential for myocarditis to evolve into dilated cardiomyopathy (DCM) is well established [9]. Moreover, in roughly 10% of patients with clinical DCM, myocarditis is identified on EMB. Many speculate that a subset of idiopathic DCM cases may be the late-term manifestation of asymptomatic viral myocarditis.

Imaging techniques, such as echocardiography and magnetic resonance imaging, can be useful techniques in guiding biopsies, but they are currently no substitute for EMB. EMB can provide 1) a definitive diagnosis of myocarditis, 2) the most likely etiology, 3) surveillance of inflammatory cardiomyopathy, and 4) confirmation of cardiac involvement by systemic disease (e.g. collagen-vascular disease, vasculitis).

Immunohistochemistry may be useful in specifically characterizing inflammatory infiltrates. The most common antibodies used are CD45, CD3, CD20, CD4, CD8, and CD68.

To further investigate potential viral myocarditis, additional material should be obtained at the time of EMB. These include additional fragments of snap-frozen or RNA-later preserved tissue and peripheral blood collected in EDTA or citrate. Molecular analyses, such as polymerase chain reaction (PCR), should be performed on both samples for proper interpretation of the results. Currently, molecular studies appear to be the most fruitful at identifying viral etiologic agents. Knowledge of the incidence of disease in the patient's community is essential. In general, however, the following viruses are of primary consideration: adenovirus, cytomegalovirus, Epstein–Barr virus, enterovirus, influenza virus A and B, herpes simplex virus 1 and 2, parvovirus B19, human herpesvirus 6, rhinovirus, and hepatitis C virus [10].

Idiopathic dilated cardiomyopathy (DCM)

DCM is a disease characterized by ventricular dilatation, myocardial fibrosis, cardiac myocyte death, and systolic dysfunction. DCM is relatively common and may present at any age. Clinically, DCM may manifest as congestive heart failure, arrhythmias, thromboemboli, and sudden cardiac death.

The diagnosis of DCM is made when other pathology, such as valvular heart disease, hypertension, and coronary artery disease have been excluded. Histologic findings in DCM include interstitial and replacement fibrosis, myocyte nuclear enlargement, myocyte vacuolization, and irregular, hyperchromatic "boxcar" nuclei. All of these findings are non-specific and not diagnostic of DCM. Therefore, the utility of EMB is limited to the exclusion of other myocardial diseases, such as active myocarditis and infiltrative disorders.

It is estimated that 30–50% of DCM are familial [11]. Numerous disease genes have been identified, encoding a diverse variety of proteins involved in heterogeneous pathways including calcium handling, nuclear envelope proteins, membrane-scaffolding, and sarcomeric structures. Inheritance is usually autosomal dominant, though X-linked variants have been described. Histologically these variants cannot be distinguished from each other or from the sporadic form of DCM. Advancing molecular techniques, such as whole-exome sequencing, may be employed to determine a specific diagnosis [12].

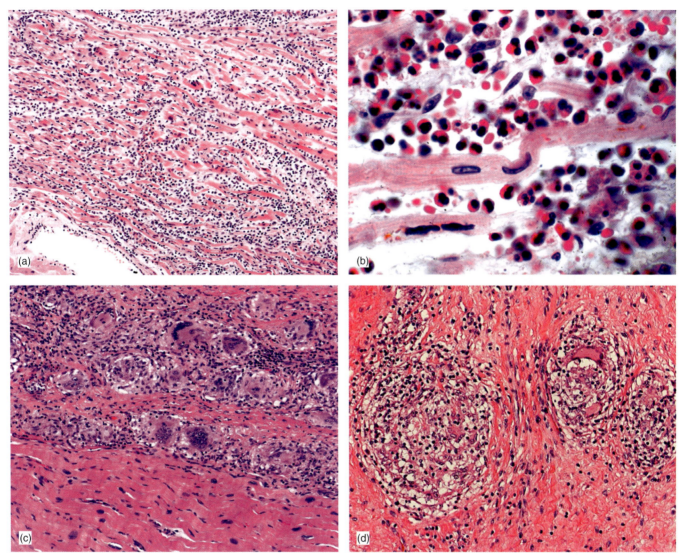

Fig. 16.1 Myocarditis: **(a)** lymphocytic myocarditis from a patient who died suddenly and unexpectedly; **(b)** eosinophilic myocarditis from a patient who died after taking sulfonamide antibiotic for 1 week; **(c)** giant cell myocarditis from a patient with acute onset of cardiogenic shock; and **(d)** discrete non-necrotizing granuloma from a patient with cardiac sarcoidosis (all H&E, a 40x, b 200x, c 100x, and d 100x).

Hypertrophic cardiomyopathy (HCM)

HCM is an autosomal dominant, hereditary disease of the myocardium characterized by hypertrophy of the left (and occasionally right) ventricle. The disease genes encode sarcomeric proteins; specific mutations are detectable by commercially available molecular diagnostic kits. The disease has a peculiar predilection for the interventricular septum, often leading to subvalvular obstruction of the left ventricular outflow tract (hence the moniker, "hypertrophic obstructive cardiomyopathy," or HOCM). Despite this predilection, hypertrophy may also be present in the free wall ("concentric" HCM). In unusual cases, the interventricular septum may even be spared.

The histologic hallmarks of HCM are myocyte hypertrophy, myocyte disarray, interstitial and replacement fibrosis, and thickening of the walls of the intramural vessels

(Fig. 16.2a). These findings may be focal; therefore, accurate histologic diagnosis is subject to significant sampling error. The diagnosis of HCM is predominantly made by clinical, non-invasive techniques, such as electrocardiogram (ECG), echocardiogram, and molecular testing. EMB is not recommended in the diagnostic work-up of HCM. Since the histologic features mentioned, including disarray, may be seen in endomyocardial biopsies as a normal finding, the diagnosis of HCM by EMB is discouraged.

Idiopathic restrictive cardiomyopathy (RC)

RC is a primary disorder of the myocardium causing impaired filling of the ventricles, leading to heart failure with restrictive physiology. Systolic function is generally normal and there is no increase in myocardial wall thickness. While widely considered an idiopathic cardiomyopathy, RC has been associated with

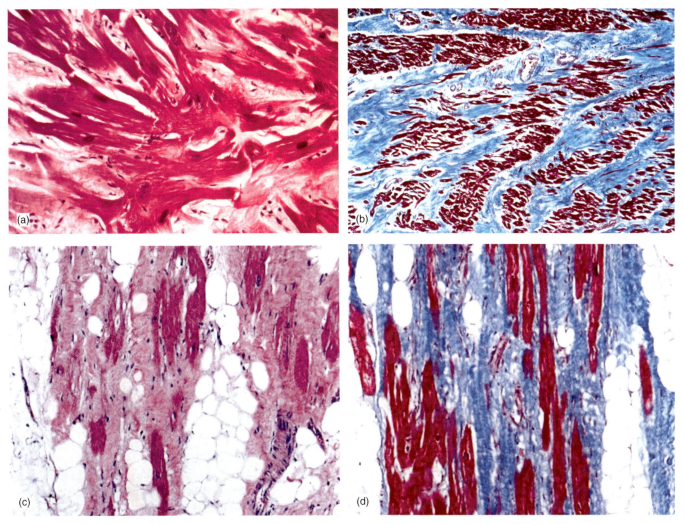

Fig. 16.2 Cardiomyopathies: **(a)** disarray characteristic of hypertrophic cardiomyopathy (H&E, 400x); **(b)** marked interstitial fibrosis of myocardium from patient with idiopathic restrictive cardiomyopathy (trichrome stain x100); **(c)** and **(d)** infiltration of right ventricular free wall by adipose and collagenous tissue characteristic of arrhythmogenic right ventricular cardiomyopathy (c H&E 100x, d trichrome stain 100x).

mutations in genes encoding sarcomeric proteins. The diagnosis is made when restrictive heart failure is observed clinically, in the absence of pericardial disease or other causes of restriction.

There are no histologic features characteristic of RC. Non-specific findings may include interstitial fibrosis and myocardial disarray (Fig. 16.2b). However, the presence of normal myocardium does not preclude the diagnosis. EMB is not generally indicated. However it may be useful when infiltrative or storage diseases need to be excluded. Furthermore, there are data suggesting that, in patients with severe restriction, judicious use of EMB may result in fewer unnecessary thoracotomies to rule out pericardial disease [13].

Arrhythmogenic right ventricular cardiomyopathy (ARVC)

ARVC is a rare disorder of the heart muscle characterized by fibrofatty replacement of the myocardium, usually involving the right ventricle. At least 50% of cases are familial. Mutations

in desmosomal proteins, such as plakoglobin and desmoplakin, are found to be responsible. Most mutations have autosomal dominant inheritance patterns, though notable autosomal recessive syndromes (e.g. Naxos disease, Carvajal syndrome) exist [14]. Clinically, ARVC may present with systolic dysfunction, mimicking DCM. However, as the name implies, ARVC is exceedingly arrhythmogenic and is an important cause of sudden death, particularly in young athletes.

Evaluation of patients with suspected ARVC most frequently involves non-invasive diagnostic modalities, such as ECG, echocardiogram, and magnetic resonance imaging (MRI). However, right ventricle EMB may be employed if alternative testing is inconclusive. The disease tends to spare the interventricular septum, so EMB of the right ventricular free wall, a considerably more dangerous approach, may be required. Complementary use of image guidance or electro-anatomic mapping may increase diagnostic accuracy.

Histologically, focal findings of ARVC are fibrous or fibrofatty replacement of the myocardium and myocardial atrophy

(Fig. 16.2c and d). The presence of fatty tissue in the myocardium is not diagnostic, as some myocardial fat is a normal finding (especially in the anterolateral apical right ventricular free wall). Cardiac myocyte vacuolization, hypertrophy, and inflammation may be seen, though these findings are non-specific. Histochemical stains demonstrating collagen (e.g. Masson trichrome, Movat) may be helpful in highlighting fibrofatty replacement.

The role of immunofluorescence and immunohistochemistry in the diagnosis of ARVC is still being determined. Antibodies to plakoglobin and other desmosomal proteins may demonstrate disease in myocardial tissue with no morphologic abnormality present by H&E microscopy, eliminating the need for targeted free wall EMB. As with the other inherited cardiomyopathies, the use of molecular diagnostic modalities may play an important role in the diagnosis of ARVC.

Peripartum cardiomyopathy (PPCM)

PPCM is a pregnancy-associated myocardial disease characterized by unexplained left ventricular dilatation, systolic dysfunction, and congestive heart failure. The peripartum period, in this context, can reasonably be defined as the interval between the last month of pregnancy and five months postpartum [15]. The diagnosis of PPCM relies on the exclusion of alternative etiologies of heart failure.

The role of EMB in the diagnosis of PPCM is unclear. Histologic findings in PPCM are non-specific. Cardiac myocytes may display nuclear enlargement, hyperchromatic "boxcar" nuclei, and vacuolization. Interstitial and replacement fibrosis may be present. In the absence of a clinical correlation with pregnancy, PPCM may be indistinguishable from DCM.

Histologically, EMB of patients with PPCM may reveal varying degrees of myocarditis. The clinical significance of this is controversial. In one systematic review, Ntusi *et al.* revealed that the reported prevalence of myocarditis on EMB in patients with PPCM ranged from 0 to 100% [16]. This "discrepancy" from study to study illustrates the astronomic institutional variation in the definition of PPCM, definition of myocarditis, prevalence of myocarditis, utilization of EMB, patient demographics, etc... Nevertheless, the finding of myocarditis on EMB may be irrelevant, as some data suggest no difference in clinical outcome [17].

Storage diseases

Metabolic diseases due to congenital enzyme deficiencies frequently have cardiac manifestations, such as ventricular hypertrophy, dilatation, and conduction abnormalities. However, these are systemic illnesses that are infrequently diagnosed by EMB. Nevertheless, storage diseases may have characteristic histologic and EM findings. Special stains, such as periodic acid-Schiff (PAS) and Alcian blue, may highlight the storage product. These are best performed on frozen tissue to prevent washout of the storage material. The intracellular deposits can sometimes be well visualized with EM (Fig. 16.3). A list of storage diseases with associated cardiac pathology is presented in Table 16.3. In many cases, therapy includes enzyme replacement. EMB may be used in monitoring the therapeutic effect, although skeletal muscle biopsy is usually sufficient.

Muscular dystrophies

Muscular dystrophies are inherited diseases characterized by progressive weakness and muscle atrophy. Cardiac manifestations are frequent. Furthermore, cardiac dysfunction may not correlate with the extent of skeletal myopathy. Muscular dystrophies present with cardiac phenotypes mimicking HCM, DCM, and even ARVC. A list of muscular dystrophies and their associated disease-causing genes is presented in Table 16.4.

Genetic mutation analysis is the primary diagnostic tool in evaluating muscular dystrophies. However, EMB may provide histologic, immunohistochemical, and EM findings indicative of disease. H&E findings are non-specific; myocytolysis, interstitial/replacement fibrosis, fibrofatty replacement, nuclear irregularity and enlargement, vacuolization, and myocyte hypertrophy may be present. EM shows variable features depending on the genetic aberrancy, such as non-specific membrane irregularities in dystrophin-related myopathies (Becker and Duchenne muscular dystrophy), nuclear blebs in lamin A/C-related myopathies (e.g. autosomal dominant Emery–Dreifuss muscular dystrophy, limb-girdle muscular dystrophy type 1B) and cytoplasmic granulofilamentous aggregates in desmin-related myopathies. Immunohistochemical stains for the disease proteins (e.g. dystrophin, desmin, lamin A/C) may be available to better characterize the pathology.

Mitochondrial cardiomyopathies (MICs)

Mitochondrial diseases are uncommon diseases of mutated proteins involved in the respiratory chain (also known as electron transport chain). These mutations may occur in either the mitochondrial or nuclear genomes, resulting in multiple modes of inheritance (maternal, autosomal dominant, autosomal recessive, X-linked, or sporadic). Cardiomyopathy is a frequent manifestation. The phenotype is typical hypertrophic (non-obstructive) although ventricular dilatation may be present [18]. In the setting of multiorgan syndromes, the diagnosis can be best made by genetic tests, biochemical analysis, or skeletal muscle biopsy. However, since the proteome of cardiac mitochondria is more extensive than that of many other cells [19], isolated MIC may occur. In such cases, EMB can be useful.

The H&E histology of MICs is non-specific. Myocytes are enlarged and show extensive vacuolization in the cytoplasm. Histoenzymatic stains for succinate dehydrogenase (SDH) and cytochrome C oxidase (COX) should be performed on frozen sections to render a diagnosis. Negative staining of COX in cardiac myocytes and increased SDH staining are diagnostic of MICs. EM shows proliferation of mitochondria, giant mitochondria with inclusion bodies, loss of contractile myofibrils,

Table 16.3. Examples of storage diseases affecting the heart

Storage material	Disease	Enzyme deficiency
Glycogen	Pompe's disease (GSD II)	acid maltase
	GSD type III (Cori's disease, Forbes' disease)	glycogen debranching enzyme
	Amylopectinosis (GSD IV, Andersen disease)	glycogen branching enzyme
	Danon disease	LAMP2
Sphingolipids	Fabry disease	α-galactosidase
	GM1 gangliosidoses	β-galactosidase
	Sandhoff disease (GM2 gangliosidosis)	hexosaminidase A and B
	Gaucher disease	glucocerebrosidase
	Niemann-Pick disease	sphingomyelinase, NPC1/NPC2 mutation
Mucopolysaccharides	Hurler syndrome (MPS I)	α-L iduronidase
	Hunter syndrome (MPS II)	iduronate-2-sulfatase
	Maroteaux-Lamy (MPS VI, polydystrophic dwarfism)	arylsulfatase B
Mucolipids	I-cell disease (ML II, inclusion-cell disease)	phosphotransferase
Glycoproteins	Galactosialidosis	cathepsin A

GSD = glycogen storage disease; LAMP = lysosome-associated membrane protein; NPC = Niemann-Pick disease, type C; MPS = mucopolysaccharidosis; ML = mucolipidosis

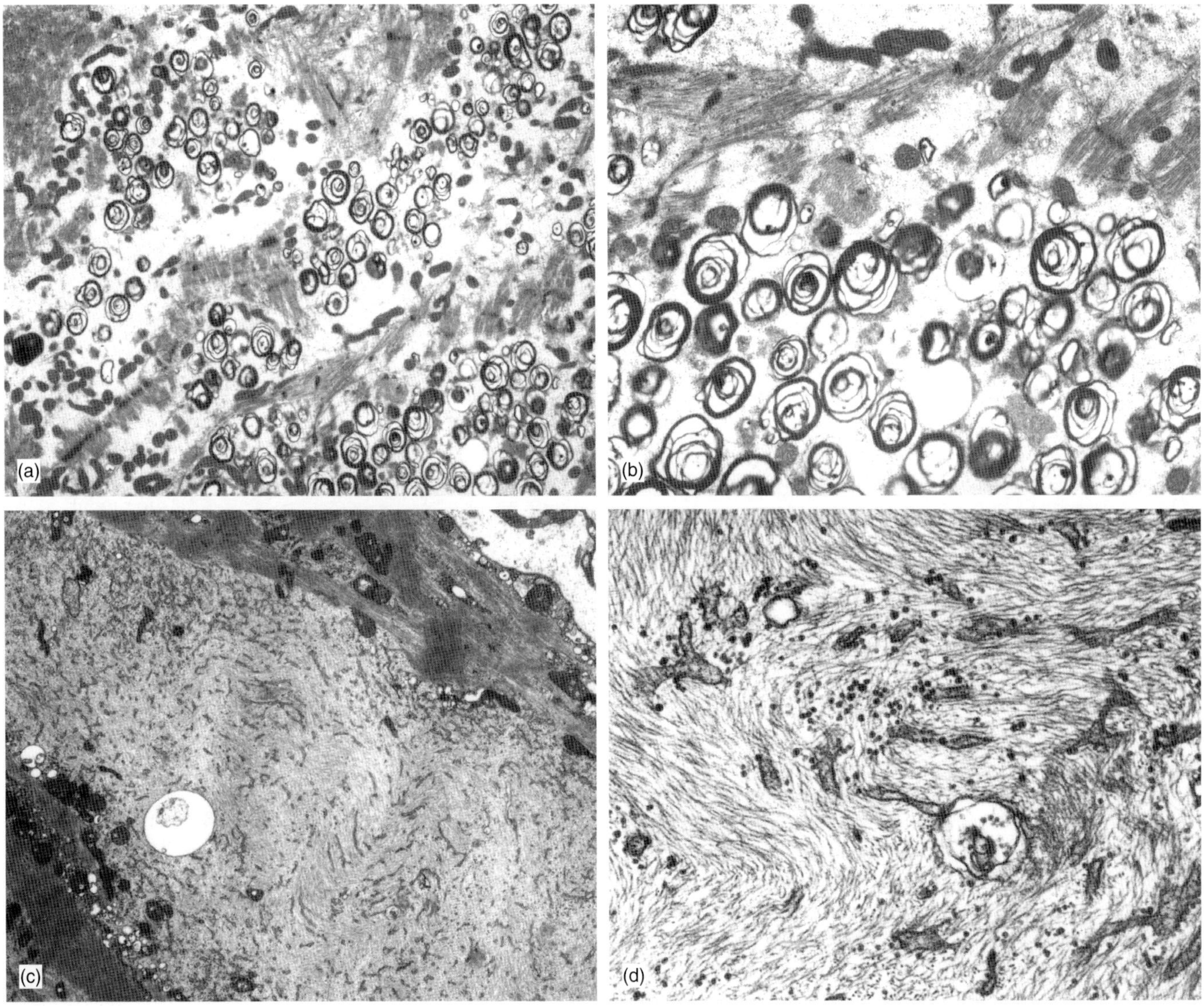

Fig. 16.3 Storage diseases, ultrastructural views: **(a and b)** concentric myelinoid inclusions seen in α-galactosidase deficiency (Fabry disease) at low and high magnification; **(c and d)** abnormal fibrillary glycogen seen in glycogen storage disease type IV (amylopectinosis/Andersen disease), low and high magnifications.

Table 16.4. Examples of muscular dystrophies in which EMB has diagnostic potential

Protein	Disease	Chromosome
Dystrophin	Duchenne muscular dystrophy	Xp21.2
	Becker muscular dystrophy	Xp21.2
	X-linked dilated cardiomyopathy	Xp21.2
Lamin A/C	Autosomal dominant Emery–Dreifuss muscular dystrophy	Xq28
	Limb-girdle muscular dystrophy, type 1B	1q21.2
	Limb-girdle muscular dystrophy, type 2B	2p13.1
Desmin	Desmin-related myofibrillar myopathy	2q.35

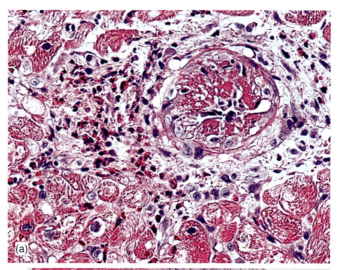

and cytoplasmic glycogen and lipid droplets. Frozen tissue for genetic analysis should be collected.

Löffler endocarditis (LE)/endomyocardial fibrosis (EMF)

LE and EMF are restrictive heart diseases characterized by fibrous thickening of the endocardium with extension to the adjacent myocardium. In advanced cases, these lesions progressively obliterate the ventricular cavities. LE and EMF are often referred to as distinct entities, both histologically and epidemiologically. However, given that the dominant feature in both entities is fibrosis of the endocardium and subendocardial myocardium, they are commonly conflated.

LE, originally described by Löffler as *endocarditis parietalis fibroplastica*[20], is a cardiac manifestation of hypereosinophilia. Tissue injury occurs as the result of degranulation of circulating eosinophils (Fig. 16.4). The hypereosinophilia may be idiopathic or secondary – it has been reported in the context of hematologic malignancies (i.e. leukemia), solid tumors associated with eosinophilia[21], Churg–Strauss disease, and, particularly in subtropical regions, helminth infection. Histologically, endomyocardial fibrosis is accompanied by mural thrombosis rich in eosinophils and eosinophilic myocarditis. LE is phasic; acute stages show primarily necrosis followed by thrombosis, whereas late stages show primarily fibrosis leading to restrictive heart failure and atrioventricular valvular dysfunction.

EMF, also called tropical endomyocardial fibrosis and Davies disease, is histologically similar to LE, but characteristically eosinophils are absent. It is nevertheless believed to be a late manifestation of hypereosinophilia. The incidence of EMF is highest in equatorial Africa, Asia, and South America. Numerous etiologies of EMF have been proposed, including infections (toxoplasmosis, helminthic parasites, malaria), allergy, malnutrition, and toxic chemicals, including thorium, serotonin, plant toxins, and vitamin D[22].

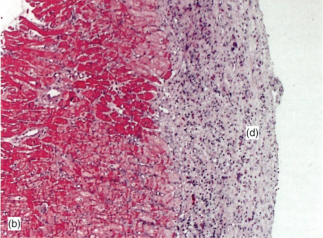

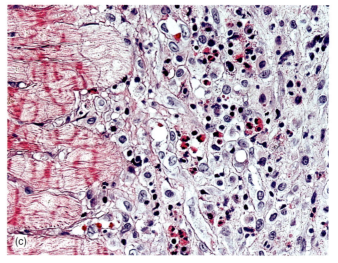

Fig. 16.4 Eosinophils in the heart: **(a)** intramyocardial artery with vasculitis and numerous eosinophils in the perivascular tissues from a patient with Churg-Strauss syndrome; **(b)** endocardium **(d)** with fibrous thickening and cellular infiltrate that at higher magnification **(c)** are shown to be eosinophils, from a patient with endomyocardial fibrosis and eosinophilia (all H&E, a 200x, b 40x, and c 200x).

A definitive diagnosis of LE/EMF in the acute/subacute phase can be made by EMB. ECG, echocardiography, and angiography may not distinguish LE/EMF from other restrictive cardiovascular diseases, such as RC and pericardial constriction [23]. EMB will demonstrate an inflammatory infiltrate rich in eosinophils, with prominent eosinophilic degranulation and endocardial thrombosis. In the chronic phase, EMB may only provide a "probable/possible" diagnosis, showing fibrous thickening of the endocardium and subendocardial myocyte injury. Clinical correlation with current or previous peripheral eosinophilia is highly suggestive.

Cardiac sarcoidosis

Sarcoidosis is a systemic granulomatous disease that predominantly affects the lymph nodes of the mediastinum and the lungs. Cardiac involvement is important to recognize, as it portends a poor prognosis. Cardiac involvement is the cause of death in roughly half of individuals with systemic sarcoidosis [3]. Early detection of cardiac disease is critical due to its treatment implications. Unfortunately, given the focal nature of the disease, EMB is positive in only 19–25% of cases in which cardiac involvement is suspected [24,25]. Nevertheless, a positive EMB warrants initiation of corticosteroid therapy and/or prophylactic implantation of a defibrillator. To improve sensitivity, electrophysiology and image-directed biopsies have been suggested.

The histologic hallmark of sarcoidosis is the well-formed, discrete, non-necrotizing granuloma – the so-called "unit granuloma" (Fig. 16.1d). Langhans and foreign body giant cells are easily identified. Inclusion bodies, such as asteroid bodies,

Schaumann (conchoid) bodies, Hamazaki-Wesenberg bodies, and centrospheres are occasionally present within the giant cells, but are non-specific [26,27]. Although a non-necrotizing granuloma is an exceedingly rare EMB finding in patients without a clinical diagnosis of sarcoidosis, other granulomatous diseases, such as giant cell myocarditis, Churg-Strauss disease, and infectious processes must be considered in the differential diagnosis. For this reason, to rule out the micro-organisms, histochemical staining for fungus (e.g. periodic acid-Schiff, Gomori methenamine silver) and acid-fast bacteria (e.g. Ziehl–Neelsen) is prudent. Sarcoidosis can be distinguished from giant cell myocarditis and Churg-Strauss disease histologically, the latter two having a prominent eosinophilic, more diffuse infiltrate and lacking discrete sarcoidal granulomas.

Cardiac amyloidosis

The term *amyloid* refers to a heterogeneous group of proteins with secondary structure characterized by extended β-pleated sheets. At least 25 amyloid proteins have been identified in human disease, a subset of which manifest as cardiac disease [28]. Characteristically, cardiac amyloidosis presents as acute or chronic heart failure with predominantly restrictive physiology. Clinical diagnosis of cardiac amyloidosis may be challenging; EMB is recommended when amyloidosis is suspected. While it has been suggested that cardiac amyloidosis can be universally recognized by sampling abdominal fat pads [29], anecdotally this method has proven to be of low yield. Table 16.5 enumerates the main amyloidoses responsible for cardiac pathology.

Table 16.5. Amyloidoses affecting the heart

	Age	Cardiac manifestation	Amyloid composition	Cause	Diagnostic testing	Immunostains	Extracardiac sites
Primary (AL) amyloidosis	55–60 years	HF, arrhythmia	Monoclonal immunoglobulin light chain	Multiple myeloma, lymphoplasmacytic lymphoma	Serum/urine protein electrophoresis	κ, λ light chains	Kidney, nerve, GI tract, liver
Secondary (AA) amyloidosis		Rare	Serum AA, β2 microglobulin	Chronic inflammatory conditions, malignancy	Target organ biopsy, synovial and bone biopsy (dialysis-related), AA antiserum staining	AA protein	Kidney
Hereditary amyloidosis		Cardiomyopathy	Mutant TTR and apolipoprotein	Mutation of TTR gene	TTR antiserum staining, genetic testing	TTR	Nervous system
Senile amyloidosis	11.5–25% of people over 80 years old	AF, conduction abnormality, HF	Wild type TTR	Ageing	TTR antiserum staining	TTR	Aorta, pulmonary arteries, and pulmonary alveolar septa
Isolated atrial amyloidosis	80–90% of people over 80 years old	AF	ANP	Ageing	ANP antiserum staining		None

AA = amyloid A; AL = amyloid light chain; HF = heart failure; AF = atrial fibrillation; GI = gastrointestinal; TTR = transthyretin; ANP = atrial natriuretic peptide

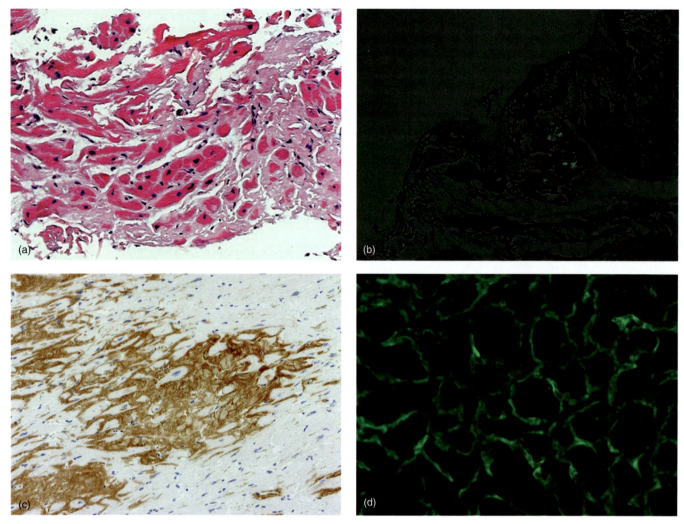

Fig. 16.5 Cardiac amyloidosis: **(a)** typical appearance as a pale, pink interstitial deposit in H&E stained sections (100x); **(b)** apple-green birefringence of Congo-red stained section (40x); **(c)** immunohistochemical stain for transthyretin from an elderly patient (100x); and **(d)** immunofluorescence stain for kappa light chains from a patient with myeloma and heart failure (200x).

Cardiac amyloidosis is an infiltrative disease caused by interstitial deposition of amyloid protein (Fig. 16.5). H&E microscopy shows amorphous, solid, eosinophilic extracellular material. This material must be distinguished from collagen and hyaline, which may appear similar. Congo red stain is famously used in making the diagnosis; under polarized light the deposits show characteristic apple-green birefringence. Masson's trichrome stain is also very helpful (and perhaps underutilized) in distinguishing amyloid from collagen; whereas collagen stains a rich blue color, amyloid appears amphophilic. Alternative histochemical stains for identifying amyloid include modified sulfated Alcian blue, crystal violet, and thioflavin T.

Subtyping of amyloid protein is critical in determining clinical management and for prognostication. Following histochemical confirmation of amyloid (i.e. Congo red, trichrome stains), an attempt at subclassification is recommended. A reasonable immunohistochemical panel would include stains for transthyretin (pre-albumin), κ and λ light chains, and amyloid-A protein. However, immunostains may be inadequate for definitive subclassification [30]. If immunofluorescence is to be employed, frozen tissue is necessary. Subtyping by protein sequencing [31] and mass spectrometry [32] can be performed at centers experienced with these techniques.

Iron overload

The normal heart contains no iron. Hence, any stainable iron in cardiac myocytes is pathologic. Heart failure secondary to iron overload is the most common cause of death in anemic patients who are transfusion-dependent [33]. Iron overload also occurs in patients with hereditary hemochromatosis, and may cause cardiac dysfunction [34]. Clinically, iron overload can present as cardiomyopathy with restrictive or dilated phenotype. Ancillary studies such as serum ferritin and MRI are effective in quantifying iron and tend to correlate with the degree of cardiac deposition [35,36]. Genetic testing is employed to identify hereditary hemochromatosis.

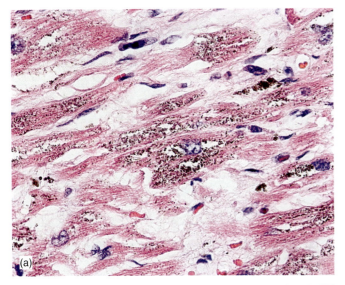

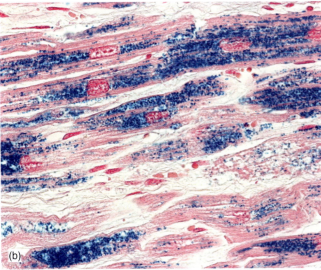

Fig. 16.6 Hemochromatosis: myocardium from patient who developed heart failure after liver transplantation: **(a)** brown pigment in myocytes (H&E 200x), and **(b)** Prussian-blue stain confirming presence of iron (200x).

However, when ancillary studies cannot provide a definitive diagnosis, EMB is indicated.

EMB of patients with unexplained DCM should be evaluated for iron deposition. If necessary, histochemical staining for iron (e.g. Prussian blue) is recommended (Fig. 16.6). EMB may also be used to monitor patients with iron overload and to verify therapeutic results. While EMB is the gold standard for evaluating cardiac iron overload, iron preferentially deposits in the sub-epicardium; biopsy of the right ventricular septum can potentially yield a false negative result due to sampling error [37].

Cardiac tumors

The majority of cardiac tumors are metastatic (10–30:1) [3,38]. Rarely neoplasms of the heart are primary, 90% of which are benign. Virtually any malignancy has the potential to metastasize to the heart. The cancers with the highest rate of cardiac involvement include pleural mesothelioma, melanoma, non-small cell lung cancer, and breast cancer [39]. Nevertheless, cardiac metastases are unusual.

Overwhelmingly, the most common primary cardiac tumor is the cardiac myxoma (Fig. 16.7). These tumors have a strong predilection for the left atrium, so much so that they are often referred to as "left atrial myxomas." Of interest, the cardiac myxoma has no histologic counterpart in other organs or tissues. Basso *et al.* found that roughly 70% of cardiac tumors biopsied were diagnosed as myxomas [40].

Papillary fibroelastoma (PFE) is the second most common benign tumor in the heart. While generally thought to be neoplastic, PFE may represent a reactive proliferation at a site of endocardial injury. PFE may be incidental and asymptomatic. However, if on the aortic valve the lesion can prolapse into the coronary ostium and cause ischemic injury. Embolism of thrombus or part of the lesion may occur [41]. PFE is usually found in the valvular endocardium; the AV is the most common site.

Other benign primary cardiac tumors include rhabdomyoma (particularly in children), fibroma, and hemangioma. Malignant primary cardiac tumors may be encountered; 95% are sarcomas, angiosarcoma being the most common [42]. Lymphomas comprise roughly 5%.

The diagnosis of cardiac tumors is primarily made clinically, using echocardiography, computed tomography, and/or magnetic resonance imaging. Preoperative biopsy, however, will facilitate the differentiation of benign and malignant lesions, as well as histologic subtype, which are critical in determining prognosis and therapy. EMB is mainly indicated for right-sided lesions; left-sided EMB is often avoided due to the risk of iatrogenic systemic embolism. Sampling errors may be minimized by the use of echocardiographic guidance.

At least three to five biopsy specimens should be formalin-fixed and paraffin embedded (2–3 mm^2 each). One or two fragments of tissue should be frozen for electron microscopy and molecular studies. Tissue collected in RPMI will allow for FISH and flow cytometric studies. Immunohistochemical studies are indicated; the specific panel chosen depends entirely on the histologic features of the tumor and clinical scenario.

Drug toxicity/hypersensitivity reactions

Drug-related cardiac injury is a potential complication of myriad routinely employed therapeutic agents. Therefore, drugs must always be considered when forming a differential diagnosis of unexplained cardiac disease. In the heart, as in most organs, drug-related pathology comes in two forms: direct toxic injury and hypersensitivity myocarditis [43,44].

Hypersensitivity myocarditis is the most common drug-related form of cardiac dysfunction. A plethora of drugs have been implicated (Table 16.6). Hypersensitivity myocarditis is idiosyncratic and independent of dose. Furthermore,

Table 16.6. Drugs associated with hypersensitivity myocarditis[39]

Acetazolamide	Carbamazepine	Heparin	Nitroprusside	Sulfadiazine
Amitriptyline	Cephalosporins	Hydralazine	Oxyphenbutazone	Sulfamethoxypyridazine
Aminophylline	Chloramphenicol	Hydrochlorothiazide	4-Aminosalicylic acid	Sulfisoxazole
Amphotericin B	Chlorthalidone	Indomethacin	Penicillin	
Ampicillin	Clozapine	Interleukin-2	Phenindione	Sulfonylureas
Azathioprine	Cyclosporine	Isoniazid	Phenylbutazone	Tetracyclines
Benzodiazepines	Digoxin	Isosorbide dinitrate	Phenytoin	Triazolam
Bumetanide	Dobutamine	Methyldopa	Spironolactone	Tricyclic antidepressants
Captopril	Furosemide	Metolazone	Streptomycin	

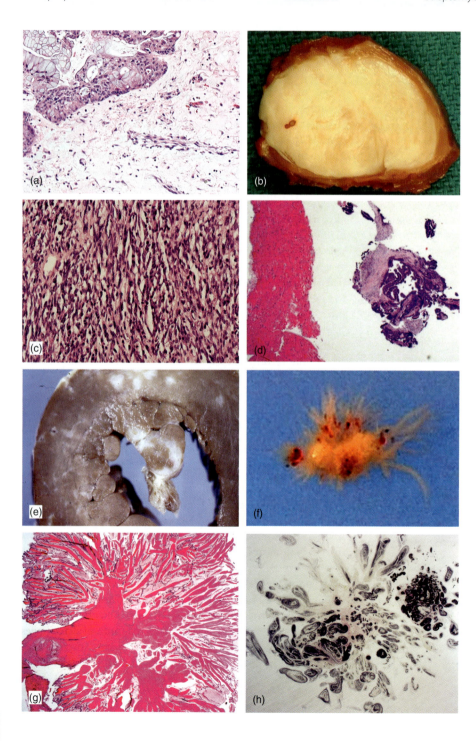

Fig. 16.7 Cardiac tumors: **(a)** unusual myxoma, with mucin positive cells as well as characteristic myxoid stroma with distinctive vasculature; **(b)** cardiac fibroma, excised from the interventricular septum of a child; **(c)** angiosarcoma from right atrium; **(d)** metastatic endometrial carcinoma to right ventricle, diagnosed by endomyocardial biopsy; **(e)** through **(h)** endocardial papillary fibroelastoma, seen attached to left ventricular papillary muscle **(e)**, underwater to demonstrate papillary hair-like projections surrounding a more solid core **(f)**, and microscopically, composed of fibroblasts, collagen and elastic fibers, and covered with hyperplastic endothelial cells **(g and h)** (a H&E 100x, c H&E 200x, d H&E 40x, g H&E 20x, and h elastic stain 20x)

Table 16.7. Drugs with known cardiotoxicity

Amphetamine	Cobalt	Interferon-α
Amsacrine	Cocaine	Interleukin-2
Anabolic steroids	Cyclophosphamide	Lead
Antimony compounds	Daunorubicin	Lithium carbonate
Antiretroviral agents	Doxorubicin	Mitomycin C
Arsenic	Emetine hydrochloride	Mitoxantrone
Catecholamines	Ethanol	Phenothiazines
Chloroquine	5-Flourouracil	

Table 16.8. ISHLT grading system for biopsy grading: acute cellular rejection

Grade 0R	No evidence of cellular rejection
Grade 1R, mild	Interstitial and/or perivascular infiltrate with up to 1 focus of myocyte injury
(1990) Grade 1A	*Perivascular infiltrates without myocyte injury*
(1990) Grade 1B	*Sparse interstitial infiltrates without myocyte injury*
Grade 2R, moderate	Two or more foci of infiltrate with associated myocyte damage
(1990) Grade 3A	*Multifocal prominent infiltrates and/or myocyte injury*
Grade 3R, severe	Diffuse infiltrate with multifocal myocyte damage ± edema ± hemorrhage ± vasculitis
(1990) Grade 3B	*Diffuse infiltrates with myocyte injury*
(1990) Grade 4	*Diffuse polymorphous infiltrate with myocyte injury ± hemorrhage ± edema ± vasculitis*

"R" indicates revised grade

hypersensitivity myocarditis frequently is caused by sensitization after prior safe use. Clinically, the reaction may be accompanied by maculopapular rash that corresponds with the initiation of pharmacologic therapy. The typical pattern of hypersensitivity myocarditis is pancarditis [45]. An inflammatory infiltrate rich in eosinophils is present. Invariably, lymphocytes, plasma cells, and histiocytes are also present. Intramyocardial vasculitis may be seen. Little or no myocardial necrosis or replacement fibrosis may be present. Clinical severity does not tend to correlate with the degree of myocardial involvement.

Numerous drugs are known for their capability of direct cardiac toxicity (Table 16.7). In contrast to hypersensitivity myocarditis, cardiac toxicity is dose dependent. The effects of the offending agent may be augmented by concomitant chemotherapy or radiation. Cardiac toxicity is not exclusively iatrogenic; street drugs, such as cocaine and methamphetamine, and environmental poisons, such as lead and arsenic, are cardiotoxic as well. There is no single pattern of cardiac toxicity, although three histologic patterns predominate: myocardial necrosis without inflammatory infiltrate; "toxic myocarditis" including mixed inflammation comprised by macrophages, neutrophils, and a small number of lymphocytes; and DCM with non-specific myocardial changes such as interstitial fibrosis, myofiber alteration, and polyploidy. EM may reveal ultrastructural changes such as lysosomal inclusions in chloroquine toxicity and sarcoplasmic vacuoles in doxorubicin (Adriamycin) toxicity. In the past, endomyocardial biopsy has been used to guide treatment with doxorubicin – plastic embedded thick sections are required to grade the effects of the drug on the myocardium.

Hypersensitivity myocarditis can usually be diagnosed by EMB when clinically suspected. As with other myocarditides, sampling error may produce false negative tests. The utility of EMB in evaluation of cardiac drug toxicity is variable, depending on the suspected agent. For drugs with a prominent reputation for cardiac toxicity, such as anthracyclines, currently clinical evaluation using echocardiography, MRI, and/or blood troponin levels may provide adequate surveillance.

Allograft rejection

Despite advances in non-invasive serologic testing, EMB remains the gold standard for allograft rejection detection and surveillance [46]. Particularly in the first year, during which acute cellular rejection (ACR) is most frequently observed, EMB is essential in determining post-transplant immunosuppressive therapy. Furthermore, the presence of antibody mediated rejection (AMR), even in the absence of clinical symptoms [47], may trigger the initiation of intravenous immunoglobulin therapy (IVIG) or plasmapheresis. Because EMB will directly impact therapeutic decision-making, the importance of effective and prompt communication between the pathologist and the cardiologist cannot be overstated.

In 1990, the International Society for Heart and Lung Transplantation (ISHLT) put forth a standardized system for grading allograft rejection [48]. The goal was to facilitate concise and effective communication between physicians and transplant centers in the context of patient care and clinical research. This system was revised in 2004 [49], resulting in a simplified classification schema that better correlates with clinical outcomes. While the revised nomenclature is preferred, it is standard practice at some institutions to report the grading of rejection using both the original and revised nomenclature.

Grading of ACR is primarily based on observed degree and pattern of inflammation and myocyte damage (Table 16.8). The inflammatory infiltrate seen in ACR is comprised predominantly of T-cell lymphocytes and macrophages (Fig. 16.8). Occasionally eosinophils are present. The presence of neutrophils may be more indicative of ischemic injury. An

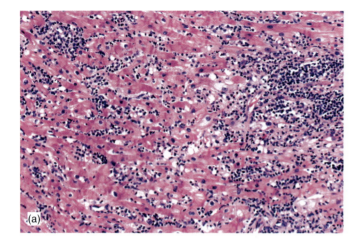

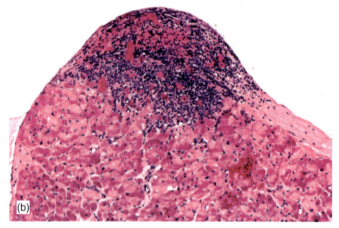

Fig. 16.8 Acute cellular rejection: **(a)** grade 2R rejection with multifocal infiltrate of mononuclear cells and with myocyte injury present (H&E 100x); and **(b)** Quilty B lesion with nodular infiltrate of lymphocytes in endocardium and underlying myocardium (H&E 40x).

infiltrate in which B-cells and/or plasma cells are increased should raise suspicion of Quilty effect (*vide infra*).

Nodular endocardial infiltrates, known as Quilty effect or Quilty lesions, are a common benign finding in allograft EMB. These lesions can be categorized as Quilty A or Quilty B according to the 1990 ISHLT criteria. However, this sub-classification was dropped in the revised ISHLT system, as the distinction between Quilty A and Quilty B is clinically irrelevant. Quilty lesions are nodular aggregates of predominantly B- and T-cell lymphocytes found in the endocardium (Quilty A), sometimes with extension into the adjacent myocardium (Quilty B). Plasma cells and associated myocyte damage may also be present. Particularly when the tissue is tangentially sectioned, Quilty lesions may mimic ACR. In such cases, deeper cut sections may reveal endocardial collagen, favoring Quilty effect. IHC is extremely helpful in distinguishing ACR from Quilty effect. ACR is predominantly a T-cell phenomenon; immunoreactivity to CD3, but not CD20, will be seen. In contrast, Quilty lesions are comprised of both T-cells and B-cells; CD3 and CD20 immunostains may demonstrate a

mixed population of T and B lymphocytes in such lesions. If the lesions are rich in T-cells, a CD68 stain to evaluate macrophages is useful – mononuclear cell staining of less than 50% favors Quilty effect.

The revised ISHLT working formulation suggests that all surveillance EMB be evaluated for histologic evidence of AMR. Histologic findings in AMR include capillary congestion, "endothelial swelling", edema, interstitial hemorrhage, acute inflammation, and thrombosis (Fig. 16.9) [50]. If these features are absent, the EMB is considered negative for AMR. However, if evidence of AMR is present on H&E microscopy, immuno-pathologic studies – IHC and/or IF – are warranted. Of note, IHC demonstrates that "endothelial swelling" may actually represent CD68 positive macrophages. The diagnostic criteria for AMR are currently in a state of evolution; in 2011 the ISHLT proposed preliminary nomenclature for pathologic AMR with special emphasis on histologic versus immuno-pathologic criteria (Table 16.9). The diagnostic histologic and immunopathologic features of AMR are enumerated in Table 16.10.

Cardiac allograft vasculopathy (CAV) is now recognized as the major factor limiting long-term graft survival in adults and children. The predominant histologic finding is fibro-muscular hyperplasia of the tunica intima of small to large coronary vessels [51]. In contrast to atherosclerosis, both intra-mural and epicardial arteries (as well as veins) may be affected. Inflammatory infiltrates may also be present, ranging from endotheliitis to marked full-thickness vasculitis. Accelerated atherosclerosis is also a component of CAV; atherosclerotic plaques are noted even in pediatric allografts. Indeed, due to low sampling of large vessels, CAV is unlikely to be seen on EMB. However, findings consistent with late ischemic injury, such as myocyte vacuolization and micro-infarcts, may suggest CAV, particularly in the clinical setting of late graft failure. Nevertheless, the current ISHLT diagnostic criteria [52] for CAV are purely clinico-radiologic and do not involve EMB.

During the peri-operative period (up to 6 weeks), early ischemic injury may be identified on EMB (Fig. 16.10). Such injury is not unexpected, given that ischemic time is unavoidable during the procurement and implantation of the donor heart ("harvesting" injury). Histologic features of early ischemic injury include contraction band necrosis, coagulative necrosis, and myocyte vacuolization. Mixed inflammatory cells – neutrophils, macrophages, lymphocytes, and eosinophils – are recruited as healing begins. When present, this inflammatory infiltrate must be distinguished from ACR. Typically, ACR features marked inflammation that is dispro-portionate to the degree of accompanying myocyte injury. Generally, the reverse is true of ischemic injury.

Post-transplant lymphoproliferative disorder (PTLD) and infections (e.g. CMV, toxoplasmosis, etc...) are rarely encountered in routine EMB. Nevertheless, identification of these entities is imperative to prevent inappropriate augmentation of immunosuppressive therapy.

Table 16.9. ISHLT proposed grading system of pathologic AMR

pAMR 0	**Negative for AMR:** No histologic or immunopathologic features of AMR
pAMR 1 (H+)	**Histopathologic AMR alone:** Histologic features of AMR present No immunopathologic features of AMR
pAMR 1 (I+)	**Immunopathologic AMR alone:** No histologic features of AMR Positive immunopathologic findings
pAMR 2	**Pathologic AMR:** Histologic features of AMR present Positive immunopathologic findings
pAMR 3	**Severe Pathologic AMR:** Histologic findings of interstitial hemorrhage, capillary fragmentation, mixed inflammatory infiltrates, edema, and endothelial cell pyknosis and/or karyorrhexis

Table 16.10. Immunohistologic features of acute antibody-mediated rejection (AMR)

Histologic evidence of acute capillary injury

Capillary endothelial changes: "swelling" or denudation with congestion
Macrophages in capillaries
Neutrophils in capillaries (more severe cases)
Interstitial edema and/or hemorrhage (more severe cases)

Immunopathologic evidence for antibody mediated injury (in the absence of OKT 3 induction)

Ig (G,M, and/or A) plus C3d and/or C4d or C1q (equivalent staining diffusely in capillaries, 2–3+), demonstrated by immunofluorescence
CD68 positivity for macrophages in capillaries (identified using CD31 or CD34), and/or C4d staining of capillaries with 2–3+ intensity by paraffin immunohistochemistry
Fibrin in vessels (optional; if present, process is reported as more severe)

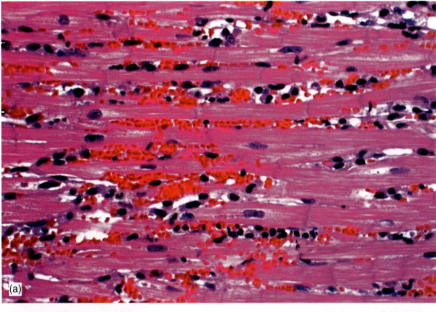

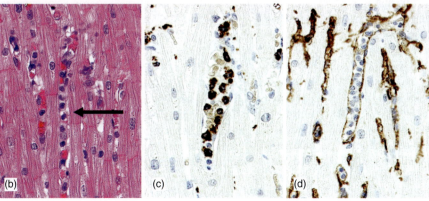

Fig. 16.9 Antibody-mediated (humoral) rejection: **(a)** severe acute case with interstitial hemorrhage and neutrophils present; **(b)** prominent cells in capillaries (arrow); **(c)** immunohistochemical stain for macrophages (CD68) showing that these cells are macrophages; and **(d)** CD31 stain form endothelial cells delineating capillaries with intraluminal macrophages typical of antibody-mediated rejection (a–d H&E 200x).

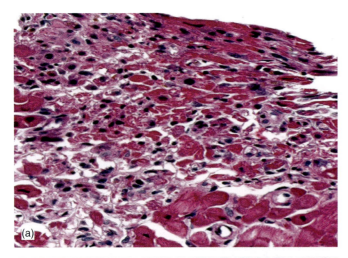

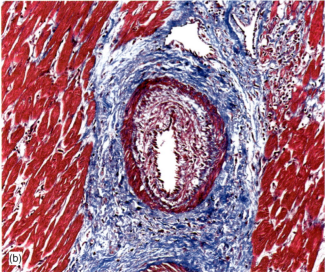

Fig. 16.10 Ischemic injury in the transplanted heart: **a)** myocardium with coagulation necrosis that can occur early after transplantation due to "harvesting" injury, or late after transplantation due to transplant vasculopathy seen in **(b)** (a H&E 200x, b trichrome stain 200x).

Cardiac valves

Introduction

Cardiac valvular disease affects approximately 100,000 people in the United States annually [53]. Excised cardiac valves are one of the more common cardiac surgical pathology specimens.

Dysfunctional cardiac valves result from either structural abnormalities and/or abnormal function of anatomically normal valves [54]. Diseased native cardiac valves may manifest dysfunctional state (stenosis and/or regurgitation) or show evidence of adherent vegetation or thrombus [54]. Sometimes valves that are anatomically normal, but dysfunctional, may be excised and reviewed in surgical pathology. With the anatomically normal valves, clinical correlation including clinical history, echocardiogram, and cardiac catheterization report is essential for accurate pathological diagnosis.

The most important information regarding the etiology of valvular dysfunction will be provided by a careful gross examination [54,55]. The microscope often reveals only non-specific changes in the end stage of a disease process, or manifestations of infection in cases of endocarditis [55]. All the components of valves must be described including numbers of cusps and leaflets as well as chordae tendineae and papillary muscles of atrioventricular valves. A photograph of the intact valve is important for documentation of gross findings.

Normal anatomy of the valves

The semilunar valves, aortic valve (AV) and pulmonary valve (PV) normally have three cusps. In the case of the AV, each cusp is named as left-coronary cusp, right-coronary cusp, or non-coronary cusp. In the case of the PV, they are the left cusp, right cusp, and anterior cusp. Of course, once the valve is excised the orientation is lost. The size of cusps is usually fairly equal, but there may be some variation.

The mitral valve (MV) has anterior and posterior leaflets. The anterior leaflet is fan-shaped; the posterior leaflet is more rectangular. The tricuspid valve (TV) has anterior, septal, and posterior leaflets. Microscopically, all valves have a distinct collagen core, the fibrosa, with a thin adjacent layer of basophilic extracellular matrix, the spongiosa. Both surfaces are covered by endothelium.

Some aging changes in the valves may occur in the absence of specific valvular diseases. The degree of the aging change differs between the valves. With aging, the mean thickness of valve leaflets increases mainly due to collagen and the extracellular matrix products [56]. As we age, the valve rings dilate too [57].

Semilunar valves in adults often have nodular thickenings, nodules of Arantii (also known as nodules of Morgagni), at the centers of the free edges of the cusps [58]. Near the closure line, fibrous thickening (Lambl's excrescences) with or without hair-like projections (Yater's whiskers) may be seen [58]. Fenestration of the cusps along the free edge is also found in semilunar valves [58]. Importantly, none of these changes are functionally significant.

Nodular thickening of the free edge of the anterior leaflet, lipid accumulation, small scars, diffuse opacity, hooding of leaflets and/or focal calcification in mitral valve occur with aging [56]. Age-related changes in the tricuspid valve are minimal.

Gross examination and sectioning

Gross examination with adequate documentation of normal and abnormal findings is essential for the evaluation of excised native valves [54]. Photographs of both the inflow and outflow surfaces are recommended.

Stenotic valves will show anatomic abnormalities. Stenosis is usually associated with fibrosis and calcification of leaflets [54]. In contrast; purely regurgitant valves may sometimes have normal leaflet anatomy [54].

Both stenosis and regurgitation can be found affecting the same valve, if there is fusion of commissures. Disease of multiple valves may be encountered particularly in post-inflammatory heart disease (rheumatic) and connective tissue diseases such as Marfan syndrome [59].

All components of the valve should be described. The dimensions of the effective orifice should be recorded if possible. More and more, valves are being repaired rather than replaced, so only fragments of leaflets may be submitted for evaluation.

Importantly, the presence of thrombus or vegetation should be mentioned [54]. If a vegetation is noted before fixation in formalin, culture of potential micro-organisms may be considered [54]. Ultrastructural examination is rarely needed, perhaps for storage disease evaluation or certain rare infections [54].

Histochemical stains

Most of the histological diagnoses will be made by H&E-staining. A Gram stain and Grocott's methenamine silver (GMS) stain are useful when vegetation or acute inflammation with organism is seen on the valve.

A Masson trichrome or Elastica van Gieson may be useful to document the degree of fibrosis and whether or not elastic tissue is present [54]. Alcian blue staining will highlight myxoid change.

Examination of different valves

Semilunar valves

Semilunar valves should be examined for incompetence or stenosis, the number of cusps, the size of cusps, commissural fusion or separation, degree of calcification and fibrosis, presence of a raphe, and defects or irregularities including fenestrations and perforations [54]. If the valve has two or three cusps, document the size of each cusp and whether they are equal or unequal [55]. After gross examination, if the valves are calcified, the entire specimen should be decalcified before sectioning [54].

Atrioventricular valves

All components should be examined and the description should include the status of leaflets, commissures, chordae, and attached papillary muscles. Document thickening, commissural fusion, irregular edges, defects, calcifications, and vegetations [54,55]. In addition the description should include whether the chordae are shortened, fused, ruptured, or normal [55]. If the specimen includes the papillary muscle, note if it is necrotic, or scarred [55].

Aortic valve disease

The aortic valve is the most frequently excised native cardiac valve. Approximately 90% of aortic valves are removed due to aortic stenosis (AS) [60]. Stenotic aortic valves always appear

Table 16.11. Aortic stenosis

Isolated pure aortic stenosis (AS):		58%
Congenital		54%
	Unicuspid	1.60%
	Bicuspid	52%
Degenerative		46%
Rare causes	Active infective endocarditis	
	Homozygous type II hyperlipoproteinemia	
	Fabry's disease	
	Systemic lupus erythematosus	
Multivalvular disease with AS:		**42%**
Post-inflammatory valve disease		100%

abnormal, while regurgitant aortic valves may or may not have some anatomic abnormality [60]. The causes of AS are limited, and AS is a chronic process. In contrast, the causes of aortic regurgitation (AR) are multiple, and AR occurs acutely or chronically [60].

Aortic stenosis (AS)

AS is the most common cause of valvular heart disease in industrialized countries [59,61–64]. AS is the most frequent indication for valve replacement surgery as there are no proven specific or effective disease-modifying medical therapies [62,64].

More than 95% of stenotic aortic valves are congenitally-malformed (unicuspid, bicuspid), "degenerative" (calcific aortic stenosis of the elderly) or post-inflammatory ("rheumatic") disease (Table 16.11 and Fig. 16.11). Rare causes of AS include infectious endocarditis, collagen vascular disease, and rarely inborn errors of metabolism such as ochronosis [60].

"Degenerative" AS, AS of the elderly, is seen in more than one-fourth of individuals over 65 years and half over 85 years [64]. The prevalence of AS increases with age. The risk factors are hypertension, diabetes, elevated plasma levels of low-density lipoprotein (LDL), and smoking [62–65]. Aortic valve calcification may be associated with calcification at other sites in the vascular system, such as coronary arteries, carotid arteries, thoracic aorta, abdominal aorta, and iliac arteries [65].

In calcific AS of the elderly, there is usually no fusion of commissures [60]. In contrast, the characteristic feature of the post-inflammatory AV is commissural fusion. Aortic cusps also show diffuse severe fibrosis [60]. Affected patients often have post-inflammatory valvular disease on the other valves, particularly the mitral valve.

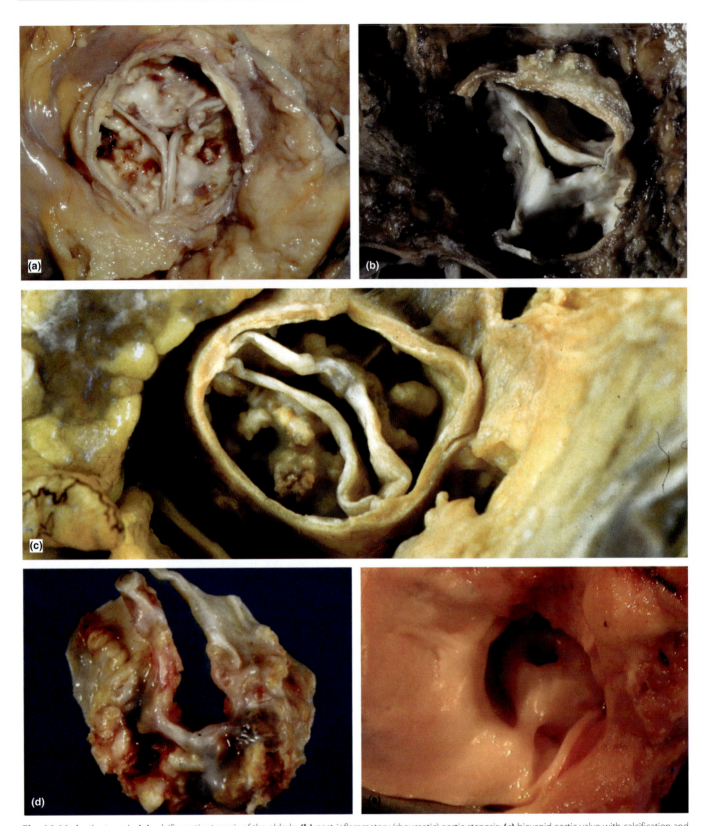

Fig. 16.11 Aortic stenosis: **(a)** calcific aortic stenosis of the elderly; **(b)** post-inflammatory (rheumatic) aortic stenosis; **(c)** bicuspid aortic valve with calcification and fibrosis; **(d)** unicommissural (exclamation point) valve; and **(e)** pyramid- or dome-shaped valve with no commissures.

Table 16.12. Bicuspid aortic valve

Frequently associated diseases of the bicuspid aortic valve (BAV)
Disease of aorta and aortic valve
aortic stenosis (fourth and fifth decades of life)
aortic regurgitation
infective endocarditis
ascending aorta dilation (20% of BAV)
ascending aorta aneurysm
coarctation of the aorta
aortic dissection
Marfan syndrome
Turner syndrome

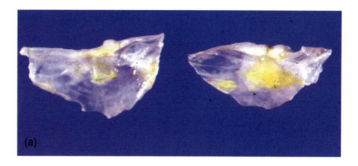

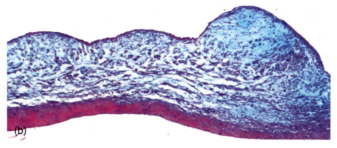

Fig. 16.12 Aortic regurgitation: **(a)** note thin transparent transilluminated leaflets in valve from patient with myxoid degeneration of aortic valve; and **(b)** histologic section showing widely expanded spongiosa layer (Alcian blue/PAS stain 40x).

Microscopically, the calcified degenerative and post-inflammatory AVs are likely to be indistinguishable from each other, with nodular calcification and fibrosis [54,55].

Bicuspid aortic valve (BAV)

BAV is the most common congenital abnormality of the heart [66,67]. The prevalence of BAV is 0.5–1.4% of the general population [66,67]. BAV may be associated with aortic stenosis, aortic regurgitation, valve dysfunction and/or infective endocarditis (IE) [67,68]. In BAV, AS occurs in the fourth and fifth decades of life, in contrast AS with tricuspid aortic valve is seen in the sixth, seventh, and eighth decades [69].

The patients with BAV may have other cardiovascular lesions: ascending aorta dilation, ascending aorta aneurysm, and coarctation of the aorta (Table 16.12). [70] Twenty percent of BAV is associated with a dilated ascending aorta [66,67,70]. Familial BAV has been reported. Underlying genetic influences have been identified with BAV [70]. Patients with BAV have increased risk for aortic aneurysm and aortic dissection even in the absence of hypertension [66,67,70]. One study showed 9 to 28% of aortic dissection in patients under 40 years old were associated with BAV [66]. The risk of the aortic dissection in people with BAV is 5–10 times higher than in individuals with trileaflet aortic valves [66,67]. Up to 30% of the patients with Turner syndrome have BAV [67].

There are variations in the orientation of the cusps with BAV. They may be right-left or anterior-posterior [60]. "Fusion" of right and left coronary cusps accounts for approximately 75% of BAV [67]. Fusion of the right and non-coronary cusps is less common, but has a higher prevalence of AS and AR, more progressive valve dysfunction, and aortic root dilation [67,70].

A false commissure, or raphe, is recognized in about 50% of BAV [60]. A right-left BAV has a raphe in the right cusp. In anterior to posterior BAV, the raphe is in the anterior cusp [60]. Histology is useful only to exclude endocarditis.

Distinguishing an acquired bicuspid valve from a congenital bicuspid valve is sometimes difficult [54]. A careful gross examination is most useful, since the microscopic appearance will be indistinguishable. An acquired bicuspid valve is usually due to distortion from post-inflammatory valvular disease. One of the apparent valve leaflets will appear twice the size of the other. Fusion of the commissures may be apparent in acquired BAV [54]. The raphe is a fibrous/calcified bar of tissue that extends from the base of the cusps to the aortic wall. The free margin of the valve cusps are not involved [54]. The aorta with BAV may show abnormalities of the aortic media, so-called "cystic medial degeneration" [67].

Unicuspid aortic valve

Unicuspid AV is rare, and seen in 0.075% of the general population, more often in males. There are two types of unicuspid aortic valve. One is an acommissural valve, the other is a unicommissural valve [60]. Unicuspid AVs are inherently stenotic at birth, and account for about 3% of excised stenotic AV [60].

An acommissural valve does not have any commissure or lateral attachments. The valve shows a volcano-like, pyramid structure. A unicommissural AV has an "exclamation point"-shaped orifice and one lateral attachment [60].

Aortic regurgitation (AR)

AR is less common than AS, but there are many more causes. AR results from either abnormalities of the aortic leaflets and/or dilation of the aortic root (Fig. 16.12). The causes of AR include congenitally abnormal valves such as bicuspid AV (13–28%), rheumatic valve disease (6–26%), IE (10–37%), aortic root-related causes (8–26%), trauma, prolapse secondary to ventricular septal defect, or myxoid degeneration (Table 16.13) [59,69,71–73]. Post-inflammatory (rheumatic) AR is generally associated with disease of the MV [73]. Myxoid

Table 16.13. Aortic regurgitation

Isolated aortic regurgitation (AR): 73%		
Disease of the valve cusps	Infective endocarditis	10–37%
	Post-inflammatory valve disease	6–38%
	Bicuspid	10–28%
	Floppy valve (prolapse)	2–3%
	Myxoid degeneration	36%
Disease of the aorta	Marfan syndrome; Aortic dissection; Ankylosing spondylitis; Collagen vascular disease	4–7%
	Aortitis	0.3–6%
Multivalvular disease with AR: 27%		
Post-inflammatory valve disease		71%
Infective endocarditis		23%

Table 16.14. Mitral stenosis

Isolated pure mitral stenosis (MS): 66%	
Post-inflammatory valve disease	100%
Rare causes Mitral annular calcification Fabry's disease Hurler-Scheie syndrome Whipple's disease	
Multivalvular disease with MS: 34%	
Post-inflammatory valve disease	100%

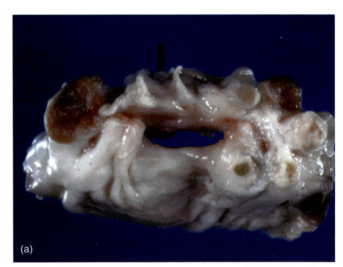

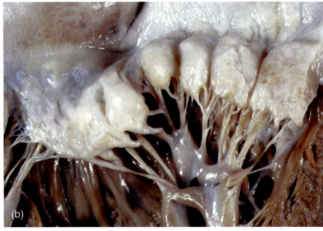

Fig. 16.13 Mitral stenosis/regurgitation: **(a)** this valve, characteristic of post-inflammatory (rheumatic) disease, shows fibrous thickening, fusion, and shortening of chordae with a fixed orifice resulting in stenosis and regurgitation; and **(b)** this valve with myxomatous degeneration caused pure mitral regurgitation.

degeneration affects any cardiac valve, with the most important being the MV. Myxoid degeneration of the AV is less common, but may result in significant AR [74]. Aortic root dilation may be secondary to Marfan syndrome, aortic dissection, collagen vascular disease, aortitis, or may be associated with hypertension and aging [69,73,75].

Post-inflammatory AR shows commissural fusion, fibrosis, and calcific deposits [73]. The aortic valve excised for AR may be grossly normal if the pathologic process is due to the disease of the aortic root [54].

Mitral valve disease

Mitral valve disease includes mitral valve regurgitation (MR), mitral stenosis (MS), mitral annular calcification (MAC), and mitral valve prolapse (MVP) (Fig. 16.13). Mitral valve disease affects 1–2% of the adult population, resulting in nearly 3,000 deaths in the United States [53].

Mitral stenosis (MS)

MS is almost always a post-inflammatory (rheumatic) disease [53,69]. MAC may rarely cause MS (Table 16.14). Other rare causes of MS include Fabry's disease, Hurler–Scheie syndrome, and Whipple's disease [72].

In developed countries, as the incidence of acute rheumatic fever is decreasing, the frequency of excised stenotic mitral valves has also decreased [75]. However, rheumatic fever and

rheumatic (post-inflammatory) heart disease are still highly prevalent in developing countries. Rheumatic fever is still the major cause of cardiovascular morbidity and mortality in young people [76]. Up to 30 million children and young adults have chronic rheumatic heart disease worldwide and there are approximately 250,000 deaths per year worldwide [77].

Stenotic mitral valves are always anatomically abnormal [75]. MS due to post-inflammatory valvular disease demonstrates diffuse fibrous thickening of leaflets and commissural fusion [72,75]. There is narrowing of the valve orifice, which often has the shape of the "fish mouth orifice" that is stenotic and regurgitant [77]. Chordae tendineae display chordal fusion and shortening [72,77].

Usually post-inflammatory MS is seen in the chronic phase. Microscopically, the normal leaflet layers are distorted. Leaflets are composed of dense collagen, elastic tissue, and calcific deposits [72]. In the acute phase, fibrinoid necrosis is seen. Aschoff Nodules may be found in the myocardial interstitium. Aschoff Nodules are rare within valvular tissue [72].

Mitral regurgitation (MR)

MR is the second most frequent valve disease after AS [59]. MR affects more than two million people in the US and nearly 10% of the population aged 75 years and older [78,79]. MR has many causes. The most common cause of MR is myxomatous degeneration of the mitral valve, including the mitral valve prolapse syndrome (MVP), accounting for about 70% of cases [69,75,79]. The prevalence of MVP increases with aging; most patients with MVP are over 50 years old [53,80,81].

The European Society of Cardiology has issued guidelines that classify MR as primary (organic) and secondary (functional) [82]. Primary MR is due to structural abnormalities of the mitral valve itself [75]. The causes of primary MR include myxomatous degeneration, rheumatic fever, active or healed IE, or collagen vascular disease (Table 16.15) [69,78]. Functional MR is caused by geometric distortion and enlargement of the left ventricle, such as with end-stage ischemic heart disease or DCM [54,79]. The mitral annulus may be dilated. Abnormalities of the orientation and function of the papillary muscles may be seen [82].

The myxomatous mitral valve is characterized by elongation or rupture of the chordae tendineae, with subsequent leaflet prolapse and increased leaflet thickness due to increased basophilic extracellular matrix [53,79–81,83]. However, ruptured mitral chordae tendineae are seen not only in myxomatous degeneration, but also in post-inflammatory disease and IE. Ruptured chordae may show a "corkscrew" or "pigtail" configuration [54].

Papillary muscle dysfunction is mainly seen secondary to atherosclerotic coronary disease. If the specimen includes the papillary muscles, old or, less commonly, recent infarction may be present [54].

Mitral valve prolapse (MVP)

MVP, also called primary myxomatous degeneration or floppy valve disease, is excursion of one or both leaflets above the plane of the annulus during systole [79,84]. MVP is a common cardiac valvular abnormality in industrialized countries [83], seen

Table 16.15. Mitral regurgitation

Isolated mitral regurgitation (MR): 73%	
Mitral valve prolapse (floppy valve)	38–70%
Papillary muscle dysfunction	11–30%
(secondary to ischemic heart disease etc.)	
Post-inflammatory valve disease	1–22%
Acute/healed infective endocarditis	2–6%
Spontaneous rupture of the chordae tendineae	
Functional MR (left ventricular dilation or genetic distortion of the valve)	
Rare causes Mitral annular calcification Marfan syndrome (dilation of annular circumference); trauma	
Multivalvular disease with MR: 27%	
Infective endocarditis	79%
Mitral valve prolapse (floppy valve)	13.50%
Post-inflammatory disease	13.50%

in 6–17% of adults [53,80]. The mean age of patients is 56–59 years old. The cause and progression of MVP is unclear. Surgical repair or valve replacement are the major treatment options. Less invasive, catheter-based procedures aimed to constrict the valve annulus or connect the valve leaflets using clips or sutures, are being developed.

MVP is characterized by floppy thickened leaflets with elongated or ruptured chordae tendineae [53,80,81]. Myxomatous degeneration is present. Microscopic findings are collagen disorganization, elastic fiber fragmentation, abundant proteoglycans, and increased spongiosa layer thickness [53,81].

Mitral annular calcification (MAC)

Severe MAC with encroachment into the orifice is an uncommon cause of functional MS and is uncommonly observed in surgical pathology specimens. MAC is rarely found under the age of 40 years; the incidence increases with age. Young adults may demonstrate MAC in the case of a concomitant connective tissue disorder, such as Marfan syndrome, or disorders of calcium metabolism [65]. The prevalence of MAC is 8.5% among people over 50 years old [85]. It is considerably more common in women over the age of 65 years. In addition, heavy calcification is seen more frequently in women [58,85,86]. Rarely MAC extends into the conduction system causing atrioventricular block [86,87].

Microscopic findings will be non-specific. About half of the cases show non-specific chronic inflammatory changes adjacent to calcific deposits. Foreign body giant cells are seen in

Table 16.16. Tricuspid stenosis

Tricuspid stenosis (TS)	
Post-inflammatory valve disease	90%
Rare causes	
Carcinoid heart disease	
Congenital heart disease	
Ebstein's anomaly	
Complex congenital heart disease	
Shortened chordae and/or fused commissure	
Infective endocarditis	
Fabry's disease	
Whipple's disease	
Giant blood cyst	

Table 16.17. Tricuspid regurgitation

Isolated tricuspid regurgitation (TR)
Anatomically abnormal valves
Ebstein's anomaly
Infective endocarditis
Floppy valve
Carcinoid disease
Papillary muscle dysfunction
Marfan syndrome
Functional TR
Multivalvular disease with TR
Post-inflammatory valvular disease
Floppy valve

Table 16.18. Pulmonary stenosis

Pulmonary stenosis (PS)	
Congenital disease	95%
Isolated congenital pulmonary valve	
Acommissural, dome-shaped	
Dysplastic	
Bicuspid	
Associated with other congenital heart disease	
Bicuspid	
Three-cuspid	
Acommissural, dome-shaped	
Acquired PS	
Carcinoid disease	
Post-inflammatory valve disease	
Infective endocarditis	

about 6% of cases [85]. There is usually no evidence of previous endocarditis.

Tricuspid valve diseases

Excision of the tricuspid valve (TV) is rare, making up approximately 1% of operatively excised native cardiac valves [88]. The TV is usually removed for IE, congenital malformations, or carcinoid heart disease [54]. Cultures should be performed for cases with visible or suspected infection [54].

Tricuspid stenosis (TS)

More than 90% of TS is due to post-inflammatory disease. Post-inflammatory TS is almost always associated with disease of other valves [59,89]. Rare causes of TS include carcinoid heart disease, congenital malformations, IE, metabolic or enzymatic abnormalities (Fabry's disease, Whipple's disease), and giant blood cyst (Table 16.16) [89]. Congenital malformations causing

TS are most commonly seen in infants. Ebstein's anomaly may cause TS, but is usually associated with tricuspid regurgitation (TR). Post-inflammatory TS shows diffuse fibrous thickening of the leaflets, fused commissures, and thickened chordae tendineae [89].

Tricuspid regurgitation (TR)

TR occurs in post-inflammatory valvular disease, IE, Ebstein's anomaly, valve prolapse, congenital anomaly, carcinoid heart disease, papillary muscle dysfunction, and Marfan syndrome [88]. Functional TR is due to annular dilation (Table 16.17) [54,89]. Underlying causes are pulmonary hypertension (cor pulmonale) and pulmonary stenosis [59,89]. TR is due to post-inflammatory disease in approximately 40% of cases [88].

Post-inflammatory TR displays diffuse fibrous thickening, fused commissures, and mildly thickened, fused chordae tendineae. Findings in TR due to myxomatous degeneration include marked dilation of the annulus, increased leaflet area, and chordal rupture – microscopic findings are similar to those observed in MVP [88].

Pulmonary valve disease
Pulmonary stenosis

Approximately 95% of excised stenotic pulmonary valves (PVs) are in association with congenital malformations, such as Teratology of Fallot, double outlet right ventricle, and univentricular atrioventricular connection (Table 16.18) [91]. Isolated congenital PV stenosis can be classified into two types, dome-shaped acommissural and dysplastic. The acommissural PV appears dome-shaped with central aperture and severe fibrous thickening of the valve cusps. Dysplastic congenital PVs will have three identifiable cusps, but the cusps are generally distorted by nodular, mucoid-appearing tissue. The valve annulus is usually small in dysplastic PV [91]. Acquired pulmonary stenosis is rare; a notable cause is carcinoid heart disease (discussed separately). Post-inflammatory PS shows commissural fusion and diffuse fibrous thickening of cusps; it is

Table 16.19. Pulmonary regurgitation

Pulmonary regurgitation (PR)
Anatomically abnormal valve cusps
Congenital malformation
Post-inflammatory valve disease
Carcinoid disease
Trauma
Infective endocarditis
Anatomically normal valve
Elevated pulmonary artery systolic pressure
Marfan syndrome

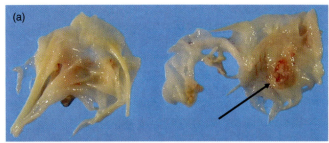

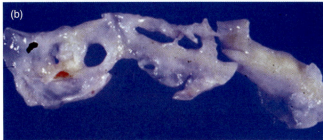

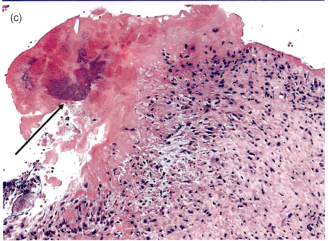

Fig. 16.14 Infective endocarditis: **(a)** active bacterial endocarditis with vegetation (arrow) and destruction of leaflet; **(b)** healed endocarditis resulting in numerous perforations of the valve leaflets; and **(c)** microscopic section showing vegetation with bacteria (arrow) and inflammation and destruction of the underlying leaflet.

invariably associated with post-inflammatory disease of other cardiac valves [91].

Pulmonary regurgitation

Pulmonary valve regurgitation may be associated with congenital malformations, post-inflammatory disease, carcinoid heart disease, trauma or IE [91]. If the regurgitation is caused by elevated pulmonary artery pressure, the valve leaflets may be anatomically normal [91] (Table 16.19).

Endocarditis

Infective endocarditis (IE) is a microbial infection of an endocardial surface [92,93]. The prevalence of IE at autopsy has been reported to be 1.3%, and has remained relatively constant throughout the years [94,95]. Up to one-third of patients with IE have pre-existing valvular disease such as bicuspid AV or MVP [94,96]. The predominant pathogen is *Staphylococcus aureus* [93–98]. Fungal endocarditis is less common, but results in larger vegetations and greater destruction of the tissue [96]. Prosthetic valve endocarditis is difficult to eradicate; often there are serious, sometimes lethal complications [99].

IE may be left-sided or right-sided. Left-sided IE is more common [95,96]. Right-sided IE is seen more often in intravenous drug users or patients with pulmonary artery catheterization [95,96,98]. IE is associated with vegetations and destruction of the architecture of valves (Fig. 16.14). The infection may involve surrounding cardiac structures. Acute endocarditis may cause perforations of the leaflets and rupture of chordal tendineae [75]. In the chronic phase, fibrous thickening of valves, leaflet perforations, and/or ruptured chordae tendineae may be seen [73]. Vegetations harboring bacterial colonies or fungal hyphae may be present [99]. Micro-organisms are frequently detectable in both treated and untreated endocarditis. Gram stain, for bacteria, and PAS or GMS stain, for fungi, are recommended [96].

Non-bacterial thrombotic endocarditis (NBTE), also called "marantic" endocarditis, is a sterile, thrombotic vegetation of heart valves. NBTE is usually first diagnosed at autopsy [100]. The mitral and aortic valves are most commonly involved [101]. NBTE is mostly found in patients with some underlying disease, such as metastatic malignancy, especially adenocarcinomas, disseminated intravascular coagulation (DIC), antiphospholipid syndrome (APS) or disorders characterized by hypercoagulability [100–102].

NBTE occurs on the inflow valvular surfaces (atrial surfaces of the mitral and tricuspid valves, ventricular surfaces of the aortic and pulmonic valves) [101]. NBTE is superficial with no destruction of underlying valve tissue or inflammatory reaction [101,102]. The vegetations in NBTE are fragile and easily removed from valves (Fig. 16.15). Histologically, NBTE is composed of deposits of fibrin and platelets seen along the lines of closure of the affected valves [101,102].

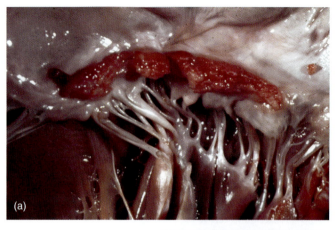

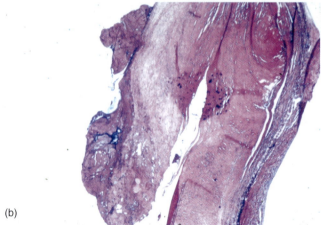

Fig. 16.15 Non-bacterial thrombotic endocarditis: **(a)** gross appearance of thrombi on the line of mitral valve closure with no destruction of the leaflet; and **(b)** histologic section with bland thrombus (T) (Alcian blue/PAS stain 20x).

Carcinoid heart disease

Carcinoid tumors are neuroendocrine malignancies most commonly seen in the gastrointestinal tract; the appendix and the terminal ileum are predominant sites [103]. Carcinoid tumors may secrete large amounts of vasoactive substances, including serotonin, that are usually inactivated in the liver and lung [104]. If released into portal circulation, for example, these substances are metabolized by the liver and do not enter systemic circulation. Carcinoid heart disease occurs when neuroendocrine tumors metastasize to the liver or other organs, releasing vasoactive hormones into systemic venous and/or arterial circulation [104]. Clinical manifestation of carcinoid syndrome includes flushing, diarrhea, and bronchospasm [103]. Usually only the right-sided valves are affected. However, the left side may be involved in the presence of a right-to-left shunt or when there is distant metastasis to the lungs or heart [104]. Carcinoid heart disease typically results in TV regurgitation and, less commonly, stenosis. A combination of stenosis and regurgitation is seen in the PV [105].

Carcinoid fibrous plaques are seen on the surface of the valvular cusps and/or the endocardial surface of the cardiac

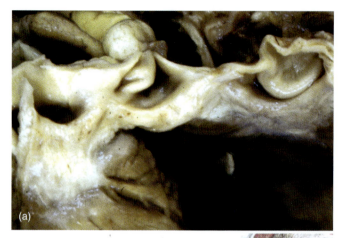

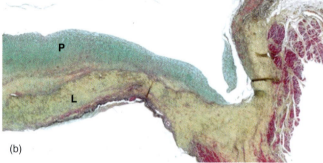

Fig. 16.16 Pulmonic valve with carcinoid valvular disease: **(a)** gross appearance of carcinoid valvular disease with thickening of leaflets and fusion of commissures; and **(b)** microscopic section showing "plaque" (P) of collagen on surface of valve leaflet (L) (Movat pentachrome stain 40x).

chambers [103,104]. Microscopically the valve is usually intact and covered by the "carcinoid plaque" (Fig. 16.16) [103,104]. Carcinoid plaques are composed of a proliferation of myofibroblasts with collagen deposition, smooth muscle cells, myxoid matrix, neovascularization and inflammation [103–105]. Valve leaflets are thickened, rigid, and reduced in area [89]. The chordae tendineae are thickened, shortened, and white [89].

The explanted heart

A relatively new surgical pathology specimen, only at centers that perform heart transplantation, is the explanted heart. The surgically-removed heart differs from the heart at autopsy. Some portions, if not most, of both atria are missing, as they are left in the patient to be connected to the donor heart. Since these patients are "end-stage" before transplantation, the heart may show sequelae of previous surgery and come with various forms of hardware and/or grafts, such as pacemakers, artificial valves, defibrillators, arterial and venous bypass grafts, stents, and/or ventricular assist devices. Although more complicated than the usual autopsy heart, the approach is much the same.

The most common entities encountered will be atherosclerotic coronary artery disease, cardiomyopathies, congenital malformations, and status post palliative repairs. Discussions of these entities are found in other sections of this chapter.

Below is a methodology for examination of the explanted heart in patients who have undergone heart transplantation. Hearts may be examined and dissected in the fresh state or after overnight fixation. Initial evaluation of the fresh heart is indicated if cultures or molecular/genetic studies are to be performed, or if a gross staining method, such as triphenyltetrazolium chloride staining (TTC) is to be used to demonstrate necrosis of myocardium [106]. If atria are closed, opening them and perhaps cutting one transverse slice off of the ventricles at the apex will facilitate penetration of fixative. Containers should be large enough to accommodate adequate fixative and to prevent distortion of the heart during fixation. Stuffing the chambers with paper towels will help to maintain the shape of the heart during fixation.

The epicardial surface should be examined for regions of fibrosis or fibrinous exudate. A mention should be made of the amount of epicardial fat present. The relationship of the great vessels should be determined (normally aorta is posterior and to the right). Normal atrial situs should be confirmed (right appendage wedge-shaped, left appendage finger-shaped). The course and texture of the coronary arteries should be determined. If the coronary arteries are calcified, they can be dissected off the heart at this point and placed in fixative/decalcification solution overnight prior to cutting at 2–3 mm intervals. If stents are present in the coronary arteries one should attempt to determine gross patency. There are methods for dissolving stents in situ to allow routine processing [107], or coronaries can be sent to reference laboratories that will cut thick sections of the arteries with stents in place [108]. The superior and inferior venae cavae are opened to view the interior of the right atrium and the atrial surface of the tricuspid valve. The pulmonary veins are connected with cuts to reveal the inside of the left atrium and the atrial surface of the mitral valve. This allows viewing of the atrioventricular valves with minimal dissection, so if there are vegetations present meaningful cultures may be obtained. The heart should have already been separated from the great vessels, leaving about 1 cm of aorta and pulmonary artery attached. At this time, all four cardiac valves should have been viewed. If there is a severe stenotic valvular lesion, the usual dissection may be modified to leave the involved valve intact.

The heart is then breadloafed from apex to the mid ventricular level at approximately 1.5 to 2 cm intervals to give a good view of the myocardium at different sites and at different levels. If lesions are observed, they can be described as to their location and extent, so terms such as anterior, lateral, posterior and septal, and subendocardial and transmural, should be applied. Lesions may show coagulation necrosis, fibrosis, and/or hemorrhage in the myocardium. There are gross techniques for detecting acute myocardial necrosis, such as TTC technique [106]. If such techniques are available, cross sections of the ventricles may be incubated in TTC to facilitate demonstration of early myocardial necrosis. Very early necrosis may not be visible to the naked eye; however, the affected myocardium may be soft compared to adjacent myocardium due to tissue edema.

At this point, the heart can be opened according to blood flow. Some pathologists prefer to make the initial cuts posteriorly adjacent to the septum. I prefer lateral cuts at the obtuse and acute margins of the heart, as the heart tends to be easier to view after such cuts. Accordingly, using a pointed knife or large scissors, the right atrium and right ventricle are cut laterally down to the apex. The next cut is anterior, as close to the interventricular septum as possible. At this point, any findings in the right atrium, tricuspid valve, or right ventricle may be described.

Moving to the left side of the heart, a similar lateral cut is made through the left atrium and mitral valve to the lateral portion of the ventricle. This allows a nice view of the mitral valve with its usual fan-shaped anterior leaflet. The posterior leaflet will have been cut through by this initial lateral cut. If the tricuspid or mitral valves have been replaced or have annular rings, the lateral cuts cannot be performed. In this event, more transverse slices should be made than usual, extending closer to the atrioventricular valve level, so the outflow surfaces of the valves may be examined. The final cut is anterior, and again, as close to the septum as possible. A common error is to cut through the mitral valve in attempting to open the aorta. Care should be taken to keep the knife or scissors to the medial side of the mitral valve, again as close to the septum as possible, parallel to the anterior descending coronary artery. Sometimes the last cut should be curved towards the right side of the heart to more easily expose the aortic valve.

Following fixation and decalcification, the coronary arteries should be cut at 2–3 mm intervals to attempt to detect and semi-quantitate the degree of luminal narrowing, whether there are any lesions, and whether these lesions consist of plaque, thrombosis, or both. If obvious plaque hemorrhage or plaque rupture is present, this is an important finding that should be mentioned. Of note, there are marked dimensional changes between life and death, particularly due to lack of pressure in the postmortem coronary arteries. Accordingly a common error among pathologists is to over-estimate the amount of narrowing due to the lack of distention of coronary arteries in the postmortem state. Of note, typically more than 75–80% of cross-sectional luminal narrowing is necessary to cause any hemodynamic compromise to blood flow in the coronary arteries in the resting state. Ventricular wall thickness should be measured. This measurement can be done most consistently approximately 1 cm below the pulmonic valve and on the posterolateral wall of the left ventricle, approximately 1 cm below the mitral valve. Typically trabeculae carneae muscles are not included in this measurement. The heart should be accurately weighed, only after any clot has been removed. Although other measurements such as ventricular dimensions or valve circumferences are less meaningful once the heart is no longer in the patient, these are typically done and recorded as part of the protocol.

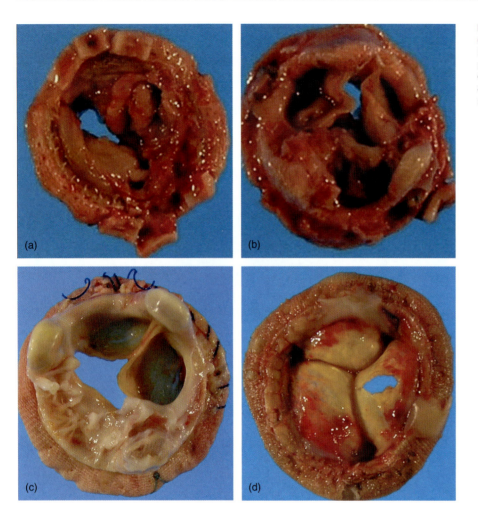

Fig. 16.17 Bioprosthetic valves: **(a and b)** inflow **(a)** and outflow **(b)** surfaces of porcine bioprosthetic valve with bacterial endocarditis; **(c)** porcine bioprosthetic valve with pannus formation on outflow surface causing bioprosthetic stenosis; and **(d)** porcine bioprosthetic valve with perforation of leaflet causing regurgitation.

Prostheses/devices

Substitute cardiac valves

Surgically implanted substitute cardiac valves have been in clinical use for over 50 years. These valves have been of various designs and composed of a variety of synthetic materials and mammalian tissues [109]. New valves and modifications to existing valves are continually being introduced into clinical practice. The general surgical pathologist cannot be expected to recognize all of the specific valves that have been in clinical use.

However, all valves have common components that can be described generically. All valves have a fixation ring, or some mechanism to attach to the heart. These usually consist of a metallic material covered by cloth. The internal and external diameter of the fixation ring should be recorded. In some newer designs for percutaneous implantation, there may be a metallic mesh with hooklets framing the leaflets. All valves have some type of occluder. There are some occluders composed entirely of tissue, consisting of valve leaflets and often

attached aortic wall. In the case of bioprosthetic tissue valves, this could be fixed cadaveric human tissue, bovine pericardium, or porcine aortic valve. In the past, synthetic occluders may have been a silicone or metallic ball, a single disc or a bileaflet disc. Some of the ball and disc occluders may have been made of silicone, but current valves use pyrolytic carbon, a hard, durable black material. The occluder should be described. All valves have to have some housing or support for the occluder. This could be some type of cage or hinge, or in the case of tissue valves, aortic wall with or without some vertical struts (Fig. 16.17). All substitute valves, like native valves, have an inflow or outflow surface that may be abnormal.

The major advantage of synthetic valves is that they are durable; however, patients usually require anticoagulation. The major advantage of tissue valves is that patients often do not require anticoagulation. However, tissue valves will degenerate with time. All substitute valves are susceptible to thrombosis and infection – so called "prosthetic endocarditis" (Figs. 16.17 and 16.18). All thrombi or vegetations should be sectioned to

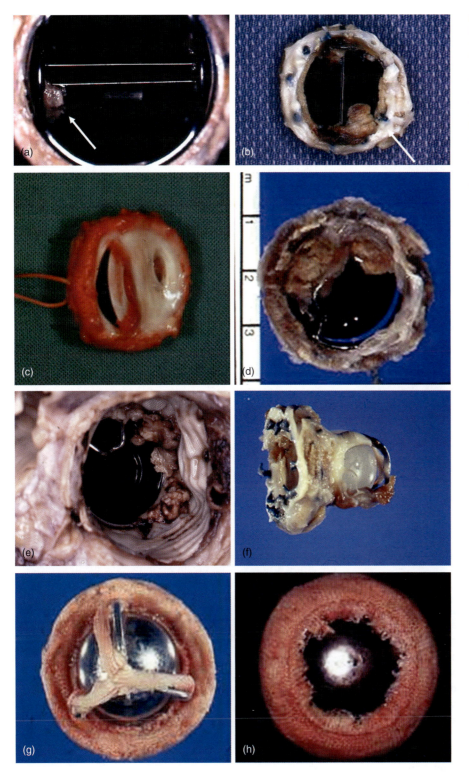

Fig. 16.18 Mechanical prosthetic valves: **(a and b)** St. Jude valves with recent thrombus (a – arrow), and organized thrombus (b – arrow) on hinge area, interfering with function of the prosthesis; **(c)** older version of Bjork-Shiley valve with silicone disc stuck in a partially open and closed position due to pannus formation; **(d and e)** more recent version of Bjork-Shiley valve with similar prosthetic valve dysfunction due to recent thrombus; **(f)** older Starr-Edwards valve with silicone poppet stuck in open position by pannus and thrombus; and **(g and h)** more recent Starr-Edwards valve with titanium poppet with cloth wear. Displaced cloth may interfere with function and even embolize to the brain and other organs.

attempt to identify acute inflammation and/or organisms. Tissue valves are susceptible to degeneration. Indeed, many tissue valves will have to be replaced usually 10 to 15 years after implantation. Tears, most often at commissural attachment sites, perforations, and calcifications occur and should be documented grossly and histologically. It is a good idea to photograph all explanted substitute valves.

Even grossly normal tissue valves will have microscopic abnormalities, such as host inflammatory cell infiltrates, mural thrombi, and degenerative changes of collagen.

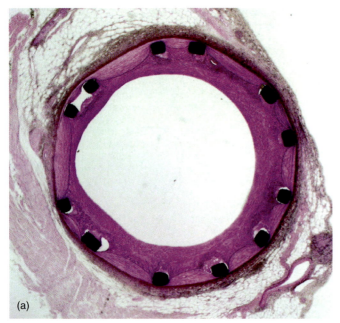

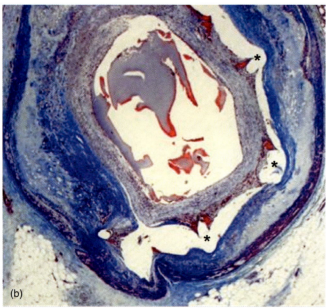

Fig. 16.19 Stents: **(a)** coronary artery with stent, processed and embedded in plastic and cut with stent in place showing neointima over stent struts (black) (methylene blue stain x12.5); and **(b)** stented section of coronary artery from which stent was removed prior to processing, showing site of stent struts (*) (trichrome stain 12.5x).

Ventricular assist devices

Ventricular assist devices, or VADs, have revolutionized the treatment of end-stage heart failure and have extended the lives of heart failure patients. VADs were originally intended to be a "bridge" to transplantation, but some have been implanted for years, and serve as "destination therapy" for patients who are not heart transplant candidates. These devices may be partially or completely implanted in the body. They may be used to support the right or left ventricle. They all have common parts. They all have some type of pump of various designs that may have been inside or outside of the body. There must be a power supply to the pump, and there must be conduits that attach somewhere at the great vessels, or in the heart, to remove blood returning to the heart and then to return blood from the pump back to the arterial system. There may or may not be an artificial valve within the conduits.

The surgical pathologist should describe the parts received and the model name, number, and serial number, present somewhere on the device. The general surgical pathologist cannot examine the internal parts of the pump where thrombi may form. Infection can occur, usually where lines or conduits enter or leave the body. Attempts should be made to look for thrombi or vegetations in conduits or on valves, if present [110].

Other medical devices

In addition to artificial heart valves and VADs, there are a host of existing devices, and devices under development, for intracardiac use. The most common are pacemakers with leads implanted in one or more cardiac chambers. There are also implantable defibrillators, atrial and ventricular septal defect closure devices, atrial appendage occluders, and various stents for intracoronary use, or to keep defects open in certain patients with congenital defects. These devices have similar potential complications, the most common being thrombosis and infection. In the case of stents, "restenosis" due to thrombosis and/or neointimal formation also occurs (Fig. 16.19). Tissue submitted on leads of devices, or on the surfaces of devices, should be sampled to document thrombosis and to rule out infection. Evaluation of stents is covered in the section on the explanted heart.

References

1. Sakakibara S, Konno S, *et al.* Endomyocardial biopsy. *Japanese Heart Journal* 1962; 3: 537.

2. Caves PK, Stinson EB, Billingham ME, Rider AK, Shumway NE. Diagnosis of human cardiac allograft rejection by serial cardiac biopsy. *Journal of Thoracic and Cardiovascular Surgery* 1973; 66: 461.

3. Leone O, Veinot JP, Angelini A, Baandrup UT, Basso C, Berry G, *et al.* Consensus statement on endomyocardial biopsy from the Association for European Cardiovascular Pathology and the Society for Cardiovascular Pathology. *Cardiovascular Pathology: the official journal of the Society for Cardiovascular Pathology* 2012; 21: 245–74.

4. Aretz H, Billingham M, Edwards W, Factor S, Fallon J, Fenoglio JJ, *et al.* Myocarditis. A histopathologic definition and classification. *Am J Cardiovasc Path* 1987; 1: 3–14.

5. Sagar S, Liu PP, Cooper LT. Myocarditis. *Lancet* 2012; 379: 738–47.

6. McCarthy RE, Boehmer JP, Hruban RH, Hutchins GM, Kasper EK, Hare JM, *et al.* Long-Term outcome of fulminant myocarditis as compared with acute (nonfulminant) myocarditis. *New England Journal of Medicine* 2000; 342: 690–5.

7. Sanders GE, Giles TD. Cardiovascular complications of collagen-vascular diseases. *Curr Treat Options Cardiovasc Med* 2002; 4: 151–9.

8. Kane GC, Keogh KA. Involvement of the heart by small and medium vessel vasculitis. *Curr Opin Rheumatol* 2009; 21: 29–34.

9. Kawai C. From myocarditis to cardiomyopathy: mechanisms of inflammation and cell death: learning from the past for the future. *Circulation* 1999; 99: 1091–100.

10. Calabrese F, Thiene G. Myocarditis and inflammatory cardiomyopathy: microbiological and molecular biological aspects. *Cardiovasc Res* 2003; 60: 11–25.

11. Watkins H, Ashrafian H, Redwood C, Watkins H, Ashrafian H RC. Inherited cardiomyopathies. *N Engl J Med* 2011; 364: 1643–56.

12. Norton N, Li D, Hershberger RE. Next-generation sequencing to identify genetic causes of cardiomyopathies. *Curr Opin Cardiol* 2012; 27: 214–20.

13. Schoenfeld MH, Supple EW, Dec GW, Fallon JT, Palacios IF. Restrictive cardiomyopathy versus constrictive pericarditis: role of endomyocardial biopsy in avoiding unnecessary thoracotomy. *Circulation* 1987; 75: 1012–17.

14. Basso C, Corrado D, Marcus FI, Nava A, Thiene G. Arrhythmogenic right ventricular cardiomyopathy. *Lancet* 2009; 373: 1289–300.

15. Karaye KM, Henein MY. Peripartum cardiomyopathy: A review article. *International Journal of Cardiology* 2013; 164:33–8.

16. Ntusi NBA, Mayosi BM. Aetiology and risk factors of peripartum cardiomyopathy: a systematic review. *International Journal of Cardiology* 2009; 131: 168–79.

17. Felker GM, Jaeger CJ, Klodas E, Thiemann DR, Hare JM, Hruban RH, *et al.* Myocarditis and long-term survival in peripartum cardiomyopathy. *American Heart Journal* 2000; 140: 785–91.

18. Limongelli G, Tome-Esteban M, Dejthevaporn C, Rahman S, Hanna MG, Elliott PM. Prevalence and natural history of heart disease in adults with primary mitochondrial respiratory chain disease. *European Journal of Heart Failure* 2010; 12: 114–21.

19. Taylor SW, Fahy E, Zhang B, Glenn GM, Warnock DE, Wiley S, *et al.* Characterization of the human heart mitochondrial proteome. *Nature Biotechnology* 2003; 21: 281–6.

20. Löffler W, *et al.* Endocarditis parietalis fibroplastica mit Bluteosinophilie. *Schweiz Med Wochenschr* 1936; 65: 817–20.

21. Jaski BE, Goetzl EJ, Said JW, Fishbein MC. Endomyocardial disease and eosinophilia. Report of a case. *Circulation* 1978; 57: 824–7.

22. Bukhman G, Ziegler J, Parry E. Endomyocardial fibrosis: still a mystery after 60 years. *PLoS Neglected Tropical Diseases* 2008; 2: e97.

23. Chopra P, Narula J, Talwar KK, Kumar V, Bhatia ML. Histomorphologic characteristics of endomyocardial fibrosis: an endomyocardial biopsy study. *Human Pathology* 1990; 21: 613–16.

24. Uemura A, Morimoto S, Hiramitsu S, Kato Y, Ito T, Hishida H. Histologic diagnostic rate of cardiac sarcoidosis: evaluation of endomyocardial biopsies. *American Heart Journal* 1999; 138: 299–302.

25. Ardehali H, Howard DL, Hariri A, Qasim A, Hare JM, Baughman KL, *et al.* A positive endomyocardial biopsy result for sarcoid is associated with poor prognosis in patients with initially unexplained cardiomyopathy. *American Heart Journal* 2005; 150: 459–63.

26. Baro C, Butt CG. Hamazaki-Wesenberg bodies in sarcoidosis. *Lab Med Bull Pathol* 1969; 10: 281.

27. Uehlinger E. The sarcoid tissue reaction: The origin and significance of inclusion bodies. Differential diagnosis with particular delineation from tuberculosis. *Acta Medica Scandinavica* 1964; 176: 7–13.

28. Westermark P, Benson MD, Buxbaum JN, Cohen AS, Frangione B, Ikeda S-I, *et al.* Amyloid: toward terminology clarification. Report from the Nomenclature Committee of the International Society of Amyloidosis. *Amyloid: the international journal of experimental and clinical investigation: the official journal of the International Society of Amyloidosis* 2005; 12: 1–4.

29. Crotty TB, Li C-Y, Edwards WD, Suman VJ. Amyloidosis and endomyocardial biopsy: Correlation of extent and pattern of deposition with amyloid immunophenotype in 100 cases. *Cardiovascular Pathology* 1995; 4: 39–42.

30. Collins AB, Smith RN, Stone JR. Classification of amyloid deposits in diagnostic cardiac specimens by immunofluorescence. *Cardiovascular Pathology: the official journal of the Society for Cardiovascular Pathology* 2009; 18: 205–16.

31. Benson MD, Breall J, Cummings OW, Liepnieks JJ. Biochemical characterisation of amyloid by endomyocardial biopsy. *Amyloid: the international journal of experimental and clinical investigation: the official journal of the International Society of Amyloidosis* 2009; 16: 9–14.

32. Vrana JA, Gamez JD, Madden BJ, Theis JD, Bergen HR, Dogan A. Classification of amyloidosis by laser microdissection and mass spectrometry-based proteomic analysis in clinical biopsy specimens. *Blood* 2009; 114: 4957–9.

33. Kremastinos DT, Farmakis D, Aessopos A, Hahalis G, Hamodraka E, Tsiapras D, *et al.* Beta-thalassemia cardiomyopathy: history, present considerations, and future perspectives. *Circulation. Heart Failure* 2010; 3: 451–8.

34. Pietrangelo A. Hereditary hemochromatosis – A new look at an old disease. *New England Journal of Medicine* 2004; 350: 2383–97.

35. Lombardo T, Tamburino C, Bartoloni G, Morrone ML, Frontini V, Italia F, *et al.* Cardiac iron overload in thalassemic patients: an endomyocardial biopsy study. *Annals of Hematology* 1995; 71: 135–41.

36. Wood JC. Diagnosis and management of transfusion iron overload: The role of imaging. *Am J Hematol* 2007; 82: 1132–5.

37. Olson LJ, Edwards WD, McCall JT, Ilstrup DM, Gersh BJ. Cardiac iron

deposition in idiopathic hemochromatosis: Histologic and analytic assessment of 14 hearts from autopsy. *Journal of the American College of Cardiology* 1987; 10: 1239–43.

38. Roberts WC. Primary and secondary neoplasms of the heart. *The American Journal of Cardiology* 1997; 80: 671–82.

39. Bussani R, De-Giorgio F, Abbate A, Silvestri F. Cardiac metastases. *Journal of Clinical Pathology* 2007; 60: 27–34.

40. Basso C, Valente M, Poletti A, Casarotto D, Thiene G. Surgical pathology of primary cardiac and pericardial tumors. *European journal of cardio-thoracic surgery: official journal of the European Association for Cardio-thoracic Surgery* 1997; 12: 730–7; discussion 737–8.

41. Jha NK, Khouri M, Murphy DM, Salustri A, Khan JA, Saleh MA, *et al.* Papillary fibroelastoma of the aortic valve–a case report and literature review. *Journal of Cardiothoracic Surgery* 2010; 5: 84.

42. Burke A, Virmani R. Tumors of the Heart and Great Vessels. In: *Atlas of Tumor Pathology*, 3rd Series, fascicle 16. Washington, DC: Armed Forces Institute of Pathology 1996, p. 231.

43. Butany J, Ahn E, Luk A. Drug-related cardiac pathology. *Journal of Clinical Pathology* 2009; 62: 1074–84.

44. Monsuez J-J, Charniot J-C, Vignat N, Artigou J-Y. Cardiac side-effects of cancer chemotherapy. *International Journal of Cardiology* 2010; 144: 3–15.

45. Burke AP, Saenger J, Mullick F, Virmani R. Hypersensitivity myocarditis. *Arch Pathol Lab Med* 1991; 115: 764–9.

46. Pham MX, Teuteberg JJ, Kfoury AG, Starling RC, Deng MC, Cappola TP, *et al.* Gene-expression profiling for rejection surveillance after cardiac transplantation. *N Engl J Med* 2010; 362: 1890–900.

47. Kobashigawa J, Crespo-Leiro MG, Ensminger SM, Reichenspurner H, Angelini A, Berry G, *et al.* Report from a consensus conference on antibody-mediated rejection in heart transplantation. *J Heart Lung Transplant* 2011; 30: 252–69.

48. Billingham ME, Cary NR, Hammond ME, Kemnitz J, Marboe C, McCallister HA, *et al.* A working formulation for the standardization of nomenclature in the diagnosis of heart and lung

rejection: Heart Rejection Study Group. The International Society for Heart Transplantation. *J Heart Transplant* 1990; 9: 587–93.

49. Stewart S, Winters GL, Fishbein MC, Tazelaar HD, Kobashigawa J, Abrams J, *et al.* Revision of the 1990 working formulation for the standardization of nomenclature in the diagnosis of heart rejection. *J Heart Lung Transplant* 2005; 24: 1710–20.

50. Fishbein G, Fishbein M. Morphologic and immunohistochemical findings in antibody-mediated rejection of the cardiac allograft. *Hum Immunol* 2012; 73: 1213–17.

51. Lu W-H, Palatnik K, Fishbein GA, Lai C, Levi DS, Perens G, *et al.* Diverse morphologic manifestations of cardiac allograft vasculopathy: A pathologic study of 64 allograft hearts. *J Heart Lung Transplant* 2011; 30: 1044–50.

52. Mehra MR, Crespo-Leiro MG, Dipchand A, Ensminger SM, Hiemann NE, Kobashigawa JA, *et al.* International Society for Heart and Lung Transplantation working formulation of a standardized nomenclature for cardiac allograft vasculopathy-2010. *J Heart Lung Transplant* 2010; 29: 717–27.

53. Leong SW, Soor GS, Butany J, Henry J, Thangaroopan M, Leask RL. Morphological findings in 192 surgically excised native mitral valves. *The Canadian Journal of Cardiology* 2006; 22: 1055–61.

54. Stone JR, Basso C, Baandrup UT, Bruneval P, Butany J, Gallagher PJ, *et al.* Recommendations for processing cardiovascular surgical pathology specimens: a consensus statement from the Standards and Definitions Committee of the Society for Cardiovascular Pathology and the Association for European Cardiovascular Pathology. *Cardiovascular pathology: the official journal of the Society for Cardiovascular Pathology* 2012; 21: 2–16.

55. Roberts WC, Morrow AG. Cardiac valves and the surgical pathologist. *Archives of Pathology* 1966; 82: 309–13.

56. Sahasakul Y, Edwards WD, Naessens JM, Tajik a J. Age-related changes in aortic and mitral valve thickness: implications for two-dimensional echocardiography based on an autopsy study of 200 normal human hearts. *The*

American Journal of Cardiology 1988; 62: 424–30.

57. Chida K, Ohkawa S, Watanabe C, Shimada H, Sugiura M. A morphological study of the normally aging heart. *Cardiovascular Pathology* 1994; 3: 1–7.

58. Pomerance A. Ageing changes in human heart valves. *British Heart Journal* 1967; 29: 222–31.

59. Vahanian A, Baumgartner H, Bax J, Butchart E, Dion R, Filippatos G, *et al.* Guidelines on the management of valvular heart disease: The Task Force on the Management of Valvular Heart Disease of the European Society of Cardiology. *European Heart Journal* 2007; 28: 230–68.

60. Waller B, Howard J, Fess S. Pathology of aortic valve stenosis and pure aortic regurgitation a clinical morphologic assessment – part I. *Clinical Cardiology* 1994; 17: 85–92.

61. Iung B, Cachier A, Baron G, Messika-Zeitoun D, Delahaye F, Tornos P, *et al.* Decision-making in elderly patients with severe aortic stenosis: why are so many denied surgery? *European Heart Journal* 2005; 26: 2714–20.

62. Shah PK. Should severe aortic stenosis be operated on before symptom onset? Severe aortic stenosis should not be operated on before symptom onset. *Circulation* 2012; 126: 118–25.

63. Goldbarg SH, Elmariah S, Miller MA, Fuster V. Insights into degenerative aortic valve disease. *Journal of the American College of Cardiology* 2007; 50: 1205–13.

64. O'Brien KD. Epidemiology and Genetics of Calcific Aortic Valve Disease. *Journal of Investigative Medicine* 2007; 55: 284–91.

65. Allison MA, Cheung P, Criqui MH, Langer RD, Wright CM. Mitral and aortic annular calcification are highly associated with systemic calcified atherosclerosis. *Circulation* 2006; 113: 861–6.

66. Michelena HI, Khanna AD, Mahoney D, Margaryan E, Topilsky Y, Suri RM, *et al.* Incidence of aortic complications in patients with bicuspid aortic valves. *JAMA: Journal of the American Medical Association* 2011; 306: 1104–12.

67. Braverman AC. Aortic involvement in patients with a bicuspid aortic valve. *Heart (British Cardiac Society)* 2011; 97: 506–13.

68. Schoen FJ. Surgical pathology of removed natural and prosthetic heart valves. *Human Pathology* 1987; 18: 558–67.

69. Carabello BA, Crawford FA. Valvular heart disease. *New England Journal of Medicine* 1997; 337: 32–41.

70. Fernandes S, Khairy P, Graham DA, Colan SD, Galvin TC, Sanders SP, *et al.* Bicuspid aortic valve and associated aortic dilation in the young. *Heart (British Cardiac Society)* 2012; 98: 1014–19.

71. Allen WM, Matloff JM, Fishbein MC. Myxoid degeneration of the aortic valve and isolated severe aortic regurgitation. *American Journal of Cardiology* 1985; 55: 439–44.

72. Waller B, Howard J, Fess S. Pathology of mitral valve stenosis and pure mitral regurgitation–Part I. *Clinical Cardiology* 1994; 17: 330–6.

73. Waller B, Howard J, Fess S. Pathology of aortic valve stenosis and pure aortic regurgitation: A clinical morphologic assessment – Part II. *Clinical Cardiology* 1994; 17: 150–6.

74. Allen WM, Matloff JM, Fishbein MC. Myxoid degeneration of the aortic valve and isolated severe aortic regurgitation. *American Journal of Cardiology* 1985; 55: 439–44.

75. Adachi O, Saiki Y, Akasaka J, Oda K, Iguchi A, Tabayashi K. Surgical management of aortic regurgitation associated with takayasu arteritis and other forms of aortitis. *The Annals of Thoracic Surgery* 2007; 84: 1950–3.

76. Marijon E, Mirabel M, Celermajer DS, Jouven X. Rheumatic heart disease. *Lancet* 2012; 379: 953–64.

77. Chandrashekhar Y, Westaby S, Narula J. Mitral stenosis. *Lancet* 2009; 374: 1271–83.

78. Enriquez-Sarano M, Akins CW, Vahanian A. Mitral regurgitation. *Lancet* 2009; 373: 1382–94.

79. Ghoreishi M, Dawood M, Stauffer CE, Gammie JS. Mitral regurgitation: current trends in diagnosis and management. *Hospital Practice* 2011; 39: 181–92.

80. Tresch DD, Doyle TP, Boncheck LI, Siegel R, Keelan MH, Olinger GN, *et al.* Mitral valve prolapse requiring surgery. Clinical and pathologic study. *American Journal of Medicine* 1985; 78: 245–50.

81. Gupta V, Barzilla J, Mendez J. Abundance and location of proteoglycans and hyaluronan within normal and myxomatous mitral valves. *Cardiovascular Pathology* 2009; 18: 191–7.

82. Ciarka A, Van de Veire N. Secondary mitral regurgitation: pathophysiology, diagnosis, and treatment. *Heart (British Cardiac Society)* 2011; 97: 1012–23.

83. Freed LA, Benjamin EJ, Levy D, Larson MG, Evans JC, Fuller DL, *et al.* Mitral valve prolapse in the general population: the benign nature of echocardiographic features in the Framingham Heart Study. *Journal of the American College of Cardiology* 2002; 40: 1298–304.

84. Grau JB, Pirelli L, Yu P-J, Galloway AC, Ostrer H. The genetics of mitral valve prolapse. *Clinical Genetics* 2007; 72: 288–95.

85. Pomerance A. Pathological and clinical study of calcification of the mitral valve ring. *Journal of Clinical Pathology* 1970; 23: 354–61.

86. Fulkerson PK, Beaver BM, Auseon JC, Graber HL. Calcification of the mitral annulus: etiology, clinical associations, complications and therapy. *The American Journal of Medicine* 1979; 66: 967–77.

87. Ohkawa S. Histopathology of the conduction system (Japanese). *Journal of Arrhythmia* 2000; 16: 312–29.

88. Waller B, Howard J, Fess S. Pathology of tricuspid valve stenosis and pure tricuspid regurgitation – Part II. *Clinical Cardiology* 1995; 18: 167–74.

89. Waller B, Howard J, Fess S. Pathology of tricuspid valve stenosis and pure tricuspid regurgitation – Part I. *Clinical Cardiology* 1995; 102: 97–102.

90. Waller B, Howard J, Fess S. Pathology of tricuspid valve stenosis and pure tricuspid regurgitation–Part III. *Clinical Cardiology* 1995; 18: 225–30.

91. Waller B, Howard J, Fess S. Pathology of pulmonic valve stenosis and pure regurgitation. *Clinical Cardiology* 1995; 50: 45–50.

92. Horstkotte D, Follath F, Gutschik E, Lengyel M, Oto A, Pavie A, *et al.* Guidelines on prevention, diagnosis and treatment of infective endocarditis executive summary; the task force on infective endocarditis of the European society of cardiology. *European Heart Journal* 2004; 25: 267–76.

93. Wang A. The changing epidemiology of infective endocarditis: the paradox of prophylaxis in the current and future eras. *Journal of the American College of Cardiology* 2012; 59: 1977–8.

94. Rahimtoola SH. The year in valvular heart disease. *Journal of the American College of Cardiology* 2007; 49: 361–74.

95. Fernández Guerrero ML, Álvarez B, Manzarbeitia F, Renedo G. Infective endocarditis at autopsy: a review of pathologic manifestations and clinical correlates. *Medicine* 2012; 91: 152–64.

96. Atkinson JB, Virmani R. Infective endocarditis: Changing trends and general approach for examination. *Human Pathology* 1987; 18: 603–8.

97. Watkin R, Sandoe J. British Society of Antimicrobial Chemotherapy (BSAC) guidelines for the diagnosis and treatment of endocarditis: what the cardiologist needs to know. *Heart (British Cardiac Society)* 2012; 98: 757–9.

98. Hecht SR, Berger M. Right-sided endocarditis in intravenous drug users. Prognostic features in 102 episodes. *Annals of Internal Medicine* 1992; 117: 560–6.

99. Atkinson JB, Virmani R. Infective endocarditis: Changing trends and general approach for examination. *Human Pathology* 1987; 18: 603–8.

100. Rogers LR, Cho ES, Kempin S, Posner JB. Cerebral infarction from non-bacterial thrombotic endocarditis. Clinical and pathological study including the effects of anticoagulation. *The American Journal of Medicine* 1987; 83: 746–56.

101. Lopez JA, Ross RS, Fishbein MC, Siegel RJ. Nonbacterial thrombotic endocarditis: a review. *American Heart Journal* 1987; 113: 773–84.

102. Silbiger JJ. The valvulopathy of non-bacterial thrombotic endocarditis. *The Journal of Heart Valve Disease* 2009; 18: 159–66.

103. Bhattacharyya S, Davar J, Dreyfus G, Caplin ME. Carcinoid heart disease. *Circulation* 2007; 116: 2860–5.

104. Gustafsson BI, Hauso O, Drozdov I, Kidd M, Modlin IM. Carcinoid heart disease. *International Journal of Cardiology* 2008; 129: 318–24.

105. Bernheim AM, Connolly HM, Hobday TJ, Abel MD, Pellikka PA. Carcinoid

heart disease. *Progress in Cardiovascular Diseases* 2007; 49: 439–51.

106. Fishbein M, Meerbaum S, Rit J. Early phase acute myocardial infarct size quantification: validation of the triphenyl tetrazolium chloride tissue enzyme staining technique. *American Heart Journal* 1981; 101: 593–9.

107. Bradshaw SH, Kennedy L, Dexter DF, Veinot JP. A practical method to rapidly dissolve metallic stents. *Cardiovascular Pathology* 2009; 18: 127–33.

108. Rippstein P, Black M, Boivin M. Comparison of processing and sectioning methodologies for arteries containing metallic stents. *Journal of Histochemistry and Cytochemistry* 2006; 54: 673–81.

109. Schoen FJ. Cardiac valves and valvular pathology: Update on function, disease, repair, and replacement. *Cardiovascular Pathology* 2005; 14: 189–94.

110. Schoen FJ. Approach to the analysis of cardiac valve prostheses as surgical pathology or autopsy specimens. *Cardiovascular Pathology* 1995; 4: 241–55.

Chapter 17

Morphologic alterations of serous membranes of the mediastinum in reactive and neoplastic settings

Aliya N. Husain, MD, and Thomas Krausz, MD

Introduction

Histologic analysis of mesothelial lesions with the aim to arrive at a clinically meaningful diagnosis is a frequent task for the pathologist. This is not simply a picture-matching exercise, but, in order to avoid diagnostic pitfalls, requires not only application of reproducible morphologic criteria in the clinical context but also understanding of mesothelial cell biology. Mesothelial cells have the potential to exhibit a broad phenotypic spectrum both in reactive and neoplastic settings. Mesothelial cells have a rich morphologic repertoire in response to injury and can switch their phenotype from epithelioid to transitional to spindle, requiring pathologists to become familiar with their variable features in non-neoplastic conditions. Indeed, they present a morphologic continuum reflecting a variety of dynamic physiologic/pathophysiologic changes in the context of development, metabolism, repair, and epithelial-to-mesenchymal transition. This chapter will focus on the main histologic features and differential diagnosis of reactive and benign neoplastic mesothelial proliferations compared to those of malignant mesothelioma in the light of current understanding of key molecular alterations, which have an impact not only on phenotype but also on prognosis. Critical assessment of the usefulness of various immunohistochemical markers will be discussed in the context of the differential diagnosis of specific entities.

Although the diagnosis of mesothelioma occurring in the thoracic cavities is usually based on histologic examination of pleural and, less frequently, on pericardial biopsies, the following eventualities justify its discussion in the context of mediastinal surgical pathology:

1) Surgical pathology of neoplasms or other lesions occurring in the mediastinum requires knowledge of the boundaries of that area. The mediastinum is limited bilaterally by the mediastinal parietal pleura and extends from the diaphragm inferiorly to the level of the thoracic inlet superiorly. There is also a close association with the pericardium. It follows that primary diffuse pleural mesotheliomas often involve the mediastinal pleura (37%) and pericardial mesotheliomas often infiltrate the mediastinal structures. Detailed description of the anatomy of the three major compartments of the mediastinum is provided in Chapter 1.

2) Rarely localized malignant mesotheliomas may present as anterior, middle, or posterior mediastinal masses with appropriate clinical symptoms differing from those of conventional pleural mesothelioma (discussed below).

3) Malignant pleural mesothelioma may metastasize to mediastinal lymph nodes or may present with mediastinal lymphadenopathy [1,2]. However, pathologists need to be aware that the presence of mesothelial cells in mediastinal (and intra-abdominal) lymph nodes does not necessarily represent metastatic mesothelioma as benign mesothelial cells, or hyperplastic mesothelial aggregates in lymph nodes are well documented [3-8]. This should not be too surprising in view of better known other benign inclusions in lymph nodes (glandular inclusion, nevus cell nests, decidua). Benign mesothelial cells in lymph nodes usually occur in the setting of chronic effusion, serosal inflammation, or reaction to other conditions. They must be distinguished not only from metastatic mesothelioma but also from carcinoma and melanoma.

4) Epithelioid hemangioendothelioma (and to a lesser extent epithelioid angiosarcoma) of the pleura or of the mediastinum is not infrequently misdiagnosed as malignant epithelioid mesothelioma [9-14]. Even though the phenotype of the tumor cells may closely mimic epithelioid mesothelial cells, the myxohyaline matrix of the former together with the distinctive immunohistochemical profiles (be aware that D2–40 is positive in both and cytokeratin may be focally expressed by epithelioid vascular tumors) of each tumor type usually help to solve the differential diagnostic problem.

---

*Figures are hematoxylin and eosin (H&E) stain unless otherwise specified. IHC = immunohistochemical.

Pathology of the Mediastinum, ed. Alberto M. Marchevsky and Mark R. Wick. Published by Cambridge University Press.
© Cambridge University Press 2014.

5) Synovial sarcoma, one of the histologic mimics of malignant mesothelioma, may occur primarily in the mediastinum, pleura, or pericardium [15–19].

6) Thymoma, one of the most frequent primary mediastinal neoplasms, may not only show histologic overlap with malignant mesothelioma (type A with sarcomatoid and type B with epithelioid mesothelioma) but may also present as a primary pleural tumor with either localized or diffuse growth pattern (pseudomesotheliomatous growth pattern) [20,21].

Mesothelium: structure, function, repair

The mesothelium consists of a monolayer of specialized cells (mesothelial cells), which lines the entire surface of serous cavities (pleural, pericardial, and peritoneal) and covers the organs contained within these cavities. Embryologically, it develops from the mesodermal tissue around 14 days of gestation, with cells gradually differentiating from cuboidal cells to flattened mesothelial cells. In adults, the serous cavities are lined by two basic mesothelial cell types, flat and cuboidal, based on differences in size, shape, cell organelles, and membrane specialization [22]. Intermediate/transitional forms also exist. The flattened mesothelial cells have a large apical surface, approximately 20 μm in horizontal diameter and ill-defined intercellular boundaries. The cuboidal mesothelial cells have a relatively smaller surface area, approximately 8 μm in horizontal diameter. The mesothelial cells are characterized by long, frequently branching, microvilli on their free surfaces, which are best appreciated on ultrastructural study. The microvilli are more numerous on the surface of cuboidal cells than on the flattened mesothelial cells. The apical cell membrane of the cuboidal cells forms deep invaginations between neighboring cells, a feature corresponding to the intercellular

spaces (windows) often seen in cytology specimens between mesothelial cells. Polarized mesothelial cells have well developed cell-cell junctional complexes including tight junctions located towards their luminal aspect, adherens junctions, gap junctions, and desmosomes. The mesothelial cells also express E-, N-, and P-cadherins, but unlike true epithelia, N-cadherin predominates.

Mesothelial cells rest on a thin basement membrane, beneath which there are elastic fibers and a connective tissue stroma containing blood vessels, lymphatics, resident inflammatory cells, and fibroblast-like cells (Fig. 17.1a and b). The key functions of the mesothelial layer were traditionally thought to provide a non-adhesive, slippery surface to facilitate intracoelomic movement and to provide a protective barrier against physical damage and invading organisms. However, the mesothelium is now recognized as a dynamic cell membrane with a number of physiologic functions including fluid and solute transport, immune surveillance, fibrinolysis and the production of extracellular matrix molecules, proteases, cytokines and growth factors. The mesothelium is bathed in a small amount of serosal fluid that is similar to an ultrafiltrate of plasma and contains some blood proteins, resident inflammatory cells, sugars, various enzymes including amylase and lactate dehydrogenase, and is also rich in hyaluronic acid. The volume and composition of the serosal fluid corresponds to the pathologic states, such as infection, serositis (pleuritis, pericarditis, and peritonitis), trauma and neoplastic infiltrate. Published data suggest that the mesothelium lining each body cavity responds as a single unit to changes in serosal fluid composition.

The mesothelium is a slowly renewing tissue with <0.5% of cells undergoing mitosis at any one time in normal conditions. However, mitotic activity usually greatly increases following various injuries/stimulation. It has been demonstrated that 30–80% of mesothelial cells at the wound edge and on the

(a)

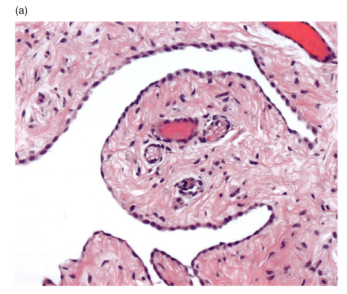

(b)

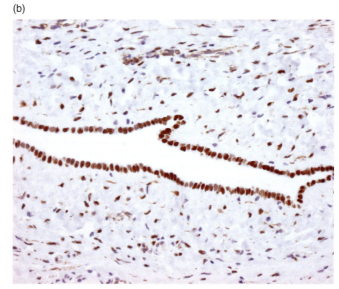

Fig. 17.1 (a) Normal serosa with a single layer of cuboidal to flat mesothelial cells and submesothelium with blood vessels and fibroblast-like cells (200x); **(b)** IHC stain for WT-1 shows nuclear positivity in normal mesothelial and submesothelial cells.

opposing surface begin DNA synthesis within 48 hours of injury. Loss of contact inhibition may be one trigger for this rapid increase in cell proliferation but soluble mediators released from inflammatory and injured cells may also play an important stimulatory role. The mechanism of regeneration is still not fully elucidated. The historical view was that dividing mesothelial cells spread over the injured area from the periphery but this view was challenged when it was found that the rate of healing was the same regardless of the size of the injured area. Mesothelial repair is strikingly different from other epithelial-like surfaces as re-growth appears diffusely across the injured surface whereas in true epithelia, healing occurs solely from the wound edges as sheets of cells. Various mechanisms of regeneration were proposed subsequently including the postulated existence of submesothelial cell layer, which would proliferate and differentiate in response to mesothelial injury. However, the suggestion that the newly formed mesothelium originates from multipotential precursor cells of the submesothelium has been challenged by some investigators [23,24]. Foley-Comer et al. [25] demonstrated that mesothelial cells distant from the wound and on opposing surfaces also proliferate, detach from the basement membrane into the serosal fluid, and settle on the wound surface. These attached cells subsequently proliferate and scatter to repopulate the injured area. The concept that repair of serosal tissue involves increased mesothelial proliferation at sites not only at the edge of the wound but also distant to it, suggests diffuse activation of the mesothelium in response to mediators or cells released into the serosal fluid or via cell to cell communication.

Under normal conditions in humans, the physiological pleural fluid is formed in apical parts of the parietal pleural capillaries according to Starling forces and is drained mostly by lymphatic stomata which seem to be exclusively found on the parietal side and are most numerous in the mediastinal and diaphragmatic areas. The parietal stomata possess valve-like structures that ensure unidirectional flow of fluid out of the pleural space and are probably also important in volume control of the pleural fluid. Currently there is no conclusive answer to the question whether an intact pleural space has any useful function. There is an intriguing fact of nature that elephants do not have a pleural space after birth because the normal pleural space, which is present in the fetal elephant, is obliterated by fibrous tissue in late gestation (a kind of "congenital pleurodesis"). It has been suggested that this peculiar anatomy developed because the animal can snorkel at depth, and this behavior subjects the microvessels in the parietal pleura to a very large transmural pressure. Also, similar distribution of the pressures occurs when the animal raises water inside its trunk prior to drinking. Accordingly, the fetal lung development and gradual pleural space obliteration reflects the adaptations required for snorkeling in adult life [26,27]. It is suggested that the elephant has an aquatic ancestry and the trunk may have developed for snorkeling. So the elephant does not need to worry about pleural effusion and pneumothorax and veterinary pathologists specializing in elephant pathology perhaps

do not need to know about pleural mesothelial cells and pleural mesotheliomas.

Both epithelial and mesenchymal characteristics of mesothelial cells

Mesothelial cells share characteristics of both epithelial and mesenchymal cells. Epithelial characteristics include polygonal shape, presence of cytokeratin intermediate filaments (cytokeratin 6, 8, 18, and 19), tight junctions, expression of cadherins, and the ability to secrete basement membrane [28]. They also exhibit mesenchymal characteristics such as presence of vimentin, desmin (Fig. 17.2) and upon stimulation, alpha smooth muscle actin. Accordingly, mesothelial cells have the ability to change their phenotype (from polygonal to spindle) comparable to changes seen during embryonic development in the form of epithelial-to-mesenchymal transition (EMT). This observation has implications for our understanding not only of repair but also of the morphologically diverse phenotypes (epithelioid, biphasic, sarcomatoid) of malignant mesothelioma [29,30]. Interestingly, after several passages in culture, mesothelial cells lose their epithelioid, polygonal phenotype and cytokeratin expression and adopt a spindled, fibroblast-like phenotype. Incubation of mesothelial cells with the wound repair and pro-fibrotic mediator transforming growth factor-ß1 (TGF-ß1) induced EMT in mesothelial cells and up-regulated smooth muscle actin and type I collagen expression, consistent with myofibroblastic differentiation [31]. The data indicate that the mesothelium is a likely source of fibrogenic cells during serosal inflammation/fibrosis and wound healing and may play an important role in the formation of serosal adhesions. Mesothelial cells also undergo EMT during continuous ambulatory peritoneal dialysis with the induction of the transcription factor Snail and a dramatic down-regulation of E-cadherins and cytokeratins [32]. During cardiogenesis,

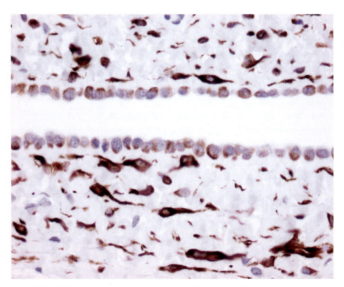

Fig. 17.2 IHC stain for desmin shows cytoplasmic positivity in mesothelial and submesothelial cells.

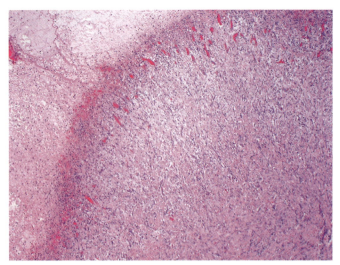

Fig. 17.3 Organizing fibrinous pleuritis shows characteristic zonation with fibrin at top left, granulation tissue underneath it, and fibrosis at bottom right.

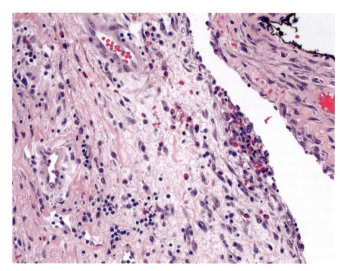

Fig. 17.4 Eosinophilic pleuritis in a 24-year-old with spontaneous pneumothorax.

the epicardium (mesothelium) undergoes epithelial-to-mesenchymal transformation, and migrates into the myocardium. These epicardium-derived cells differentiate into interstitial fibroblasts, coronary smooth muscle cells, and perivascular fibroblasts [33].

The epithelial-to-mesenchymal transition, initially recognized as an essential mechanism for embryonic development, is nowadays regarded as a key player in additional physiologic and pathologic processes such as wound healing and tumor progression, including metastasis. EMT is a complex genetic program, which implies the acquisition of migratory phenotype with the loss of cadherin-mediated cell-cell adhesion and apical-basal polarity. This causes the normal epithelial or mesothelial cells to dissociate from their neighbors and migrate. Several transcription factors have been described as key inducers of EMT, including members of the Snail superfamily (Snail1 and Snail2) [34], the basic helix-loop-helix family (bHLH), and the two zinc-finger E-box-binding homeobox factors (ZEB1 and ZEB2). There are a number of well-described signaling pathways that control the expression of Snail factors, but the regulation of the expression of bHLH and ZEB factors is less well known [35,36]. Non-coding RNAs (microRNAs) especially the miR-200 family are emerging as central players in gene expression regulation through the targeting of the mRNAs of the cadherin repressors ZEB1 and ZEB2 [30,37,38].

Inflammatory/reactive lesions of the serosal membranes

I. Pleuritis: The term pleuritis refers to both fibrinous and inflammatory reactions in the pleura. *Fibrinous or serofibrinous pleuritis* can be caused by a variety of underlying conditions which are often non-infectious (lung infarct, uremia, rheumatoid arthritis, systemic lupus erythematosus, post-operative, and metastases) or may be

infectious (pneumonia, lung abscess, systemic infections). Presence of zonation (fibrin, granulation tissue, and underlying fibrosis) from surface to deep part (Fig. 17.3) is very helpful in differentiating it from desmoplastic mesothelioma (discussed below). Eosinophilic pleuritis is commonly seen after pneumothorax (Fig. 17.4).

Pleural infections secondary to bacterial or mycotic seeding lead to purulent exudate which usually becomes localized (*empyema* or pus in the pleural cavity). If unresolved after antibiotic therapy, it is surgically excised. On histologic examination, there are numerous degenerating neutrophils admixed with fibrin and macrophages. It is unusual to find the causative organisms in the specimen. In an immunocompromised host, gram and fungal (GMS or PAS) stains may be helpful.

II. Fibrous pleurisy: Pleural thickening may be localized or diffuse and often the end result of fibrinous pleurisy. These patients usually have a history of pleural effusion, either long standing or repeated episodes. Pleural plaques are unusual in the mediastinal pleura (more common on the diaphragm and chest wall). Occasionally the mediastinal pleura is biopsied which shows fibrosis and varying amounts of chronic inflammation (Fig. 17.5) with or without organizing fibrin. The blood vessels are uniformly distributed and parallel. The collagen fibers tend to also be parallel and run in the same direction in the section. Again, the main differential is from sarcomatoid mesothelioma, especially the desmoplastic variant, which is discussed below.

III. Pericarditis: This may be fibrinous (Fig. 17.6) (myocardial infarction, post-cardiac surgery, chronic renal failure, connective tissue diseases), purulent (infections), chronic (non-specific chronic inflammation seen after surgery, trauma, chemoradiation), or constrictive (seen in any long-standing cause of pericardial effusion, or as a complication of radiation). The surgical pathologist will see these lesions when a portion of pericardium is surgically

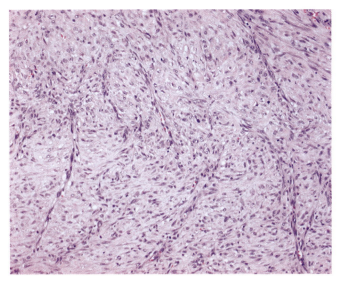

Fig. 17.5 Fibrous pleurisy with richly vascularized reactive submesothelial cells. Note that the capillaries are mostly parallel to each other.

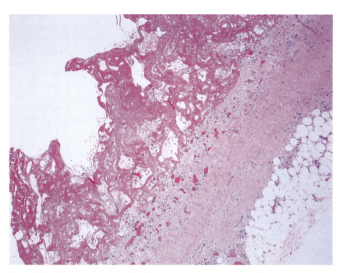

Fig. 17.6 Fibrinous pericarditis. There is a densely eosinophilic layer of fibrin on the surface with congested capillaries in the connective tissue underneath.

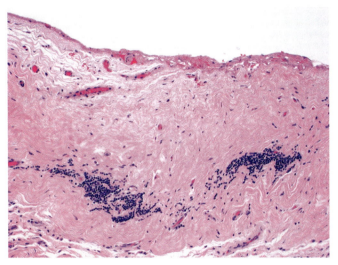

Fig. 17.7 Dense pericardial fibrosis and chronic inflammation are present in this specimen obtained from a 35-year-old female with pericardial effusion undergoing pericardial window.

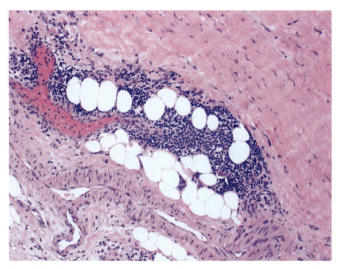

Fig. 17.8 This 65-year-old had a pericardial window done which showed focal lymphocytic infiltrates. IHC stains demonstrated monoclonality for B-cells. This was the first presentation of chronic lymphocytic leukemia in this patient.

excised to form a pericardial window. The most common findings are dense fibrosis with small foci of lymphocytic infiltration (Fig. 17.7). One should keep in mind that malignancies can rarely be the first presentation in the pericardium (Fig. 17.8). Rare cases of primary pericardial sarcomatoid mesothelioma have been described [39].

IV. Granulomatous inflammation: This may be first diagnosed on a surgical biopsy of serosal membranes or may be part of the underlying involvement of lung and/or lymph nodes.

i) *Tuberculosis:* Rarely, the serosal membranes may be the first to be biopsied in a patient with tuberculosis of the chest. Typically necrotizing granulomas are seen (Fig. 17.9), but on a limited biopsy only, necrosis may not be evident. Special stains and microbial cultures are invaluable for definite diagnosis.

ii) *Sarcoidosis:* Secondary involvement of the pleura occurs in about 10% of sarcoid patients with pulmonary disease. Well-formed non-necrotizing granulomas are present; however, focal necrosis can also be seen (Fig. 17.10). Stains for acid-fast bacilli and fungus must be performed routinely.

iii) *Rheumatoid nodule:* Rarely, pleural involvement by rheumatoid disease may manifest as a granuloma with palisaded histiocytes around fibrin.

iv) *Foreign body giant cell reaction:* This is most often seen as a reaction to talc pleurodesis commonly performed to control recurrent pleural effusions. There is a marked chronic inflammatory response with lymphocytes, fibrosis and numerous multinucleated

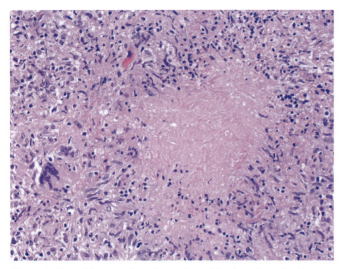

Fig. 17.9 Necrotizing granuloma in a patient with tuberculous pleuritis.

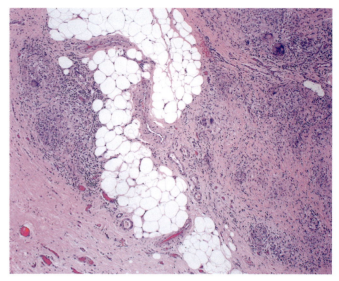

Fig. 17.10 Pleural involvement by sarcoidosis. Well-formed non-necrotizing granulomas are present in the pleura in this patient with pulmonary sarcoidosis.

(a)   (b)

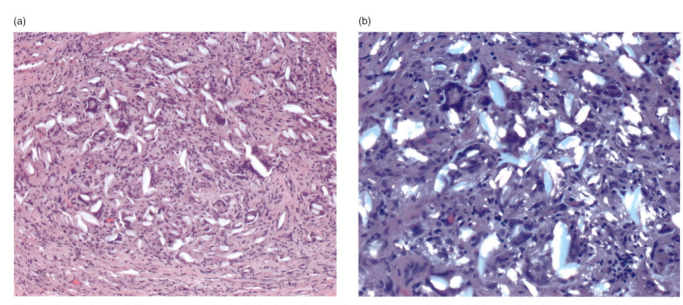

Fig. 17.11 Talc pleurodesis. There are multiple foreign body giant cells containing crystalline material **(a)**, which is strongly birefringent under polarized light **(b)**.

giant cells that have engulfed strongly birefringent talc crystals (Fig. 17.11). Pleurectomy specimens will often have both talc pleurodesis and malignant mesothelioma.

V. Mesothelial hyperplasia: A variety of injuries can cause mesothelial hyperplasia. These include effusions (both pleural and pericardial), chronic inflammation, and post-operative repair. The mesothelial cells may form papillae, tubules, or sheets (Fig. 17.12a–d) without forming an expansile nodule or invading pre-existing structures such as fat and adjacent organs. There may be prominent nucleoli, multinucleation, and mitoses; however, there are no atypical mitoses and little or no necrosis. There is a variable mixture of mesothelial cells and histiocytes/

macrophages (referred to as mesothelial/monocytic incidental cardiac excrescences "MICE" when seen in the heart or pericardium) (Fig. 17.13a and b) [40,41]. Occasionally, markedly reactive mesothelial cells can be found in lymphatics and lymph nodes and must not be misdiagnosed as evidence of malignancy (Fig. 17.14a–c). On small biopsies, the main differential is from malignant mesothelioma and metastatic carcinoma. Correlation with clinical and radiological features is always helpful. If these show a mass and the biopsy does not, then sampling may be the problem. On the other hand, if there is no mass, the presence of florid mesothelial proliferation must be interpreted with caution (Fig. 17.15).

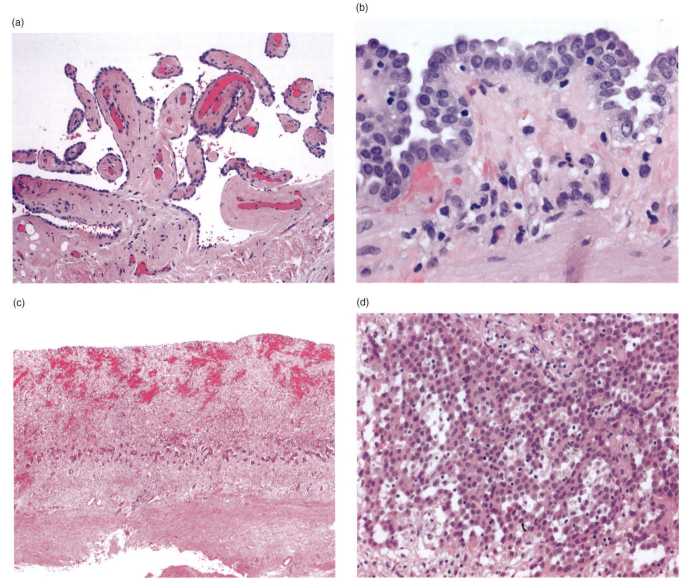

Fig. 17.12 Mesothelial hyperplasia: **(a)** incidental pericardial finding of small papillae covered by a single layer of bland cuboidal mesothelial cells; **(b)** reactive mesothelium with some crowding of cells, small nucleoli, and a mitotic figure; **(c)** linear arrangement of reactive mesothelium forming tubules as seen here is very useful in excluding malignancy; **(d)** sheet of hyperplastic mesothelial cells which appear uniform but may be difficult to differentiate from epithelioid malignant mesothelioma.

Cystic lesions of the serosal membranes

I. Pericardial cyst: This is a simple cyst, lined by a single layer of mesothelial cells which are morphologically similar to normal pericardial mesothelium (Fig. 17.16a and b). These cells stain for all the mesothelial markers (calretinin, WT-1, D2–40, and CK5/6). The wall of the cyst consists of dense connective tissue which is rather hypocellular and tends to lack inflammation.

II. Multilocular mesothelial inclusion cyst: This is a rare lesion of the pericardium or the pleura, which is multicystic, and lined by cuboidal to hyperplastic mesothelial cells. There is often a history of prior

surgery or inflammatory process leading to the concept that this is most likely a reactive, incidental finding. In contrast, a multilocular cystic mesothelioma presents as a bulky mass, which may recur and may be neoplastic. It is discussed further below with other mesothelial lesions.

Neoplastic lesions of the serosal membranes
Diffuse malignant mesothelioma

Malignant mesothelioma is a neoplasm derived from mesothelial cells, native cells of the serous cavities, and may affect the

(a)

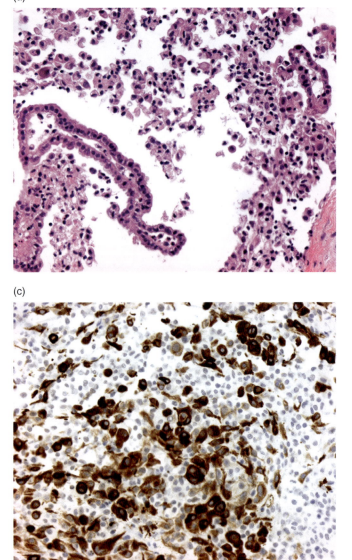

(b)

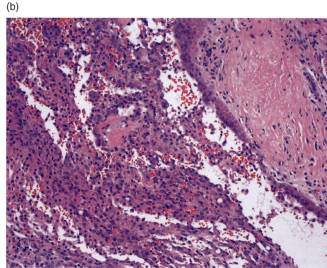

(c)

Fig. 17.13 Mesothelial/monocytic incidental cardiac excrescences "MICE": **(a)** there is a mixture of reactive mesothelial cells and macrophages; **(b)** there is a sheet of cells which are difficult to identify on H&E alone; **(c)** the mesothelial cells stain strongly with keratin 5/6 while the admixed histiocytes are negative.

pleura, pericardium, peritoneum, or the tunica vaginalis. Histologically they can be epithelioid, sarcomatoid, or biphasic (Table 17.1). Small cell and transitional types have also been described.

Despite extensive literature on the topic, the diagnosis of malignant mesothelioma remains challenging especially on small biopsies. This is because mesothelioma is well known for its phenotypic heterogeneity both from case to case and also within a single tumor. The various architectural patterns frequently combining both epithelial and mesenchymal differentiation are typical and underline the capacity of mesothelioma to mimic other neoplasms, notably adenocarcinomas and sarcomas. The definitive diagnosis is usually based on histologic examination of adequate biopsies. However, several studies have shown that while open pleural biopsy has over 95% sensitivity for the diagnosis of diffuse

malignant mesothelioma, it has much lower specificity (56%) in determining the histologic subtype, especially non-epithelioid subtypes when compared with the final diagnosis on pleurectomy or extrapleural pneumonectomy specimens [42,43]. This is because mesotheliomas histologically are heterogeneous tumors, hence different patterns in varying proportions can be observed in a given tumor within a type (all epithelioid versus epithelioid and sarcomatoid). Therefore, the result regarding subtypes of the initial biopsy should be carefully weighed in the treatment stratification.

Also, one has to consider that mesotheliomas often present with recurrent serous effusions that are usually sent for cytological examination. Even though the cytological features of malignant mesothelioma have been described over 50 years ago and further refined in several subsequent papers, there is

(a)

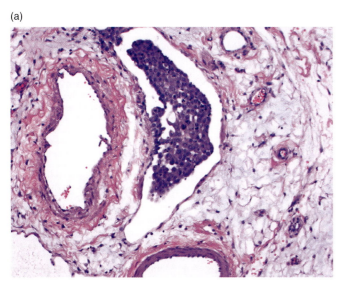

(b)

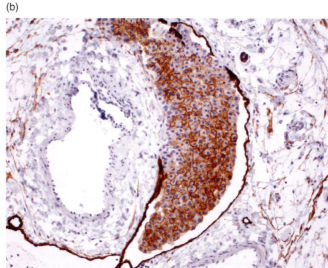

(c)

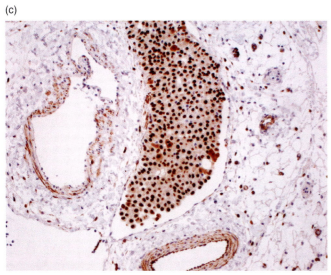

Fig. 17.14 Reactive mesothelial cells within a lymphatic from pericardial window in a 21-year-old with pericardial effusion: **(a)** H&E, **(b)** D2–40 which highlights the lymphatic endothelium, and **(c)** WT-1.

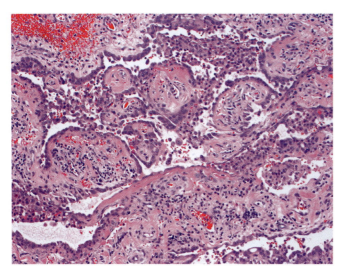

Fig. 17.15 Marked mesothelial hyperplasia seen in the pericardium, removed during an aortic dissection repair.

still doubt as to the ability of the cytopathologic modality to establish a definitive diagnosis of malignant mesothelioma. The published sensitivity of cytological diagnosis of mesothelioma ranges between 32–76%. This broad range of sensitivity is probably related to sampling rather than interpretation, though one has to accept that there is a broad morphologic overlap between reactive mesothelial cells and malignant cells of mesothelioma. The absence of one of the key histologic diagnostic features of malignant mesothelioma, invasion of pre-existing tissue (not granulation tissue), is not present in exfoliative cytological specimen. To achieve correct cytological diagnosis it is important to obtain an adequate amount of well preserved fluid which has to be prepared to ensure satisfactory cell concentration followed by quality smears (direct, cytospin, thin-layer) and cell block. In expert hands the predictive value of a positive diagnosis of malignant mesothelioma in serous effusions is 100%.

However, not all mesotheliomas yield effusions and the sarcomatoid mesotheliomas are virtually never diagnosed on effusion cytology. In such cases, FNA combined with core biopsy or open biopsy for histology is necessary to establish the diagnosis.

The main subclassification into epithelioid, sarcomatoid, and mixed has the most prognostic significance; however, recent literature supports subclassification into histologic patterns, some of which have better or worse outcomes as discussed below.

a. **Epithelioid mesothelioma:** It is the most common histologic type of malignant mesothelioma and has the best overall prognosis as compared to sarcomatoid and mixed mesotheliomas [43,44]. Epithelioid malignant mesotheliomas are, in general, remarkable for their deceptive blandness (Fig. 17.17). Most of the tumor cells are cuboidal to polygonal with little variation from one to another. This is partly due to the monotonous, round nuclei containing usually single nucleoli (Fig. 17.18). In a number of cases the nucleoli are large (macronucleoli) but in others they are

Table 17.1. 2004 World Health Organization histologic classification of mesothelioma

Epithelioid

Sarcomatoid
  Desmoplastic

Biphasic

Other tumors of mesothelial origin
  Well-differentiated papillary mesothelioma
  Localized malignant mesothelioma
  Adenomatoid tumor

inconspicuous. In general, mitoses are difficult to find. In most cases the cytoplasm is abundant and interestingly, increases further with nuclear enlargement, resulting in a relatively constant nuclear/cytoplasmic ratio between individual tumor cells contributing further to the bland histologic features. In the majority of the cases the texture of the cytoplasm is rather dense, especially around the nucleus, due to the rich intermediate filament content (cytokeratin and vimentin). In addition, cytoplasmic vacuolation (Fig. 17.19a and b), prominently or subtly, may be observed in some of the tumor cells. This is due to accumulation of hyaluronic acid, glycogen or lipid, which, when prominent, results in *signet-ring* (Fig. 17.20a–c), *clear cell* (Fig. 17.21a and b) or *lipid-rich* (Fig. 17.22a–c) *variants of malignant epithelioid mesothelioma*, respectively. Rarely, even cytoplasmic hemosiderin may be seen (not to be erroneously interpreted as melanin, hence misdiagnosing a mesothelioma as metastatic melanoma) (Fig. 17.23). Few cases of malignant mesothelioma with cytoplasmic hyaline globules staining positive for periodic acid-Schiff (PAS) with and without diastase digestion [45] and mesotheliomas with intracytoplasmic crystalloid structures have also been described [46]. These cytoplasmic characteristics do not have any demonstrated clinical significance but are important for the pathologist to be aware of in order to make the correct diagnosis of malignant mesothelioma. Also, the differential diagnosis and composition of the IHC stain panel will depend on the specific differential diagnosis of the case.

Some cases are composed of sheets of large, polygonal tumor cells with sharp cell borders, abundant glassy eosinophilic or amphophilic cytoplasm, and round vesicular nuclei with prominent nucleoli (Fig. 17.24a and b), reminiscent of deciduoid reaction (*deciduoid malignant mesothelioma*). Ordonez has

(a)

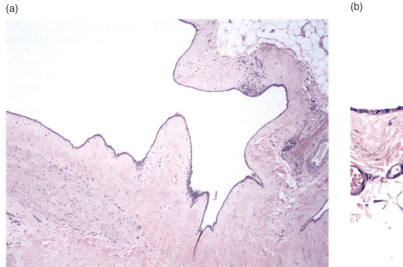

(b)

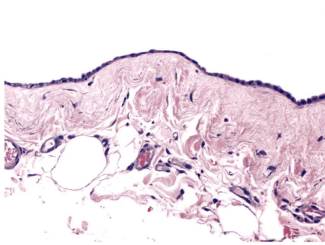

Fig. 17.16 Pericardial cyst with a single layer of cuboidal mesothelial cells and connective tissue in the wall, **(a)** low power and **(b)** high power.

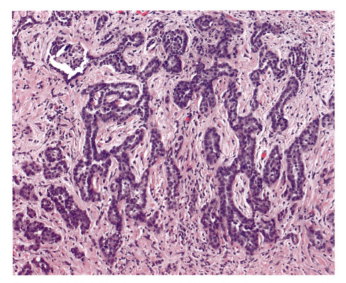

Fig. 17.17 Epithelioid malignant mesothelioma with trabecular pattern. Note the relatively bland and uniform tumor cells.

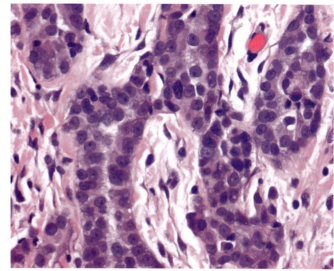

Fig. 17.18 High power of Fig. 17.18 shows single nucleoli in most of the tumor cells.

(a)

(b)

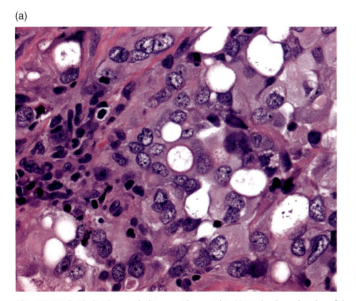

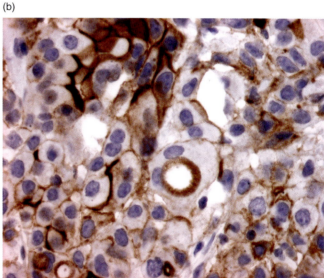

Fig. 17.19 Epithelioid mesothelioma with vacuoles. Note the fuzzy border of the vacuole which would correspond ultrastructurally to microvilli, **(a)** H&E and **(b)** D2–40 stains.

reported 21 cases of deciduoid mesothelioma and found that there is a high-grade subgroup that has a highly aggressive clinical behavior. These patients have a mean survival of seven months as compared to the usual deciduoid tumors, with a mean survival of 23 months. The high-grade tumors are composed of cells with a wide variation in their size and shape, frequent loss of cell cohesion, marked nuclear atypia (Fig. 17.25) and high mitotic activity [47].

Rare epithelioid mesotheliomas are poorly differentiated and composed of either sheets of relatively small cells (*small cell mesothelioma*) (Fig. 17.26) [48], plump spindle to round cells with features overlapping between epithelioid to sarcomatoid cells (transitional mesothelioma) (Fig. 17.27a and b) or high

grade/pleomorphic cells (*pleomorphic epithelioid mesothelioma*). Kadota *et al.* found that the pleomorphic subtype is a predictor of aggressive behavior with no survival difference from biphasic or sarcomatoid diffuse malignant mesothelioma, hence suggested that it may be best regarded as a sarcomatoid pattern rather than a subtype of epithelioid malignant mesothelioma [49]. In order to be considered pleomorphic, the tumor must have more than 10% of the cells with marked nuclear pleomorphism with frequent tumor giant cells and atypical mitoses (Fig. 17.28a and b).

In contrast to the bland cytomorphology, epithelioid mesothelioma has a rich architectural repertoire varying between cases and not infrequently within the same tumor.

(a)

(b)

(c)

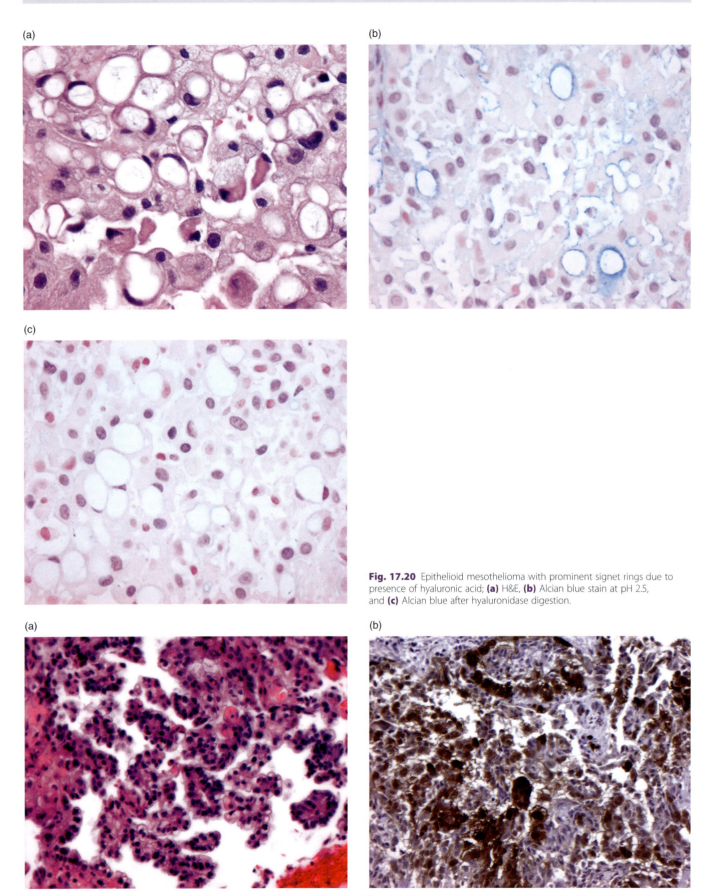

Fig. 17.20 Epithelioid mesothelioma with prominent signet rings due to presence of hyaluronic acid; **(a)** H&E, **(b)** Alcian blue stain at pH 2.5, and **(c)** Alcian blue after hyaluronidase digestion.

(a)

(b)

Fig. 17.21 Epithelioid mesothelioma with clear cell features that would raise the differential diagnosis of renal clear cell carcinoma; **(a)** H&E and **(b)** calretinin stains.

(a)

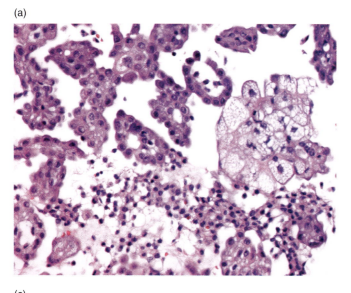

(b)

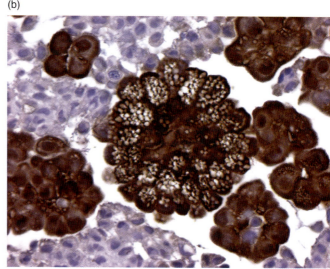

(c)

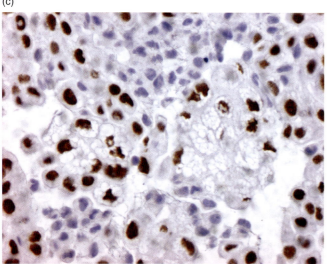

Fig. 17.22 Epithelioid mesothelioma with some lipid rich cells containing fine intracytoplasmic vacuoles; **(a)** H&E, **(b)** calretinin, and **(c)** WT-1 stains. Note that not all cells stain with mesothelial markers; the negative cells are likely histiocytes.

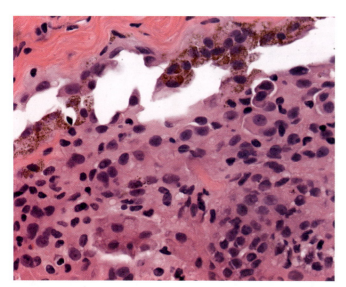

Fig. 17.23 Intracytoplasmic hemosiderin is prominent in this case with florid mesothelial hyperplasia.

The most well-recognized patterns are: solid, tubulopapillary (Fig. 17.29), acinar (Fig. 17.30), micropapillary (Fig. 17.31a and b), adenomatoid (microglandular/microcystic) (Fig. 17.32), adenoid cystic, cystic and cribriform (Fig. 17.33a–c). Of these, the micropapillary pattern (without central fibrovascular core) has a higher incidence of lymphatic invasion and lymph node metastases. The tubulopapillary and acinar patterns have the best prognosis and account for the relatively few cases of long-term survival reported in the literature.

Among the three major subtypes of malignant mesothelioma, epithelioid is the most prevalent and has the best prognosis. Considering the broad histologic spectrum of epithelioid mesothelioma and the rarity of specific subtypes, it is not surprising that there are only a few generally agreed upon histologic prognostic factors to further stratify clinical outcomes in pleural epithelioid diffuse malignant mesothelioma. There are rare publications on the usefulness of MIB-1 labeling index in pleural mesothelioma [50,51] and mitotic count as well as

(a)

(b)

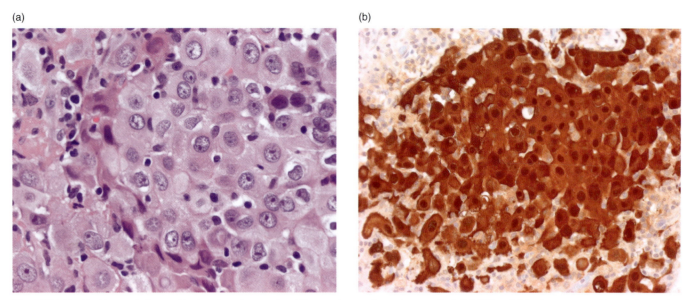

Fig. 17.24 Deciduoid mesothelioma with abundant glassy eosinophilic cytoplasm and prominent nucleoli; **(a)** H&E, and **(b)** calretinin stains. Note darker nuclear stain than the cytoplasm in the latter, which is a characteristic staining pattern of mesothelial cells.

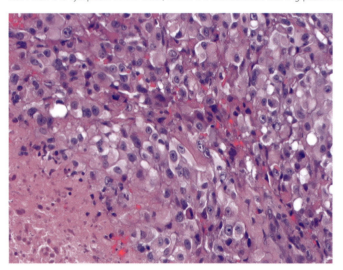

Fig. 17.25 High-grade deciduoid mesothelioma with focal necrosis and more atypia than is usually seen in the typical deciduoid mesothelioma.

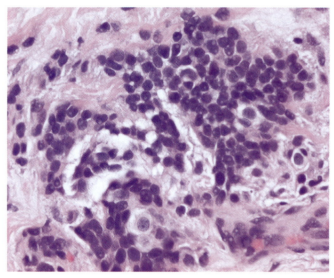

Fig. 17.26 Small cell mesothelioma with scant cytoplasm and most cells with inconspicuous, if any, nucleoli.

(a)

(b)

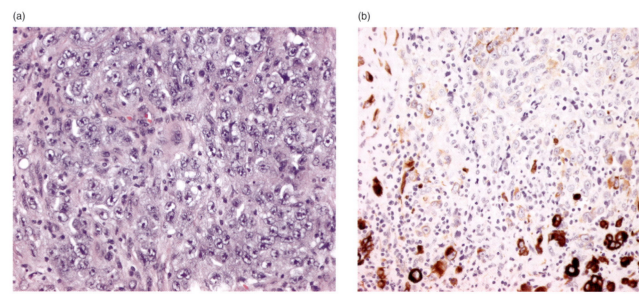

Fig. 17.27 Transitional mesothelioma is composed of sheets of cells that are not clearly epithelioid nor sarcomatoid. The cytoplasmic borders are indistinct and there are prominent nucleoli **(a)**. IHC stain for CAM5.2 demonstrates loss of keratin in the transitional area whereas it is present in the more epithelioid area at the bottom **(b)**.

(a)

(b)

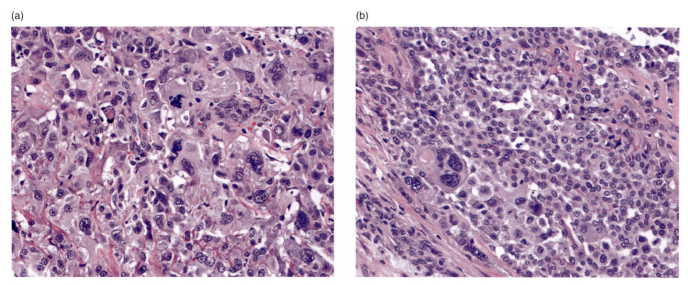

Fig. 17.28 Pleomorphic epithelioid mesothelioma has large bizarre cells with atypical mitosis and multinucleated giant cells **(a)**. These features are present in only part of the tumor **(b)**.

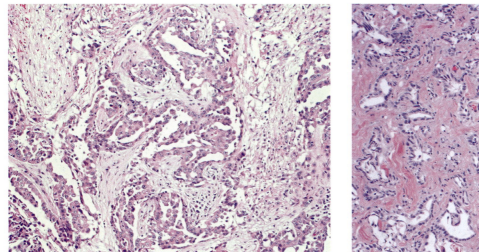

Fig. 17.29 Epithelioid malignant mesothelioma showing tubulopapillary growth pattern.

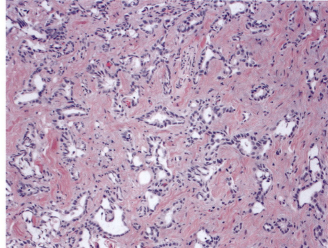

Fig. 17.30 Acinar pattern of epithelioid mesothelioma. The relatively bland tumor cells form angulated and branching gland-like structures.

(a)

(b)

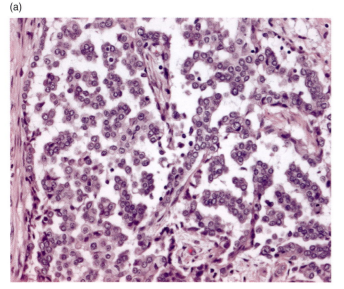

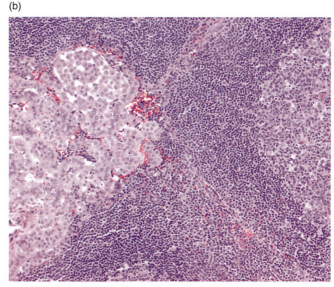

Fig. 17.31 Micropapillary variant of epithelioid mesothelioma showing **(a)** papillary projections without central fibrovascular cores and **(b)** lymph node metastasis.

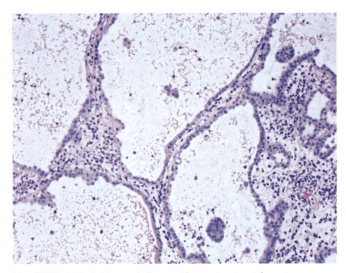

Fig. 17.32 Epithelioid mesothelioma with prominent cyst formation.

histomorphologic parameters in peritoneal mesothelioma [52]. More recently, Kadota *et al.* [53], studying a large series of pleural epithelioid malignant mesotheliomas of stage I–IV have found that nuclear grading, similarly to many other cancer types (i.e. breast, renal cell, and bladder carcinoma), is a strong predictor of survival. Multivariate analysis showed nuclear atypia and mitotic count (Fig. 17.34) as independent prognostic factors and these two factors were utilized to create a three-tier nuclear grade score. This approach stratified patients into three distinct prognostic groups: nuclear grade I (median overall survival=28 months), nuclear grade II (median overall survival=14 months), nuclear grade III (median overall survival=5 months). Hopefully further studies will confirm that, similarly to many other cancer types, nuclear grading is a useful, reproducible, and cost-effective prognostic tool in predicting clinical outcome and time of recurrence than the currently available clinicopathologic factors.

(a)

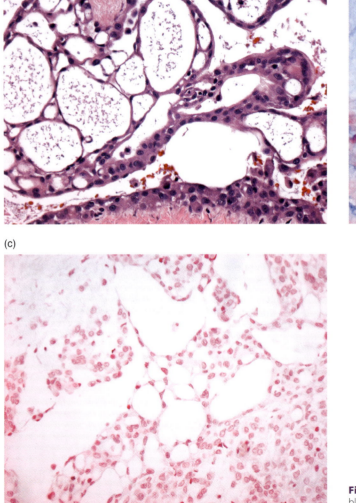

(b)

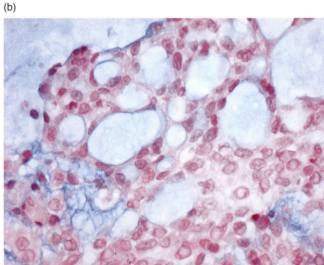

(c)

Fig. 17.33 Cribriform pattern of epithelioid mesothelioma; **(a)** H&E, **(b)** Alcian blue at pH 2.5, and **(c)** Alcian blue after hyaluronidase digestion.

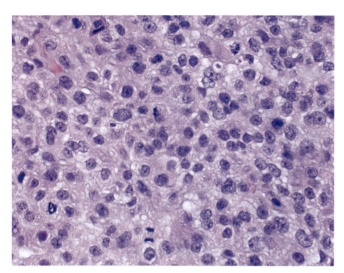

Fig. 17.34 Epithelioid mesothelioma with high mitotic count. At least four mitotic figures can be identified in this high power.

Differential diagnosis: One of the main differential diagnostic considerations of malignant epithelioid mesothelioma is *metastatic carcinoma*, especially adenocarcinoma. The application of mesothelial (Calretinin, WT-1, D2–40, cytokeratin 5/6) and epithelial (CEA, MOC31, Ber-EP4, BG8, CD15, PAX8, and TTF-1) immunocytochemical markers are often helpful to make the distinction between adenocarcinomas and mesotheliomas [54]. It is important to remember that some mesothelial markers are also expressed by selected carcinomas (WT-1 in serous carcinomas; calretinin and cytokeratin 5/6 in squamous cell and urothelial carcinomas). The expression of p40 (which is more specific but equally sensitive as p63) by squamous cell carcinomas but not by mesotheliomas helps to distinguish the two. Klebe *et al.* [55] found that a panel of three antibodies was sufficient in most cases to diagnose, or exclude, epithelioid mesothelioma. Labeling for calretinin and lack of labeling for BG8 were sufficient for definite correlation with a diagnosis of malignant mesothelioma and CD15 provided further differentiating information in some cases (renal cell carcinoma is usually positive).

The other main differential diagnostic task is to distinguish malignant mesothelioma from *mesothelial hyperplasia/atypical mesothelial hyperplasia*. A variety of methods have been attempted in an effort to distinguish between reactive and malignant mesothelial lesions, however, in practice such distinction depends more on morphologic expertise than any foolproof ancillary tests like expression of EMA, telomerase, p53 or GLUT-1 in mesothelioma and desmin in reactive mesothelial cells.

However, there is emerging data that homozygous deletion of 9p21 locus harboring gene CDKN2A (p16) in up to 74% of malignant mesotheliomas has both diagnostic and prognostic value. Demonstration of CDKNA2 (p16) deletion by FISH is particularly useful diagnostically in separating benign from malignant mesothelial proliferations of serous fluids and small

biopsy specimens [56]. Application of this assay certainly improves the accuracy of diagnosis of malignant mesotheliomas. Cases with CDKNA2 deletion usually also have loss of p16 protein expression. According to some studies loss of p16 immunoreactivity has the same prognostic significance as homozygous deletion of p16, while other studies showed about 23% discrepancy between FISH and immunohistochemistry. Loss of p16 immunoexpression in the absence of 9p21 deletion may be the result of point mutation or methylation. Best survival was observed in patients where the tumor showed p16 immunoreactivity and lack of p16 deletion [57]. MTAP resides in the same gene cluster of 9p21 region and is co-deleted in the majority of CDKNA2 (p16) deleted cases. CDKNA2 and MTAP deletions in peritoneal mesotheliomas are correlated with loss of p16 protein expression and poor survival [58].

b. **Sarcomatoid malignant mesothelioma:** Sarcomatoid mesotheliomas have worse prognosis than epithelioid mesotheliomas, with a six months median survival compared to ten months for biphasic and 16 months for epithelioid mesotheliomas [59]. Sarcomatoid mesotheliomas consist of more than 90% spindle-shaped neoplastic cells. Similarly to epithelioid mesotheliomas, sarcomatoid mesotheliomas have a broad range of histologic appearances and combinations of different patterns may be found in the same tumor [44]. Apart from the conventional sarcomatoid mesothelioma, desmoplastic mesothelioma, mesothelioma with heterologous differentiation and lymphohistiocytoid mesothelioma are recognized. Among the largest reported series of 324 cases, 145 (44%) were conventional, 70 (21%) were sarcomatoid with desmoplastic areas, 110 (34%) were desmoplastic, 8 (2%) were heterologous, and 2 (<1%) were lymphohistiocytoid [60].

Conventional sarcomatoid mesothelioma is a sarcoma-like malignant neoplasm, which is composed of closely packed spindle cells either arranged in a haphazard or fasciculated to storiform fashion (Fig. 17.35a and b). Nuclei are often hyperchromatic with moderate pleomorphism but they may be deceptively bland. The main differential in the former are various sarcomas involving the chest wall/pleura or pleural fibrosis in the latter. Less cellular areas often alternate with frankly sarcomatoid highly cellular foci. The presence of bland necrosis is a helpful diagnostic sign; so is the invasion of the chest wall, diaphragm, or lung parenchyma. Most sarcomatoid mesotheliomas are broad-spectrum keratin positive but in some cases keratin expression is only focal (Fig. 17.36) and rare keratin negative examples, especially mesotheliomas with heterologous differentiation, may occur. It is important to remember that reactive mesothelium (both epithelioid and spindle) is also keratin positive. However, keratin immunostain is very helpful to highlight invasive foci of malignant mesothelioma (Fig. 17.37).

Desmoplastic mesothelioma is a variant of sarcomatoid mesothelioma which grossly is similar to other histologic types

(a)

(b)

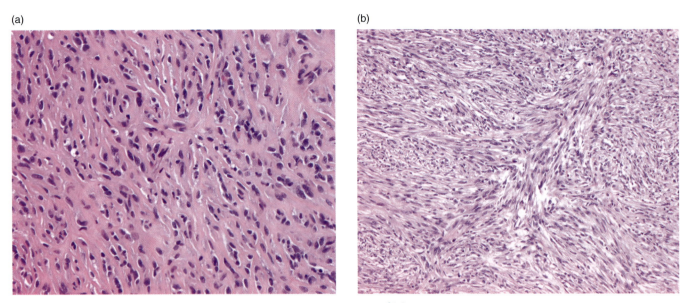

Fig. 17.35 Sarcomatoid mesothelioma with spindle cells arranged in **(a)** haphazard and **(b)** fasciculated patterns.

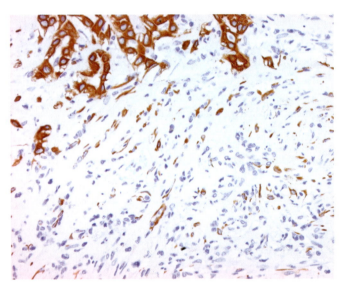

Fig. 17.36 Keratin staining is only focal in the sarcomatoid part (lower right) and diffuse in the epithelioid part (upper left) of this biphasic mesothelioma.

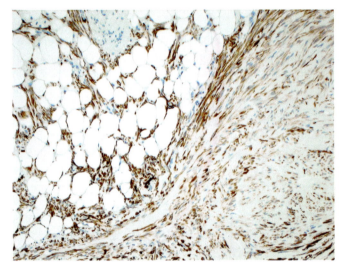

Fig. 17.37 Keratin (CAM5.2) staining highlights sarcomatoid mesothelioma invading fat.

of mesothelioma. By definition, it consists of paucicellular, densely hyalinized neoplastic tissue, which should occupy more than 50% of the tumor [61]. It occurs most frequently on the pleura while occurrence at other serosal sites, such as the pericardium, is rare [39]. Histologically, it shows a markedly thickened collagenized/hyalinized pleura of low cellularity, where the deceptively bland neoplastic spindle cells which are arranged in a storiform or 'patternless pattern' of Stout, mimicking benign fibrous pleurisy, which is the main differential diagnosis. Because of the morphologic overlap with fibrosing pleuritis, a definitive histologic diagnosis of desmoplastic malignant mesothelioma, in addition to the basic morphology, requires one of the following features: invasion of adipose tissue (Fig. 17.38), muscle, bone or lung, bland necrosis

(Fig. 17.39), overtly sarcomatous cellular foci (Fig. 17.40), or distant metastasis. Bland necrosis is a sharply demarcated eosinophilic necrotic focus which, in contrast to many other forms of necrosis, shows very little or no karyorrhexis or inflammatory reaction. The presence of "expansile stromal nodules" also supports the diagnosis of desmoplastic mesothelioma over a benign condition. Expansile stromal nodules are of low cellularity with a pushing border exhibiting different tinctorial characteristics from the surrounding stroma (Fig. 17.41). One also has to be careful not to mistake the so-called "fake fat phenomenon" (Fig. 17.42) for real fat invasion [62]. The diagnosis of desmoplastic malignant mesothelioma is often difficult especially on a small biopsy specimen, as the diagnostic foci are widely scattered, therefore it often requires open biopsy [63]. Finding homozygous deletion of p16

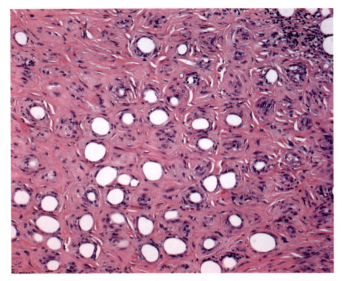

Fig. 17.38 Desmoplastic mesothelioma invading and encircling fat cells.

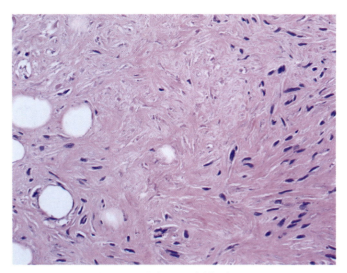

Fig. 17.39 Desmoplastic mesothelioma with bland necrosis.

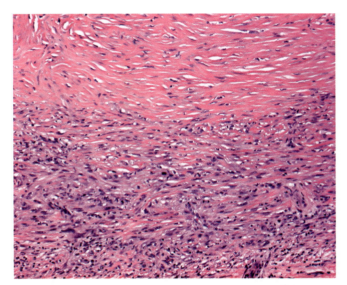

Fig. 17.40 Desmoplastic mesothelioma with variable cellularity from hypocellular to frankly sarcomatous areas.

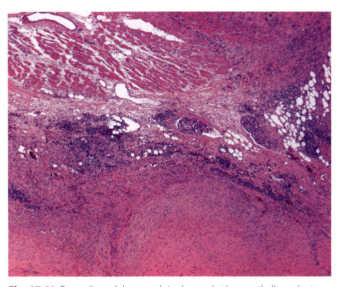

Fig. 17.41 Expansile nodular growth in desmoplastic mesothelioma (note skeletal muscle in upper part of picture).

(FISH test can be performed on formalin fixed paraffin embedded tissue) is diagnostic [64]. Rarely, desmoplastic mesothelioma presents with metastasis (bone, lung etc.) with histological features similar to the primary neoplasm. These metastatic foci are also keratin positive.

Lymphohistiocytoid mesothelioma: lymphohistiocytoid malignant mesothelioma was originally described as a variant of sarcomatoid mesothelioma, but the tumor cells are only rarely spindly but rather polygonal with pale, less dense cytoplasm than one would see in epithelioid mesotheliomas, hence the descriptive "histiocytoid" designation [65]. Lymphohistiocytoid mesothelioma typically has a diffuse, dense chronic inflammatory infiltrate (lymphocytes, plasma cells and sometimes eosinophils) obscuring the underlying proliferation of neoplastic mesothelial cells. The mesothelial cells do not form distinct structures but are arranged in sheets, ill-defined nests, or in a dispersed fashion. In our opinion, the appearance of these 'histiocytoid' mesothelial cells is between epithelioid and transitional mesothelioma (Fig. 17.43). They are negative for lymphoid/histiocytic markers but usually express virtually all the mesothelial markers. The importance of this rare type of malignant mesothelioma is the diagnostic difficulty in recognizing the "hiding" neoplastic mesothelial proliferation and distinguishing it from a variety of benign and malignant lymphoproliferative conditions [66]. It has a better prognosis than sarcomatoid mesothelioma and some would consider it to be better classified as a variant of epithelioid mesothelioma.

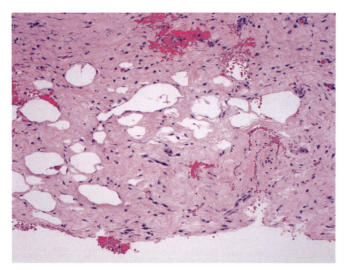

Fig. 17.42 "Fake fat" is seen here as irregular air spaces, likely an artifact of biopsy, in a 3-year-old patient with pleural fistula.

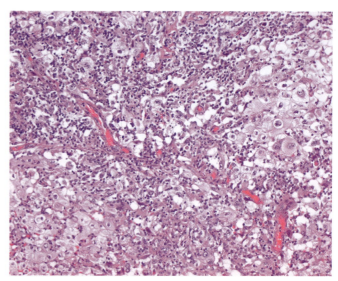

Fig. 17.43 Histiocytoid mesothelioma with intermixed large tumor cells and reactive small lymphocytes.

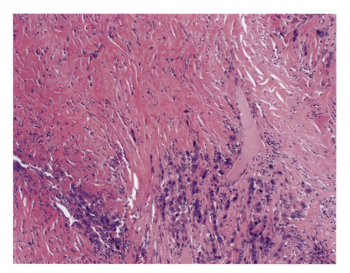

Fig. 17.44 Sarcomatoid mesothelioma with desmoplastic (upper) and transitional (lower) features.

c. **Biphasic mesothelioma:** Is a mixed epithelioid and sarcomatoid mesothelioma. Biphasic mesothelioma should have at least 10% of both epithelioid and sarcomatoid components in order to be diagnosed as such [59]. Tumors with less than 10% sarcomatoid component have a prognosis similar to epithelioid mesothelioma whereas those with about 10–30% sarcomatoid component have an intermediate prognosis. Thus, the pathologist needs to include the amount of sarcomatoid component in the surgical pathology report. One must remember, though, that the amount of sarcomatoid component is generally underestimated on biopsy when compared to resection specimens.

Transitional mesothelioma: the term "transitional mesothelioma" is applied to some of those malignant mesotheliomas where the neoplastic cells exhibit a plump fusiform to round phenotype and as a result, on the plane of the histologic section, it is difficult to determine whether the tumor is epithelioid or sarcomatoid. Some authors regarded this type of mesothelioma as "poorly differentiated" mesothelioma. Transitional mesothelioma is usually seen in the context of biphasic or sarcomatoid mesothelioma (Fig. 17.44). Even in cases where "transitional" is the dominant phenotype, the behavior is usually similar to that of sarcomatoid mesothelioma.

Differential diagnosis: The histological differential diagnosis of sarcomatoid and biphasic mesothelioma includes reactive pleural fibrosis, a variety of sarcomas and sarcomatoid carcinomas. Sarcomatoid mesothelioma usually does not shed diagnostically relevant cells to effusions or when it does the atypical cells are few and more likely to exhibit an epithelioid rather than a spindle phenotype. In sarcomatoid mesotheliomas most of the mesothelial immunocytochemical markers are down-regulated or absent. However D2–40 expression is often observed. Interestingly, the tumor cells from "transitional" types of mesotheliomas, even though they exhibit an epithelioid phenotype, may also have reduced expression of mesothelial markers, including keratins. Cytokeratin expression like CAM5.2 is very useful to differentiate the spindle-shaped tumor cells of sarcomatoid mesothelioma from most sarcomas. The majority of sarcomatoid mesotheliomas do express this marker in contrast to keratin 5/6 which is usually lost. Keratin immunoreactivity, including CAM5.2, does not differentiate between pleural fibrosis and sarcomatoid mesotheliomas, as it is expressed by a varying number of lesional cells of both. To distinguish the spindle cells of pleural fibrosis from those of sarcomatoid mesothelioma, in most cases, is virtually impossible on cytological grounds. It is important to know that a small percentage of sarcomatoid mesotheliomas may be keratin-negative. In such cases the mesothelial nature of the neoplasm is "hidden" and close clinicopathologic and imaging correlation is necessary to make the correct diagnosis of sarcomatoid mesothelioma. The differential diagnosis of sarcomatoid and biphasic mesotheliomas on FNA samples usually includes synovial sarcomas, which may present as primary pleural, pericardial, or mediastinal tumors. The spindle cell component of synovial sarcomas is morphologically different than the spindle cells of sarcomatoid mesothelioma. The tumor cells of synovial sarcoma have very little cytoplasm and consequently the aspirated cell groups are crowded. Also the nuclei of synovial sarcoma are relatively small and show evenly distributed chromatin pattern compared to the larger spindle cells with vesicular nuclei of sarcomatoid mesothelioma. FNA smears of synovial sarcomas often also show a large number of "naked" nuclei. The keratin expression in the spindle tumor cells of synovial sarcomas is limited to a few cells. Both monophasic and biphasic synovial sarcomas may immunoreact with the mesothelial marker Calretinin (more frequently in the spindle cells), but in contrast to mesotheliomas they also stain with carcinoma markers, like BerEP4 and show no immunoreactivity to WT-1 [67]. TLE1 had been shown to be a specific marker for synovial sarcoma and diagnostically useful. However, recent data indicate a limited value of this marker in distinguishing malignant mesothelioma from synovial sarcoma, as it is expressed in a varying percentage of the tumor cells of many mesotheliomas regardless of histomorphological subtype [68].

Localized malignant mesothelioma of the pleura, pericardium, and mediastinum

Localized malignant mesothelioma is a rare form of malignant mesothelioma characterized grossly and on imaging by a discrete, solitary, circumscribed mass arising either from the visceral or parietal pleura. Extremely rare examples of localized malignant mesothelioma of the pericardium and mediastinum have also been described. It occurs both in men and women and the age range consists of those in their 40s to 70s. These neoplasms can be sessile or pedunculated, variable in size, from a few to 10 cm [44]. Histologically and immunohistochemically they are comparable to all major forms of diffuse malignant mesothelioma. In contrast to diffuse malignant mesotheliomas, which may present with a dominant mass, localized malignant mesotheliomas do not have an adjacent diffuse component. It follows that some of these tumors can be completely excised with recurrence-free survival of patients. However, other examples may recur after excision and may metastasize [69]. The largest reported series of 23 cases included 21 pleural and 2 peritoneal examples. After surgical excision of the tumor, 10 of 21 patients with follow-up were alive without evidence of disease from 18 months to 11 years. Patients who died had developed local recurrence and metastases, but none had diffuse spread. Localized malignant mesotheliomas should be separated from diffuse malignant mesotheliomas as the former has a different biologic behavior and far better prognosis [70].

Crotty *et al.* [71] have described a case of localized mediastinal desmoplastic malignant mesothelioma, which was masquerading as sclerosing mediastinitis. The patient died postoperatively. Bierhoff and Pfeifer [72] have documented a case of localized malignant mesothelioma arising from a benign mediastinal mesothelial cyst. The patient developed metastases in the adrenal glands and the brain. Occurrence of localized malignant mesothelioma in the anterior [73], posterior [74], and middle mediastinum [75] are also on record. The latter case was a lymphohistiocytoid malignant mesothelioma and was assumed to have arisen from the pericardium. The tumor was completely resected, but local recurrence developed after one year and the patient died of disease two years later. Dysphagia only occurs in 1.4% of pleural malignant mesotheliomas [76] and is very rare as the initial symptom [77]. Malignant mesothelioma is a rare cause of malignant pseudoachalasia [78]. Hayama *et al.* [79] described an additional example of malignant mesothelioma of the posterior mediastinum, which caused dysphagia.

Other tumors of mesothelial origin (benign mesothelial tumors and mesothelial tumors of uncertain malignant potential) of the pleura and pericardium

a. **Adenomatoid tumor:** Adenomatoid tumors are benign mesothelial lesions usually arising in the genitourinary tract. Most frequently they present as incidental small indurated masses, generally less than 2 cm in greatest dimension. Extragenital adenomatoid tumors have also been described in locations such as adrenal gland [80], liver [81–85], heart [86,87] and mediastinum [88]. Pleural adenomatoid tumors are very rare with only five cases documented in the English literature to date [89–92]. Adenomatoid tumors are composed of small tubular, cystic, and vascular-like spaces lined by cuboidal or flattened mesothelial cells or single cells in a fibromyxoid stroma (Fig. 17.45). When cystic structures dominate,

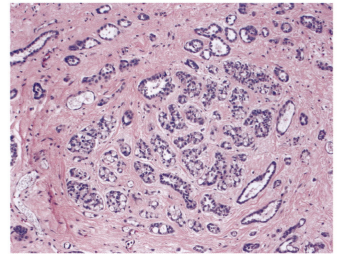

Fig. 17.45 Adenomatoid tumor of the pericardium, incidental finding in this patient.

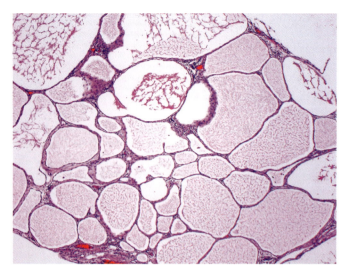

Fig. 17.46 Benign multicystic mesothelioma is composed of variable-sized cysts lined by flattened mesothelial cells.

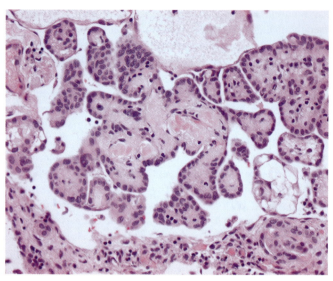

Fig. 17.47 Well-differentiated papillary mesothelioma is composed of papillary structures lined by a single layer of bland mesothelial cells.

differentiating it from benign multicystic mesothelioma can be problematic. Individual cells have eccentric vesicular nuclei, eosinophilic cytoplasm, and cytoplasmic vacuolization. Nucleoli are small and mitotic figure is difficult to find.

The main differential diagnosis is the adenomatoid variant of malignant mesothelioma. However, most adenomatoid tumors are relatively small and localized in contrast to diffuse malignant mesothelioma with the appropriate clinical and imaging data. Weissferdt et al.[93] emphasized that no invasive growth should be identified in true adenomatoid tumors. In the genital tract, however, one should not over-interpret the presence of smooth muscle cells among the cells of adenomatoid tumor as destructive invasion. Adenomatoid tumors with cystic change may show morphologic overlap with benign multicystic mesothelioma (see below). Adenomatoid tumors express virtually all the mesothelial immuno-markers. The differential diagnosis also includes epithelioid hemangioendothelioma, which apart from D2–40 does not immunoreact with other mesothelial markers.

b. **Benign multicystic mesothelioma:** Benign multicystic mesothelioma occurs most frequently in young to middle-aged women in the peritoneum. A few cases in men and very rare examples in other locations, including the pleura and pericardium have been documented[94]. Grossly, they are large, bulky, and consist of multiple fluid-filled cysts that have thin translucent walls. Histologically, the variable-sized cysts are lined by flattened or cuboidal bland mesothelial cells (Fig. 17.46). The cysts are separated by edematous fibrous vascularized septae containing some chronic inflammatory cells, fibrin deposits, and entrapped mesothelial cells. The term 'multilocular inclusion cyst' reflects the view of some that multicystic mesothelioma is a reactive rather than a neoplastic lesion.

c. **Well-differentiated papillary mesothelioma (WDPM):** Most cases of this entity have been documented on the

peritoneum in women[95] of reproductive age group with no history of asbestos exposure and, less frequently, in the tunica vaginalis of men[96]. Historically, documentation of the occurrence of WDPM on the pleura and pericardium was limited to a few case reports[97]. However, following the publications of two series, WDPM of the pleura has become a well-established entity[98,99].

The key problem pathologists have to face, similar to other serosal sites, is how to differentiate a malignant mesothelioma with papillary architecture from WDPM. Distinguishing the two has both prognostic and therapeutic implications. The other issue is that the original morphologic criteria of WDPM[100] have been expanded in the literature without the support of long-term clinical follow-up. Strictly defined, a WDPM is a localized solitary tumor showing an exclusively papillary architecture in which the papillae are lined by a single layer of bland cuboidal mesothelial cells (Fig. 17.47)[95,96,100,101]. Such tumors, if completely excised, are expected to follow a benign clinical course. However, subsequent descriptions in the literature of more complex architectural patterns of growth including tubulopapillary, cribriform, corded and even solid areas, has led to controversy regarding both the terminology and the biologic behavior and has caused diagnostic uncertainty for the practicing pathologists. This controversy is further enhanced by some publications where cases with focal/superficial invasion were not excluded from the morphologic spectrum of WDPMs[98,99]. The authors admit that the follow-up in the two cases with focal invasion was relatively short[98]. Goldblum and Hart[102], examining six cases of incidental, small and localized peritoneal mesothelial neoplasms with benign follow-up preferred to use the diagnostic term of "localized mesothelioma" or "localized mesothelioma of low-grade malignancy" rather than WDPM. Brimo et al.[96], studying tunica vaginalis mesotheliomas, proposed that mesothelial tumors, which are more complex histologically than the classic well-differentiated papillary mesotheliomas, and yet are not overtly histologically malignant, be classified as "mesotheliomas of uncertain malignant potential". We agree with Goldblum et al.[102] and Brimo et al.[96] that it is imperative that most, if not all, of the lesion(s) be removed before a diagnosis of WDPM is rendered.

The largest series of pleural WDPM to date[99] included 11 men and 13 women, with an age range of 31 to 79 years (average age of 60 years). Eleven of the 24 patients had a history of mostly occupational asbestos exposure. One patient with no history of asbestos exposure had breast carcinoma who underwent radiotherapy to the chest on the same side as her diagnosed WDPM seven years later. Most of the patients presented with the history of dyspnea and recurrent pleural effusion. Only one case was discovered incidentally. Chest radiograph and CT scan revealed unilateral free-flowing pleural effusion, in some cases accompanied by thin focal pleural thickening (9 of 24 patients). Pleural nodularity and sometimes encasement of the lung appeared with progression of disease. Thoracoscopy in six patients revealed multiple small/millimeter nodules on the parietal and/or visceral pleura. Twenty-two patients had thoracoscopic pleural biopsy and two patients surgical open lung biopsy.

For inclusion in this study, "all cases had to show a relatively uniform superficial spreading of papillary formations with very limited or no invasion". Invasion was present in ten cases at the time of diagnosis but was limited to the submesothelial layers and no involvement of either adipose tissue or subpleural alveoli. The papillae had thin or broad (stout) myxoid fibrovascular cores and were lined by a single layer of bland, flattened, or cuboidal mesothelial cells with focal subnuclear vacuolation. Mitotic activity was absent. In contrast, diffuse malignant mesothelioma usually shows an admixture of papillary and solid patterns where the mesothelial cells exhibit some atypia with enlarged nuclei and few mitotic figures. In addition, the papillae in diffuse malignant mesothelioma frequently show a back-to-back arrangement without stout fibrovascular cores. The other differential diagnostic consideration is atypical mesothelial hyperplasia. According to the authors the papillae in atypical mesothelial hyperplasia are thinner with collagenized/hyalinized cores containing prominent vessels in contrast to the more delicate smaller vessels haphazardly distributed in myxoid cores of WDPM. All the cases of WDPM in this study showed diffuse linear membranous immunostaining for epithelial membrane antibody.

The authors emphasize that the patients with WDPM showed prolonged survival, often several years or even decades. Seventeen patients were alive with disease, including 11 with survival longer than two years and three with follow-up periods between five and ten years. Ten-year survival was 30.8%. In two patients with no evidence of invasion in the initial biopsy, a ten-year symptom-free interval was observed before dissemination and death. The histologic features at the time of progression were those of conventional epithelioid mesothelioma. The survival ranged from 36 to 180 months

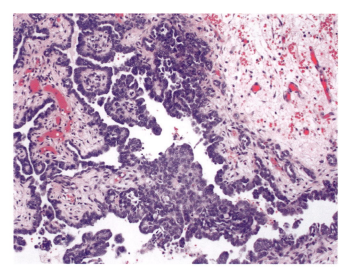

Fig. 17.48 Papillary mesothelioma with superficial invasion into underlying stroma mimicking well-differentiated papillary mesothelioma.

with an average of 74 months as compared with 10 months for 1248 paired patients with diffuse malignant mesothelioma. It appears from this study that the presence or absence of superficial invasion had no impact on disease progression.

In conclusion, the vast majority of published cases of WDPM at various anatomic sites behaved in a benign or indolent fashion. However, some cases have pursued a more aggressive course, resulting in death after the development of diffuse malignant mesothelioma. In our opinion, part of the problem is that the classic diagnostic criteria (small localized lesions with exclusively papillary pattern and no invasion) have been expanded in several studies, therefore, perhaps not surprisingly, some of the cases progressed to malignant mesothelioma. Those cases which are diagnosed on the basis of the classic criteria are expected to behave in a benign fashion (benign papillary mesothelioma). Multiple tumors with areas of more complex or solid areas or even superficial invasion (Fig. 17.48) should be regarded with great caution and not be classified as benign as they may follow a progressive clinical course even though there are reports of patients with widespread WDPMs with conventional histologic features that have behaved in a benign fashion[100]. Cases with invasion into the subpleural lung parenchyma and/or adipose tissue, in our opinion, should not be regarded as WDPM but malignant mesothelioma[103]. Clearly studies of more cases occurring at various serosal sites with long clinical follow-up combined with molecular pathologic data are needed to confidently distinguish benign localized papillary mesotheliomas from those WDPMs which are likely to have a slowly progressive course. Until such data are available, we agree with Brimo et al.[96] that WDPMs with more complex architecture can be classified as "mesotheliomas of uncertain malignant potential" and, as always, histologic findings must be correlated with clinical and imaging data.

Given the lack of any universally accepted treatment for mesothelioma, the short life expectancy and the need for definitive diagnosis in order to support claims for asbestos exposure compensation, the responsibility of the pathologist is onerous. The correlation between clinical history, radiographic/imaging and pathologic findings is a must for correct diagnosis. As the diagnosis of mesothelioma during life is often based on limited histological material, a multimodal diagnostic approach using routine and special stains, along with immunocytochemistry and sometimes electron microscopy is recommended. Guidelines for pathologic diagnosis of malignant mesothelioma have been published by the International Mesothelioma Interest Group [54], for the management of pleural malignant mesothelioma by the European Respiratory Society and European Society of Surgeons Task Force [104], and for peritoneal mesothelioma the guidelines reviewed by Chua *et al.* [105]. Pathologists play an important role in the management of malignant mesothelioma.

Mesenchymal tumors

There are rare case reports of primary benign mesenchymal tumors and sarcomas of the mediastinal pleura and pericardium. These include solitary fibrous tumor, epithelioid hemangioendothelioma, angiosarcoma, synovial sarcoma, solitary fibrous tumor, calcifying tumor of the pleura, and desmoplastic round cell tumor. These are discussed in detail in Chapter 13.

Lymphoproliferative disorders

There is more likely to be secondary involvement by nodal, bone marrow, or extra-nodal diseases since primary lymphoproliferative disorders of the pleura and pericardium are rare. The normal serosal membrane has only a few lymphoid cells. There may be a florid lymphoid or plasma cell infiltrate in conditions such as chronic infections and connective tissue diseases. IHC stains will show a mixed population of B and T-cells which is very helpful in excluding malignancy.

Primary effusion lymphoma occurs in HIV-infected patients and may involve one or multiple serosal cavities. The infiltrating tumor cells are large, pleomorphic, with deeply basophilic cytoplasm and prominent nucleoli. They are of null-phenotype (lack B- and T-cell markers) or aberrantly express CD3. Clonal rearrangements of immunoglobulin genes are seen on molecular genetic studies, confirming that these tumors are indeed of B-cell origin. Demonstration of human herpesvirus 8/Kaposi sarcoma herpesvirus viral genome is possible and diagnostic in all cases. In addition, most cases are co-infected with Ebstein-Barr virus [66].

Metastases to the pleura and pericardium

Metastases to mediastinal serosal membranes are much more common than a primary tumor such as malignant mesothelioma; however this is a very important differential diagnosis as discussed above. Electron microscopy is possible but is generally no longer easily available except in specialized centers. Even more sensitive and specific antibodies are becoming commercially available. Thus, IHC panels in differentiating various carcinomas, melanoma and sarcomas from mesothelioma and other rare tumors are very useful. There are several recent publications regarding the various antibodies available. The 2012 update in mesothelioma diagnosis guidelines by IMIG pathologists has tables listing the antibodies according to differential diagnosis and usefulness of the antibody [54]. Selection of which antibodies to use depends on the individual case, the differential diagnosis, the laboratory's experience and sensitivity and specificity of the antibody.

References

1. Sugarbaker DJ, Flores RM, Jaklitsch MT, Richards WG, Strauss GM, Corson JM, et al. Resection margins, extrapleural nodal status, and cell type determine postoperative long-term survival in trimodality therapy of malignant pleural mesothelioma: results in 183 patients. *J Thorac Cardiovasc Surg* 1999 Jan;117(1):54–63; discussion 63–5.

2. Kahi CJ, Dewitt JM, Lykens M, LeBlanc JK, Chappo J, McHenry L, et al. Diagnosis of a malignant mesothelioma by EUS-guided FNA of a mediastinal lymph node. *Gastrointest Endosc* 2004 Nov;60(5):859–61.

3. Clement PB, Young RH, Oliva E, Sumner HW, Scully RE. Hyperplastic mesothelial cells within abdominal lymph nodes: mimic of metastatic ovarian carcinoma and serous borderline tumor–a report of two cases associated with ovarian neoplasms. *Mod Pathol* 1996 Sep;9(9):879–86.

4. Colby TV. Benign mesothelial cells in lymph node. *Adv Anat Pathol* 1999 Jan;6(1):41–8.

5. Parkash V, Vidwans M, Carter D. Benign mesothelial cells in mediastinal lymph nodes. *Am J Surg Pathol* 1999 Oct;23(10):1264–9.

6. Moonim MT, Ng WW, Routledge T. Benign metastasizing mesothelial cells: a potential pitfall in mediastinal lymph nodes. *J Clin Oncol* 2011 Jun 20;29(18):e546–8.

7. Argani P, Rosai J. Hyperplastic mesothelial cells in lymph nodes: report of six cases of a benign process that can stimulate metastatic involvement by mesothelioma or carcinoma. *Hum Pathol* 1998 Apr;29(4):339–46.

8. Suarez Vilela D, Izquierdo Garcia FM. Embolization of mesothelial cells in lymphatics: the route to mesothelial inclusions in lymph nodes? *Histopathology* 1998 Dec;33(6):570–5.

9. Lin BT, Colby T, Gown AM, Hammar SP, Mertens RB, Churg A, et al. Malignant vascular tumors of the serous membranes mimicking mesothelioma. A report of 14 cases. *Am J Surg Pathol* 1996 Dec;20(12):1431–9.

10. Zhang PJ, Livolsi VA, Brooks JJ. Malignant epithelioid vascular tumors of the pleura: report of a series and literature review. *Hum Pathol* 2000 Jan;31(1):29–34.

11. Bahrami A, Allen TC, Cagle PT. Pulmonary epithelioid hemangioendothelioma mimicking mesothelioma. *Pathol Int* 2008 Nov;58(11):730–4.

12. Yanagi S, Sakamoto A, Tsubouchi H, Imai K, Imazu Y, Miyoshi K, et al. A case of pulmonary epithelioid hemangioendothelioma that required differentiation from malignant mesothelioma. *Nihon Kokyuki Gakkai Zasshi* 2010 May;48(5):385–90.

13. Carassai P, Caput M. Report of a case of epithelioid hemangioendothelioma of the anterior mediastinum metastatic to pleura. *Pathologica* 2010 Jun;102(3):112–14.

14. Hart J, Mandavilli S. Epithelioid angiosarcoma: a brief diagnostic review and differential diagnosis. *Arch Pathol Lab Med* 2011 Feb;135(2):268–72.

15. Witkin GB, Miettinen M, Rosai J. A Biphasic tumor of the mediastinum with features of synovial sarcoma. A report of four cases. *Am J Surg Pathol* 1989 Jun;13(6):490–9.

16. Suster S, Moran CA. Primary synovial sarcomas of the mediastinum: a clinicopathologic, immunohistochemical, and ultrastructural study of 15 cases. *Am J Surg Pathol* 2005 May;29(5):569–78.

17. Essary LR, Vargas SO, Fletcher CD. Primary pleuropulmonary synovial sarcoma: reappraisal of a recently described anatomic subset. *Cancer* 2002 Jan 15;94(2):459–69.

18. Begueret H, Galateau-Salle F, Guillou L, Chetaille B, Brambilla E, Vignaud JM, et al. Primary intrathoracic synovial sarcoma: a clinicopathologic study of 40 t(X;18)-positive cases from the French Sarcoma Group and the Mesopath Group. *Am J Surg Pathol* 2005 Mar;29(3):339–46.

19. Cheng Y, Sheng W, Zhou X, Wang J. Pericardial synovial sarcoma, a potential for misdiagnosis: clinicopathologic and molecular cytogenetic analysis of three cases with literature review. *Am J Clin Pathol* 2012 Jan;137(1):142–9.

20. Attanoos RL, Galateau-Salle F, Gibbs AR, Muller S, Ghandour F, Dojcinov SD. Primary thymic epithelial tumours of the pleura mimicking malignant mesothelioma. *Histopathology* 2002 Jul;41(1):42–9.

21. Vural M, Abali H, Oksuzoglu B, Akbulut M. An atypical presentation of thymoma with diffuse pleural dissemination mimicking mesothelioma. *Cancer Invest* 2006 Oct;24(6):615–20.

22. Michailova KN, Usunoff KG. Serosal membranes (pleura, pericardium, peritoneum). Normal structure, development and experimental pathology. *Adv Anat Embryol Cell Biol* 2006;183:i–vii, 1–144.

23. Mutsaers SE, Whitaker D, Papadimitriou JM. Mesothelial regeneration is not dependent on subserosal cells. *J Pathol* 2000 Jan;190(1):86–92.

24. Mutsaers SE. The mesothelial cell. *Int J Biochem Cell Biol* 2004 Jan;36(1):9–16.

25. Foley-Comer AJ, Herrick SE, Al-Mishlab T, Prele CM, Laurent GJ, Mutsaers SE. Evidence for incorporation of free-floating mesothelial cells as a mechanism of serosal healing. *J Cell Sci* 2002 Apr 1;115(Pt 7):1383–9.

26. West JB. Snorkel breathing in the elephant explains the unique anatomy of its pleura. *Respir Physiol* 2001 May;126(1):1–8.

27. West JB, Fu Z, Gaeth AP, Short RV. Fetal lung development in the elephant reflects the adaptations required for snorkeling in adult life. *Respir Physiol Neurobiol* 2003 Nov 14;138(2–3):325–33.

28. Yanez-Mo M, Lara-Pezzi E, Selgas R, Ramirez-Huesca M, Dominguez-Jimenez C, Jimenez-Heffernan JA, et al. Peritoneal dialysis and epithelial-to-mesenchymal transition of mesothelial cells. *N Engl J Med* 2003 Jan 30;348(5):403–13.

29. Schramm A, Opitz I, Thies S, Seifert B, Moch H, Weder W, et al. Prognostic significance of epithelial-mesenchymal transition in malignant pleural mesothelioma. *Eur J Cardiothorac Surg* 2010 Mar;37(3):566–72.

30. Fassina A, Cappellesso R, Guzzardo V, Dalla Via L, Piccolo S, Ventura L, et al. Epithelial-mesenchymal transition in malignant mesothelioma. *Mod Pathol* 2012 Jan;25(1):86–99.

31. Yang AH, Chen JY, Lin JK. Myofibroblastic conversion of mesothelial cells. *Kidney Int* 2003 Apr;63(4):1530–9.

32. Strippoli R, Benedicto I, Perez Lozano ML, Cerezo A, Lopez-Cabrera M, del Pozo MA. Epithelial-to-mesenchymal transition of peritoneal mesothelial cells is regulated by an ERK/NF-kappaB/Snail1 pathway. *Dis Model Mech* 2008 Nov–Dec;1(4–5):264–74.

33. Winter EM, Gittenberger-de Groot AC. Epicardium-derived cells in cardiogenesis and cardiac regeneration. *Cell Mol Life Sci* 2007 Mar;64(6):692–703.

34. Sivertsen S, Hadar R, Elloul S, Vintman L, Bedrossian C, Reich R, et al. Expression of Snail, Slug and Sip1 in malignant mesothelioma effusions is associated with matrix metalloproteinase, but not with cadherin expression. *Lung Cancer* 2006 Dec;54(3):309–17.

35. Horio M, Sato M, Takeyama Y, Elshazley M, Yamashita R, Hase T, et al. Transient but not stable ZEB1 knockdown dramatically inhibits growth of malignant pleural mesothelioma cells. *Ann Surg Oncol* 2012 Jul;19 Suppl 3:S634–45.

36. Merikallio H, Paakko P, Salmenkivi K, Kinnula V, Harju T, Soini Y. Expression of snail, twist, and Zeb1 in malignant mesothelioma. *APMIS* 2013 Jan;121(1):1–10.

37. Cano A, Nieto MA. Non-coding RNAs take centre stage in epithelial-to-mesenchymal transition. *Trends Cell Biol* 2008 Aug;18(8):357–9.

38. Korpal M, Lee ES, Hu G, Kang Y. The miR-200 family inhibits epithelial-mesenchymal transition and cancer cell migration by direct targeting of E-cadherin transcriptional repressors ZEB1 and ZEB2. *J Biol Chem* 2008 May 30;283(22):14910–14.

39. Tateishi K, Ikeda M, Yokoyama T, Urushihata K, Yamamoto H, Hanaoka M, et al. Primary malignant sarcomatoid mesothelioma in the pericardium. *Intern Med* 2013;52(2):249–53.

40. Ray R, Kumar N, Gupta R, Mridha AR, Tyagi JS, Kumar AS. Mesothelial/monocytic incidental cardiac excrescences (MICE) with tubercular aortitis: report of the first case with brief review of the literature. *J Clin Pathol* 2010 Sep;63(9):853–5.

41. Erinanc H, Gunday M, Saba T, Ozulku M, Sezgin A. Lesion of aggregated monocytes and mesothelial cells: mesothelial/monocytic incidental cardiac lesion. *Case Rep Pathol* 2013;2013:836398.

42. Bueno R, Reblando J, Glickman J, Jaklitsch MT, Lukanich JM, Sugarbaker DJ. Pleural biopsy: a reliable method for determining the diagnosis but not

subtype in mesothelioma. *Ann Thorac Surg* 2004 Nov;78(5):1774–6.

43. Arrossi AV, Lin E, Rice D, Moran CA. Histologic assessment and prognostic factors of malignant pleural mesothelioma treated with extrapleural pneumonectomy. *Am J Clin Pathol* 2008 Nov;130(5):754–64.

44. Churg A, Cagle PT, Roggli VL (eds). *Tumors of the Serosal Membranes. Atlas of Tumor Pathology.* Series 4, Fascicle 3. Silver Spring, MD: ARP Press; 2006.

45. Cavazza A, Moroni M, Bacigalupo B, Rossi G, De Marco L, Fedeli F. Malignant epithelioid mesothelioma of the pleura with hyaline globules. *Histopathology* 2003 Nov;43(5):500–1.

46. Ordonez NG. Mesotheliomas with crystalloid structures: report of nine cases, including one with oncocytic features. *Mod Pathol* 2012 Feb;25(2):272–81.

47. Ordonez NG. Deciduoid mesothelioma: report of 21 cases with review of the literature. *Mod Pathol* 2012 Nov;25(11):1481–95.

48. Ordonez NG. Mesotheliomas with small cell features: report of eight cases. *Mod Pathol* 2012 May;25(5):689–98.

49. Kadota K, Suzuki K, Sima CS, Rusch VW, Adusumilli PS, Travis WD. Pleomorphic epithelioid diffuse malignant pleural mesothelioma: a clinicopathological review and conceptual proposal to reclassify as biphasic or sarcomatoid mesothelioma. *J Thorac Oncol* 2011 May;6(5):896–904.

50. Beer TW, Buchanan R, Matthews AW, Stradling R, Pullinger N, Pethybridge RJ. Prognosis in malignant mesothelioma related to MIB 1 proliferation index and histological subtype. *Hum Pathol* 1998 Mar;29(3):246–51.

51. Comin CE, Anichini C, Boddi V, Novelli L, Dini S. MIB-1 proliferation index correlates with survival in pleural malignant mesothelioma. *Histopathology* 2000 Jan;36(1):26–31.

52. Cerruto CA, Brun EA, Chang D, Sugarbaker PH. Prognostic significance of histomorphologic parameters in diffuse malignant peritoneal mesothelioma. *Arch Pathol Lab Med* 2006 Nov;130(11):1654–61.

53. Kadota K, Suzuki K, Colovos C, Sima CS, Rusch VW, Travis WD, *et al.*

A nuclear grading system is a strong predictor of survival in epithelioid diffuse malignant pleural mesothelioma. *Mod Pathol* 2012 Feb;25(2):260–71.

54. Husain AN, Colby T, Ordonez N, Krausz T, Attanoos R, Beasley MB, *et al.* Guidelines for Pathologic Diagnosis of Malignant Mesothelioma: 2012 Update of the Consensus Statement from the International Mesothelioma Interest Group. *Arch Pathol Lab Med* 2013 May; 137(5):647–67.

55. Klebe S, Nurminen M, Leigh J, Henderson DW. Diagnosis of epithelial mesothelioma using tree-based regression analysis and a minimal panel of antibodies. *Pathology* 2009 Feb;41(2):140–8.

56. Illei PB, Ladanyi M, Rusch VW, Zakowski MF. The use of CDKN2A deletion as a diagnostic marker for malignant mesothelioma in body cavity effusions. *Cancer* 2003 Feb 25;99(1):51–6.

57. Dacic S, Kothmaier H, Land S, Shuai Y, Halbwedl I, Morbini P, *et al.* Prognostic significance of p16/cdkn2a loss in pleural malignant mesotheliomas. *Virchows Arch* 2008 Dec;453(6):627–35.

58. Krasinskas AM, Bartlett DL, Cieply K, Dacic S. CDKN2A and MTAP deletions in peritoneal mesotheliomas are correlated with loss of p16 protein expression and poor survival. *Mod Pathol* 2010 Apr;23(4):531–8.

59. Travis WD. Sarcomatoid neoplasms of the lung and pleura. *Arch Pathol Lab Med* 2010 Nov;134(11):1645–58.

60. Klebe S, Brownlee NA, Mahar A, Burchette JL, Sporn TA, Vollmer RT, *et al.* Sarcomatoid mesothelioma: a clinical-pathologic correlation of 326 cases. *Mod Pathol* 2010 Mar;23(3):470–9.

61. Wilson GE, Hasleton PS, Chatterjee AK. Desmoplastic malignant mesothelioma: a review of 17 cases. *J Clin Pathol* 1992 Apr;45(4):295–8.

62. Churg A, Cagle P, Colby TV, Corson JM, Gibbs AR, Hammar S, *et al.* The fake fat phenomenon in organizing pleuritis: A source of confusion with desmoplastic malignant mesotheliomas. *Am J Surg Pathol* 2011 Dec; 35(12):1823–9.

63. Mangano WE, Cagle PT, Churg A, Vollmer RT, Roggli VL. The diagnosis

of desmoplastic malignant mesothelioma and its distinction from fibrous pleurisy: a histologic and immunohistochemical analysis of 31 cases including p53 immunostaining. *Am J Clin Pathol* 1998 Aug;110(2):191–9.

64. Chiosea S, Krasinskas A, Cagle PT, Mitchell KA, Zander DS, Dacic S. Diagnostic importance of 9p21 homozygous deletion in malignant mesotheliomas. *Mod Pathol* 2008 Jun;21(6):742–7.

65. Henderson DW, Attwood HD, Constance TJ, Shilkin KB, Steele RH. Lymphohistiocytoid mesothelioma: a rare lymphomatoid variant of predominantly sarcomatoid mesothelioma. *Ultrastruct Pathol* 1988;12(4):367–84.

66. Attanoos R. Lymphoproliferative conditions of the serosa. *Arch Pathol Lab Med* 2012 Mar;136(3):268–76.

67. Miettinen M, Limon J, Niezabitowski A, Lasota J. Calretinin and other mesothelioma markers in synovial sarcoma: analysis of antigenic similarities and differences with malignant mesothelioma. *Am J Surg Pathol* 2001 May;25(5):610–17.

68. Matsuyama A, Hisaoka M, Iwasaki M, Iwashita M, Hisanaga S, Hashimoto H. TLE1 expression in malignant mesothelioma. *Virchows Arch* 2010 Nov;457(5):577–83.

69. Crotty TB, Myers JL, Katzenstein AL, Tazelaar HD, Swensen SJ, Churg A. Localized malignant mesothelioma. A clinicopathologic and flow cytometric study. *Am J Surg Pathol* 1994 Apr;18(4):357–63.

70. Allen TC, Cagle PT, Churg AM, Colby TV, Gibbs AR, Hammar SP, *et al.* Localized malignant mesothelioma. *Am J Surg Pathol* 2005 Jul;29(7):866–73.

71. Crotty TB, Colby TV, Gay PC, Pisani RJ. Desmoplastic malignant mesothelioma masquerading as sclerosing mediastinitis: a diagnostic dilemma. *Hum Pathol* 1992 Jan;23(1):79–82.

72. Bierhoff E, Pfeifer U. Malignant mesothelioma arising from a benign mediastinal mesothelial cyst. *Gen Diagn Pathol* 1996 Jun;142(1):59–62.

73. Tagliamonti JA, Yannopoulos K, Kryle LS. Malignant epithelial mesothelioma of the anterior mediastinum. *N Y State J Med* 1984 Mar;84(3 Pt 1):127–9.

74. Togashi K, Hosaka Y, Sato K. Sarcomatoid pleural mesothelioma presenting as posterior mediastinal tumor with dysphagia. *Kyobu Geka* 2007 Jan;60(1):49–52.

75. Akamoto S, Ono Y, Ota K, Suzaki N, Sasaki A, Matsuo Y, et al. Localized malignant mesothelioma in the middle mediastinum: report of a case. *Surg Today* 2008;38(7):635–8.

76. Ruffie P, Feld R, Minkin S, Cormier Y, Boutan-Laroze A, Ginsberg R, et al. Diffuse malignant mesothelioma of the pleura in Ontario and Quebec: a retrospective study of 332 patients. *J Clin Oncol* 1989 Aug;7(8):1157–68.

77. Johnson CE, Wardman AG, McMahon MJ, Cooke NJ. Dysphagia complicating malignant mesothelioma. *Thorax* 1983 Aug;38(8):635–6.

78. Liu W, Fackler W, Rice TW, Richter JE, Achkar E, Goldblum JR. The pathogenesis of pseudoachalasia: a clinicopathologic study of 13 cases of a rare entity. *Am J Surg Pathol* 2002 Jun;26(6):784–8.

79. Hayama M, Maeda H. A rare cause of dysphagia: malignant pleural mesothelioma in the posterior mediastinum. *Ann Thorac Surg* 2010 Oct;90(4):1358–61.

80. Travis WD, Lack EE, Azumi N, Tsokos M, Norton J. Adenomatoid tumor of the adrenal gland with ultrastructural and immunohistochemical demonstration of a mesothelial origin. *Arch Pathol Lab Med* 1990 Jul;114(7):722–4.

81. Hoffmann M, Yedibela S, Dimmler A, Hohenberger W, Meyer T. Adenomatoid tumor of the adrenal gland mimicking an echinococcus cyst of the liver–a case report. *Int J Surg* 2008 Dec;6(6):485–7.

82. Hayes SJ, Clark P, Mathias R, Formela L, Vickers J, Armstrong GR. Multiple adenomatoid tumours in the liver and peritoneum. *J Clin Pathol* 2007 Jun;60(6):722–4.

83. Nagata S, Aishima S, Fukuzawa K, Takagi H, Yonemasu H, Iwashita Y, et al. Adenomatoid tumour of the liver. *J Clin Pathol* 2008 Jun;61(6):777–80.

84. Adachi S, Yanagawa T, Furumoto A, Fujino S, Doi R, Dono K, et al. Adenomatoid tumor of the liver. *Pathol Int* 2012 Feb;62(2):153–4.

85. Kim JB, Yu E, Shim JH, Song GW, Kim GU, Jin YJ, et al. Concurrent hepatic adenomatoid tumor and hepatic hemangioma: a case report. *Clin Mol Hepatol* 2012 Jun;18(2):229–34.

86. Natarajan S, Luthringer DJ, Fishbein MC. Adenomatoid tumor of the heart: report of a case. *Am J Surg Pathol* 1997 Nov;21(11):1378–80.

87. Tursi M, Martinetti M, Gili S, Muscio M, Gay L, Crudelini M, et al. Myocardial adenomatoid tumor in eight cattle: evidence for mesothelial origin of bovine myocardial epithelial inclusions. *Vet Pathol* 2009 Sep;46(5):897–903.

88. Plaza JA, Dominguez F, Suster S. Cystic adenomatoid tumor of the mediastinum. *Am J Surg Pathol* 2004 Jan;28(1):132–8.

89. Ikuta N, Tano M, Iwata M, Ishiguro H, Nishiura T, Inagaki T, et al. A case of adenomatoid mesothelioma of the pleura. *Nihon Kyobu Shikkan Gakkai Zasshi* 1989 Dec;27(12):1540–4.

90. Kaplan MA, Tazelaar HD, Hayashi T, Schroer KR, Travis WD. Adenomatoid tumors of the pleura. *Am J Surg Pathol* 1996 Oct;20(10):1219–23.

91. Handra-Luca A, Couvelard A, Abd Alsamad I, Launay O, Larousserie F, Walker F, et al. Adenomatoid tumor of the pleura. Case report. *Ann Pathol* 2000 Sep;20(4):369–72.

92. Minato H, Nojima T, Kurose N, Kinoshita E. Adenomatoid tumor of the pleura. *Pathol Int* 2009 Aug;59(8):567–71.

93. Weissferdt A, Kalhor N, Suster S. Malignant mesothelioma with prominent adenomatoid features: a clinicopathologic and immunohistochemical study of 10 cases. *Ann Diagn Pathol* 2011 Feb;15(1):25–9.

94. Morita S, Goto A, Sakatani T, Ota S, Murakawa T, Nakajima J, et al. Multicystic mesothelioma of the pericardium. *Pathol Int* 2011 May;61(5):319–21.

95. Malpica A, Sant'Ambrogio S, Deavers MT, Silva EG. Well-differentiated papillary mesothelioma of the female peritoneum: a clinicopathologic study of 26 cases. *Am J Surg Pathol* 2012 Jan;36(1):117–27.

96. Brimo F, Illei PB, Epstein JI. Mesothelioma of the tunica vaginalis: a series of eight cases with uncertain malignant potential. *Mod Pathol* 2010 Aug;23(8):1165–72.

97. Sane AC, Roggli VL. Curative resection of a well-differentiated papillary mesothelioma of the pericardium. *Arch Pathol Lab Med* 1995 Mar;119(3):266–7.

98. Butnor KJ, Sporn TA, Hammar SP, Roggli VL. Well-differentiated papillary mesothelioma. *Am J Surg Pathol* 2001 Oct;25(10):1304–9.

99. Galateau-Salle F, Vignaud JM, Burke L, Gibbs A, Brambilla E, Attanoos R, et al. Well-differentiated papillary mesothelioma of the pleura: a series of 24 cases. *Am J Surg Pathol* 2004 Apr;28(4):534–40.

100. Daya D, McCaughey WT. Well-differentiated papillary mesothelioma of the peritoneum. A clinicopathologic study of 22 cases. *Cancer* 1990 Jan 15;65(2):292–6.

101. Travis WD, Brambilla E, Müller-Hermelink HK, Harris CC (eds). *Pathology and Genetics: Tumours of the Lung, Pleura, Thymus and Heart.* Lyon, France: IARC; 2004.

102. Goldblum J, Hart WR. Localized and diffuse mesotheliomas of the genital tract and peritoneum in women. A clinicopathologic study of nineteen true mesothelial neoplasms, other than adenomatoid tumors, multicystic mesotheliomas, and localized fibrous tumors. *Am J Surg Pathol* 1995 Oct;19(10):1124–37.

103. Torii I, Hashimoto M, Terada T, Kondo N, Fushimi H, Shimazu K, et al. Well-differentiated papillary mesothelioma with invasion to the chest wall. *Lung Cancer* 2010 Feb;67(2):244–7.

104. Scherpereel A, Astoul P, Baas P, Berghmans T, Clayson H, de Vuyst P, et al. Guidelines of the European Respiratory Society and the European Society of Thoracic Surgeons for the management of malignant pleural mesothelioma. *Eur Respir J* 2010 Mar;35(3):479–95.

105. Chua TC, Yan TD, Morris DL. Surgical biology for the clinician: peritoneal mesothelioma: current understanding and management. *Can J Surg* 2009 Feb;52(1):59–64.

Index

abscess, 19, 27, 216
acetylcholine receptor (AChR) autoantibodies,
    myasthenia gravis, 56, 67, 276
    detection of, 69
    laboratory tests for, 276–7
acquired immunodeficiency syndrome (AIDS), 56
acute cellular rejection (ACR), 297–8
acute myocardial infarction (AMI), 280
    clinical laboratory studies, 280–1
    necrosis markers, 280
adenocarcinoma, 333
adenomatoid tumor, 337–8
adenosquamous carcinoma of the thymus, 108
allograft rejection, 297–8
alveolar soft part sarcoma (ASPS), 254–5
amyloidosis, cardiac, 293–4
anaplastic carcinoma of the thymus, 112
anaplastic large cell lymphoma (ALCL), 206–8
anaplastic lymphoma kinase (ALK), 208
angina, 280
angiolipoma, 243
angiomatoid carcinoid, 140
angiomyolipoma, 256
angiosarcoma, 237–9
anterior mediastinum, 3
    masses, 4–8
antibody mediated rejection (AMR), 297–9
aortic injury, 15–17
aortic valve (AV), 300–4
arrhythmogenic right ventricular cardiomyopathy (ARVCM), 282, 289–90
Askin tumors, 233
atrioventricular valves, examination, 301

autoimmune polyendocrinopathy candidiasis ectodermal dystrophy (APECED), 68
Autoimmune Regulator (AIRE) gene, 45

basaloid squamous cell carcinoma of the mediastinum (BSCC), 109
B-cell lymphomas. See lymphomas
benign cystic teratoma (BCT), 220–1
bicuspid aortic valve (BAV), 303
biliary atresia, 56
biopsy
    endomyocardial (EMB), 285–300
    germ cell tumor diagnosis, 148
    indications, 272–3
    parathyroid lesions, 174
    thymoma diagnosis, 89–90
biphasic mesothelioma, 336–7
Bochdalek hernia, 11
bone marrow allograft recipients, 56
brain natriuretic peptide (BNP), 281–2
bronchogenic cysts, 11, 158, 214–15
Bruton's X-linked hypogammaglobulinemia, 54
Burkitt lymphoma, 203–4

carcinoid
    angiomatoid, 140
    combined with thymolipoma, 143
    oncocytic, 140
    pigmented, 139
    spindle cell, 139
    with mucinous stroma, 139–40
    with sarcomatoid changes, 143
carcinoid heart disease, 308
cardiac allograft vasculopathy (CAV), 298
cardiac amyloidosis, 293–4
cardiac myxoma, 295

cardiac sarcoidosis, 293
cardiac toxicity, 297
cardiac valves, 300–8, see also specific valves
    anatomy, 300
    endocarditis, 307
    examination, 300–1
    histochemical stains, 301
    regurgitation, 301
    stenosis, 300
    substitute valves, 310–11
cardiomyopathies, 282–3
    arrhythmogenic right ventricular cardiomyopathy (ARVCM), 282, 289–90
    dilated (DCM), 287–8
    genetic tests, 282–3
    hypertrophic (HCM), 282, 288
    mitochondrial (MIC), 290–2
    peripartum (PPCM), 290
    restrictive (RC), 289
Castleman's disease, 11
catecholaminergic polymorphic ventricular tachycardia (CPVT), 283
chemodectoma, 15
children, thymomas, 94–5
chondrosarcoma, 249
    extraskeletal mesenchymal, 249–50
    extraskeletal myxoid (EMC), 250
chordoma, 255
choriocarcinoma, 163–4
    differential diagnosis, 154, 163–4
    immunohistochemistry, 164
clear-cell carcinoma of the thymus, 108
clear-cell sarcoma of soft tissue (CCST), 257–8
clear-cell sugar tumor (CCST), 256
clinical diagnosis, 270–2
combined thymoma and thymic carcinoma, 81
composite paraganglioma-neuroblastoma (PG-NB), 180

congenital heart disease (CHD), 283
congenital infantile fibrosarcoma, 240–2
congestive heart failure, 281–2
coronary artery disease, 280
Cushing's syndrome, 132
    clinical laboratory studies, 278
cystic hygromas, 218, 234
cysts, see mediastinal cysts; specific cysts

dedifferentiation, 245
desmoid-type fibromatosis (DTF), 237
desmoplastic small round cell tumor (DSRCT), 254
Di George's syndrome, 54
diaphragmatic hernia, 13
diffuse large B-cell lymphoma (DLBCL), 200–2
    EBV-positive, 205
dilated cardiomyopathy (DCM), 287–8
duplication cysts, 11
dysgammaglobulinemia, 56
dysphagia, 26
dyspnea, 26, 65

Echinococcus granulosus, 216
ectopic thymic tissue, 38
ectopic thyroid tissue, 280
embryonal carcinoma, 162–3
    differential diagnosis, 163
    immunohistochemistry, 163
endocarditis, 307
endomyocardial biopsy (EMB), 285–300
    allograft rejection, 297–8
    arrhythmogenic right ventricular cardiomyopathy (ARVC), 289–90
    cardiac amyloidosis, 293–4
    cardiac sarcoidosis, 293
    cardiac tumors, 295

dilated cardiomyopathy (DCM), 287–8
endomyocardial fibrosis (EMF), 293
hypersensitivity myocarditis, 297
iron overload, 295
Löffler endocarditis (LE), 293
mitochondrial cardiomyopathies (MIC), 290–2
muscular dystrophies, 290, 292
myocarditis, 285–7
peripartum cardiomyopathy (PPCM), 290
restrictive cardiomyopathy (RC), 289
storage diseases, 290
endomyocardial fibrosis (EMF), 292–3
enteric cysts, 158, 215
ependymoma, 234
epithelial-to-mesenchymal transition (EMT), 319–20
epithelioid hemangioendothelioma, 235–7, 317
epithelioid large cell tumors, 261
epithelioid mesothelioma, 326–33
Epstein–Barr virus (EBV)
diffuse large B-cell lymphoma and, 205
thymoma association, 68
esophageal abnormalities, 11
cancer, 11
cysts, 215
dilatation, 11
varices, 11
esophageal perforation, 19
mediastinitis and, 25–6
Ewing sarcoma family of tumors (ESFT), 233
explanted heart, 308–10
extramedullary hematopoiesis, 15
extraosseous osteosarcoma (EOS), 251
extraskeletal mesenchymal chondrosarcoma, 249–50
extraskeletal myxoid chondrosarcoma (EMC), 250

fibrosarcoma, 237–40
congenital infantile, 240–2
fibrosing mediastinitis, 19
fibrous pleurisy, 320
foregut embryology, 212
foreign body giant cell reaction, 322

galectin-3, 282
ganglioneuroma, 233
gastroenteric cysts (GECs), 215

germ cell tumors, 7–8, 106, 146
choriocarcinoma, 163–4
clinical features, 148
clinical laboratory studies, 277–8
prognostic factors, 278
diagnosis, 148
differential diagnosis, 120, 154
distribution of histologic subtypes, 149–51
postpubertal female patients, 151
postpubertal male patients, 149–50
prepubertal patients, 151
embryonal carcinoma, 162–3
epidemiology, 149
genetics, 149
location, 146–7
metastatic, 165
mixed, teratomatous components, 157
pathogenesis theories, 148
seminomas, 151–5
somatic-type malignancy of germ cell tumor origin, 157
staging, 151
teratomas, 155–8
yolk sac tumors, 158–62
Glanzmann-Riniker disease, 54
glomerulonephritis, 69
goblet cell carcinoma, 143
goiter, 8, 185
Good's syndrome, 68
graft-versus-host disease (GVHD), 56
granular cell tumor (GCT), 226
granulocytic sarcoma, 208
granuloma
cardiac sarcoidosis, 293
sclerosing mediastinitis, 28–9
excision, 31
granulomatous inflammation, 321–2
Graves disease, 280
gray zone lymphoma, 203

Hassall's corpuscles, 40–1, 43
heart disease, 280,
see also cardiac valves; cardiomyopathies
acute coronary syndromes, 281
allograft rejection, 297–8
carcinoid, 308
cardiac amyloidosis, 293–4
cardiac sarcoidosis, 293
catecholaminergic polymorphic ventricular tachycardia (CPVT), 283
clinical laboratory studies, 280–1
congenital heart disease (CHD), 283

congestive heart failure, 281–2
drug toxicity/hypersensitivity reactions, 295–7
endomyocardial fibrosis (EF), 292–3
explanted heart, 308–10
genetic tests, 282–3
iron overload, 294–5
Löffler endocarditis (LE), 292–3
myocarditis, 285–7
prostheses/devices, 310–12
substitute valves, 310–11
ventricular assist devices, 312
storage diseases, 291
tumors, 295
hemangioendothelioma
epithelioid, 235–7
kaposiform, 237
hemangioma, 219, 235
hemangiopericytoma, 251–3
hernia
diaphragmatic, 13
hiatal, 11
heterologous thymomas, 81
hiatal hernia, 11
hibernoma, 243
hila, 3
Histoplasma capsulatum, 10, 19
histoplasmosis, 28–9
Hodgkin's lymphoma, 8, 120, 202–3
differential diagnosis, 153
nodular lymphocyte predominant (NLPHL), 202–3
overlapping features, 203
human herpesvirus 8 (HHV-8), 205
human immunodeficiency virus (HIV), 56
hydatid cyst, 216
hypercalcemia, 170, 174
laboratory investigation, 278–9
hyperparathyroidism, 170, 278
hypersensitivity myocarditis, 295–7
hypertrophic cardiomyopathy (HCM), 282, 288
hypertrophic osteoarthropathy, 69
hypogammaglobulinemia, 54

IgG4-related sclerosing disease, 31–3
immunodeficiency syndromes see also specific syndromes
congenital, 54–5
thymic dysplasia, 55–6
thymoma association, 68
infective endocarditis, 307
inflammatory myofibroblastic tumor (IMT), 242

infraaortic area, 1
infraazygous area, 1
injury, 15–17
aortic, 15–17
esophageal perforation, 19
tracheobronchial, 19
intermediate filament typing, 183
iron overload, 294–5

Kaposi sarcoma, 237
kaposiform hemangioendothelioma, 237
Kasabach-Merritt phenomenon, 237
keratinizing squamous cell carcinoma of the thymus (KSCC), 106
Klinefelter syndrome, 149

Lambert–Eaton syndrome (LES), 66, 67, 277
Langerhan cell histiocytosis (LCH), 209
leiomyoma, 248
leiomyosarcoma (LMS), 248
lipoblastoma, 243–4
lipoblastomatosis, 243
lipofibroadenoma, thymus gland, 85
lipoma, 243
lipomatosis, 243
liposarcoma, 244–6
Löffler endocarditis (LE), 292–3
lymph nodes, 8
calcified, 8
histoplasmosis, 29
granulomatous infections, 30
metastases, 10
size, 8
lymphadenopathy, 8–11
lymphangioleiomyomatosis (LAM), 256–7
lymphangioma, 218–19, 234–5
lymphangiomatosis, 235
lymphoblastic lymphoma, 206
lymphocyte-depleted thymoma with atypia, 80–1
lymphocyte-rich thymomas, 74–6
with atypia, 77–9
with spindle cells, 76–7
lymphoepithelioma-like thymic carcinoma (LETC), 106–7
lymphoid hyperplasia, 7
lymphomas, 8, 199–200 see also Hodgkin's lymphoma; non-Hodgkin's lymphoma
anaplastic large cell lymphoma (ALCL), 206–8
B-cell lymphoma, unclassifiable, 204
Burkitt, 203–4
differential diagnosis, 120, 153

lymphomas (cont.)
diffuse large B-cell lymphoma
(DLBCL), 200–2
EBV-positive, 205
low grade, 200
lymphoblastic, 206
overlapping features, 203
peripheral T-cell, 208
plasmablastic, 205
primary effusion, 205–6, 340
primary mediastinal large B-
cell lymphoma (PMLBL),
200–2
lymphorrhages, 219

malignant peripheral nerve
sheath tumors (MPNST),
230–1
malignant rhabdoid tumor
(MRT), 260
mediastinal cysts, 11, 211,
see also specific cysts
acquired cystic lesions,
216–23
infectious and
postinflammatory lesions,
216
congenital cystic lesions,
211–16
embryology, 211–12
cystic change in solid
neoplasms, 221–2
in thymomas, 70–1
primary cystic neoplasms,
218–20
mediastinal germ cell tumors,
see germ cell tumors
mediastinal hemorrhage, 33
mediastinitis, 19–22, 25, 282
acute, 19, 25–7
clinical findings, 25–7
etiology, 25
pathology, 27
treatment, 27
chronic, 19–22, 27–31,
see also sclerosing
mediastinitis
laboratory findings, 282
mediastinum, 1
anatomy, 2
classifications, 1–3
compartments, 3
disorders, 276
injury, 15–17
megakaryoblastic leukemia, 161
melanoma
differential diagnosis, 122, 153
malignant, 122
sarcomatoid, 258
metastatic, 153
melanotic neuroectodermal
tumor of infancy, 233
meningocele, 215, 258
mesenchymal chondrosarcoma,
249–50

mesenchymal tumors, 226, 340,
see also specific tumors
differential diagnosis, 260–2
mesenchymoma, 258
mesothelial cells, 318–20
epithelial-to-mesenchymal
transition (EMT),
319–20
mesothelial hyperplasia,
322, 333
mesothelial lesions, 317
mesothelioma, 122–3
benign multicystic, 338
biphasic, 336–7
classification, 326
deciduoid, 327
desmoplastic, 333–5
differential diagnosis, 122–3,
333, 336–7
diffuse malignant, 323–37
epithelioid, 326–33
pleomorphic, 327
localized malignant, 337
lymphohistiocytoid, 335
sarcomatoid, 335
small cell, 327
transitional, 336
well-differentiated papillary
(WDPM), 338–40
mesothelium, 318–19
metastases, 119–20
cardiac, 295
differential diagnosis, 119–20,
162, 333
lymph nodes, 10
metastatic germ cell tumors,
165
to serosal membranes, 340
micronodular lymphoid-rich
thymic carcinoma
(MLRTC), 113–15
micronodular thymoma, 83–4
middle mediastinum, 3
masses, 8–13
mitochondrial cardiomyopathies
(MICs), 290–2
mitral valve (MV), 300, 304–6
annular calcification (MAC),
305–6
prolapse (MVP), 305
regurgitation (MR), 305
stenosis (MS), 304–5
Morgagni hernia, 11
mucinous carcinoma of the
thymus, 113
muco-cutaneous candidiasis, 68
mucoepidermoid carcinoma of
the thymus, 108
mucosa-associated lymphoid
tissue (MALT), 200
Mullerian cysts, 219
multicystic mesothelial
proliferation of
borderline malignancy
(MMPBM), 220

multilocular mesothelial
inclusion cyst, 323
multilocular thymic cysts
(MTCs), 157–8, 216–18
proliferating, 217
multinodular thyroid
hyperplasia, 187
multiple endocrine neoplasia
(MEN), 131–2
parathyroid tumors and, 170
muscular dystrophies, 290
endomyocardial biopsy, 292
myasthenia gravis (MG), 43,
56–8
clinical laboratory studies,
276–7
adult MG panel, 276–7
MG/Lambert–Eaton
syndrome panel, 277
pediatric MG panel, 277
thymoma MG panel, 277
congenital myasthenia
syndromes, 57
serum autoantibody detection,
69
thymic follicular hyperplasia,
57
thymoma association, 58,
66–7, 69
pathogenesis, 67
prognostic signficance, 67
thymoma characteristics, 85
myeloid sarcoma, 208
myelolipoma, 244
myocarditis, 285–7
endomyocardial biopsy,
285–7
giant cell, 287
hypersensitivity, 295–7
myogenic neoplasms, 246–8
myoglobin assay, 280
myxoma, cardiac, 295

natriuretic hormone testing,
281–2
Naxos syndrome, 282
nephrotic syndrome, 69
neurilemmoma, 226
neuroblastoma, 15, 231–2
neuroendocrine carcinomas of
the thymus (NEC), 131,
181, 183
classification, 131
combined with other tumors,
143
differential diagnosis, 174
grade III, 140–3
large cell carcinoma variant,
141–3
small cell carcinoma variant,
140–1
treatment, 143
with other thymic
carcinoma components,
143

grades I and II, 131–9
angiomatoid carcinoid, 140
carcinoid with mucinous
stroma, 139–40
differential diagnosis, 138
histochemical and
immunohistochemical
features, 135–7
imaging findings, 132
oncocytic carcinoid, 140
pathology, 132
pigmented carcinoid, 139
prognosis, 138
spindle cell carcinoid, 139
treatment, 138
typical and atypical tumors,
131–2
ultrastructural features,
137–8
with grades I–III features, 143
neuroendocrine tumors, clinical
laboratory studies, 278
neuroenteric cysts, 11
neurofibroma, 15, 229–30
Nezelof's syndrome, 54
nodular lymphocyte
predominant Hodgkin's
lymphoma (NLPHL),
202–3
non-bacterial thrombotic
endocarditis (NBTE), 307
non-Hodgkin's lymphoma, 8,
120
non-keratinizing squamous cell
carcinoma of the thymus
(NKSCC), 106
non-seminomatous germ cell
tumors, 7–8

oncocytic carcinoma, 140

pancreatic pseudocysts, 216
papillary adenocarcinoma of the
thymus, 108
papillary fibroelastoma (PFE),
295
paragangliomas, 15, 174–81
aorticosympathetic, 175
branchiomeric, 175
clinical characteristics, 177
composite paraganglioma-
neuroblastoma (PG-NB),
180
genetic findings, 180–1
histology, 178–80
historical considerations, 176–7
immunohistology, 183–4
macroscopic features, 177–8
prognosis, 184
radiographic findings, 177
treatment, 185
ultrastructural features,
181–3
parathyroid gland embryology,
212

parathyroid hormone (PTH), 170, 183
parathyroid tumors, 212
  adenomas, 173–4
    clinical laboratory studies, 278–9
  carcinomas, 174
  clinical features, 170
  cysts, 212
  cytogenetic findings, 175
  cytology, 38–43
  histology, 38–43
  historical considerations, 169–70
  immunohistology, 183–4
  lipoadenomas, 174
  macroscopic features, 170–1
  parathyroid hyperplasia, 173–4
  prognosis, 184
  radiographic findings, 170
  treatment, 185
  ultrastructural features, 181–3
pemphigus erythematosus, 68
pemphigus vulgaris, 68
pericardial cysts, 11, 215, 323
pericarditis, 321
peripartum cardiomyopathy (PPCM), 290
peripheral nerve sheath tumors, 226–31
  malignant tumors, 230–1
  neurofibroma, 15, 229–30
  schwannoma, 15, 226–9
peripheral T-cell lymphomas, 208
perivascular epithelioid cell tumor (PEComa), 255–7
perivascular spaces, 42
pigmented carcinoid, 139
placental site trophoblastic tumor, 164–5
plasmablastic lymphoma, 205
pleomorphic adenoma (PA), 194–5
pleomorphic undifferentiated tumors, 262
  sarcoma (MFH), 240
pleuritis, 320
pleuropericardial membranes, 212
popcorn-cells, 203
posterior mediastinum, 3
  masses, 13–19
primary effusion lymphoma, 205–6
primary mediastinal large B-cell lymphoma (PMLBL), 200–2
primary thymic carcinoma (PTC), 5–6, 104–6,
  see also thymic carcinoma
  adenosquamous carcinoma, 108

adjunctive pathological findings, 115–19
anaplastic carcinoma, 112
basaloid squamous cell carcinoma (BSCC), 109
clear-cell carcinoma, 108
clinical findings, 106
differential diagnosis, 119–23
  germ cell tumors, 120
  malignant melanoma, 122
  mesothelioma, 122–3
  metastatic mediastinal carcinomas, 119–20
  sarcoma, 122
etiology, 106
keratinizing squamous cell carcinoma (KSCC), 106
lymphoepithelioma-like thymic carcinoma (LETC), 106–7
management, 125–6
micronodular lymphoid-rich carcinoma (MLRTC), 113–15
mucinous carcinoma, 113
mucoepidermoid carcinoma, 108
non-keratinizing squamous cell carcinoma (NSCC), 106
papillary adenocarcinoma, 108
rhabdoid carcinoma, 113
sarcomatoid carcinoma, 109–12
staging, 123–5
thymoma differentiation, 104–6
prosthetic endocarditis, 310
pulmonary thrombosis, 30
pulmonary valve (PV), 300, 306–7
  regurgitation, 307
  stenosis, 306–7

Quilty effect, 298

red cell aplasia, 68
Reed–Sternberg (RS) cells, 202
respiratory distress, 25
respiratory system embryology, 211–12
restrictive cardiomyopathy (RC), 289
reticular dysgenesis, 54
rhabdoid thymic carcinoma, 113
rhabdomyoma, 248
rhabdomyomatous thymoma, 84
rhabdomyosarcoma (RMS), 246–8
rheumatic fever, 304
rheumatoid nodule, 321

sarcoidosis, 10, 321
  cardiac, 293
sarcomas, 122

alveolar soft part sarcoma, 254–5
arising in germ cell neoplasms, 258
clear-cell sarcoma of soft tissue, 257–8
differential diagnosis, 122
Ewings sarcoma family of tumors (ESFT), 233
Kaposi, 237
myeloid, 208
of germ cell tumor origin, 159–61
pleomorphic undifferentiated, 240
synovial, 253–4, 318
sarcomatoid malignant melanoma, 258
sarcomatoid mesothelioma, 335
sarcomatoid thymic carcinoma, 109–12
schwannoma, 15, 226–9
  cellular, 228
  melanotic, 227–8
sclerosing mediastinitis, 19, 27–31, see also IgG4-related sclerosing disease
sclerosing thymoma, 84
semilunar valves, 300
  examination, 301
seminomas, 7, 151–5
  differential diagnosis, 153–4, 162, 164
  immunohistochemistry, 154–5
  postpubertal male patients, 149–50
serum thymic factor (FTS), 44
severe combined immunodeficiency syndrome (SCID), 54–5
Sipple's syndrome, 132
small round cell tumors, 261
smooth muscle tumors, 248
solitary fibrous tumor (SFT)-hemangiopericytoma, 251–3
spindle cell tumors, 261
  carcinoid, 139
  lipoma, 243
  thymomas, 73–4
    with atypia, 80
    with prominent papillary and pseudo-papillary features, 85
ST2 marker, 282
storage diseases, 290–1
succinic dehydrogenase (SDHB) mutations, 180–1
superior mediastinum, 3
superior vena cava syndrome, 30
supraaortic area, 1
supraazygous area, 1
synovial sarcoma, 253–4, 318
systemic lupus erythematosus (SLE), 56

T-cell development, 41, 44–5
T-cell rich B-cell lymphoma (TCRBCL), 203
teratomas, 7, 143, 148, 155–8
  benign cystic teratoma (BCT), 220–1
  differential diagnosis, 157–8
  immature, 156–7
  mature, 155–6
  postpubertal female patients, 151
  postpubertal male patients, 149–50
  prepubertal patients, 151
thoracic inlet, 1
thymic carcinoma, 71,
  see also neuroendocrine carcinomas of the thymus (NEC); primary thymic carcinoma (PTC)
  arising from pre-existing lesion, 115
  combined thymoma and thymic carcinoma, 81
  cytopathologic features, 115
  differential diagnosis, 153
    lymphomas, 120
thymic humoral factor, 43
thymic hyperplasia, 7
thymolipoma, 7, 259
  combined with carcinoid, 143
thymoliposarcoma, 259–60
thymomas, 5, 65, 318
  associated conditions, 66
  autoimmune disorders and, 68–9
  bone disorders and, 69
  children, 94–5
  classification, 71–3
  clinical features, 65–7
  combined thymoma and neuroendocrine carcinoma, 143
  combined thymoma and thymic carcinoma, 81
  cytogenetic and molecular analysis, 89
  degenerative changes, 86, 221
  diagnosis on biopsy specimens, 89–90
  differential diagnosis, 53, 104–6, 153
  endocrine disorders and, 69
  epidemiology, 65
  Epstein–Barr virus association, 68
  hematologic disorders and, 68
  heterologous thymomas, 81
  hormone receptors, 87
  imaging techniques, 69
  immunodeficiency syndromes and, 68
  intermediate-grade malignant thymic epithelial lesions, 79–81
  location, 65

thymomas (cont.)
  low-grade malignant thymic
      epithelial neoplasms, 73–9
  lymphocyte-depleted thymoma
      with atypia, 80–1
  lymphocyte-rich thymomas,
      74–6
    with atypia, 74–9
    with spindle cells, 76–7
  micronodular thymoma, 83–4
  microscopic, 70
  myasthenia gravis association,
      58, 66–7
    pathogenesis, 67
    prognostic significance, 67
    serum autoantibody
        detection, 69
    thymoma characteristics, 85
  nuclear DNA content, 87
  other neoplasms and, 69
  pathology, 69–71
  prognosis, 93–4, 96
  renal disorders and, 69
  rhabdomyomatous thymoma,
      84
  sclerosing thymoma, 84
  secretory activity, 87
  spindle cell thymomas, 73–4

  with atypia, 80
  with prominent papillary
      and pseudo-papillary
      features, 85
  staging, 90–1
  treatment, 91–3
  ultrastructural features, 86–7
  with monster atypical cells, 85
  with prominent glandular
      differentiation, 84–5
  with pseudosarcomatous
      stroma, 81–2
thymopoiesis, 44–5
thymopoietin, 43
thymosin, 43
thymulin, 44
thymus gland, 4–5, 37
  anatomy, 37
  ectopic thymic tissue, 38
  embryology, 37–8, 212
  follicular hyperplasia (FH),
      52–4, 57
  histology, 38–43
  hormones, 43–4
  immunity and, 44–5
    immunologic self-tolerance,
        45
    T-cell development, 41, 44–5

  immunodeficiency syndromes
      and, 54–6,
      see also specific syndromes
    congenital syndromes, 54–5
    thymic dysplasia, 55–6
  innervation, 42
  involution, 45–6
    pathological, 51
  lipofibroadenoma, 85
  myasthenia gravis and, 56–8
    congenital myasthenia
        syndromes, 57
    germinal center density
        significance, 58
  soft tissue neoplasms, 259–60
  true thymic hyperplasia
      (TTH), 52–3
  weights by age, 38, 45, 52
thyroid tumors, 185–94
  adenomas, 185–7
  carcinomas, 185–94
    follicular, 185, 189
    medullary, 187, 189–93
    papillary, 185, 188
  goiter, 8, 185
tracheobronchial injury, 19
tricuspid valve (TV), 300, 306
troponin assays, 280–1

tuberculosis, 10, 321
tuberous sclerosis complex
    (TSC), 255

unicuspid aortic valve, 303
unilocular thymic cysts (UTCs),
    212–13

ventricular assist devices,
    312

well-differentiated papillary
    mesothelioma (WDPM),
    338–40
Wermer's syndrome, 132
Wiscott–Aldrich syndrome, 55

yolk sac tumors, 158–62
  differential diagnosis, 154,
      162–3
  hematopoietic neoplasm
      association, 161–2
  immunohistochemistry,
      162
  postpubertal male patients,
      150
  prepubertal patients, 151
  sarcomatoid, 159–61

TERMS AND CONDITIONS OF USE

1. License

(a) Cambridge University Press grants the customer a non-exclusive license to use this CD-ROM either (i) on a single computer for use by one or more people at different times or (ii) by a single user on one or more computers (provided the CDROM is used only on one computer at one time and is always used by the same user).

(b) The customer must not: (i) copy or authorize the copying of the CD-ROM, except that library customers may make one copy for archiving purposes only, (ii) translate the CD-ROM, (iii) reverseengineer, disassemble, or decompile the CD-ROM, (iv) transfer, sell, assign, or otherwise convey any portion of the CD-ROM from a network or mainframe system.

(c) The customer may use the CD-ROM for educational and research purposes as follows: material contained on a simple screen may be printed out and used within a fair use/fair dealing context; the images may be downloaded for bona fide teaching purposes, but may not be further distributed in any form or made available for sale. An archive copy of the product may be made where libraries have this facility, on condition that the copy is for archiving purposes only and is not used or circulated within or beyond the library where the copy is made.

2. Copyright

All material within the CD-ROM is protected by copyright. All rights are reserved except those expressly licensed.

3. Liability

To the extent permitted by applicable law, Cambridge University Press accepts no liability for consequential loss or damage of any kind resulting from use of the CD-ROM or from errors or faults contained in it.